Sports Nutrition for Health Professionals

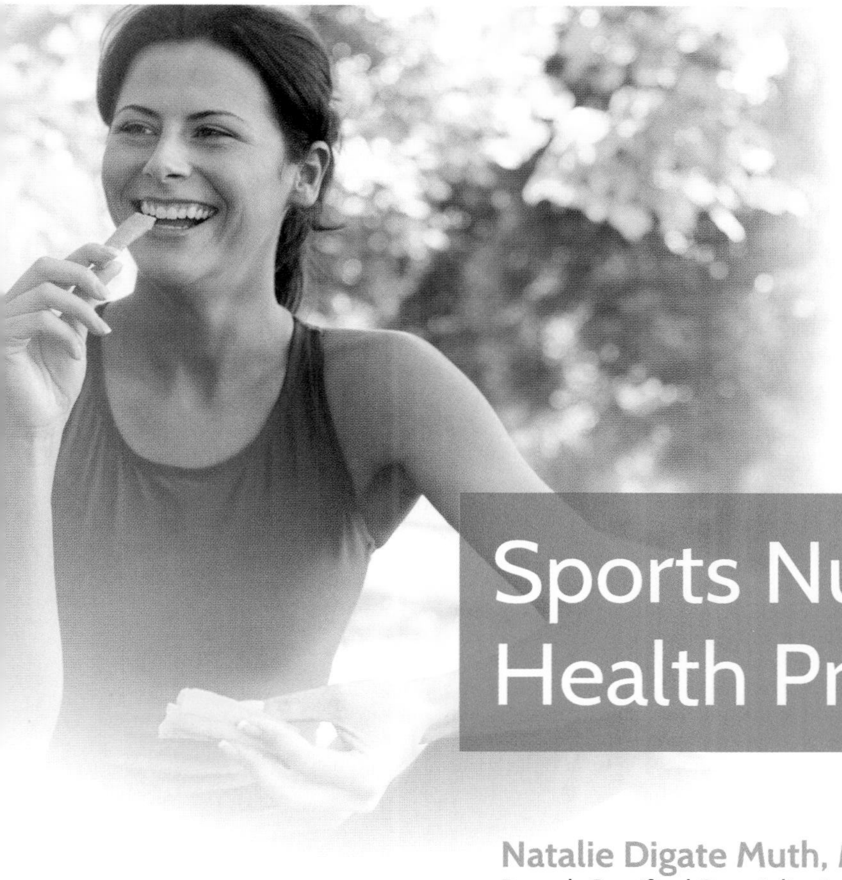

Sports Nutrition for Health Professionals

Natalie Digate Muth, MD, MPH, RD, CSSD, FAAP
Board-Certified Specialist in Sports Dietetics
Board-Certified Pediatrician
Fellow of the American Academy of Pediatrics
Diplomate of the American Board of Obesity Medicine
Senior Advisor for Healthcare Solutions, American Council on Exercise, San Diego, CA
Pediatrician, Children's Primary Care Medical Group, Vista, CA

F.A. Davis Company • Philadelphia

F. A. Davis Company
1915 Arch Street
Philadelphia, PA 19103
www.fadavis.com

Printed in the United States of America

Last digit indicates print number: 10 9 8 7 6 5 4 3 2

Publisher: Quincy McDonald
Director of Content Development: George W. Lang
Developmental Editor: Patricia Gillivan
Art and Design Manager: Carolyn O'Brien

Library of Congress Cataloging-in-Publication Data

Muth, Natalie Digate, author.
Sports nutrition for health professionals / Natalie Digate Muth.
p. ; cm.
Includes bibliographical references and index.
ISBN-13: 978-0-8036-2955-4
ISBN-10: 0-8036-2955-9
I. Title.
[DNLM: 1. Sports Nutritional Physiological Phenomena. 2. Athletic Performance–physiology. 3. Sports Nutritional Sciences. QT 261]
RA781
613.7'1–dc23
2013048220

To Bob, for his enduring patience and support

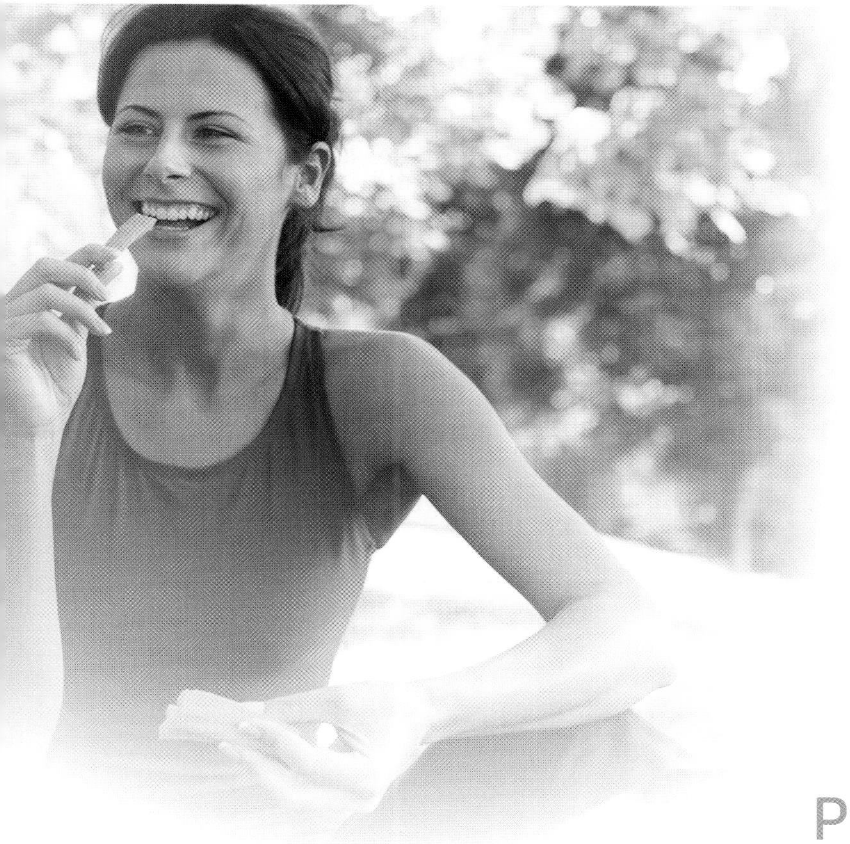

Preface

Over the past decade, the field of sports nutrition has grown substantially. With the improved quantity and quality of sports nutrition research, increased attention to nutrition among recreational and professional athletes alike, and a blossoming interest in the field among college students, sports nutrition programs in universities and colleges across the United States have expanded significantly. At the same time, the demand for a comprehensive, up-to-date, and practical sports nutrition resource for non-nutrition majors has grown.

This text, *Sports Nutrition for Health Professionals*, merges the basic principles and latest evidence-based knowledge and scientific understanding of sports nutrition with real-world practical applications and examples that health professional students must master to help their current and future clients to optimize athletic performance and overall satisfaction and success with sports and physical activity. Chapters are intended to be practical and application-based while still including all of the essential background and scientific information a student needs to fully understand the field of sports nutrition. While the text incorporates topic areas included in the content outline for registered dietitians who are board-certified specialists in sports dietetics (CSSD), the text is geared toward allied health professionals working with a diverse population of active individuals.

The information and tools contained in this text serve as a resource to those professionals working with elite and recreational athletes, fit and active non-athletes, and the newly active population. The major objective of this text is to provide students with a comprehensive understanding of sports nutrition in a format that is easy to digest, recall, and apply. To meet this objective, the text includes the following features:

- The stories of six clients— a professional triathlete, a recreational bodybuilder, a high school basketball player, a marathon runner, an active octogenarian, and an overweight middle-aged woman training to hike the Grand Canyon—are weaved throughout the text. These six sample clients are used to illustrate major principles and take-home points contained within the text. The sample clients are evaluated by a variety of health professionals and undergo a series of assessments and self-administered tests to evaluate and optimize their nutritional status. Readers are given access to these assessments and tests and are encouraged to use them to evaluate their own nutritional status.
- Speed Bumps—or review questions highlighting the major points of the preceding several paragraphs—to help students stop and comprehend what they just read.
- A Key Points Summary at the end of each chapter that distills the main learning points from the chapter into a succinct list of critical take-home points.

- Ten multiple choice questions that assess the student's comprehension of the chapter's main points.
- Communication Strategies boxes, in which students practice taking the information they've just learned and effectively sharing it with clients, colleagues, and the general public.
- Evaluating the Evidence boxes, in which students learn to think critically to understand, interpret, and use the results of peer-reviewed research studies.

Sports Nutrition for Health Professionals promises to serve as a comprehensive, yet easy-to-read and practical textbook for allied health professional students interested in sports nutrition. Ultimately, after completing a sports nutrition course based upon this textbook, students not only will understand the physiological basis of sports nutrition, but also will be able to clearly articulate how to apply the physiology to real-life situations and interactions with their clients.

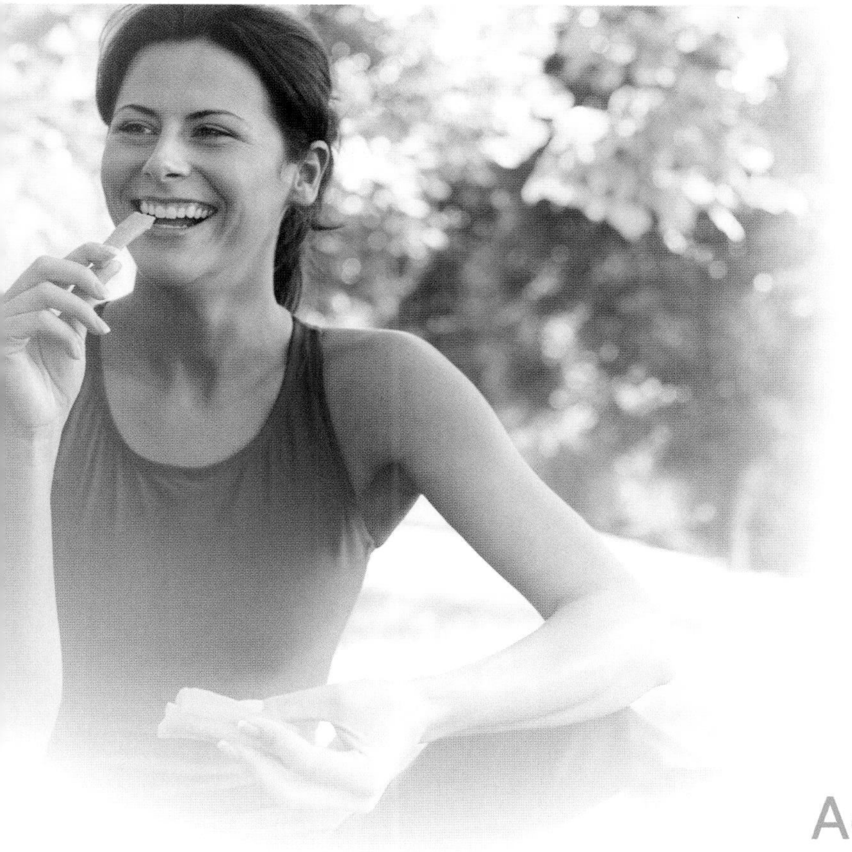

Acknowledgments

As I set out to develop a practical sports nutrition text containing all of the necessary scientific background paired with easy-to-digest and apply information, tools, and resources, I had no idea of the magnitude of such a project. I am grateful for the many people who helped me over the past four years to turn this vision into this completed sports nutrition text. Without them, there is no way that I would have come to this point in the process, in expressing my heartfelt thanks for a project completed.

First, to Cedric Bryant, the Chief Science Officer at the American Council on Exercise, who nominated me for such a project and had faith in my abilities to convert complex scientific information into an easily digestible and practically useful text for students. I hope that this text has lived up to that vision. Also, to Quincy McDonald at F.A. Davis, who believed in me and offered me the great privilege to author my first textbook. Thank you for taking a chance on me.

No words can adequately express my gratitude to Pat Gillivan, my developmental editor, who so beautifully edited this text, coordinated contributors and reviewers, assured quality of the information, and gently nudged me to stay on track through a long and laborious process that at times felt overwhelming. I am grateful for her countless hours, energy, and commitment to this project.

I am grateful to the contributors who helped to enhance the chapters' content and readability and ensured the accuracy and quality of the content. These contributors graciously lent their insights and skills to enhancing the value of the text to students. My sincerest appreciation to Diana Castellanos, PhD, RD, who contributed to Chapters 1 and 2; Michelle Futrell, MA, ATC, SCAT, who contributed to Chapter 3; Dana Angelo White, MS, ATC, RD, who co-authored Chapter 5; Michelle Murphy Zive, MS, RD, who contributed greatly to the text with her help for Chapters 4, 6, 7, 8, and 12; Monica Grages, MS, RD, LD, who authored Box 9-1; Sabrena Merrill, MS, who authored the multiple choice questions for Chapters 3, 4, and 9–16; and Bethany Pianca, BS, RD who helped with several features and sample answers for much of the text.

A special thank you to the external reviewers who assured the accuracy and quality of the information. They carefully evaluated each chapter and provided extremely valuable feedback and recommendations to improve the quality of the text.

Finally, thank you to my husband, Bob, and my children, Thomas and Mariella. They have continued to show support, patience, and ongoing sacrifice through the entire process from vision to publication of this project. I thank them for the many free nights and spare moments they uncomplainingly allowed me to finish just one more feature, work on that final chapter, tie up loose ends, and otherwise nurture this project to completion.

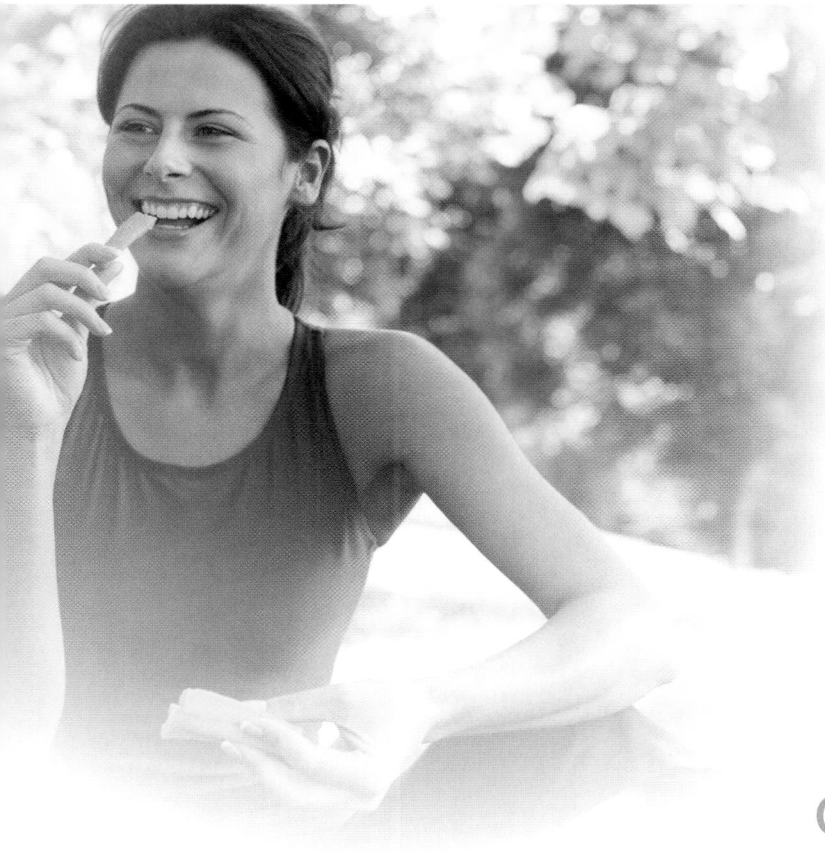

Contributors

Diana Castellanos, PhD, RD
Assistant Professor
Marywood University
Scranton, PA
CHAPTERS 1 AND 2

Michelle Futrell, MA, ATC, SCAT
Director of Undergraduate Academic Services
Senior Instructor Health & Human Performance
College of Charleston
Charleston, SC
CHAPTER 3

Monica Grages, BS, MS, RD, LD
Graduate Research Assistant
Laboratory for Elite Athlete Performance
Georgia State University
Atlanta, GA
BOX 9-1

Sabrena Merrill, MS
Exercise Scientist
ACE-Certified Personal Trainer, Health Coach, and Group Fitness Instructor
PRACTICAL APPLICATIONS, CHAPTERS 3, 4, 9–16

Bethany Pianca, BS, RD
San Francisco State University
SELECT SAMPLE ANSWERS AND FEATURES

Dana Angelo White, MS, ATC, RD
Assistant Clinical Faculty
Quinnipiac University
Hamden, CT
CHAPTER 5

Michelle Murphy Zive, MS, RD
Principal Investigator, Communities Putting Prevention to Work (UC San Diego Interventions only) and *Network for a Healthy California*
Division of Child Development and Community Health
University of California, San Diego
San Diego, CA
CHAPTERS 4, 6, 7, 8, 12 ANCILLARIES

Michelle Futrell, MA, ATC, SCAT
Director of Undergraduate Academic Services
Senior Instructor Health & Human Performance
College of Charleston
Charleston, SC
TESTBANK

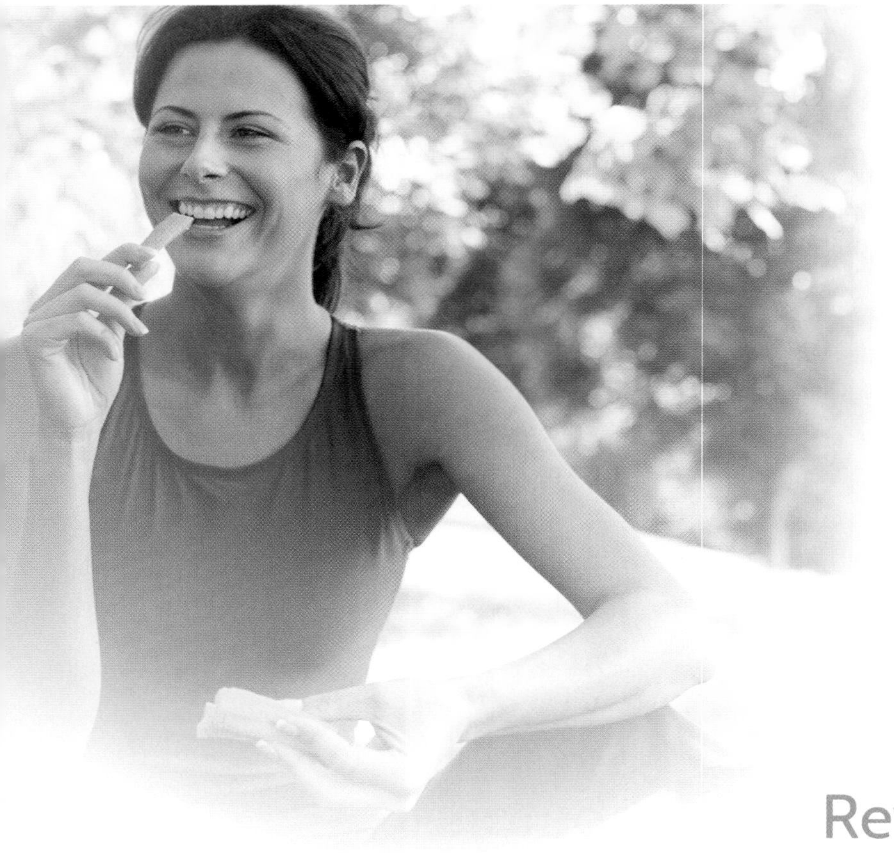

Reviewers

Carolyn Albright, PhD
Assistant Professor
Human Movement Sciences
Immaculata University
Immaculata, PA

Jessica Bachman, PhD, MPH, RD
Assistant Professor
Nutrition and Dietetics
Marywood University
Scranton, PA

Thomas E. Ball, PhD
Professor
Kinesiology
DePauw University
Greencastle, IN

Diana K. Castellanos, PhD, RD
Assistant Professor
Nutrition and Dietetics
Marywood University
Scranton, PA

Melissa Chabot, MS, RD, CDN
Nutrition Undergraduate Coordinator
Exercise and Nutrition Sciences
SUNY at Buffalo
Buffalo, NY

Resa M. Chandler, PhD
Associate Professor of Exercise Science and Coordinator of Exercise Science Major
Exercise Science
Brevard College
Brevard, NC

Kristine L. Clark, PhD, RD, FACSM
Director of Sports Nutrition, Assistant Professor of Nutrition Science
Intercollegiate Athletics and Nutritional Sciences
The Pennsylvania State University
University Park, PA

Lisa A. Farley, EdD
Assistant Professor
Physical and Health Education
Butler University
Indianapolis, IN

Jennifer Farrell, MS, RD
Research Associate in Nutrition
Nutrition, Food and Exercise Science
The Florida State University
Tallahassee, FL

Philip D, Ford, PhD, ATC, PES
Program Director and Associate Professor, Applied Exercise Science
Exercise and Sport Science
Azusa Pacific University
Azusa, CA

Sharon Frandsen, MS
Adjunct Instructor
Kinesiology
Albion College
Albion, MI

Michelle Futrell, MA, ATC, SCAT
Director of Undergraduate Academic Services, Senior Instructor in Health and Human Performance
College of Charleston
Charleston, SC

Janeen R. Hull, BS, MS, CSCS
Faculty, Instructor
Fitness Technology and Physical Education
Portland Community College
Portland, OR

Alexandra Kazaks, PhD, RD, CDE, ACSM
Assistant Professor
Nutrition and Exercise Science
Bastyr University
Kenmore, WA

June Kloubec, PhD
Associate Professor
Nutrition and Exercise Science
Bastyr University
Kenmore, WA

Robert G. LeFavi, PhD, CSCS
Professor
Health Sciences
Armstrong Atlantic State University
Savannah, GA

Simin Levinson, MS, RD
Lecturer
Nutrition
Arizona State University
Phoenix, AZ

Fred L. Miller, III, PhD, ACSM-HFS
Assistant Professor
Kinesiology
Anderson University
Anderson, IN

Adam Parker, PhD
Assistant Professor
Kinesiology
Angelo State University
San Angelo, TX

Charles J. Pelitera, MS, CSCS
Assistant Professor
Kinesiology
Canisius College
Buffalo, NY

Rachel E. Scherr, PhD
Postdoctoral Scholar
Nutrition
UC Davis
Davis, CA

Jay D. Seelbach, PhD, ACSM, ETT, HRI
Professor of Kinesiology, Director of Human Performance Lab
Kinesiology
Anderson University
Anderson, In

Steven R. Snowden, PhD, ATC, LAT
Associate Professor
Kinesiology
Angelo State University
San Angelo, TX

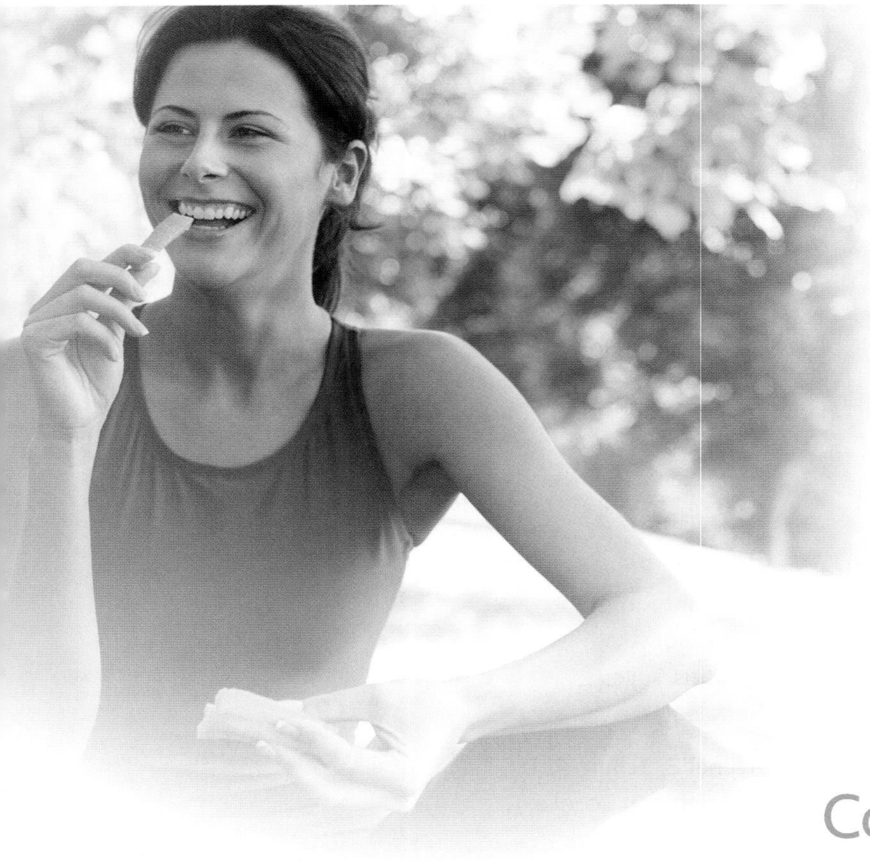

Contents

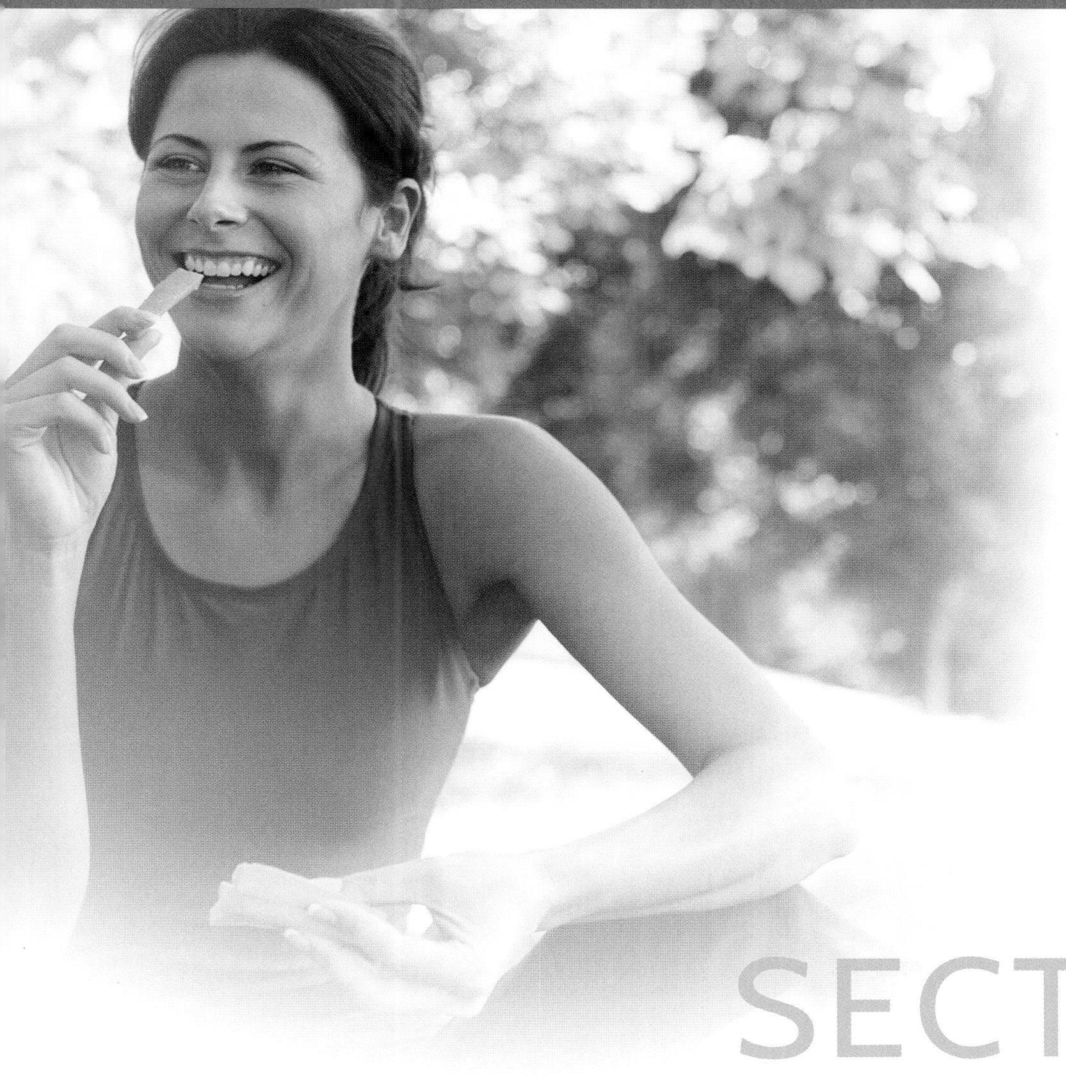

SECTION 1

From Food to Fuel

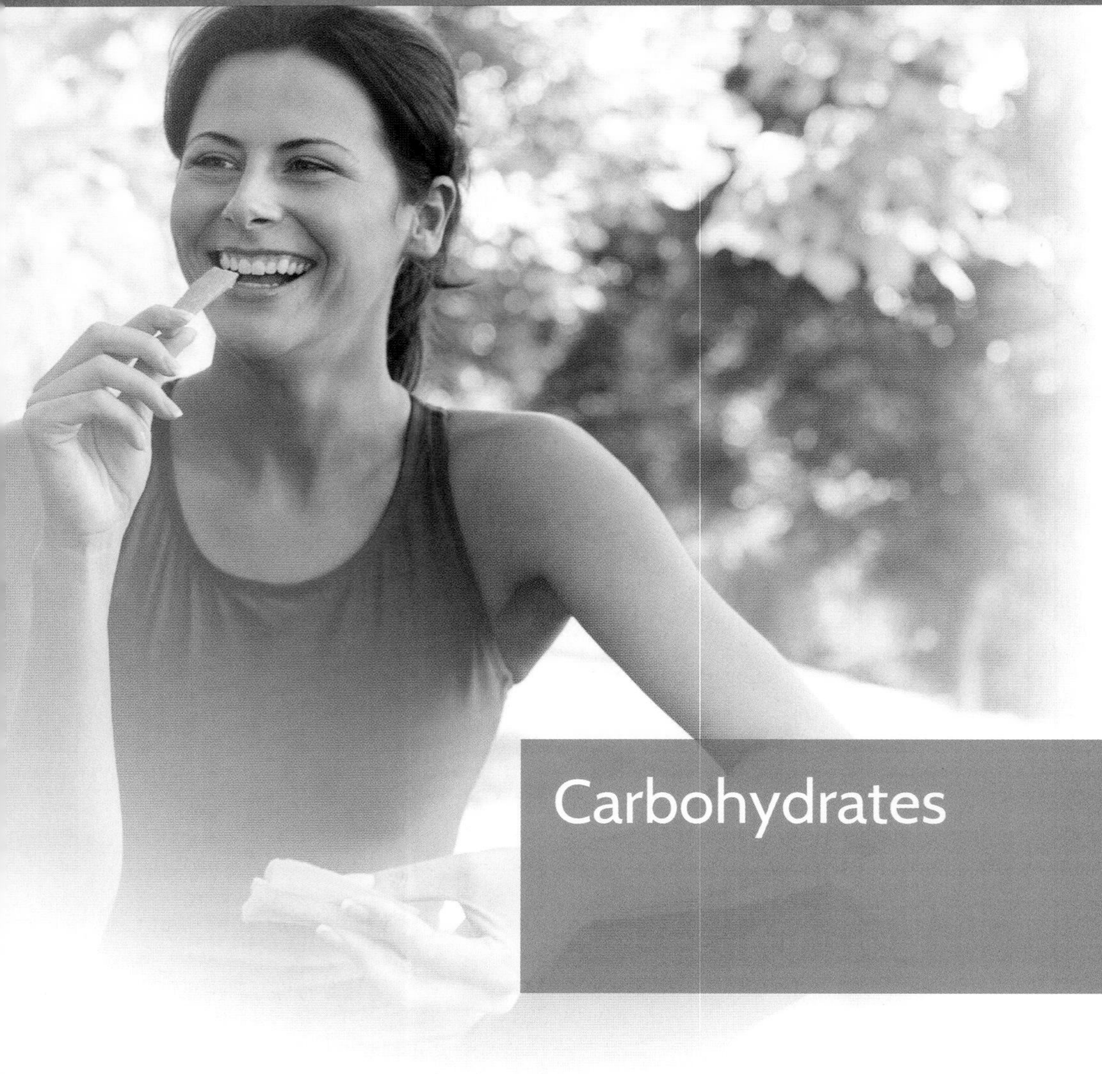

CHAPTER 1

Carbohydrates

CHAPTER OUTLINE

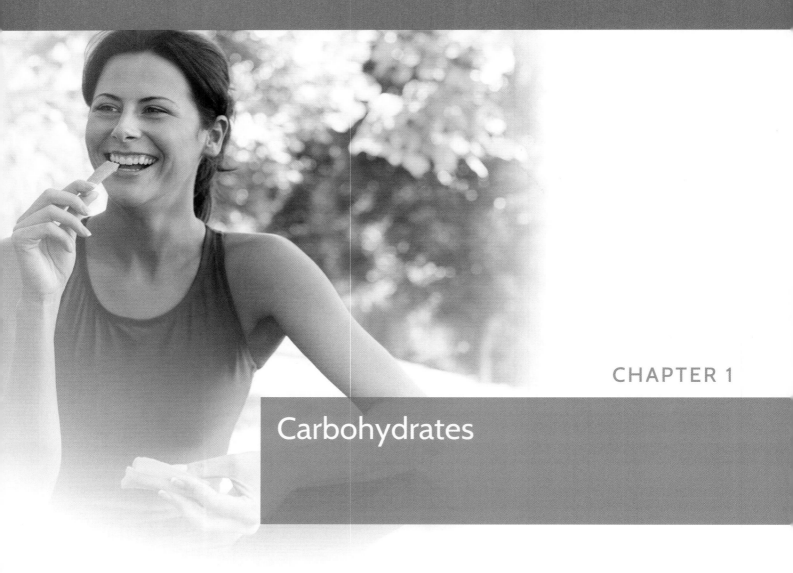

LEARNING OBJECTIVES

After studying this chapter, the reader should be able to:

1.1 Describe the roles of carbohydrate in the body.

1.2 Identify food sources containing carbohydrates.

1.3 Explain the factors that constitute a high-quality carbohydrate.

1.4 Briefly describe the process of carbohydrate digestion and absorption.

1.5 Outline the process of carbohydrate metabolism.

1.6 Define and describe glycemic index.

1.7 List several benefits of a high-fiber diet.

1.8 List various types of carbohydrates and their effect on athletic performance, weight management, and overall health.

KEY TERMS

absorption The transfer of nutrients from the digestive system into the blood supply.

acceptable macronutrient distribution range (AMDR) The range of intake for a macronutrient that is associated with decreased risk of chronic disease while providing sufficient intake of essential nutrients.

adenosine triphosphate (ATP) The body's usable energy source.

amylopectin A polysaccharide highly branched chain of glucose molecules that is easily digested.

amylose A polysaccharide made of glucose molecules bound together in a linear chain that is mostly resistant to digestion.

bolus A food and saliva digestive mix that is swallowed and further digested in the stomach and small intestine.

brush border The site of nutrient absorption in the small intestine. Enterocyte cells line the small intestine and have microvilli. The microvilli are closely packed together and resemble the bristles of a brush. The enterocyte cells secrete enzymes and proteins that assist with nutrient digestion and absorption.

calorie The amount of energy needed to increase 1 kilogram of water by 1 degree Celsius. It is used to measure the amount of energy in a food available after digestion.

carbohydrate A macronutrient made of carbon, hydrogen, and oxygen; the body's preferred energy source.

cellulose A low viscosity starch made of long chains of glucose; a structural component of the cell wall in plants that is indigestible to humans.

chyme A partially digested mass of food formed in the stomach and released into the duodenum of the small intestine.

complex carbohydrates Oligosaccharides and polysaccharides; multiple monosaccharides joined by glycosidic bonds; takes more time to digest than a simple carbohydrate.

dietary fiber Nondigestible carbohydrates and lignins that are obtained naturally from plant foods.

digestion The process of breaking down food into units small enough for absorption.

disaccharide A simple carbohydrate; two monosaccharides bound together. Maltose, sucrose and lactose are all disaccharides.

duodenum The approximately 1-foot long first portion of the small intestine where the majority of chemical digestion of food occurs.

enzymes Proteins that speed up the rate of chemical reactions.

esophagus A muscular tube extending from the mouth to the stomach.

fructooligosaccharide A category of oligosaccharides that are mostly indigestible, may help to relieve constipation, improve triglyceride levels, and decrease production of foul-smelling digestive byproducts.

fructose The sweetest of the monosaccharides, found in varying levels in different types of fruits.

functional fiber Nondigestible carbohydrates that have been isolated from foods and added to food products, and have a potentially beneficial effect on human health.

galactose A monosaccharide, a component of lactose.

gastric emptying The process by which food is emptied from the stomach into the small intestine.

glucagon A hormone secreted by the pancreas that stimulates glucose release from the liver when blood glucose levels are low.

gluconeogenesis The formation of glucose from noncarbohydrate substances.

glucose The predominant monosaccharide in nature and the basic building block of most other carbohydrates.

glycemic index A measurement of the amount of increase in blood sugar after eating particular foods.

glycemic load A measure of a consumed carbohydrate's overall effect on blood glucose levels; equal to the glycemic index multiplied by the number of grams consumed divided by 100.

glycogen A polysaccharide that is a highly branched chain of glucose molecules. The chief carbohydrate storage material in animals formed and stored in the liver and muscle.

glycosidic bond A link between two sugar molecules. The two molecules share an oxygen atom.

high viscosity fiber See *soluble fiber.*

hypoglycemia Low blood glucose (≤ 70 mg/dL); characterized by symptoms such as tiredness, weakness, shaking, fast heart rate, and feeling nervous.

ileum The final portion of the small intestine, which is approximately 12 feet in length; where absorption of vitamin B12, bile salts, and digestive products not already absorbed in the jejunum occurs.

insoluble fiber Fiber that does not bind with water and adds bulk to the diet (includes cellulose, hemicellulose, and lignins found in wheat bran, vegetables, and whole grain breads and cereals); important for proper bowel function and reducing symptoms of constipation.

insulin A hormone secreted by the pancreas that is required for the transport of glucose from blood into tissues.

jejunum The middle portion of the small intestine, which is approximately 8 feet in length; where much of food absorption occurs.

lactase The enzyme required to digest lactose.

lactose A disaccharide made of glucose and galactose; the principal sugar found in milk.

lactose intolerance A condition in which a person does not make enough of the enzyme lactase required to break down the sugar lactose, resulting in gastrointestinal symptoms such as abdominal cramps, bloating, diarrhea, and flatulence when lactose is ingested.

large intestine Connects the small intestine to the anus; absorbs most of the fluid from waste products and serves as a storage site for fecal waste; includes three portions: the cecum, colon, and rectum.

CALCULATIONS

1 gram of carbohydrate = 4 calories

Glycemic load = glycemic index × grams of carbohydrate consumed/100

liver A large vital organ inside the body which plays a major role in metabolism including protein synthesis, glycogen storage, and production of chemicals necessary for digestion; other functions include detoxification and purification and breakdown of red blood cells.

low viscosity fiber See *insoluble fiber.*

maltose A disaccharide of two glucose molecules bound together; found in malt beverages, chocolate malts, and beer.

monosaccharide The simplest form of carbohydrate (glucose, galactose, and fructose); it cannot be digested any further.

oligosaccharide A complex carbohydrate, a chain of approximately three to ten monosaccharides.

pancreas A vital organ that is both a digestive organ, secreting pancreatic juice containing digestive enzymes that assist the absorption of nutrients and the digestion in the small intestine, and an endocrine organ that releases important hormones including insulin, glucagon, and somatostatin.

peristalsis The process by which muscles in the esophagus push food to the stomach through a wave-like motion.

polysaccharide A complex carbohydrate, long chain of monosaccharides. There are three categories: starch, fiber, and glycogen.

portal circulation The circulation of blood directly from the small intestine to the liver via the portal vein.

recommended dietary allowance (RDA) The amount of nutrient known to be adequate to meet the nutritional needs of nearly all healthy persons.

saliva A secretion from the salivary glands that begins digestion; consists of water, salts, and enzymes.

simple carbohydrate Monosaccharides and disaccharides.

small intestine The three-segment portion of the digestive system between the stomach and large intestine that is responsible for the majority of digestion and absorption of swallowed foods.

soluble fiber A type of fiber that forms gel in water; may help prevent heart disease and stroke by binding bile and cholesterol, diabetes by slowing glucose absorption, and constipation by holding moisture in stools and softening them; includes gums, pectin, and psyllium seeds.

starch Plant carbohydrate found in grains and vegetables.

sucrose A disaccharide formed by glucose and fructose linked together; also known as table sugar.

sugar Chemically speaking it may refer to simple carbohydrates (mono and disaccharides), or it may refer to table sugar or sucrose.

villi Folds or finger-like projections of the small intestine that increase surface area for digestion and absorption.

INTRODUCTION

Carbohydrates serve as the body's preferred energy source and help to fend off the fatigue and exhaustion that threatens the end of a prolonged workout. In recent years there has been a backlash against carbohydrates in popular diets, lay media stories, and now to some extent even in the scientific literature. While carbohydrates such as refined **sugars** can pose health problems, healthful carbohydrates chosen in appropriate amounts and at the appropriate times can benefit athletic performance, weight management, and optimal health.

CARBOHYDRATE FUNCTION

Carbohydrates serve several essential functions in the human body. As the body's preferred energy source, carbohydrates are ideally suited to provide fuel for the body's many metabolic functions, including that required for normal brain function. When carbohydrates are readily available, the body does not need to break down protein for fuel. This protein sparing allows protein to be used to build muscle and other important body tissues and structures rather than for energy. Furthermore, carbohydrates can be used for energy during anaerobic and aerobic exercise and are required to efficiently break down fat. In addition, fiber, an important type of carbohydrate, improves digestive health and cholesterol levels. Carbohydrates play other important roles, including satiety, providing flavor and sweet taste to foods, and serving as signaling molecules for essential biological reactions.

CARBOHYDRATE STRUCTURE

Carbohydrates are built from chains of **monosaccharides**. Monosaccharides are made of carbon, hydrogen, and oxygen molecules, hence the abbreviation CHO. They are bound together to form larger carbohydrate compounds such as **disaccharides, oligosaccharides**, and **polysaccharides**. Carbohydrates are categorized into two categories: simple and complex. Simple carbohydrates include monosaccharides and disaccharides and complex carbohydrates include the oligosaccharides and polysaccharides. Most carbohydrates provide 4 **calories** per gram; however, as discussed in this chapter, dietary fiber, a form of complex carbohydrates, contributes fewer calories per gram.

Simple Carbohydrates

Monosaccharides

Three monosaccharides found in nature can be absorbed and used by humans: glucose, fructose, and galactose. **Glucose** is the predominant monosaccharide in nature and the basic building block of most other carbohydrates. **Fructose** is the sweetest of the monosaccharides and is found in varying levels in different types of fruits. **Galactose** is most often bound to glucose to form the disaccharide **lactose**, the principal sugar found in milk. Furthermore, monosaccharides can be bound together by a **glycosidic bond** to form disaccharides, oligosaccharides, or polysaccharides.

After being consumed, all carbohydrates are eventually digested to monosaccharides and absorbed into the bloodstream. The cells in the body use the monosaccharide form of glucose for energy. The other two monosaccharides, fructose and galactose, must be converted to glucose to be used by the cells for energy.

Disaccharides

Three disaccharides found in food are lactose, sucrose, and maltose. Lactose, which is a glucose molecule and galactose molecule bound together, is found in dairy products such as milk, yogurt, and ice cream. **Sucrose** (table sugar) is formed by glucose and fructose, and **maltose** (malt sugar) is two glucose molecules bound together.

The human preference for sweet tastes is innate. This preference has inspired food manufacturers to add sucrose and a variety of other sweeteners to food products to enhance consumer appeal. Most caloric sweeteners (meaning they provide calories) are disaccharides. Raw sugar, granulated sugar, brown sugar, powdered sugar, and turbinado sugar (Sugar in the Raw) are all forms of sucrose. Honey is a natural form of sucrose that is made from plant nectar and harvested by honeybees, which secrete an enzyme that hydrolyzes sucrose to glucose and fructose. Other natural caloric sweeteners include molasses, agave nectar, and maple. Corn sweeteners, such as corn syrup and high fructose corn syrup, are commonly used in commercially processed foods such as sodas, baked goods, and some canned products (see Evaluating the Evidence).

Weight- and calorie-conscious consumers have long used low-calorie sweeteners to enhance food flavors. Sorbitol, which is used in many diet products, is produced from glucose and found naturally in some berries and fruits. It is absorbed by the body at a slower rate than sugar. Noncaloric sweeteners—which are calorie-free because the body cannot metabolize them—also are used to add sweet taste to foods and beverages. In the United States, these sweeteners are regulated by the Food and Drug Administration (FDA). Aspartame, also known as Equal in packaged sweetener and NutraSweet in foods and beverages; Acesulfame K, which is called Sunett in cooking products and Sweet One as a tabletop sweetener; saccharin; sucralose (Splenda); and neotame are all approved for use in the United States. While early studies found that certain sweeteners may cause bladder cancer in laboratory rats,[1,2] subsequent studies have not confirmed this finding.[3,4] Sugar extracted from the stevia plant is

EVALUATING THE EVIDENCE

Does High Fructose Corn Syrup Really Make You Overweight?

High fructose corn syrup (HFCS) first made its debut into the American food supply around 1970 when it accounted for about 0.5% of total sweetener use. It is produced when corn syrup undergoes processing to convert glucose to fructose. By the mid-2000s, almost half of all sweetened foods were sweetened with HFCS. HFCS makes up a large proportion of added sweeteners in beverages and processed and packaged foods including many canned foods, cereals, baked goods, desserts, flavored and sweetened dairy products, candy, and fast food. Two forms of HFCS are used in the U.S. food supply: HFCS-55, which is found mostly in carbonated beverages and is 55% fructose, 41% glucose, and 4% glucose polymers; and HFCS-42, which is found mostly in processed foods and contains slightly less fructose (42% fructose, 53% glucose, and 5% glucose polymers).[25] Food manufacturers prefer fructose to sucrose because it is less expensive. Corn subsidies and other policies aimed at increasing corn production led to corn prices that are lower than the cost of producing sugar. High tariffs on imported sugar cane add to the cost of sweetening with pure sugar.

Publication of several animal studies and human studies showed that HFCS may contribute to obesity, insulin resistance, diabetes, and decreased feelings of fullness after consumption. Health advocates and the media became alarmed that HFCS may contribute to negative health outcomes, including the surge in obesity. Recent large-scale human studies have not shown increased risk of overweight, obesity, or metabolic disorders like diabetes when HFCS is consumed in reasonable amounts.[26] However, the number of long-term high-quality controlled studies is limited. This is not to say that clients can eat unlimited amounts of HFCS without risk of ill consequence; rather, HFCS probably does not increase health risk *more than* sugar or other sweeteners. But the typical American still consumes greater than 10% of daily calories from added sugars.[25,27] That's about an extra 200 calories per day of empty calories, which provide minimal nutritional value. Add it up and the typical American eats about 20 pounds worth of added sugar over the course of a year. Manufacturers add HFCS to foods that would not typically contain sugar such as breads, crackers, juices, and yogurt to increase shelf-life and enhance flavor.

Anyone trying to lose or control their weight or curb risk of insulin resistance or diabetes should aim to minimize consumption of HFCS as well as other added sugars, including sucrose (table sugar) and other caloric sweeteners. As clients carefully scan ingredient lists they will soon find that it doesn't matter whether they eat foods and drinks with sucrose, high fructose corn syrup, or any of the other many added sugars–trying to cut added sugars in the diet is a major challenge.

1. What is your opinion of high fructose corn syrup after reading this summary?
2. More research needs to be done to fully understand the effects of high fructose corn syrup on health. Using the scientific method, define a question, develop a hypothesis, and propose a theoretical study to evaluate the effects of high fructose corn syrup on a health outcome.

The Scientific Method

1. Define a question
2. Gather information and resources (observe)
3 Form a hypothesis
4. Test the hypothesis through experimentation and data collection
5. Analyze the data
6. Interpret the data and draw conclusions
7. Publish results

now a widely available natural alternative to artificial sweeteners (see Emerging Trends). Studies are mixed on whether consumption of noncaloric sweeteners assists with weight control.[7,32]

Complex Carbohydrates

Oligosaccharides and Polysaccharides

An oligosaccharide is a chain of approximately three to ten simple sugars. **Fructooligosaccharides**, a category of oligosaccharides found naturally in some fruits and vegetables and commercially produced as a reduced-calorie sweetener, are mostly indigestible. These oligosaccharides help relieve constipation, improve triglyceride levels, and decrease production of foul-smelling digestive byproducts.[5]

Polysaccharides can consist of hundreds of monosaccharides bound together. There are three categories of polysaccharides: starch, fiber, and glycogen. Plants such as different grains and vegetables make **starch**,

EMERGING TRENDS

IN STORES NOW: STEVIA, THE ALL-NATURAL PLANT-BASED SWEETENER

Once limited to the health-food market as an unapproved herb, the plant-derived sweetener known as stevia is now widely available and rapidly replacing artificial sweeteners in consumer products. Thirty times sweeter than sugar and with no effect on blood glucose and little aftertaste, stevia sales are predicted to reach about $700 million in the next few years according to the agribusiness finance giant Rabobank.

Stevia's history goes back to ancient times. Grown naturally in tropical climates, stevia is an herb in the chrysanthemum family that grows wild as a small shrub in Paraguay and Brazil, though it can easily be cultivated elsewhere. Paraguayans have used stevia as a food sweetener for centuries, while other countries, including Brazil, Korea, Japan, China, and much of South America, also have a shorter, though still long-standing, record of stevia use. There are over 100 species of stevia plant, but one stands out for its excellent properties as a sweetener: *Stevia rebaudiana*, which contains the compound rebaudioside A, the sweetest-flavored component of the stevia leaf. Rebaudioside A chemically acts very similar to sucrose in onset, intensity, and duration of sweetness and is free of aftertaste. Most stevia-containing products contain mostly extracted Rebaudioside A with some proportion of stevioside, which is a white crystalline compound present in stevia that tastes 100 to 300 times sweeter than table sugar.[28]

Though widely available throughout the world, in 1991 stevia was banned in the United States due to early studies that suggested the sweetener may cause cancer. A follow-up study refuted the initial study and in 1995 the FDA allowed stevia to be imported and sold as a food supplement, but not as a sweetener. Several companies argued to the FDA that stevia should be categorized similarly to its artificial sweetener cousins as "generally recognized as safe (GRAS)." Substances that are considered GRAS have been determined to be safe through expert consensus, scientific review, or widespread use without negative complications. They are exempt from the rigorous approval process required for food additives. In December 2008, the FDA declared stevia GRAS, and allowed its use in mainstream U.S. food production.[29] It has taken food manufacturers a few years to work out the right stevia-containing recipes, but stevia is now present in a number of foods and beverages in the United States, such as Gatorade's G2, VitaminWater Zero, SoBe Lifewater Zero, Crystal Light, and Sprite Green. Around the world it has been used in soft drinks, chewing gums, wines, yogurts, candies, and many other products. Stevia powder can also be used for cooking and baking (in markedly decreased amounts compared to table sugar due to its high sweetness potency).

Stevia is marketed under the trade names of Truvia (Coca-Cola and agricultural giant Cargill), PureVia (Pepsi-Cola and Whole Earth Sweetener Company), and SweetLeaf (Wisdom Natural Brands). The three sweeteners are essentially the same product, though they contain slightly different proportions of rebaudioside A and stevioside. FDA classification of the high-purity Rebaudioside M (Reb M) as GRAS cleared Coke to launch a new product called Coca-Cola Life, a 100-calorie sugar- and stevia-sweetened soft drink. Presumably, Pepsi will follow suit.

Though stevia is most likely as safe or more so than artificial sweeteners, few long-term studies have been done to document its health effects in humans. A review conducted by toxicologists at UCLA, which was commissioned by nutrition advocate Center for Science in the Public Interest, raised concerns that stevia could contribute to cancer.[28] The authors noted that in some test tube and animal studies stevioside (but not rebaudioside A) caused genetic mutations, chromosome damage, and DNA breakage. These changes presumably could contribute to malignancy, though no one has actually studied if these compounds cause cancer in animal models. Notably, initial concerns that stevia may reduce fertility or worsen diabetes seem to have been put to rest after studies showed no negative outcomes. In fact, one study of human subjects showed that stevia may improve glucose tolerance. Another found that stevia may induce the pancreas to release insulin, thus potentially serving as a treatment for type 2 diabetes.[29] After artificial sweeteners were banned in Japan over 40 years ago, the Japanese began to sweeten their foods with stevia. Since then, they have conducted over 40,000 clinical studies on stevia and concluded that it is safe for human use. But still, there is a general lack of long-term studies on stevia's use and effects.

Stevia's sweet taste and all-natural origins make it a popular sugar substitute. With little long-term outcomes data available on the plant extract, it is possible that stevia in large quantities could have harmful effects. However, it seems safe to say that when consumed within the acceptable range (4 mg/kg of body weight),[29] stevia may be an exceptional natural plant-based sugar substitute.

which is an energy source for the plant and provides carbohydrates for animals that consume the plant. There are two types of starch: amylose and amylopectin. **Amylose** is a small, linear molecule of tightly packed glucose molecules that is mostly resistant to digestion. **Amylopectin** is a larger, highly branched chain of glucose molecules that is easily digested. Because starches are longer than disaccharides and oligosaccharides, they take longer to digest. Still, humans are easily able to break down and digest starches with specific enzymes. However, the rest of the plant, which is formed largely of the carbohydrate **cellulose** and other fibers, is indigestible because humans do not produce the necessary enzymes to break the glycosidic bonds found in these polysaccharides (though some fiber does undergo fermentation in the large intestine, providing a small amount of energy for normal gut bacterial growth). While other carbohydrates contain 4 calories per gram, fiber probably contributes about 1.5 to 2.5 calories per gram.[6]

Animals, including humans, also produce a polysaccharide called **glycogen**. Glycogen is a large, highly branched chain of glucose molecules. Glycogen is made and stored in the **liver** and muscle and is a source of energy for the body.

SPEED BUMP

1. Describe the different categories of carbohydrates.

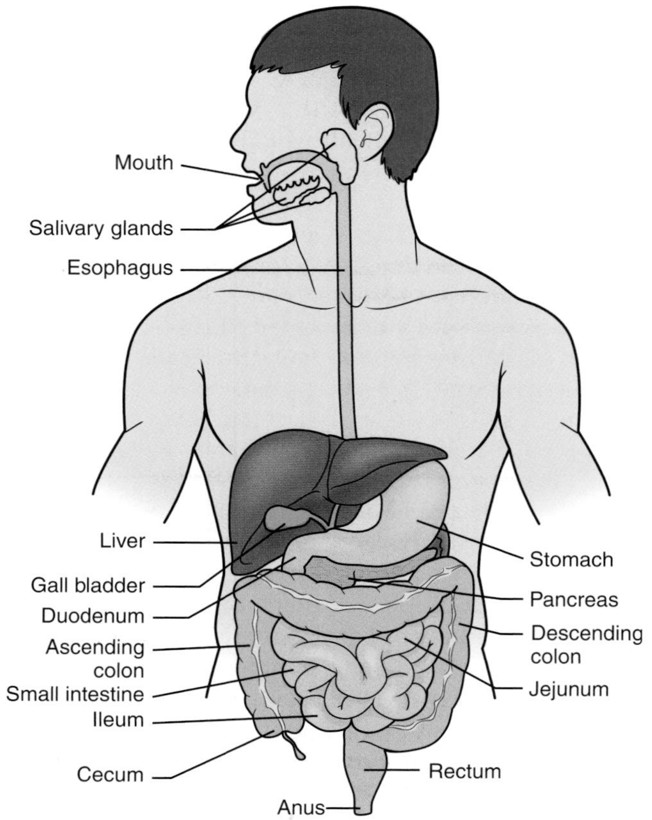

Figure 1-1. Carbohydrate digestion and absorption.

CARBOHYDRATE DIGESTION AND ABSORPTION

The body has a remarkable ability to transform a food into its individual nutrients through the process of **digestion** (Fig. 1-1). Digestion of the carbohydrate components of a food begins in the mouth. **Saliva** is released from the salivary glands. Saliva contains **enzymes**, such as salivary *a*-amylase, which cleaves large polysaccharides into oligosaccharides and disaccharides. With swallowing, the **bolus** of food passes through the throat into the **esophagus**. Muscles in the esophagus push the bolus into the stomach in a wave-like motion called **peristalsis**.

In the stomach, peristalsis continues and churns the bolus with gastric juices, forming a substance called **chyme**. However, these gastric juices have a very low pH, inhibiting enzymes that break apart glycosidic bonds found between monosaccharides. The chyme, containing partially digested carbohydrates, moves into the **small intestine**, which is composed of the duodenum, jejunum, and ileum, for further enzymatic digestion (Fig. 1-2). Once in the **duodenum**, the approximately 1-foot long first portion of the small intestine, the **pancreas** releases enzymes that help to cleave the glycosidic bonds between monosaccharides, therefore breaking the oligosaccharides and polysaccharides into smaller parts (Fig. 1-3). Also, bicarbonate is released from the pancreas to produce a more alkaline environment in which the enzymes can function. From there, the chyme passes to the second and third portions of the small intestine, the **jejunum** and **ileum**. Together comprising about 20 feet of convoluted intestine, the jejunum and ileum are where final digestion and most nutrient **absorption** occur.

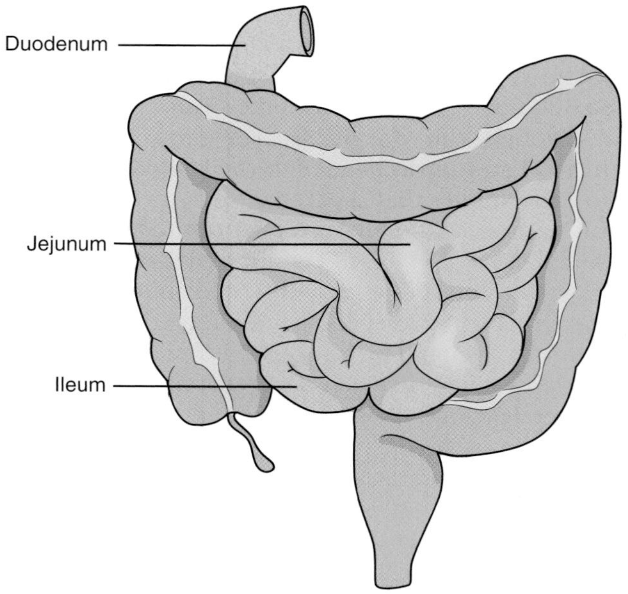

Figure 1-2. The small intestine is composed of the duodenum, jejunum, and ileum.

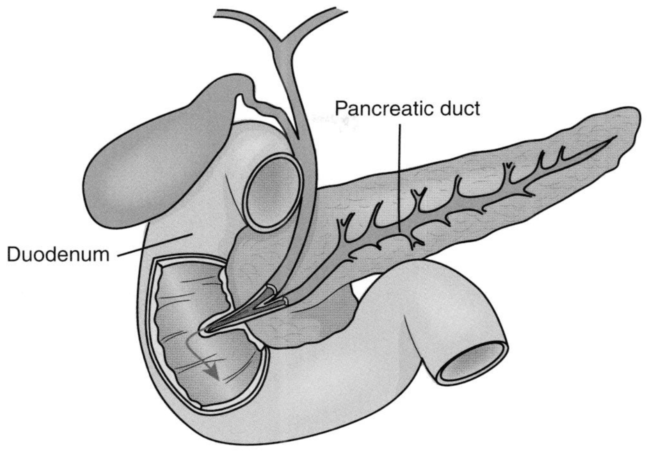

Figure 1-3. Enzymes flow through the pancreatic duct to the duodenum, where they cleave to the glycosidic bonds between monosaccharides, breaking them into smaller parts.

In the small intestine there are **villi** and **microvilli** that create a **brush border** (Fig. 1-4)—an ideal environment for final digestion and absorption. Within this border, enzymes are released that complete the digestion of most carbohydrates. For example, the enzyme **lactase** digests lactose into its component parts, the monosaccharides glucose and galactose. **Lactose intolerance** results from a deficiency in the enzyme lactase. This inability to break down lactose causes symptoms like abdominal cramps, bloating, diarrhea, and flatulence (Fig. 1-5). Other carbohydrates are broken down into monosaccharides by various brush border enzymes including maltase, *a*-dextrinase, sucrase, and trehalase. The monosaccharides are then absorbed through the microvilli, the tiny finger-like projections on the villi of the intestinal brush border into the bloodstream.

Nutrients cross the brush border into the blood in different ways depending on how well they dissolve in water (solubility), their size, and their relative concentration. Once sugars are absorbed into the bloodstream, they are delivered directly to the liver (known as **portal circulation**) for processing and distribution of nutrients to the rest of the body. Fructose and galactose are converted into glucose in the liver. Glucose either enters the bloodstream for use by the cells or is converted into glycogen or fat. The use of glucose is determined by the needs of the body.

Undigested carbohydrates such as fiber continue to move from the small intestine into the large intestine. In the **large intestine**, some fiber is digested for energy by bacteria, which also produces gas. Most of the fiber continues through the intestine and is excreted, adding bulk to the feces and protecting against constipation.

CARBOHYDRATE METABOLISM

If energy is needed, glucose is transported into the cells where it is metabolized. End products of glucose metabolism are carbon dioxide, water, and **adenosine triphosphate** (ATP). ATP is the body's usable energy source. Chapter 6 describes the process of breaking glucose down to make energy through the processes of aerobic and anaerobic glycolysis.

Carbohydrates consumed in the diet that are not immediately used for energy are stored in the liver and muscle as glycogen. Approximately 90 grams of glycogen is stored in the liver. About 150 grams of glycogen is stored in muscle, though this amount can be increased with physical training and carbohydrate loading.[8] Because glycogen contains many water molecules, it is large and bulky and therefore unsuitable for long-term energy storage. Thus, if a person continues to consume more carbohydrates than the body can use or store, the body will convert the excess carbohydrates into fat for long-term storage.

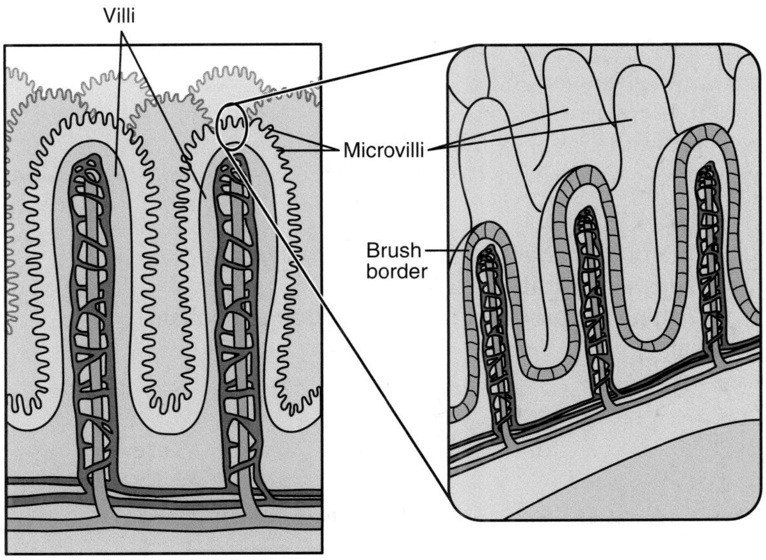

Figure 1-4. Enzymes are released in the brush border to complete digestion of most carbohydrates.

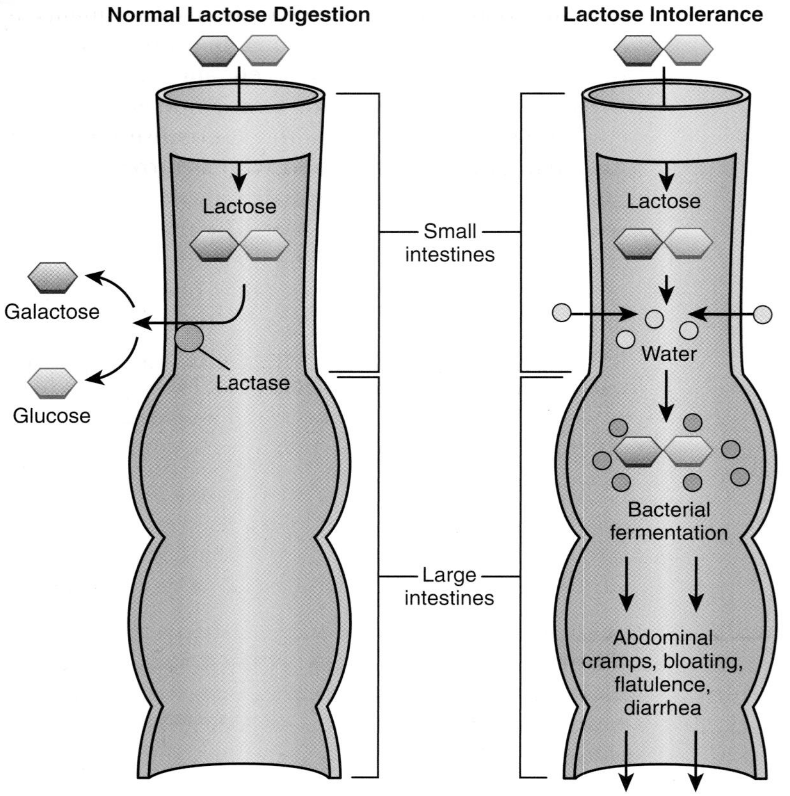

Figure 1-5. Lactose intolerance.

Hormone Regulation

Two hormones responsible for blood glucose regulation are **insulin** and **glucagon**. Both are produced in the pancreas. When a meal is consumed and blood glucose levels begin to rise, insulin is released into the blood. Insulin aids cells in the uptake of glucose, therefore maintaining a desirable blood glucose level (70 to 110 mg/dl).[8] When blood glucose begins to decrease (between periods of food consumption or during exercise), glucagon is released. One way glucagon works to increase blood glucose levels is through regulating the breakdown of glycogen into glucose. Once glycogen has been broken down into glucose, it is released into the bloodstream, increasing blood glucose levels. As glycogen decreases, glucagon metabolizes fat from storage for fuel to help conserve glycogen and maintain blood glucose levels. When there is an abundance of sugar available and glycogen stores are maximized, insulin promotes the conversion of carbohydrates into fat for long-term storage.

SPEED BUMP

2. **Briefly describe the process of carbohydrate digestion and absorption.**
3. **Outline the process of carbohydrate metabolism.**

GENERAL CARBOHYDRATE RECOMMENDATIONS

The **acceptable macronutrient distribution ranges** (AMDR) are set for carbohydrates, fat, and protein. The AMDR is the range associated with reduced risk for chronic diseases while still providing adequate intake of nutrients such as vitamins and minerals. Those whose diets fall outside the AMDR have a higher risk for developing a chronic disease or nutrient deficiency.[6] The AMDR for carbohydrates is 45% to 65% of total calories. The **recommended dietary allowance** (RDA), the amount of nutrient known to be adequate to meet the nutritional needs of nearly all healthy persons, for carbohydrates is 130 grams per day. This is a minimum requirement based on the amount of carbohydrates needed by the brain daily. Therefore, for energy maintenance the body needs more than 130 grams per day.[6] For example, a person following the AMDR who consumes 2,000 calories needs approximately 225 to 325 grams per day. The Academy of Nutrition and Dietetics and the American College of Sports Medicine also provide a g/kg of body weight method to calculate carbohydrate need for athletes. The formula is 6 to 10 g/kg (2.7 to 4.5 g/lb) of body weight per day depending on their total daily energy expenditure, type of exercise performed, gender, and environmental conditions to maintain blood glucose levels during exercise and to replace muscle glycogen.[9]

CARBOHYDRATE QUALITY

Most athletes recognize that carbohydrates are essential to fuel optimal athletic performance, but fad diets have given the general population the impression that carbohydrates are "bad" when it comes to weight control and overall health (see Myths and Misconceptions). This is not the case, as long as high-quality, minimally processed carbohydrates are consumed in appropriate portion sizes.

It used to be that carbohydrate quality was determined based on whether the carbohydrate was classified as a **simple carbohydrate** (mono- or disaccharides) like table sugar or a **complex carbohydrate** (oligo- and polysaccharides) like brown rice. This classification branded simple carbohydrates as nutrient-poor and "unhealthy" and complex carbohydrates as more nutrient-dense and "healthy." The belief was that digestion rate, and thus postprandial effect on blood glucose, was based primarily on the length of the carbohydrate chain, with short chains causing a more pronounced blood glucose response and long chains causing only a small bump in blood glucose. Today, carbohydrate quality is better determined by considering the food's nutrient value, effect on blood glucose levels, and extent of processing. While no one scale or formula determines carbohydrate quality, many health experts use **glycemic index** (GI) and **glycemic load** (GL) as proxies.[10]

Myths and Misconceptions

Carbohydrates Are Bad for Your Health and Your Waistline

The Myth

Carbohydrates make you gain weight. And, by the way, if you eat too many carbohydrates, you also increase your risk of developing type 2 diabetes.

The Logic

The digestion of carbohydrates to monosaccharides leads to a spike in blood glucose. In response, the body releases more of the fat-promoting hormone insulin. High insulin levels may lead to weight gain as well as type 2 diabetes.

The Science

Not all carbohydrates are created equal, although all carbohydrates do ultimately get broken down into glucose. Depending on a carbohydrate's glycemic index, extent of processing, and other foods consumed at the same time, the blood glucose response varies. While a growing body of research suggests that carbohydrates that have a lesser effect on blood glucose (such as low glycemic index carbohydrates) are better for overall health, including the risk of type 2 diabetes,[15] when it comes to weight gain, the research has not confirmed that increased carbohydrate type or consumption leads to increased weight[24,30,31] (when overall caloric consumption is maintained). Time and again researchers studying the effects of various diets of differing macronutrient composition on weight have found the same result: it does not matter where the calories come from, it only matters how many total calories a person consumes in a day. If dieters eat fewer calories than they expend—whether those calories come from carbohydrates, protein, or fat—they will lose weight.

Glycemic Index and Glycemic Load

Glycemic index ranks carbohydrates based on their blood glucose response: high-glycemic index foods enter the bloodstream rapidly, causing a large glucose spike (Fig. 1-6). This rapid increase in glucose stimulates release of insulin and a subsequent insulin spike. Insulin promotes glucose uptake in muscle cells and fat deposition in adipose tissue. From 2 to 4 hours after consumption of a high-glycemic index meal, residual effects from high insulin levels can cause a rapid drop in blood sugar and **hypoglycemia**.[11] Low-glycemic index foods such as nonstarchy vegetables, whole fruit, whole grains, and legumes are digested more slowly and cause a smaller glucose increase and a small boost in blood insulin levels (Table 1-1). Highly processed, refined starches and sugar tend to have a higher glycemic index and have been associated with negative health consequences such as heart disease and diabetes.[12] Although valuable, the glycemic index does not account for the caloric amount consumed of one product. For example, carrots have a higher glycemic index than a candy bar.

Glycemic index is based on a reference amount of carbohydrate (50 g). Glycemic load (GL) accounts for portion size (GL = GI × grams of carbohydrate/100). Notably, a food can have a high glycemic index but a low glycemic load. For example, while carrots have a high glycemic index, to actually eat 50 grams of carrot, a person would need to eat 4 cups of the vegetable. Because the typical serving size is approximately one-half cup, the glycemic load is small. Also, carbohydrate-containing foods that are also moderate to high in fat or protein, fiber, and other nutrients and that are minimally processed may have a high glycemic index but a low glycemic load. Table 1-2 lists the glycemic index and glycemic load of commonly eaten carbohydrates.[13]

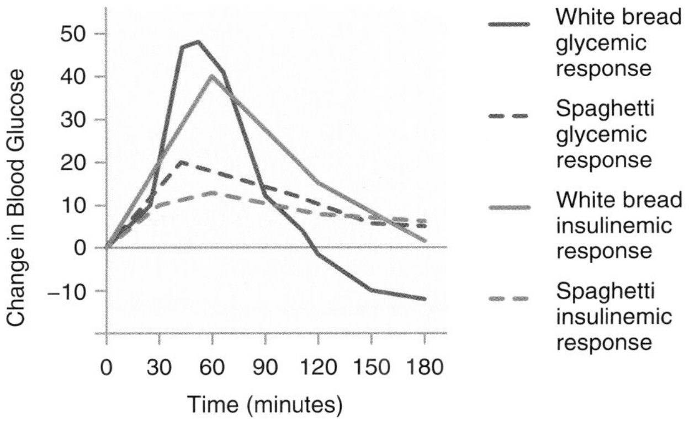

Figure 1-6. Blood glucose and insulin response after high- and low-glycemic carbohydrates.

Table 1-1. Factors That Reduce Glycemic Index

INTRINSIC	EXTRINSIC
High amylose:amylopectin ratio	Protective insoluble fiber and coat as in whole intact grains
Intact grain/large particle size	Viscous fibers
Intact starch granule	Enzyme inhibitors
Raw starch	Raw foods (vs. cooked foods)
Physical interaction with fat or protein	Minimal food processing Reduced ripeness in fruit Minimal (compared to extended) storage

Table 1-2. Glycemic Index and Glycemic Load of Representative Foods[8,10]

FOOD	GLYCEMIC INDEX	GLYCEMIC LOAD	CARBOHYDRATE CALCULATION
Carrots	92	4.6	1 cup = 5 g
Corn flakes	80	12	¾ cup = 15 g
White rice	72	10.8	⅓ cup cooked = 15 g
White bread	69	10.3	1 slice = 15 g
Brown rice	66	9.9	½ cup cooked = 15 g
Raisins	64	9.6	2 Tbsp = 15 g
Bananas	62	9.3	1 small = 15 g
White pasta	50	7.5	½ cup cooked = 15 g
Oatmeal	49	7.4	½ cup cooked = 15 g
Sweet potatoes	48	7.2	½ cup = 15 g
Whole wheat pasta	42	6.3	½ cup = 15 g
Oranges	40	6	1 small = 15 g
Apples	39	5.9	1 small = 15 g
Skim milk	46	5.5	1 cup = 12 g
Lentils	29	4.4	½ cup = 15 g
Low fat yogurt	14	2.1	1 cup = 15 g

Glycemic load = Glycemic Index × CHO (g) per serving/100.
Glucose = reference = 100.
*Note: Glycemic load is based on the *amount* of carbohydrate consumed. If more than 1 serving of carbohydrate is consumed, the glycemic load will increase proportionally.

A growing body of research supports that eating a diet with the majority of carbohydrates of lower glycemic load may offer health benefits including weight control, decreased risk of diabetes and heart disease, and reduced morbidity in individuals with chronic diseases including diabetes and heart disease.[11,12,14–19] Furthermore, foods with a low glycemic load are commonly nutrient dense, meaning they provide more nutrients per calorie. For example, 16 ounces of soda has about the same amount of carbohydrates as two medium-sized apples, though the glycemic load of the soda is much higher. The two apples provide more vitamins, minerals, and fiber compared to the soda, making the apples more nutrient dense.

Fiber

In addition to considering a carbohydrate's glycemic index or load, an important consideration when evaluating carbohydrate quality is the food's fiber content.

Fiber is classified as **functional fiber** and **dietary fiber**. Together, dietary and functional fiber comprise "total fiber."

Functional Fiber

Functional fiber is defined as an isolated nondigestible carbohydrate that may have beneficial physiological effects in humans. Functional fiber is typically available as both natural and synthetic dietary supplements, which claim to offer such benefits as improved gastrointestinal symptoms, weight loss, reduced cholesterol, and colon cancer prevention, among other claims. On the food label, *functional fiber* shows up as isolated, nondigestible plant (e.g., resistant starch, pectin, and gums), animal (e.g., chitin and chitosan), or commercially produced (e.g., resistant starch, polydextrose, inulin, and indigestible dextrins) carbohydrates. It is typically *added* to foods.

Dietary Fiber

Dietary fiber is the fiber naturally found in certain foods. It is further classified as **high viscosity** and **low viscosity**. **High viscosity fibers** (typically those that also are referred to as **soluble fiber**) include gums (found in foods like oats, legumes, guar, and barley), pectin (found in foods like apples, citrus fruits, strawberries, and carrots), and psyllium seeds. These fibers slow **gastric emptying**, or the passage of food from the stomach into the intestines. Consequently, once mixed with digestive juices they become gel-like, causing an increased feeling of fullness. Also, the delayed gastric emptying slows the release of sugar into the bloodstream, which may help attenuate insulin resistance. High viscosity fibers also can interfere with the absorption of fat and cholesterol and the recirculation of cholesterol in the liver, which may decrease cholesterol levels.[20] **Low viscosity fibers** (previously referred to as **insoluble fiber**) such as cellulose (found in whole wheat flour, bran, and vegetables), hemicellulose (found in whole grains and bran), and lignin (found in mature vegetables, wheat, and fruit with edible seeds like strawberries and kiwi) play an important role in increasing fecal bulk and provide a laxative effect.

Clearly, fiber serves many important and beneficial roles in the human body.[20–22] Still, the average American consumes far less than the recommended 14 grams per 1,000 calories consumed per day—or the approximately 25 to 35 grams per day for most adults. (Children over the age of 2 should eat their age plus 5 grams per day).[6] With increased consumption of fruits, vegetables, legumes, and whole grains, most Americans could easily achieve this fiber goal (Table 1-3).

Table 1-3. Fiber Content of Commonly Consumed Foods

FOOD	SERVING SIZE	TOTAL DIETARY FIBER (g/SERVING)
Fruits		
Apple, raw, with skin	1 apple	3.3
Banana, raw	1 banana	3.1
Figs, dried	2 figs	3.7
Peaches, dried, sulfured, uncooked	3 halves	3.2
Pear	1 pear	5.1
Vegetables		
Broccoli, raw	½ cup	1.2
Carrots, raw	½ cup	1.5
Celery, raw	1 stalk	0.6
Peas, green, canned	½ cup	3.5
Sweet potato, baked in skin	1 potato	4.8
Legumes		
Beans, baked, canned, plain or vegetarian	½ cup	5.2
Beans, kidney, canned	½ cup	6.9
Lentils, cooked	½ cup	7.8
Peas, split, cooked	½ cup	8.2

Continued

Table 1-3. Fiber Content of Commonly Consumed Foods–cont'd

FOOD	SERVING SIZE	TOTAL DIETARY FIBER (g/SERVING)
Grains		
Bread, whole wheat	1 slice	1.9
Bread, white	1 slice	0.6
Cereal, oatmeal, cooked	1 cup	4.0
Cereal, raisin bran	1 cup	6.8
Cereal, shredded wheat	2 biscuits	5.5
Crackers, whole wheat	4 crackers	1.7
Muffin, oat bran	1 muffin	2.6

Source: Adapted from USDA National Nutrient Database for Standard Reference, Release 20. A complete list of foods can be accessed at www.nal.usda.gov/fnic/foodcomp/Data/SR20/nutrlist/sr20a291.pdf.

SPEED BUMP

4. Explain the factors that constitute a high-quality carbohydrate.
5. Define and describe glycemic index and glycemic load.
6. List several benefits of a high-fiber diet.

CARBOHYDRATES AND ATHLETIC PERFORMANCE

Athletes need the right types and amounts of food before, during, and after exercise to maximize the energy available to fuel optimal performance. Typically, these foods need to be high in carbohydrates. Carbohydrates are readily and efficiently broken down by the body to the monosaccharide glucose, the body's preferred energy source. During exercise, when energy is needed, glucose that is stored in muscle, floating in the bloodstream, and/or stored in the liver can be directed to the working cell where it is converted into ATP. If glucose or glycogen is limited, then **gluconeogenesis** occurs. This entails the conversion of a nonglucose substance such as protein or glycerol (three carbon molecule) into glucose. To inhibit gluconeogenesis and spare protein, it is crucial that an athlete consumes enough carbohydrates to fuel performance. Moreover, athletes who do not consume sufficient carbohydrates may be unable to work at an optimal performance level. Refer to Chapter 7 for a detailed discussion of the importance of carbohydrate intake before, during, and after intense or prolonged physical activity.

CARBOHYDRATES AND WEIGHT MANAGEMENT

Some weight loss diets may advocate severely restricted carbohydrate intake. However, the proportion of macronutrients consumed is not as important as the total caloric intake versus caloric expenditure. If more calories are consumed in a day than are burned through physical activity and the body's metabolic processes, then a person will gain weight. Similar to excess protein or fat consumption, any excess carbohydrates that are consumed in the diet beyond what the body can immediately use (as free glucose or stored as glycogen) can be converted to fat and stored primarily in adipose tissue. Foods that are high in fiber tend to be more filling and may help to reduce caloric intake and contribute to weight loss.[21]

If dieters who severely restrict carbohydrates lose large amounts of weight shortly after starting the diet, the majority of this weight loss comes from loss of water. Glycogen requires water for storage. When these glycogen stores are broken down in response to carbohydrate deprivation, the body excretes water. In the long term, there is no difference in sustained weight loss in dieters on low-carbohydrate diets versus high-carbohydrate diets [23,24] (see Communication Strategies). Chapter 15 describes nutrition and weight management in more detail.

COMMUNICATION STRATEGIES

You have been working with a 44-year-old moderately active and overweight woman who shared her goal to run a half marathon by her 45th birthday, which is 5 months away. She tells you she has made significant changes to her diet, including eliminating all highly refined carbohydrates. She expresses frustration because, although she has been working with you for the past 4 weeks, she says that she has not lost any weight and she does not feel that running a mile is any easier than when she started. She tells you that she is ready to give up on this program and that this will be her last week working with you.

Consider the following communication model, adapted from Holli and Cabrese's *Communication and Education Skills for Dietetics Professionals* (Fig. 1-7):

1. Summarize the client's *explicit* verbal message. What is the *implicit* verbal message?
2. Based on the verbal message above, what nonverbal messages do you expect the client to have given?
3. Summarize how you feel in response to this verbal message from the client.
4. How do you think you would reflexively respond to this statement? What kind of nonverbal feedback do you think you might send?
5. What might be some sources of *psychological* (such as bias, prejudice, close-mindedness) or *physical* (such as room and environmental factors, physiological state of communicators, noise) interference from this interaction?

Although you perceived this statement from your client as an attack, before you respond defensively and risk further damaging the relationship, you tell your client that you can understand her frustration and would like to schedule a follow-up phone call to discuss her concern in more detail and develop an action plan. In the meantime, you decide to look up some characteristics of effective communication. You learn that effective verbal communication should be:

- Descriptive, with a clear and objective statement of the issue at hand rather than evaluative by providing a label or attacking the other person
- Problem-oriented, with objective identification of the main challenges rather than manipulative in trying to get the other person to adopt your point of view
- Provisional, with suggestions for how to overcome barriers treated simply as ideas rather than dogmatic in which advice is stated as if it is mandatory
- Egalitarian, with the health professional on equal ground with the client, rather than superior and dictated by authority or rank
- Empathic, in which the provider tries to relate to the client's feelings and experiences rather than neutral and without regard to the client's feelings

6. Given your understanding of what comprises effective communication, detail how you might respond to this client's concerns.

SPEED BUMP

7. List various types of carbohydrates and their effect on athletic performance and weight management.

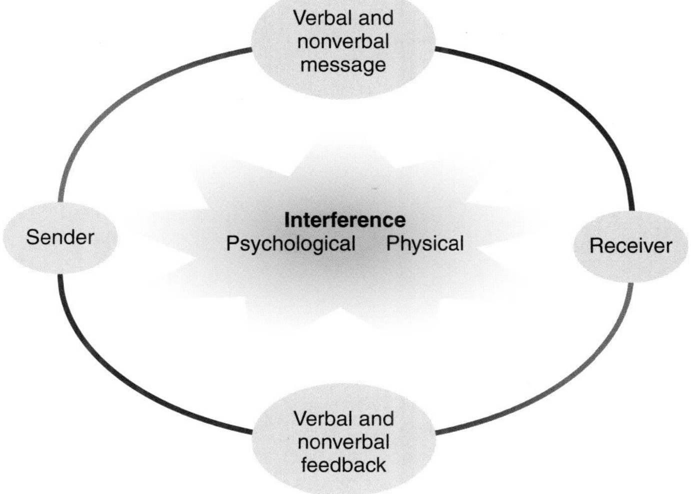

Figure 1-7. Interpersonal communication model. *Reprinted with permission from* Communication and Education Skills for Dietetic Professionals, *5th edition, 2008, by Betsy B. Holli, Julie O'Sullivan Maillet, Judith A. Beto, & Richard J. Calabrese. Philadelphia: Wolters Kluwer Health.*

CHAPTER SUMMARY

Carbohydrates are essential for optimal athletic performance. They also are important to maintain good health, especially those carbohydrates that are high in fiber and low in glycemic load.

KEY POINTS SUMMARY

1. Carbohydrates serve many important functions in the body such as providing energy to fuel activity, sparing protein catabolism, facilitating good cardiovascular and digestive health (from fiber), and providing flavor to foods.
2. Carbohydrates are made of long chains of monosaccharides. All carbohydrates can be converted to glucose in the body and used to provide or store energy. Carbohydrates are stored as glycogen (a capacity of about 90 grams in the liver and 150 grams in the muscle). Any carbohydrates consumed beyond what the body can use or store as glycogen can be converted to fat.
3. Carbohydrates provide 4 calories per gram, except for fiber, which passes through the body largely unabsorbed. Fiber provides 1.5 to 2.5 calories per gram.
4. Natural and artificial sweeteners are made of carbohydrates and are added to foods to increase palatability. Nonnutritive sweeteners contain 0 calories per gram while nutritive sweeteners contain 4 calories per gram.
5. Most people should consume 45% to 65% of total calories from carbohydrates. Athletes need near the higher end with the recommendation from the American College of Sports Medicine and the Academy of Dietetics and Nutrition of 6 to 10 g/kg of body weight (or 2.7 to 4.5 g/lb of body weight) per day based on total energy expenditure, exercise type, gender, and environmental conditions.
6. The highest quality carbohydrates are high in fiber and low in glycemic load.
7. Glycemic index is a measure of blood glucose response after consuming a carbohydrate. Glycemic load is based on how many grams of a particular carbohydrate of a given glycemic index are consumed.
8. High glycemic index carbohydrates are rapidly absorbed by the body and cause a spike in blood glucose and blood insulin levels. Low glycemic index carbohydrates are more slowly absorbed and cause a much smaller, more gradual increase in glucose and insulin.
9. Fiber helps to improve health by delaying gastric emptying, improving cholesterol levels, regulating bowel movements, increasing feelings of satiety, and more. Most people do not consume the recommended 14 grams of fiber per 1,000 calories consumed.
10. Carbohydrates are the body's preferred energy source during exercise. Restricting carbohydrate intake to less than the recommended amounts will negatively affect athletic performance.
11. Carbohydrates in and of themselves do not contribute to weight gain or interfere with weight loss.

PRACTICAL APPLICATIONS

1. A 13-year-old competitive gymnast and her mother have scheduled a consultation with you because the gymnast has experienced increased difficulty with her cardiovascular training over the past few months. She is constantly fatigued. She is consuming adequate calories and 60% of her calories are from carbohydrates. When asked what types of foods she consumes, she indicates that due to her busy schedule she is constantly grabbing quick items such as granola bars, chips, crackers, pretzels, and candy bars. The client's mom brings with her a copy of the gymnast's last sports physical from her pediatrician, which was completed 3 months ago and was normal, including a blood test confirming that she is not anemic. Her weight is normal for her age and height. What is the MOST LIKELY explanation for the gymnast's decreased performance?
   A. Severe restriction of dietary intake
   B. Insufficient carbohydrate intake to fuel her exercise
   C. Consumption of high glycemic index carbohydrates
   D. Overconsumption of carbohydrates

2. A healthy 55-year-old athlete tells you that every time he runs outside in the morning he initially feels great, but after about 15 minutes he frequently has to stop because he quickly becomes lightheaded and dizzy. On further questioning he tells you that he typically eats a bowl of cornflakes about 90 minutes before exercising and that he is careful to consume sips of water every 10 minutes or so during his workouts. What is the MOST LIKELY source of his symptoms?
   A. Cornflakes are a high glycemic index food possibly leading to hypoglycemia during his run.
   B. Cornflakes are a low glycemic index food possibly leading to hypoglycemia during his run.
   C. Water retention due to his intake of corn flakes.
   D. Cornflakes are a nutrient-dense food that can cause dizziness during running.

3. What is the theory behind why lower glycemic index carbohydrates may be better for health?
   A. The shorter glucose chains provide less of a spike in blood sugar.
   B. They have a lesser effect on blood insulin levels.
   C. They help to remove "bad" cholesterol from the bloodstream.
   D. The increased extent of processing allows for faster absorption.

Choose from the following answer choices for questions 4 through 7:
   a. Pancreas
   b. Small intestine
   c. Liver
   d. Mouth

4. Where does carbohydrate digestion begin?
5. This organ releases insulin in response to high blood sugar levels.
6. Where does production of glycogen occur?
7. Where does absorption of carbohydrates occur?
8. A teenage client tells you that she has frequent stomachaches, intermittent episodes of constipation, and occasional headaches. She says that she read in a magazine that a high-fiber diet might help to make her feel better. How might fiber MOST help her symptoms?
   A. A diet high in fiber will help to normalize her bowel movements.
   B. A diet high in fiber will help to delay gastric emptying and lead to feelings of fullness.
   C. A diet high in fiber will help to decrease her LDL cholesterol levels.
   D. A diet high in fiber will help to reduce her feelings of anxiety.
9. A client tells you that after reading about how good fiber is for optimal health she decided to take a fiber supplement that provides 15 grams of fiber per day. She also tries to eat ample amounts of whole grains, fruits, and vegetables. While she feels good overall, she has noticed that over the past several weeks endurance exercise has become more difficult due to frequent stomach cramps and urges to use the restroom. What is the BEST advice to provide this client?
   A. She should eliminate the fiber supplement from her diet and reassess her exercise tolerance.
   B. She should continue the same high-fiber diet and her body will acclimate within the next week.
   C. She should eliminate high-fiber foods within 1 to 3 hours prior to endurance exercise.
   D. She should consult a physician, as her problems are most likely due to an underlying disorder.
10. A 170-pound, 35-year-old male is training for a long-distance endurance event. His daily caloric needs are about 3,000 calories per day. About how many grams of carbohydrate should he eat daily for optimal performance?
   A. 100 grams
   B. 325 grams
   C. 450 grams
   D. 550 grams

Case 1 Kate, the Cross-Country Runner

Kate is a cross-country runner who wants to make sure that she is consuming sufficient carbohydrates for optimal athletic performance and to spare protein. She needs about 2,700 calories per day. Answer the following questions regarding Kate's recommended carbohydrate intake.

Carbohydrate Needs

1. Based on the AMDR for carbohydrates, how many grams of carbohydrate should Kate consume per day (provide a range)?
2. Provide four high glycemic load sources of carbohydrate that she could consume when she needs a quick energy boost.
3. Provide at least eight foods that she could consume throughout her day that are low glycemic index carbohydrate sources.

Case 2 Adele, the Active Octogenarian

Adele is an 85-year-old woman who recently moved to a retirement community after her husband died. With the move, she also decided that she would make significant lifestyle changes, starting with eating "healthier" and exercising more. One of Adele's daughters just started a low-carbohydrate diet and convinced Adele to start with her. Now Adele wonders if that was the right decision to make.

Carbohydrate Needs

1. Adele is on a very-low carbohydrate diet (about 15% of calories from carbohydrates). She eats about 1,600 calories per day. What is the difference between the amount of carbohydrates that Adele is advised to consume and how much she gets on this diet?
2. What are possible complications for Adele's exercise program resulting from her new diet?

Carbohydrates and Exercise

Adele frequently participates in water aerobics classes. Lately she says that she has had decreased energy and it is increasingly difficult to get through the class.

1. What might be some nutritional reasons why Adele has low energy?
2. How might Adele modify her diet?

Special Considerations: Low Glycemic Index Diet

Concerned about Adele's waning energy levels and her overall health, her physician requests that she abandon the very-low carbohydrate diet. He says she should try to consume a low-glycemic-load diet. Adele asks you what this means.

1. Explain how you would describe a low-glycemic-load diet to a layperson.

TRAIN YOURSELF: CARBOHYDRATE NEEDS

1. Based on your weight, what carbohydrate range do you need in a day? (Use the recommended carbohydrate intake formula for athletes by the Academy of Nutrition and Dietetics on page 10 or app.)

2. Think back to all of the food you ate in the past 24 hours. On a sheet of paper, complete a dietary recall of your intake. Input your food intake into the Supertracker.usda.gov, MyFitnessPal.com, or other online nutrition calculator or app. Approximately how many grams of carbohydrates did you eat? How does this compare to your recommended needs? How much fiber did you consume? Did you reach the recommended 14 grams per 1,000 calories? If not, what foods could you incorporate into your diet to help you increase your fiber intake?

3. Complete a sample meal and snack plan that would provide you with the recommended amount of carbohydrates.

REFERENCES

1. Hicks RM, Wakefield, J, & Chowaniec, J, Impurities in saccharin and bladder cancer. *Nature.* 1973;90(5): 1203-1214.
2. Reuber MD. Carcinogenicity of saccharin. *Environ Health Perspect.* 1978;25:173-200.
3. Takayama S, Sieber, S.M., Adamson, R.H., et al. Long-term feeding of sodium saccharin to nonhuman primates: implications for urinary tract cancer. *J Natl Cancer Inst.* 1998;90(1):19-25.
4. Carlborg FW. A cancer risk assessment for saccharin. *Food Chem Toxicol.* 1985;23(4-5):499-506.
5. Roberfroid MB. Health benefits of non-digestible oligosaccharides. *Adv Exp Med Biol.* 1997;427:211-219.
6. Institute of Medicine (U.S.). Panel on Macronutrients, Institute of Medicine (U.S.). Standing Committee on the Scientific Evaluation of Dietary Reference Intakes. *Dietary reference intakes for energy, carbohydrate, fiber, fat, fatty acids, cholesterol, protein, and amino acids.* Washington, DC: National Academies Press; 2005.
7. Tate, D.F., Turner-McGrievy, G, Lyons, E., et al. Replacing caloric beverages with water or diet beverages for weight loss in adults: main results of the Choose Healthy Options Consciously Everyday (CHOICE) randomized clinical trial. *Am J Clin Nutr,* 2012 Mar; 95(3): 555-563.
8. Mahan LK, Escott-Stump S. *Krause's Food, Nutrition, & Diet Therapy.* 12th ed. Philadelphia: W.B. Saunders; 2011.
9. Rodriguez NR, Di Marco NM, Langley S. American College of Sports Medicine position stand. Nutrition and athletic performance. *Med Sci Sports Exerc.* March 2009;41(3): 709-731.
10. Atkinson FS, Foster-Powell K, & Brand-Miller JC.. International tables of glycemic index and glycemic load values: 2008. *Diabetes Care.* 2008;31(12):2281-2283.
11. Willett W, Manson J. & Liu S. Glycemic index, glycemic load, and risk of type 2 diabetes. *Am J Clin Nutr.* 2002; 76(1):274S-280S.
12. Barclay AW, Petocz P, McMillan-Price J., et al. Glycemic index, glycemic load, and chronic disease risk—a meta-analysis of observational studies. *Am J Clin Nutr.* 2008;87(3):627-637.
13. Wolever TM, Jenkins DJ. The use of the glycemic index in predicting the blood glucose response to mixed meals. *Am J Clin Nutr.* January 1986;43(1):167-172.
14. Ludwig DS. The glycemic index: physiological mechanisms relating to obesity, diabetes, and cardiovascular disease. *JAMA.* May 8 2002;287(18):2414-2423.
15. Barclay AW, Petocz P, McMillan-Price J, et al. Glycemic index, glycemic load, and chronic disease risk—a meta-analysis of observational studies. *Am J Clin Nutr.* March 2008; 87(3):627-637.
16. Botero D, Ebbeling CB, Blumberg JB, et al. Acute effects of dietary glycemic index on antioxidant capacity in a nutrient-controlled feeding study. *Obesity (Silver Spring).* 2009;17(9):1664-1670.
17. Hu Y, Block G, Norkus EP, et al. Relations of glycemic index and glycemic load with plasma oxidative stress markers. *Am J Clin Nutr.* 2006;84(1):70-76; quiz 266-267.
18. Levitan EB, Cook NR, Stampfer MJ, et al. Dietary glycemic index, dietary glycemic load, blood lipids, and C-reactive protein. *Metabolism.* 2008;57(3):437-443.
19. Liu S, Willett WC, Stampfer MJ., et al. A prospective study of dietary glycemic load, carbohydrate intake, and risk of coronary heart disease in US women. *Am J Clin Nutr.* 2000; 71(6):1455-1461.
20. Anderson JW, Baird P, Davis RH, et al. Health benefits of dietary fiber. *Nutr Rev.* 2009;67(4):188-205.
21. Howarth NC, Saltzman E, Roberts SB. Dietary fiber and weight regulation. *Nutr Rev.* 2001;59(5):129-139.
22. Zhang C, Liu S, Solomon CG, Hu FB. Dietary fiber intake, dietary glycemic load, and the risk for gestational diabetes mellitus. *Diabetes Care.* 2006;29(10):2223-2230.
23. Dansinger ML, Gleason JA, Griffith JL, Selker HP, Schaefer EJ. Comparison of the Atkins, Ornish, Weight Watchers, and Zone diets for weight loss and heart disease risk reduction: a randomized trial. *JAMA.* January 5 2005;293(1):43-53.
24. Ebbeling CB, Leidig MM, Feldman HA, Lovesky MM, Ludwig DS. Effects of a low-glycemic load vs low-fat diet in obese young adults: a randomized trial. *JAMA.* May 16 2007;297(19):2092-2102.
25. Duffey KJ, Popkin BM. High-fructose corn syrup: is this what's for dinner? *Am J Clin Nutr.* December 2008;88(6): 1722S-1732S.
26. Rizkalla SW. Health implications of fructose consumption: a review of recent data. *Nutr Metab (Lond).* 2010;7:82.

27. Welsh JA, Sharma A, Abramson JL, et al. Caloric sweetener consumption and dyslipidemia among US adults. *JAMA.* 2010;303(15):1490-1497.
28. Kobylewski S, Eckhert CD. *Toxicology of rebaudioside A: a Review.* Los Angeles: University of California at Los Angeles; 2008.
29. Goyal SK, Samsher, Goyal RK. Stevia (Stevia rebaudiana) a bio-sweetener: a review. *Int J Food Sci Nutr.* February 2010; 61(1):1-10.
30. Sacks FM, Bray GA, Carey VJ, et al. Comparison of weight-loss diets with different compositions of fat, protein, and carbohydrates. *N Engl J Med.* February 26 2009;360(9): 859-873.
31. Bray GA, Smith SR, de Jonge L, et al. Effect of dietary protein content on weight gain, energy expenditure, and body composition during overeating: a randomized controlled trial. *JAMA.* January 4 2012;307(1):47-55.
32. Anderson, G.H., Foreyt, J., Sigman-Grents, M., Allison D.B. The use of low-calorie sweeteners by adults: impact on weight management. *J Nutr* 2012 June; 142(6): 1163S-1169S.

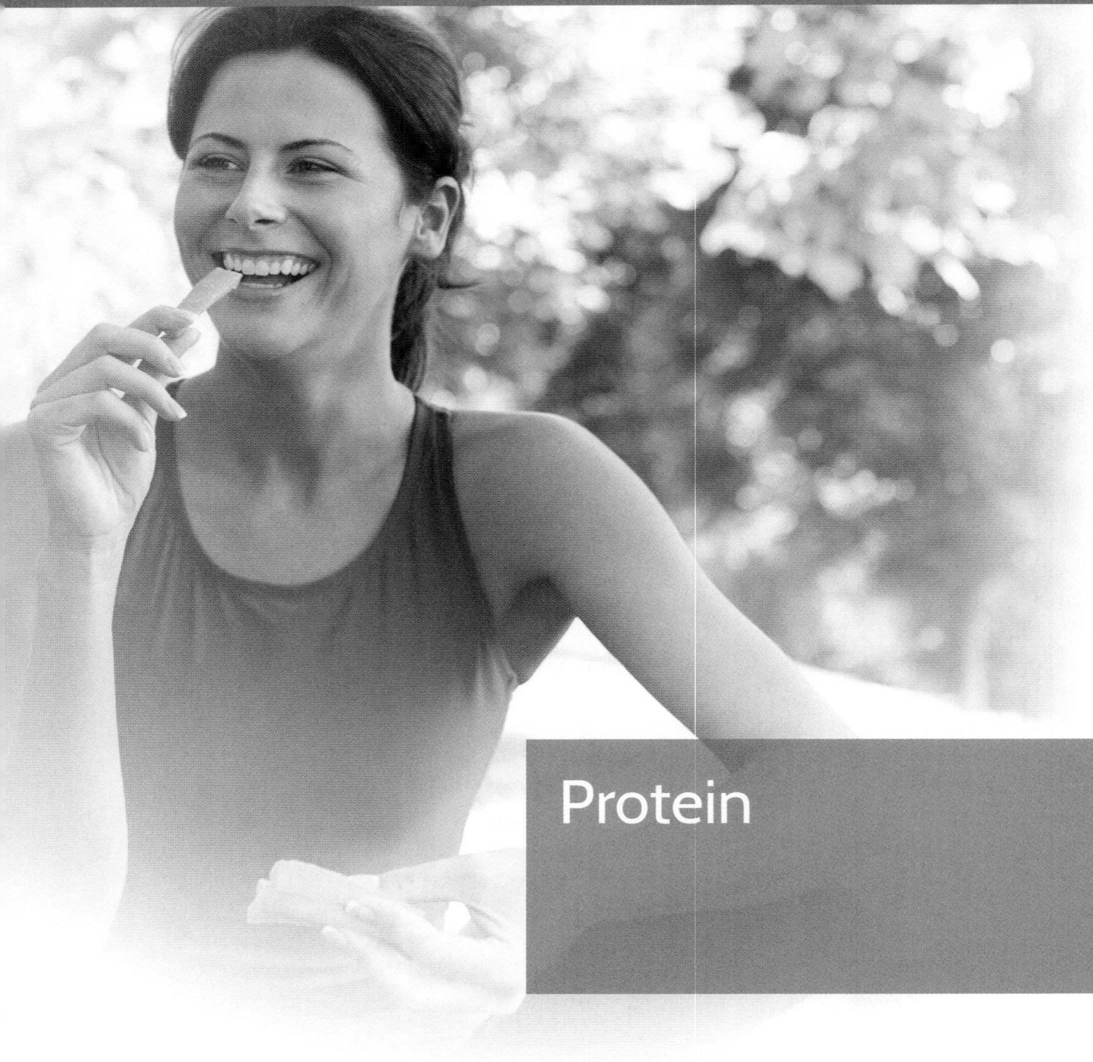

CHAPTER 2

Protein

CHAPTER OUTLINE

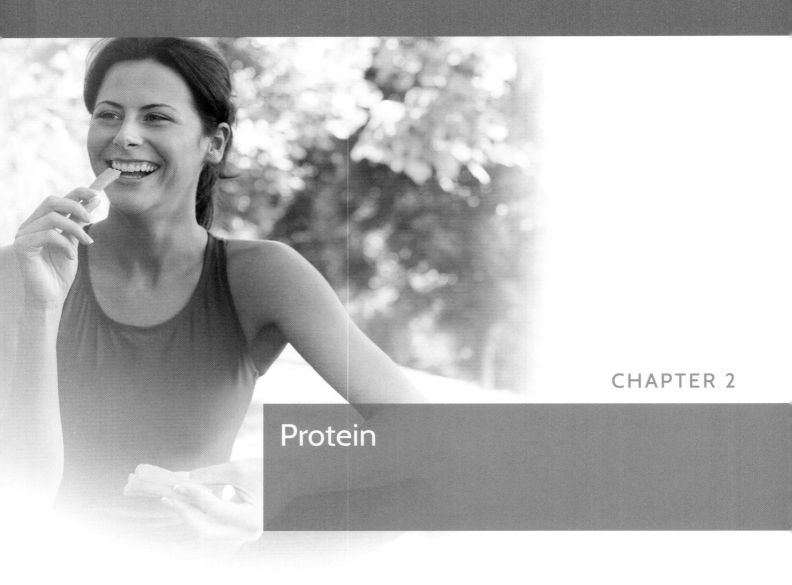

LEARNING OBJECTIVES

After studying this chapter, the reader should be able to:

2.1 Explain the factors that constitute a high-quality protein.

2.2 Briefly describe the process of protein digestion and absorption.

2.3 Outline the process of protein metabolism.

2.4 Describe several benefits and risks of a high-protein diet.

2.5 List various types of protein and their effect on athletic performance.

2.6 List several considerations when working with clients interested in adopting a high-protein diet.

KEY TERMS

alanine-glucose cycle The cycle of transporting pyruvate and nitrogen from the muscle tissues to the liver as the amino acid alanine. In the liver, the alanine unloads the nitrogen group to become pyruvate, which is converted to glucose through gluconeogenesis. This process moves the work of gluconeogenesis from the muscle to the liver.

amino acids The basic building blocks of proteins. Each amino acid has an amino- or nitrogen-containing group and a unique R chain that determines its ability to be used in various processes. Also known as peptides.

amino acid pool The amino acids available in the body to be used for protein synthesis.

anabolism The state in which the body builds and creates new tissues.

antibodies Proteins that fight infection.

bioavailability The degree to which a nutrient can be absorbed and used by the body.

branched chain amino acids Essential amino acids with a branched R chain. These amino acids are metabolized in the muscle and are thought to be important in the formation of muscle mass.

catabolism The state in which the body breaks down tissues and amino acids for fuel.

complementary protein Combining two or more limiting proteins to form a complete protein.

complete protein A food item that contains all of the essential amino acids.

deamination The process of removing a nitrogen group from an amino acid.

denaturation The process of unfolding a protein by destroying its quaternary, tertiary, and secondary structure.

dipeptide Two amino acids connected by a peptide bond.

enzymes Proteins that speed up the rate of chemical reactions.

essential amino acid An amino acid that cannot be made by the body and must be consumed in the diet.

gastrin Hormone that prepares the stomach for food digestion; secreted by the stomach and stimulates pepsin release.

hypertrophy Abnormal increase in size; excessive growth.

incomplete protein A food item that does not contain all of the essential amino acids.

lacto-ovo-vegetarian A vegetarian who consumes eggs and dairy products but does not consume meat, poultry, or fish.

lacto-vegetarian A vegetarian who consumes dairy products but does not consume eggs, meat, poultry, or fish.

micelle A compound similar to a soap sud that has a hydrophobic (water-averse) inside and a hydrophilic (water-loving) outside.

nitrogen balance The amount of nitrogen (via protein) consumed compared to the amount of nitrogen excreted. This provides information as to the person's metabolic state, muscle synthesis, muscle degradation, or equilibrium.

nonessential amino acid An amino acid that can be made by the body.

pepsin The stomach acid responsible for initiating the digestion of proteins.

peptide bonds The connections between amino acids.

polypeptide A chain of many amino acids connected by peptide bonds.

positive nitrogen balance The state in which the amount of nitrogen (via protein) consumed is greater than the amount of nitrogen excreted in feces, urine, and skin. During this time the body is building muscle protein; this occurs during pregnancy, infancy, childhood, adolescence, recovery from illness, and in response to resistance training.

protein digestibility corrected amino acid score (PDCAAS) A measure of protein quality that compares the essential amino acid composition of a reference protein with the test protein; the FDA- and WHO-endorsed method of measuring protein quality.

proteolysis The process by which proteins are broken down into simpler, soluble compounds.

proteolytic enzymes Enzymes made in the pancreas and released into the small intestine to break peptide bonds between amino acids during digestion.

recommended dietary allowance (RDA) The amount of nutrient known to be adequate to meet the nutritional needs of nearly all healthy persons.
small intestine The three-segment portion of the digestive system between the stomach and large intestine that is responsible for the majority of digestion and absorption of swallowed foods.
stomach An organ between the esophagus and small intestine that stores swallowed food, mixes the food with stomach acids, and then sends the mixture to the small intestine.
tripeptide Three amino acid chain combined by peptide bonds.

CALCULATION

1 gram of protein = 4 calories

trypsin The active form of the precursor trypsinogen, which breaks down protein chains into single amino acids, dipeptides, and tripeptides.
urea The nitrogenous byproduct of protein deamination; formed in the liver and excreted in the urine.
vegan A person who does not include any animal products in their diet. This means they do not consume meat, poultry, fish, eggs, or dairy products.
vegetarian A person who eats a plant-based diet and does not consume meat and poultry.
whey A high-quality protein; the liquid remaining after milk has been curdled and strained.
whey protein concentrate A whey protein supplement that is 25% to 89% protein by weight.
whey protein isolate A whey protein supplement that is 90% or more protein by weight; lactose free.
whey protein powder A form of whey protein that is 11% to 15% protein by weight; used as an additive in many food products.

INTRODUCTION

From athletes and body builders to dieters, weekend warriors, and the health conscious, high-protein diets and their promises of muscle gain, weight loss, and improved health appeal to a wide diversity of people. But how much and what kind of protein is best, and does the macronutrient fulfill all of its promises?

PROTEIN STRUCTURE

Proteins are composed of long chains of **amino acids** linked by peptide bonds (Fig. 2-1). The order in which the amino acids are linked together is called the primary structure. The primary structure dictates the final structure and function of a protein. The primary structure is coiled or pleated into its secondary structure. The coil or pleated strand is then looped into its tertiary structure. Multiple tertiary structures can be bound together to make the final quaternary structure. The final quaternary structure is a protein.

PROTEIN FUNCTION

Proteins form the major structural components of muscle as well as that of the brain, nervous system, blood, skin, and hair. This important macronutrient serves as the transport mechanism for iron, vitamins, minerals, fats, and oxygen within the body, and is the key to acid-base and fluid balance. **Enzymes** that speed up chemical reactions and **antibodies** that the body uses to fight infection are proteins. In situations of energy deprivation, the body can break down proteins for energy. With all of protein's essential functions, the human body is served well by consumption of the right kind and correct amount of high-quality proteins.

PROTEIN QUALITY

A specific food's protein quality is determined by assessing its essential amino acid composition, digestibility, and **bioavailability**. All proteins are made up of some combination of amino acids. There are nine **essential amino acids**, which, by definition, are amino acids that cannot be made by the body and must be consumed in the diet. The other 11 are called **nonessential amino acids** because they can be made by the body and do not need to be obtained through the diet (Table 2-1).

Generally, animal products contain all of the essential amino acids (called **complete proteins**), whereas plant foods do not and are called **incomplete proteins**. Notable exceptions include soy, quinoa, chia seeds, buckwheat, hemp, and flax seeds which are plant-based complete protein.

The **protein digestibility corrected amino acid score** (PDCAAS) is the most accepted and widely used measure of protein quality. The PDCAAS is calculated through a somewhat complex mathematical formulation that gives each protein food a score determined by its chemical score (essential amino acid content in a test protein divided by the amino acid content in a reference protein food) multiplied

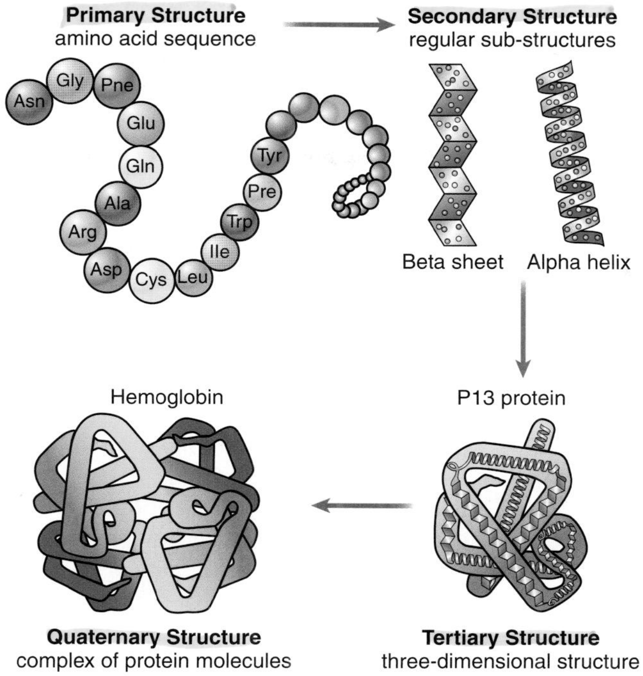

Figure 2-1. Protein structure.

by its fecal digestibility. A value of 1.0 is the highest PDCAAS score. (In reality, some proteins may have a score greater than 1.0, but physiologically the increased score is essentially the same as 1.0.) This score means that after digestion the test protein provides the body with 100% of the essential amino acids that the body needs. Casein, egg, milk, whey, and soy proteins have a score of 1.0. Beef comes in next (0.92), followed by black beans (0.75), peanuts (0.52), and wheat gluten (0.25)[1] (see Evaluating the Evidence).

Protein bioavailability is the amount of protein the body can absorb and use, which is an extension of digestibility. The more easily a food is digested, the more bioavailable it is to the body.

Animal proteins are complete proteins (have all essential amino acids), have higher PDCAAS values, and are therefore more bioavailable. That is why animal proteins are better sources of high-quality protein than plant proteins. However, an individual can boost protein quality and obtain all the essential amino acids by combining incomplete plant proteins to form a **complementary protein**. Excellent combinations include grains and legumes (rice and beans), grains and dairy (pasta and cheese), and legumes and seeds (falafel). Box 2-1 describes factors related to choosing the right protein.

SPEED BUMP

1. **Explain the factors that constitute a high-quality protein.**

Table 2-1. The Amino Acids

The pool of 20 amino acids combine to form an unlimited number of proteins, which are strings of 100+ amino acids joined together by peptide bonds. Nine essential amino acids must be consumed in the diet, while the body can produce the other 11 nonessential amino acids. All amino acids share the same general structure of a carbohydrate plus a nitrogen-based amino group; the "R" group, or amino acid side chain, is what makes each amino acid unique. Amino acids with similar "R" groups are grouped together and share similar functions.

AMINO ACID	CLASSIFICATION	METABOLIC CLASSIFICATION
Glycine	Nonessential	Glucogenic
Alanine	Nonessential	Glucogenic
Valine	Essential	Glucogenic
Leucine	Essential	Ketogenic
Isoleucine	Essential	Glucogenic/ ketogenic
Cysteine	Essential	Glucogenic
Methionine	Essential	Glucogenic
Serine	Nonessential	Glucogenic
Threonine	Essential	Glucogenic/ ketogenic
Phenylalanine	Essential	Glucogenic/ ketogenic
Tyrosine	Nonessential	Glucogenic/ ketogenic
Tryptophan	Essential	Glucogenic/ ketogenic
Proline	Nonessential	Glucogenic
Lysine	Essential	Ketogenic
Histidine	Essential	Glucogenic
Arginine	Nonessential	Glucogenic
Aspartic acid	Nonessential	Glucogenic
Glutamic acid	Nonessential	Glucogenic

PROTEIN TYPES

Whey

Whey is one of the two major milk proteins; the other is casein. **Whey** is the liquid remaining after the milk

EVALUATING THE EVIDENCE

Determining Protein Quality

Several methods are used to measure protein quality.

Name	Description	Typical Use	Rationale (i.e., why this method could be valid)	Strengths	Limitations
Protein Digestibility Correct Amino Acid Score (PDCAAS)	Calculated as the amount of the first limiting essential amino acid of the test protein (mg amino acid in 1 g of test protein) divided by the amount of the same amino acid in a reference protein multiplied by true fecal digestibility. The reference amino acids are based upon the essential amino acid requirements of preschool-age children.	Considered to be "gold standard" for determining protein quality.	Compared to the other methods, more accurately measures the correct relative nutritional value of animal and vegetable sources of protein in the diet.	Based on human amino acid requirements (albeit for a young child). Uses essential amino acid composition as the primary marker for protein quality. Objective measurement.	Measure of a single protein's quality, not of an entire diet comprised of many protein sources. Does not take into consideration the quality of intake of combined proteins (such as a grain protein combined with a white bean protein, which would give a PDCAAS of 1.0, though the individual proteins PDCAAS ranges from .50–.70). Based on requirements of preschool children, which is not representative of the adult population. Values may be > 100% but are truncated to 100% for purposes of reporting. This can create difficulties when determining a value of mixed food intakes. Takes into account fecal digestibility, while ileal digestibility is more accurate. Difficult to assess in practice (need to use reference chart).
Protein Efficiency Ratio	A rat is fed a test protein and then weight gain in grams is	Until the 1990s, was the standard by which the FDA determined	Characterizes how well a protein helps to support growth, a key	Widely recognized and utilized within the food industry.	Based on needs of rats, which are not necessarily highly correlated with

EVALUATING THE EVIDENCE—cont'd

Name	Description	Typical Use	Rationale (i.e., why this method could be valid)	Strengths	Limitations
	measured per gram of protein consumed. The calculated value is compared to 2.7, which is the standard value of casein.	recommended dietary allowances.	function of protein.		the needs of humans. Overestimates the value of some animal proteins and underestimates the value of some vegetable proteins. Underestimates the value of those proteins that may not support growth but help with maintenance.
Biological Value	Calculated by dividing the nitrogen used for tissue formation by the nitrogen absorbed from blood and multiplied by 100, which is the percentage of nitrogen utilized.	Often used in body building.	Measures how efficiently the body utilizes a protein. A higher value indicates a higher amount of essential amino acids.	Provides good measure of usability of a protein (albeit under highly controlled "laboratory" conditions).	Does not take into consideration how rapidly and effectively a protein can be digested and absorbed. High amount of variation in bioavailability of any individual food based on preparation methods and consumption of other food items. Some foods deficient in an essential amino acid can still receive a relatively high score.
Net Protein Utilization	Calculated by dividing the nitrogen used for tissue formation by the amount of nitrogen consumed and multiplied by 100.	Not commonly used anymore.	Functions similar to biological value with the addition that it takes into consideration digestibility.	Similar to biological value	Similar to biological value except that it does take digestibility into account

The FDA/WHO endorsed the PDCAAS as the most accurate and reliable method of measuring protein quality.

1. Why do you think the FDA and WHO chose the PDCAAS method as the most reliable; that is, what are its strengths compared to the other methods?
2. Describe what you think would be an "ideal" way to measure protein quality.
3. In everyday practice, how might your clients evaluate the protein quality of the foods they eat?
4. How does protein quality factor into nutritional recommendations for a recreational or competitive athlete?

Box 2-1. Choosing the Right Protein

Several factors come into play when choosing a protein source: protein quality, health benefits, dietary restrictions, cost, convenience, taste—to name just a few. While no one type of protein is best for everyone, keep these considerations in mind:

1. **Protein quality varies.** Egg, milk, and soy contain all of the essential amino acids and are easily digestible and absorbed. Fruits, vegetables, grains, and nuts are incomplete proteins and must be combined over the course of the day to ensure adequate intake of each of the essential amino acids.
2. **Protein does not exist in a vacuum.** Remember that other macronutrients also offer health benefits. While beef is a fairly good protein source, it is also high in saturated fat and calories. For example, a 6-ounce broiled porterhouse steak contains 38 grams of protein, but it also delivers 44 grams of fat, 16 of them saturated—almost three-fourths of the recommended daily intake for saturated fat. The same amount of salmon gives you 34 grams of protein and only 18 grams of fat, 4 of them saturated.
3. **Different proteins are better at different times.** Whey protein is rapidly digested, resulting in short bursts of amino acids into the blood-stream, whereas casein is slowly digested, resulting in a more prolonged release of amino acids.[26] If the goal is for amino acids to be readily available for muscle regeneration immediately following a workout, protein intake should be timed accordingly.
4. **A high-protein diet is not for everybody.** Individuals with pre-existing disease, such as kidney disease, osteoporosis, diabetes, or liver disease, should consult with their physician prior to adopting a high-protein diet.

has been curdled and strained. There are three varieties of whey—**whey protein powder, whey protein concentrate,** and **whey protein isolate**—all of which provide high levels of the essential and **branched chain amino acids** (leucine, isoleucine, and valine, which have branched side chains and are thought to be important in muscle protein synthesis), vitamins, and minerals. Whey powder is 11% to 15% protein and is used as an additive in many food products. Whey concentrate is 25% to 89% protein, whereas whey isolate is 90+% protein; both are commonly used in dietary supplements. It should be noted that while the isolate form is nearly pure whey, some of the proteins can be lost during the manufacturing process. Unlike the other whey forms, the isolate is lactose-free.[1]

Studies have found that whey protein offers numerous health benefits, some of which are highlighted in Figure 2-2.[2-4] Whey contains high levels of the amino acid leucine, which plays a particularly important role in muscle **hypertrophy** (excessive growth).[4,5] Whey is rapidly digested and absorbed and has a remarkable ability to stimulate muscle protein synthesis, even more so than other high-quality proteins such as casein and soy.[4]

Casein

Casein, which gives milk its white color, accounts for 70% to 80% of milk protein.[1] Casein exists in what is known as a **micelle**, a compound similar to soap suds

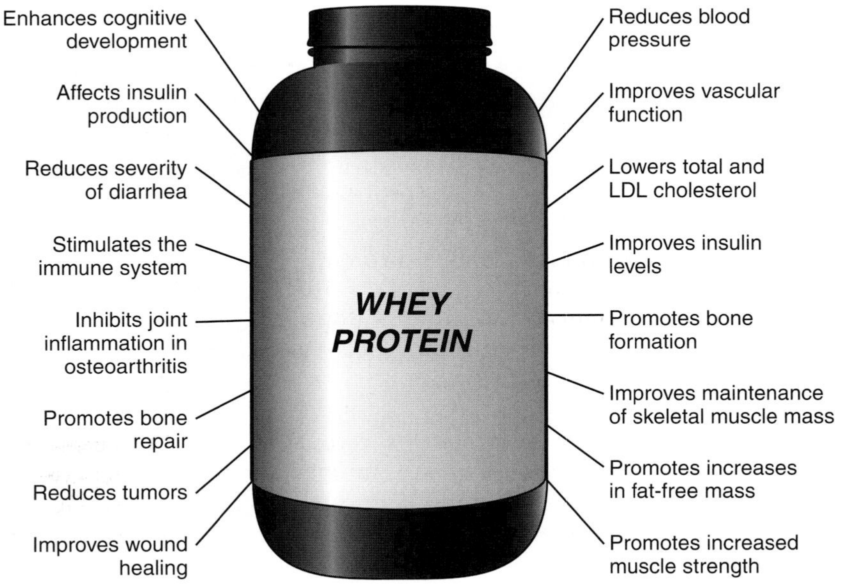

Figure 2-2. Health benefits of whey protein.

that has a hydrophobic (water-averse) inside and a hydrophilic (water-loving) outside. In the **stomach**, the micelle is broken down and casein is released. The casein released from multiple micelles then aggregates and is digested via **proteolysis**, the process by which proteins are broken down into simpler, soluble compounds. Digestion is slow due to the aggregation of casein, allowing the protein to provide a sustained slow release of amino acids into the bloodstream, sometimes lasting for hours.[1] During a resistance training workout that produces micro tears in the muscle tissues, a ready supply of amino acids is useful. Some studies suggest that combined casein and whey may produce the greatest muscular strength improvements after an intensive resistance training program.[6]

Soy

Soy is the most widely used vegetable protein. It is one of the only vegetable proteins that contains all of the essential amino acids, including a high proportion of branched chain amino acids. Similar to whey, soy proteins can be consumed in three types: flour (50% protein), which is often used in baked goods; concentrates (70% protein), which are commonly added to nutrition bars, cereals, and yogurts; and isolates (90% protein). Soy isolates are highly digestible and often added to sports drinks, health beverages, and infant formulas.[1]

Although early studies suggested that soy might decrease low-density lipoprotein (LDL) cholesterol and blood pressure, protect against breast cancer, maintain bone density, and decrease menopausal symptoms,[1] subsequent studies failed to confirm the early research. The Nutrition Committee of the American Heart Association (AHA) released an advisory warning against soy or isoflavone (a component in soy) supplementation because of a lack of benefit[7] but did recommend increased intake of soy products such as tofu, soy burgers, and soy nuts. Soy foods are thought to be heart healthy due to their high content of polyunsaturated fats, fiber, vitamins, and minerals and low levels of saturated fat.[7]

PROTEIN DIGESTION AND ABSORPTION

Protein digestion begins in the stomach with **denaturation**. Denaturing is an important process to understand in terms of protein digestion. It is the destruction of the quaternary, tertiary, and secondary structure of the protein, leaving only the primary structure, which is the sequence of amino acids connected together by peptide bonds. Adding acid, salt, or heat to meat products facilitates denaturation. This process happens in food. When a cook marinates a piece of meat in acid, the meat becomes lighter in color and has an almost "cooked" appearance. This is where the acid has denatured the proteins. The same process happens in the stomach when food mixes with hydrochloric acid. Denaturing a protein makes it more available to digestive enzymes. Vegetable protein is not as well digested as animal protein because it is less available to digestive enzymes. Furthermore, food processing can damage amino acids and reduce their availability for digestion.

As soon as the body anticipates eating (whether from external cues, like seeing or smelling food, or internal cues, like thinking of food), the stomach releases the hormone **gastrin**. The gastrin stimulates the stomach to release hydrochloric acid (Fig. 2-3). The resulting rapid acidification of the stomach denatures proteins and triggers the activation of the enzyme **pepsin**. Pepsin breaks the **peptide bonds** between amino acids to shorten long protein complex into shorter **polypeptide** chains. The stomach mixes and churns the food until it becomes chyme. It is then released in small quantities into the **small intestine** over the course of 1 to 4 hours. The pancreas then releases **proteolytic enzymes** into the small intestine. Trypsinogen, which is transformed into **trypsin** in the small intestine, is an example of a proteolytic enzyme responsible for further breaking down proteins into single amino acids or amino acids joined in twos (**dipeptide**) or threes (**tripeptide**). The dipeptides and tripeptides are absorbed into the intestinal epithelial cells, cleaved into single amino acids, and passed to the bloodstream. After being absorbed into the bloodstream, they are carried to the **liver**.

PROTEIN METABOLISM

Amino acids may be used for anabolic or catabolic functions. **Anabolism** is the state in which the body builds and creates new tissues. **Catabolism** is the state in which the body breaks down tissues and amino acids for fuel.

Anabolic

Amino acids may be used in the synthesis of new proteins. The new proteins may be structural, such as actin and myosin, or fibrous, such as collagen. They may be hormones, enzymes, or transport proteins found on cell membranes or located in the bloodstream, antibodies such as immunoglobins, or any other type of protein. When a protein is formed, DNA dictates the primary sequence. Remember that the primary sequence is a string of amino acids held together by peptide bonds. If an essential amino acid required in the primary sequence is missing, the protein is not made. If a nonessential amino acid is missing, the protein can be formed via transamination. Transamination is the transfer of the nitrogen (or amino) group from one amino acid to another compound to form a nonessential amino acid. After the primary sequence is formed, the peptide undergoes coiling and folding to

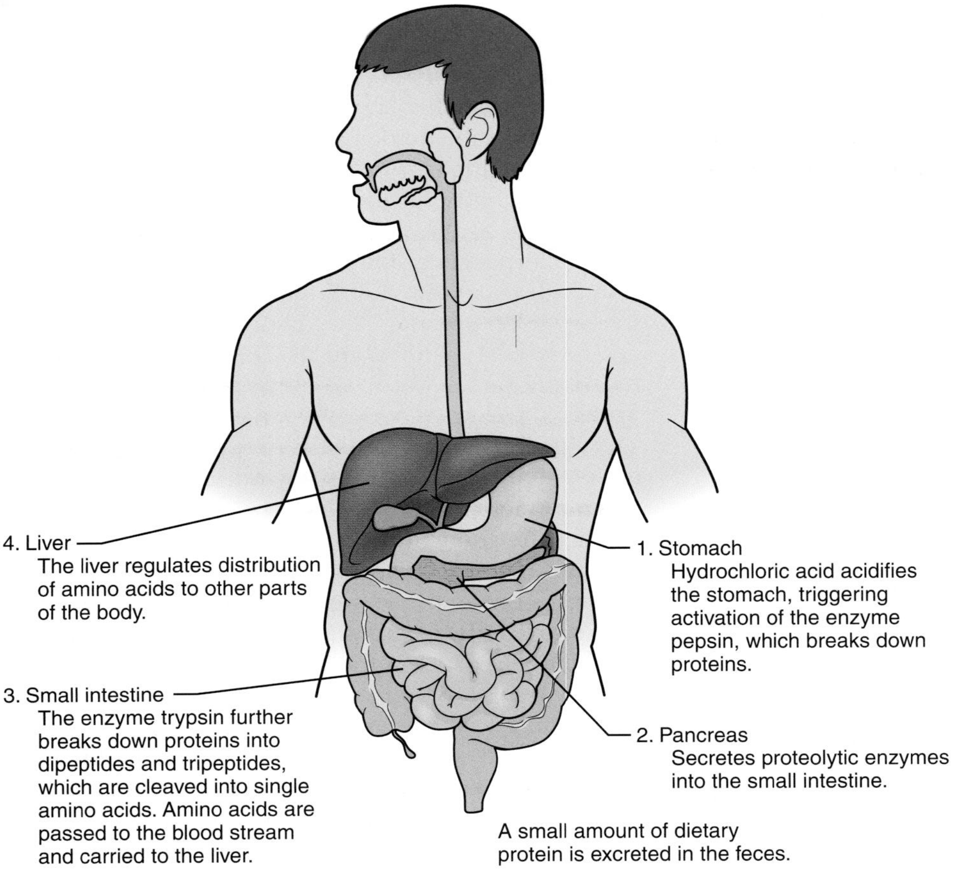
4. Liver
The liver regulates distribution of amino acids to other parts of the body.
1. Stomach
Hydrochloric acid acidifies the stomach, triggering activation of the enzyme pepsin, which breaks down proteins.
3. Small intestine
The enzyme trypsin further breaks down proteins into dipeptides and tripeptides, which are cleaved into single amino acids. Amino acids are passed to the blood stream and carried to the liver.
2. Pancreas
Secretes proteolytic enzymes into the small intestine.
A small amount of dietary protein is excreted in the feces.

Figure 2-3. Protein digestion.

form the secondary, tertiary, and quaternary structures until it becomes a functioning protein.

Catabolic

Amino acids may undergo catabolic reactions, including energy production. In the liver, the amino acid undergoes **deamination**. Deamination is the process by which the amino or nitrogen group is removed from the carbon skeleton. The nitrogen is converted to **urea** via the urea cycle. The urea is then sent from the liver to the kidneys to be excreted in urine. The carbon skeleton can be converted to glucose or ketones and metabolized for energy, or used for cholesterol or fatty acid synthesis. All carbon skeletons can be used for energy, but only glucogenic amino acids can make glucose and only ketogenic amino acids can make ketones.

Branched chain amino acids are metabolized in the muscle. Because the urea cycle occurs in the liver, the body must transport the nitrogen from the muscle to the liver. It does so via the **glucose-alanine cycle**. In the muscle, a branched chain amino acid is transaminated. The carbon skeleton is used to make energy, glucose, or fat and the nitrogen is transferred to a different carbon skeleton to make the nonessential amino acid alanine (Fig. 2-4). The alanine travels from the muscle to the liver where it is deaminated into pyruvate and nitrogen. The nitrogen enters the urea cycle and the pyruvate can enter gluconeogenesis. The new glucose

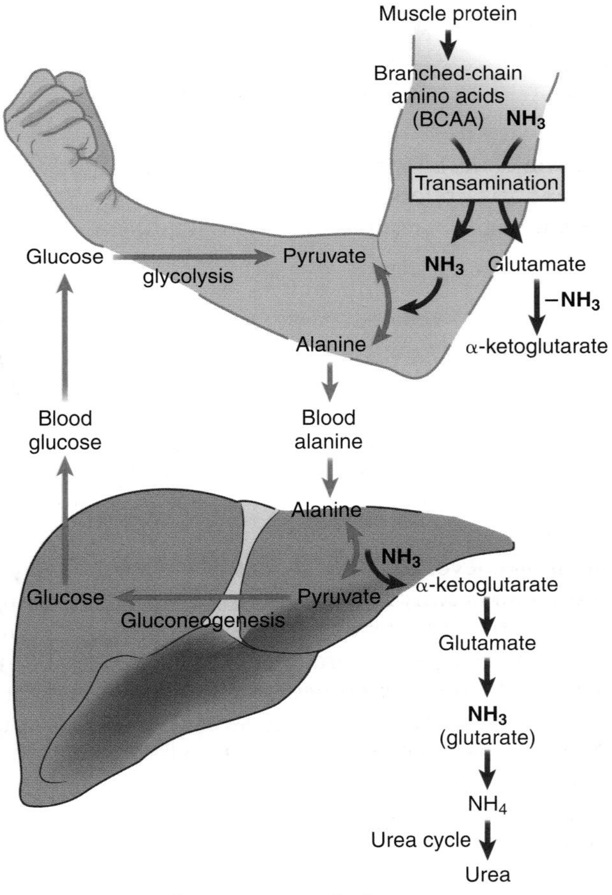
Muscle protein
Branched-chain amino acids (BCAA)
NH_3
Transamination
Glucose
glycolysis
Pyruvate
NH_3
Glutamate
$-NH_3$
α-ketoglutarate
Alanine
Blood glucose
Blood alanine
Alanine
NH_3
Glucose
Gluconeogenesis
Pyruvate
α-ketoglutarate
Glutamate
NH_3
(glutarate)
NH_4
Urea cycle
Urea

Figure 2-4. Muscle protein catabolism.

that has been made in the liver can be used in the liver or transported back to the muscle. Ultimately, this process transfers the burden of glucose production from the muscle to the liver.

Unlike carbohydrates and fat, the body does not store protein. The continuous recycling of amino acids through the removal and addition of nitrogen allows the body to carefully regulate protein balance. In a healthy body, the amount of protein ingested is exactly matched by the amount of protein excreted in feces, urine, and skin (**nitrogen balance**). The muscle tissues undergo continual breakdown and resynthesis from the cell's **amino acid pool**. Negative protein balance is when the body breaks down more protein than the amount of protein consumed (catabolism). This normally occurs during times of high stress, such as with severe infections and trauma. Positive protein balance is when protein consumed is greater than protein broken down and occurs in times of growth, such as childhood, pregnancy, recovery from illness, and in response to resistance training when overloading the muscle promotes protein synthesis (anabolism). Importantly, just because an athlete consumes a high-protein diet does not necessarily mean that he or she will be in **positive nitrogen balance** and experience muscle growth. Case in point, an endurance athlete who consumes a diet high in protein but insufficient carbohydrates to support endurance activities will rely heavily on muscle protein for fuel. As a result, more protein may be broken down than is consumed and this athlete will experience decreased athletic performance due to low blood glucose supply and worsened muscular strength and endurance due to protein catabolism (see Myths and Misconceptions).

SPEED BUMP

2. **Briefly describe the process of protein digestion and absorption.**
3. **Outline the process of protein metabolism.**

GENERAL PROTEIN RECOMMENDATIONS

Resistance training and cardiovascular exercise induce muscular and structural damage. Protein is required for the muscles and tissues to undergo the beneficial process of repairing and rebuilding. The **recommended dietary allowance** (RDA), 0.8 g/kg/day, is the *minimum* daily intake level that meets the nutrient requirements of nearly all healthy individuals. However, the Academy of Nutrition and Dietetics, Dietitians of Canada, and the American College of Sports Medicine suggest that athletes have higher protein needs than the general population and advise that endurance athletes consume about 1.2 to 1.4 g/kg (0.5 to 0.6 g/lb) of protein per day, and strength-trained athletes consume up to 1.6 to 1.7 g/kg (0.7 to 0.8 g/lb) of protein per day.[8] Conversely, the Institute of Medicine (IOM) concluded that there was no compelling scientific evidence to support active individuals increasing their daily protein intake above the RDA of 0.8 g/kg. Some who question the IOM report findings note that a variety of studies have shown that higher levels of protein intake benefit muscle mass, strength, and function; bone health; maintenance of energy balance; cardiovascular function; and wound health.[9]

Ultimately, the ideal protein consumption for athletes is still uncertain and the subject of ongoing research and evaluation. In the meantime, most experts agree it is appropriate to determine an ideal protein intake based on the acceptable macronutrient distribution range (AMDR), which is 10% to 35% of daily energy intake.[10] For example, a registered dietitian calculates that her client, John, an endurance runner, needs about 3,000 calories per day to maintain his weight and recommends that he ingest 20% of his calories from protein. Based on this recommendation he needs about 150 grams of protein/day ($3{,}000 \times 0.20 = 600$ calories/4 g = 150 g of protein). Table 2-2 shows the total protein intake at various levels of energy intake within the AMDR for protein, and Table 2-3 lists amounts of protein per serving for various foods.

Myths and Misconceptions

Excess Protein in the Diet Just Gets Excreted

The Myth
As far as weight is concerned, you can't eat too much protein. Anything beyond what your body needs you'll just get rid of in the urine.

The Logic
Because the body has little capacity to store proteins, it makes sense that anything consumed beyond what the body immediately needs will be excreted in the urine (similar to water soluble vitamins).

The Science
It is true that the body has limited ability to store protein. It is also true that a portion of the protein is excreted in the urine (the nitrogen group that shows up in urine as urea). However, the other portion of the protein (the carbon group) is converted to glucose or fat, depending on the body's current needs. Ultimately, protein consumed beyond what the body needs has the same fate as carbohydrates or fat consumed beyond what the body needs—conversion into stored fat.

BENEFITS AND RISKS OF A HIGH-PROTEIN DIET

Research is underway to best understand the benefits and risks associated with consuming more protein, including its ability to promote weight loss, improve

Table 2-2. Protein Intake (grams) at Various Levels of Energy Intake*

ENERGY INTAKE	LOW-PROTEIN DIET	AVERAGE DIET	HIGH-PROTEIN DIET	VERY HIGH PROTEIN DIET
Kcal/d	**(< 10% kcal)**	**(≈ 15% kcal)**	**(≥ 20% kcal)**	**(≥ 30% kcal)**
1,200	30	45	60	90
2,000	50	75	100	150
3,000	75	112	150	225

* Each gram of protein contains 4 calories. Protein intake is in grams per day.

Source: Reprinted with permission from St Jeor ST, Howard BV, Prewitt TE, Bovee V, Bazzarre T, Eckel RH. Dietary protein and weight reduction: a statement for healthcare professionals from the Nutrition Committee of the Council on Nutrition, Physical Activity, and Metabolism of the American Heart Association. *Circulation.* Oct 9 2001;104(15):1869-1874. Copyright ©2001 American Heart Association Inc.

Table 2-3. Amount of Protein per Serving

Grains (Approximately 1 ounce)	3 g
Nonstarchy vegetables (½ cup cooked, 1 cup raw)	2 g
Fruit	0 g
Dairy (1 cup of milk or yogurt; 1 to 1.5 ounces of cheese)	8 g
Legumes and beans (½ cup)	7 g
Meat, poultry, and fish (1 ounce)	7 g

athletic performance, and how it can be incorporated into a vegetarian diet.

Weight Loss

The once widely popular low-carbohydrate, high-protein diets, such as the Atkins and South Beach diets, may no longer be the hottest trend, but research has consistently shown that these diets are just as good for weight loss and health benefits, if not better in some cases, than the standard recommendation of a low-fat, high-carbohydrate diet.[11-13] Research indicates that high-protein diets preserve lean body mass, at least in the short-term (24 weeks), and contribute to increased satiety. Studies examining the long-term effects of these diets are limited. Low-carbohydrate, high-protein diets contribute to weight loss through several mechanisms. The initial weight loss on these diets is largely attributable to a diuretic effect of a low-carbohydrate diet, which contributes to rapid early water loss. These diets also contribute to glycogen depletion, which may be detrimental for endurance athletes, and metabolic ketosis, which leads to decreased appetite and decreased caloric intake.[14] Early studies showed that the Atkins diet produced greater weight reduction at 3 and 6 months than the other diets studied, but 1 year after starting the diet, the weight loss was the same as the other diets.[11] A randomized trial that compared Atkins, Zone, Ornish, and LEARN (similar to the Dietary Guidelines) diets found that the Atkins dieters had more weight loss and an improved health profile at 1 year.[12] The overall consensus among health experts is that it does not matter what type of diet people choose as long as they can maintain, which is difficult to do regardless of what plan they choose.[13]

Athletic Performance

Protein plays important roles in endurance and resistance training exercise. Both modes of exercise stimulate muscle protein synthesis,[15] which is further enhanced if protein is consumed around the time of physical activity.[4] Research indicates that meals and snacks consumed throughout the day, particularly foods consumed before, during, and after exercise, should be a combination of carbohydrates and protein at approximately a 3:1 ratio to encourage positive nitrogen balance and therefore muscle synthesis, hydration, and adequate energy to sustain exercise.[16] Consumption of protein immediately *after* exercise (within 15 to 30 minutes) helps in the repair and synthesis of muscle proteins.[17] Furthermore, it is recommended that 6 to 20 grams of protein be consumed with 30 to 40 grams of carbohydrates within 3 hours' post-exercise as well as immediately before exercise to encourage muscle resynthesis.[16] An example of a post-workout snack that would fall into this range would be one cup of yogurt (8 g protein; 12 g carbohydrates), one-fourth of a banana (0 g protein; 7.5 g of carbohydrates), and one slice of whole wheat toast (3 g protein; 15 g carbohydrates). Research indicates that as little as 5 to 10 grams of protein consumed immediately after exercise can promote optimal muscle repair. Protein consumption with the intake of water post-exercise also helps to restore hydration. Carbohydrates are important to pair with protein. If only protein is consumed without sufficient carbohydrates to provide the body's energy needs, then muscle synthesis may be compromised.[18,19]

Protein intake *during* exercise has been shown to be beneficial in endurance athletes, particularly branched-chain amino acids (BCAAs) to combat fatigue.[20,21] Furthermore, the ingestion of BCAAs during the recovery process has shown to increase muscle resynthesis and decrease fatigue. It is recommended that more than 45 mg/kg/day of leucine and approximately 22.5 mg/kg/day of each isoleucine and valine unnecessary be ingested by athletes daily (2:1:1 ratio).[22,23]

While these may seem like great reasons to consume high amounts of protein, protein metabolism becomes more efficient with exercise training, lending support to the IOM assertion that athletes do not have increased protein needs compared to the more sedentary population.[9] Research indicates that the ingestion of more than 2.0 g/kg/day of protein is unlikely to result in further muscle gains because the body has a limited capacity to utilize amino acids to build muscle.[24]

Vegetarianism

Vegetarians eat a plant-based diet that does not include meat and poultry. Different types of vegetarians differ in terms of what foods are restricted. For example, **lacto-ovo vegetarians** consume egg and dairy products, both of which are complete protein sources. A **lacto-vegetarian** does not consume eggs, but does consume dairy products. **Vegans** do not consume any foods that are from or contain an animal source. Therefore, in terms of protein consumption, vegetarians have more protein choices compared to vegans. However, with proper planning, vegan athletes can consume a diet containing adequate amounts of high-quality proteins. Legumes, dried beans, peas, nuts, soy, and meat alternatives provide ample protein, although only soy provides all of the essential amino acids. Vegans must consume a variety of complementary protein-rich plant foods. Plant proteins are not as readily digested as animal proteins, thus vegans and vegetarians should consume about 10% more grams of protein than the preceding recommendations.[8] That is, if an athlete consumes a 3,000-calorie diet with 20% from protein, approximately 600 calories (150 g) are from protein. A vegan or vegetarian should consume about 60 extra protein calories (15 g), for a total of 660 calories ((150 g + 15 g) $\times$ 4 calories per gram) from protein. For more information on vegetarian diets, see Chapter 16.

Protein Supplements

Protein supplements have become a popular means of increasing overall protein intake or increasing consumption of a particular protein type or amino acid. As aforementioned, research supports that BCCAs (leucine, isoleucine, valine) may enhance endurance by delaying the onset of fatigue and contribute to increased energy availability.[8] Further research supports the use of BCCAs, specifically leucine, to increase the rate of protein synthesis and decrease the rate of protein catabolism when taken after exercise.[25] The billion-dollar supplement industry has been quick to respond; leucine supplements are widely available in health food stores, with a cost upwards of $50 per container. However, because the research findings are inconsistent and little is known about the safety of these products, the Academy of Nutrition and Dietetics advises against individual amino acid supplementation and protein supplementation overall.[8] While some supplements may provide health benefits, generally speaking, consumers should purchase and use these products cautiously, as they are not closely regulated by the FDA. Importantly, no matter how safe a supplement seems, health professionals should not recommend supplements to clients unless supported by a medical diagnosis. See Chapter 10 for more information regarding supplements.

COMMUNICATION STRATEGIES

Blogging

Blogging is a way to disseminate information via the Internet. Sports nutrition information is posted on various blogs. Find three different sports nutrition blogs and do the following:

1. List the name and URL of the blog. Describe who developed the blog and the purpose of the blog.
2. Briefly summarize the information provided relating to protein.
3. Discuss whether you believe the information is accurate. Why do you think it is or is not accurate?

SPEED BUMP

4. Describe several benefits and risks of a high-protein diet.
5. List various types of proteins and their effect on athletic performance.
6. List several considerations when working with clients interested in adopting a high-protein diet.

CHAPTER SUMMARY

While a final determination has yet to be made on the best amounts, mechanisms, and methods, a large body of research supports that adequate amounts of high-quality protein can contribute to muscle gain, weight loss, and improved health.

KEY POINTS SUMMARY

1. Proteins play many critical functions in the body, including serving as the major structural component of muscle.
2. Proteins are made of long chains of amino acids. There are nine essential amino acids, including three branched chain amino acids, which play particularly important roles in muscle hypertrophy, as well as 11 nonessential amino acids.
3. Egg and milk are the highest quality proteins; they contain all essential amino acids and are easily digested and bioavailable. Whey protein is rapidly digested and best consumed shortly after exercise to facilitate muscle regeneration. Casein is released slowly into the bloodstream and is best consumed prior to exercise to minimize muscle catabolism.
4. Proteins consumed in the diet are broken down into amino acids. Amino acids are continuously recycled through the removal and addition of nitrogen groups. Monitoring an athlete's nitrogen status provides a glimpse into whether or not he or she is consuming adequate amounts of protein. The goal is for the athlete to consume more nitrogen (protein) than is excreted.
5. Perhaps the best way to determine protein needs is through the AMDR of 10% to 35% of daily energy intake. When discussing absolute numbers, there is not scientific consensus on exactly how much protein athletes need. However, the Academy of Nutrition and Dietetics and the American College of Sports Medicine recommend that endurance athletes consume 1.2 to 1.4 grams of protein per kilogram of body weight (0.5 to 0.6 g/lb) and that strength athletes consume 1.6 to 1.7 grams of protein per kilogram of body weight (0.7 to 0.8 g/lb).
6. Vegetarian athletes need about 10% more protein than their meat-eating counterparts.
7. It is best to obtain protein through whole foods. If a client is considering supplementation, he or she should be referred to a registered dietitian or his or her physician. Non-physician or registered dietitian health professionals should not endorse or recommend supplements.

PRACTICAL APPLICATIONS

1. According to the PDCAAS scale for measuring protein quality, casein and whey are among the highest quality proteins. What is it about these proteins that make them so highly rated?
   A. They contain all essential amino acids
   B. The low content of branched chain amino acids
   C. The low level of digestibility
   D. The fast rate of absorption

Choose from the following answer choices for questions 2 through 4:
A. Stomach
B. Small intestine
C. Liver
D. Pancreas

2. Where does protein digestion begin? A
3. This organ releases protein-digesting enzymes (or proteolytic enzymes) into the gut and hormones into the bloodstream. C
4. Where does transamination occur? B
5. What is the main physiological difference between whey and casein proteins?
   A. The amino acids from whey are slowly absorbed and released into the bloodstream, providing a continual supply of amino acids to build tissue while the amino acids from casein are rapidly released into the bloodstream, supplying an immediate source of amino acids to rebuild muscle tissue after a strenuous workout.
   B. The amino acids from casein are slowly absorbed and released into the bloodstream, providing a continual supply of amino acids to build tissue while the amino acids from whey are rapidly released into the bloodstream, supplying an immediate source of amino acids to rebuild muscle tissue after a strenuous workout.
   C. Though whey and casein both come from milk, the whey protein, which is the primary constituent of milk, is a higher quality protein than casein because it contains a greater proportion of essential amino acids.
   D. None of the above
6. What happens to excess protein consumed in the diet?
   A. It is transported to muscle tissues and helps to increase muscle size.
   B. It is excreted from the body.

C. It is converted to fat for storage.
D. It is converted to glucose for energy.

7. What is the most appropriate AMDR protein intake?
   A. 0.8 g/kg body weight per day
   B. 1.5 g/kg body weight per day
   C. 10% to 35% of total caloric intake
   D. ≥ 35% of total caloric intake

8. Jenna, 5′4″ and 120 lb, is a 21-year-old vegetarian college student who just began a resistance training program. She lifts weights for about
   1 hour 3 days per week. She also runs about 25 miles per week. She needs about 2,500 calories per day to maintain her current weight.
   About how many grams of protein does she need each day?
   A. 116 grams
   B. 128 grams
   C. 138 grams
   D. 145 grams

9. Your client read in a magazine that protein supplements help to increase muscle mass. He asks you if that's true, and if so, what supplements you recommend. How do you respond?
   A. Tell him that the article is not true and you recommend a diet high in fruits and vegetables combined with twice-weekly resistance training.
   B. Tell him that the article is true and you recommend supplementing with a whey protein powder immediately after a strength session.
   C. Tell him that the article is not true and you recommend he read a different, more reputable magazine and stick to his current diet.
   D. Tell him that research supports protein's role in muscle building and you recommend getting the protein from whole food sources or meeting with a registered dietitian for specific supplement recommendations.

10. An endurance athlete wants to adopt a high-protein diet without increasing total caloric intake. What is your biggest concern?
    A. She will not consume enough carbohydrates to fuel for optimal performance.
    B. She will rely too heavily on supplements to meet her protein goals.
    C. She will not be able to meet her protein goals at her current level of caloric intake.
    D. She will end up consuming too much saturated fat, which will be detrimental to her heart health.

Case 1 Kate, the Marathon Runner

Kate is an experienced 22-year-old marathon runner who is trying to qualify for the Boston Marathon. She is 5′6″ and 126 pounds. To qualify, she needs to shave 20 minutes off of her personal record (PR). She would like to develop a nutrition program that will help her achieve her goal. The marathon is in 1 month.

Protein Needs

The American College of Sports Medicine and the Academy of Nutrition and Dietetics recommend that endurance athletes consume 1.2 to 1.4 g/kg (0.5 to 0.6 g/lb) of protein per day.

1. Based on this recommendation, about how many grams of protein should Kate eat per day?

Protein Timing and Exercise

2. As an endurance athlete, what are general recommendations for protein consumption before, during, and after a prolonged endurance workout?

Special Considerations: Vegetarianism

Kate shares that she is considering adopting a vegetarian diet.

3. What is a nutritional concern in terms of adequate protein intake for vegetarian athletes?
4. How much protein will Kate need per day if she becomes a strict vegetarian? Translate this increased need into a vegetarian food item or food items.
5. What are five possible protein combinations to ensure that she consumes all of the essential amino acids.

Case 2 Eric, the Recreational Body Builder

Eric is a 31-year-old competitive body builder. He participates in body building competitions in the fall and trains the rest of the year. He is 5′11″ and weighs 184 pounds. He is currently in summer training. He is reviewing his current exercise and nutrition plan to see if he can identify any areas for improvement.

Protein Needs

The American College of Sports Medicine and the Academy of Nutrition and Dietetics recommend that strength athletes consume 1.6 to 1.7 g/kg (0.7 to 0.8 g/lb) of protein per day.

1. Based on these recommendations, about how many grams of protein should Eric eat per day?

Protein Timing and Exercise

The timing of protein intake likely plays an important role in determining extent of strength gains around the time of exercise.

2. How might Eric time his protein intake?

Special Considerations: Ergogenic Aids

3. Eric asks you if you recommend whey supplementation. How would you respond?
4. Explain how you would respond to an athlete asking your opinion of leucine supplementation.

TRAIN YOURSELF: PROTEIN NEEDS

1. Based on your weight and physical activity patterns, about how much protein do you need in a day?
2. Think back to all of the food you ate in the past 24 hours. Complete a dietary recall of your intake. Input your food intake into supertracker.usda.gov, MyFitnessPal.com, or another online nutrition calculator or app. Approximately how many grams of protein did you eat? How does this compare to your recommended needs?

Protein Timing and Exercise

3. How might you space this daily protein intake during days in which you engage in strenuous aerobic exercise? How about days in which you do heavy lifting?

Special Considerations

4. Are there any special considerations such as diets or vegetarianism you should keep in mind when considering your protein needs? If yes, describe how this unique situation affects your protein needs and protein intake. If not, make up a special consideration (one of the above or one of your own) and describe how it might affect protein needs and protein intake.

REFERENCES

1. Hoffman JR, Falvo MJ. Protein: which is best? *J Sports Sci Med.* 2004;3:118-130.
2. Pal S, Ellis V. The chronic effects of whey proteins on blood pressure, vascular function, and inflammatory markers in overweight individuals. *Obesity (Silver Spring).* July 2010; 18(7):1354-1359.
3. Pal S, Ellis V, Dhaliwal S. Effects of whey protein isolate on body composition, lipids, insulin and glucose in overweight and obese individuals. *British J Nutr.* September 2010; 104(5):716-723.
4. Hayes A, Cribb PJ. Effect of whey protein isolate on strength, body composition and muscle hypertrophy during resistance training. *Curr Opin Clin Nutr Metab Care.* January 2008;11(1): 40-44.
5. Krissansen GW. Emerging health properties of whey proteins and their clinical implications. *J Am Coll Nutr.* December 2007;26(6):713S-723S.
6. Kerksick CM, Rasmussen CJ, Lancaster SL, et al. The effects of protein and amino acid supplementation on performance and training adaptations during ten weeks of resistance training. *J Strength Cond Res / National Strength & Conditioning Association.* August 2006;20(3):643-653.
7. Sacks FM, Lichtenstein A, Van Horn L, Harris W, Kris-Etherton P, Winston M. Soy protein, isoflavones, and cardiovascular health: an American Heart Association Science Advisory for professionals from the Nutrition Committee. *Circulation.* February 21 2006;113(7):1034-1044.
8. Rodriguez NR, Di Marco NM, Langley S. American College of Sports Medicine position stand. Nutrition and athletic performance. *Med Sci Sports Exerc.* March 2009;41(3):709-731.
9. *Dietary Reference Intakes for Energy, Carbohydrate, Fiber, Fat, Fatty Acids, Cholesterol, Protein, and Amino Acids.* Washington, DC: Institute of Medicine, Food and Nutrition Board; 2005.
10. Wolfe RR, Miller SL. The recommended dietary allowance of protein: a misunderstood concept. *JAMA.* Jun 25 2008; 299(24):2891-2893.
11. Foster GD, Wyatt HR, Hill JO, et al. A randomized trial of a low-carbohydrate diet for obesity. *N Engl J Med.* May 22 2003;348(21):2082-2090.
12. Gardner CD, Kiazand A, Alhassan S, et al. Comparison of the Atkins, Zone, Ornish, and LEARN diets for change in weight and related risk factors among overweight premenopausal women: the A TO Z Weight Loss Study: a randomized trial. *JAMA.* March 7 2007;297(9):969-977.
13. Dansinger ML, Gleason JA, Griffith JL, Selker HP, Schaefer EJ. Comparison of the Atkins, Ornish, Weight Watchers, and Zone diets for weight loss and heart disease risk reduction: a randomized trial. *JAMA.* January 5 2005;293(1):43-53.
14. St Jeor ST, Howard BV, Prewitt TE, Bovee V, Bazzarre T, Eckel RH. Dietary protein and weight reduction: a statement for healthcare professionals from the Nutrition Committee of the Council on Nutrition, Physical Activity, and Metabolism of the American Heart Association. *Circulation.* October 9 2001;104(15):1869-1874.
15. Phillips SM. Dietary protein for athletes: from requirements to metabolic advantage. *Appl Physiol Nutr Metab.* December 2006; 31(6):647-654.
16. Kreider RB, Wilborn CD, Taylor L, et al. ISSN exercise and sport nutrition review: research and recommendations. *JISSN.* 2010;7(7). www.jissn.com/content/7/1/7.
17. Gibala MJ. Protein metabolism and endurance exercise. *Sports Med.* 2007;37(4-5):337-340.
18. Tipton KD, Ferrando AA, Phillips SM, Doyle D Jr, Wolfe RR. Postexercise net protein synthesis in human muscle from orally administered amino acids. *Am J Physiol Endocrinol Metab.* 1999;276:E628-E634.
19. Ivy JL, Goforth HW Jr, Damon BM, McCauley TR, Parsons EC, Price TB. Early postexercise muscle glycogen recovery is enhanced with a carbohydrate-protein supplement. *J Appl Physiol.* October 2002;93(4):1337-1344.
20. Blomstrand E. A role for branched-chain amino acids in reducing central fatigue. *J Nutr.* February 2006;136(2):544S-547S.

21. Matsumoto K, Koba T, Hamada K, et al. Branched-chain amino acid supplementation attenuates muscle soreness, muscle damage and inflammation during an intensive training program. *J Sports Med Phys Fitness*. December 2009;49(4):424-431.
22. Blomstrand E, Newsholme EA. Effect of branched-chain amino acid supplementation on the exercise-induced change in aromatic amino acid concentration in human muscle. *Acta Physiol Scand*. 1992;146(3):293-298.
23. Shimomura Y, Murakami T, Nakai N, Nagasaki M, Harris RA. Exercise promotes BCAA catabolism: effects of BCAA supplementation on skeletal muscle during exercise. *J Nutr*. 2004;134(6 Suppl):1583S-1587S.
24. Butterfield GE. Whole-body protein utilization in humans. *Med Sci Sports Exerc*. October 1987;19(5 Suppl):S157-165.
25. Blomstrand E, Eliasson J, Karlsson HK, Kohnke R. Branched-chain amino acids activate key enzymes in protein synthesis after physical exercise. *J Nutr*. January 2006;136(1 Suppl): 269S-273S.
26. Dangin M, Boirie Y, Guillet C, Beaufrere B. Influence of the protein digestion rate on protein turnover in young and elderly subjects. *J Nutr*. October 2002;132(10): 3228S-3233S.

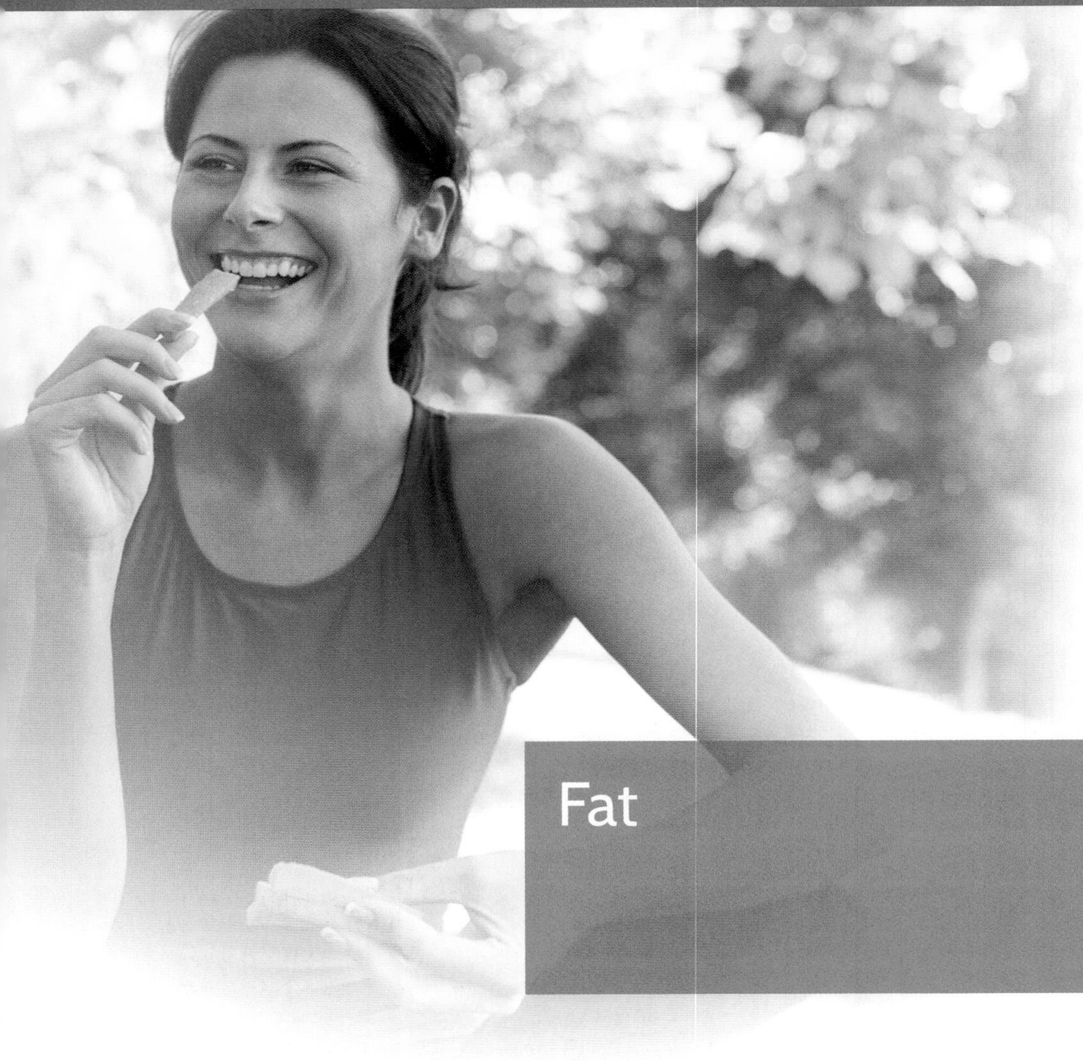

CHAPTER 3

Fat

CHAPTER OUTLINE

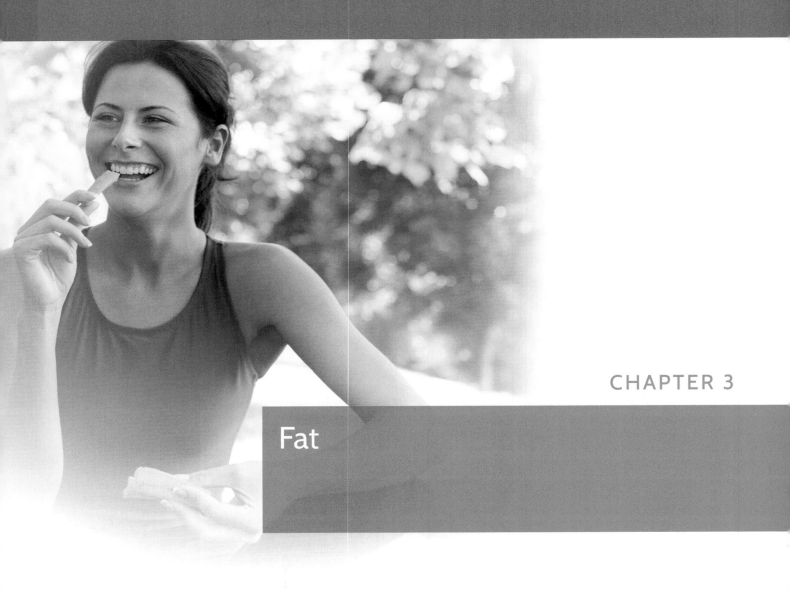

LEARNING OBJECTIVES

After studying this chapter, the reader should be able to:

3.1 List the functions of fat in the body.

3.2 Describe the difference between saturated fat, unsaturated fat, and trans fat.

3.3 Outline the process of fat digestion, absorption, and storage.

3.4 Describe the effect of various fats on health and disease risk.

3.5 Describe the effect of fat intake on athletic performance.

3.6 List several principles to share with clients when discussing fat intake.

KEY TERMS

adequate intake The amount of intake believed to cover the needs of all healthy individuals in age- and gender-specific groups; used when insufficient evidence is available to establish an RDA.

adipocyte A fat cell.

adipose tissue Fatty tissue; connective tissue made of fat cells.

androgen A hormone that stimulates or produces masculine characteristics.

angina Chest pain due to decreased blood flow resulting in inadequate supply of oxygen to the heart muscle.

atherogenic dyslipidemia A triad of increased blood concentrations of small, dense low-density lipoprotein (LDL) particles, decreased high-density lipoprotein (HDL) particles, and increased triglycerides.

atherosclerosis The accumulation of fatty material on the inner walls of the arteries, causing them to harden, thicken, and lose elasticity.

bile acids Produced by the liver and stored in the gallbladder, these acids are important in the digestion of fat. After lipid digestion, they are recycled and reused by the liver.

cardiovascular disease A term that refers to disease of the heart and vascular system.

cholecystokinin (CCK) A hormone released from the small intestine in response to the presence of amino acids and fatty acids from protein and fat digestion; stimulates the pancreas to secrete enzymes, stimulates the gallbladder to contract, and slows gastric emptying through release of gastric inhibitory peptide and secretin.

cholesterol A fat-like waxy structure found in the blood and body tissues and some animal-based foods. Cholesterol is important in metabolism as the precursor to various steroid hormones. It is transported in the body via lipoproteins. Excess cholesterol can contribute to cardiovascular disease.

chylomicron A large lipoprotein particle that transports fat from digested food from the small intestine to the liver and adipose tissue.

coronary heart disease The major form of cardiovascular disease that results when the arteries supplying the heart muscle (coronary arteries) are narrowed or completely blocked by deposits of fat and fibrous tissue.

dietary fat Fat consumed in the diet; in contrast to fat produced in the body.

dietary reference intake (DRI) A collective term used to refer to several types of reference values: recommended dietary allowance, estimated average requirement, tolerable upper intake level, and adequate intake.

eicosanoids Locally acting hormones that are made from omega-3 and omega-6 fatty acids and play roles in inflammation, fever, regulation of blood pressure, blood clotting, immunity, control of reproductive processes and tissue growth, and regulation of the sleep/wake cycle.

emulsify To break lipids into small droplets to facilitate fat digestion and absorption.

essential fatty acids Fats that are not produced by the body and must be consumed in the diet; linolenic and linoleic acids.

estrogens Substances that stimulate or produce feminine characteristics; typically refers to estrogen, estradiol, estrone, and estriol.

fat adaptation Increasing dietary fat consumption in an effort to increase fatty acid oxidation during exercise with the intent of sparing glycogen stores.

fat loading A strategy of progressively increasing percentage of fat intake to increase fatty acid oxidation and thus preserve glycogen stores for prolonged exercise.

fatty acids Long hydrocarbon chains with varying degrees of saturation with hydrogen.

gastric inhibitory peptide Protein that is released from the small intestine and functions to slow digestion by inhibiting gastric acid secretion and stimulating insulin release.

gastric lipase Enzyme released from the stomach that works with lingual lipase to digest short- and medium-chain fatty acids into partial glycerides and free fatty acids.

glucocorticoid A classification of hormones released from the adrenal cortex that protect against stress or contribute to protein and carbohydrate metabolism; the most important is cortisol.

high-density lipoprotein (HDL) Lipoprotein that contains approximately 50% protein and carries excess cholesterol from the bloodstream to the liver, where it can be prepared for excretion; also known as "good cholesterol."

hydrogenation The process of adding hydrogen atoms to unsaturated fats. This process eliminates double bonds and turns fatty acids into partially or completely saturated fats.

hyperplasia Abnormal increase in the number of cells.

intermediate-density lipoprotein (IDL) Lipoprotein that is composed of cholesterol, triglycerides, and protein, and results from the degradation of very low-density lipoprotein; transports cholesterol throughout the body.

lecithin A phospholipid that breaks down into glycerol, stearic acid, phosphoric acid, and choline; a major component of HDL.

leptin A hormone produced by adipose tissue that suppresses appetite and increases energy expenditure; levels increase with increased fat storage.

lingual lipase An enzyme released from the mouth that begins to break short- and medium-chain fatty acids into partial glycerides and free fatty acids.

lipids A fat or fat-like substance used in the body or bloodstream; includes fats, oils, waxes, sterols, and triglycerides, all of which are insoluble in water.

lipoprotein Compounds found in the bloodstream consisting of simple proteins bound to lipids including cholesterol, phospholipids, and triglycerides. Lipoproteins transport cholesterol and other lipids to and from various tissues.

lipoprotein lipase An enzyme that facilitates transport of lipid from a lipoprotein in the blood into the adipocyte or other tissue.

low-density lipoprotein (LDL) Lipoprotein that is composed of over 50% cholesterol and transports cholesterol and triglycerides from the liver and small intestines to cells and tissues; high levels are a proven cause of atherosclerosis.

lymphatic system A network of organs, lymph nodes, lymph ducts, and lymph vessels that produce and transport lymph.

mineralocorticoid A steroid hormone that regulates fluid and electrolyte retention and excretion by the kidneys; typically refers to the hormone aldosterone.

monounsaturated fatty acid A type of unsaturated fatty acid that has one double bond between carbon atoms; includes oleic acid, the main component of olive oil.

myocardial infarction The medical term for *heart attack*, which occurs when blood flow to a portion of the heart muscle is severely restricted or stopped, resulting in inadequate oxygen supply and decreased ability of the heart to pump.

oleic acid A monounsaturated fatty acid that occurs naturally in many animal and vegetable oils; improves cardiovascular health when used as a substitute for saturated fat and refined carbohydrates.

omega-3 fatty acids Named for the position of their first double bond. Alpha linolenic acid (ALA) is an essential polyunsaturated fatty acid that can be converted to eicosapentaenoic acid (EPA) and docosahexanoic acid (DHA); found in flaxseed, walnuts, dark green leafy vegetables, egg yolks, and cold water fish like tuna, salmon, mackerel, cod, crab, shrimp, and oysters. ALA, EPA, and DHA can be converted to eicosanoids.

omega-6 fatty acids Named for the position of their first double bond. Linoleic acid is an essential polyunsaturated fatty acid that can be converted to eicosanoids; found in sunflower, safflower, corn, and soybean oils.

partially hydrogenated oil An oil in which the double bonds of an unsaturated fatty acid have been chemically manipulated to create a saturated fatty acid.

phospholipid A compound with a modified glycerol backbone and two fatty acids. The molecule is water-soluble at one end and water-insoluble at the other end. These compounds form the cell-membrane structure phospholipid bilayer.

polyunsaturated fatty acids A type of unsaturated fatty acid that has two or more double bonds between carbon atoms; includes the essential fatty acids omega-6 and omega-3 fatty acids; improves heart health when used to replace saturated fats.

resistin A hormone secreted by adipose tissue that decreases cell sensitivity to insulin.

saturated fatty acids Fatty acids that contain no double bonds between carbon atoms. Foods high in saturated fatty acids are typically solid at room temperature and are from animal products such as butter and lard.

solid fats and added sugars (SoFAS) A term first introduced in the 2010 *Dietary Guidelines for Americans* that refers to a food ingredient that provides little nutritional value and should be avoided. The guidelines recommend that Americans: (1) cut back on calories from solid fats and added sugars; (2) limit foods that contain refined grains, especially refined grains that contain solid fats, added sugars, and sodium; and (3) use oils to replace solid fats whenever possible.

sphingomyelin A class of phospholipid composed of phosphoric acid, choline, sphingosine, and a fatty acid; found in high concentration in cell membranes of nervous tissues.

TNF-alpha Tumor necrosis factor; helps to regulate fat metabolism and along with other cytokines contributes to acute inflammatory reactions.

triglycerides Three fatty acids bound to a glycerol backbone. The primary form of fat storage in the body and the composition of most fats in the food supply.

CALCULATION

1 gram of fat = 9 calories

unsaturated fatty acids Fatty acids that contain one or more double bonds between carbon atoms; typically liquid at room temperature and fairly unstable, making them susceptible to oxidative damage and a shorter half life.

very low-density lipoprotein (VLDL) The least dense of all of the lipoproteins, carrying a greater ratio of lipid to protein than LDL; main transport mechanism for endogenously produced lipids.

INTRODUCTION

Athletes, dieters, and the health conscious have long been warned to avoid fat. Fat provides 9 calories per gram—2.25 times more calories than the 4 calories per gram contained in carbohydrates and protein. While its high caloric density can easily and quickly contribute to weight gain, fat serves many essential functions in the body. In fact, certain types of fat are heart-healthy and an excellent source of essential nutrients (though still calorie-dense). On the other hand, fat can contribute to obesity, cardiovascular disease, and overall poor health. Consumers need well-informed health professionals to help them choose eating plans that are rich in healthy fats and low in unhealthy fats.

FAT STRUCTURE AND FUNCTION

Lipids serve many important functions in the human body, including providing a readily available source of stored energy during times of caloric deprivation, insulation, protection of vital organs and bones, a means for absorption of the fat-soluble vitamins, precursor to hormones, and cell membrane structure, among other necessary roles. While different classes of lipids serve different functions in the body, all lipids are organic structures made up of hydrogen, carbon, and oxygen and all are insoluble in water (see Fig. 3-1). The major classes of lipids that are important for human function and are discussed in this text are **sterols,** including **cholesterol**, **fatty acids** (which are components of **phospholipids**), and **triglycerides**.

CHOLESTEROL AND STEROIDS

Sterols are a class of lipids that share a ring-like carbon structure. The most common sterol is cholesterol. Cholesterol is a fat-like, waxy substance produced in the liver and found in the cell membrane of all animal tissues, where it provides cell structure and integrity. It is also found in the adrenal glands, testes and ovaries, and liver, where it forms the building blocks of the steroid hormones and bile acids. Steroid hormones such as **glucocorticoid hormone** (cortisol) and **mineralocorticoid hormone** (aldosterone) are made in the adrenal glands. **Androgens** (testosterone) and **estrogens** (estradiol) are made in the testes and ovaries. **Bile acids** are made in the liver and sent to the gallbladder for storage. When the skin is exposed to sun, cholesterol in the epidermal layer of the skin is converted to cholecalciferol. Cholecalciferol is then converted in the body to calcitriol, the active form of vitamin D.

Cholesterol may be consumed in the diet (exogenous cholesterol) or made by the body (endogenous cholesterol). Because cholesterol is fat soluble, it needs water-soluble carrier proteins called **lipoproteins** to transport it in the bloodstream. Lipoproteins are comprised of lipids (including cholesterol, triglycerides, and phospholipids) and proteins. There are five classes of lipoproteins: **chylomicrons, very low-density lipoproteins** (VLDLs), **intermediate-density lipoproteins** (IDLs), **low-density lipoproteins** (LDLs), and **high-density lipoproteins** (HDLs).

Cholesterol is transported in the blood to the body cells primarily as LDL. LDLs are susceptible to oxidation. Oxidized LDLs distribute cholesterol to the inner linings or walls of arteries and may form a plaque and ultimately cause **atherosclerosis**. Conversely, high-density lipoproteins (HDLs) remove excess cholesterol from the arteries and carry it back to the liver, where it is excreted.

While excessive cholesterol intake may be harmful to the body, for most people consuming a diet high in cholesterol probably has little effect on overall blood cholesterol levels because the body can carefully regulate cholesterol concentration and rid itself of any excess dietary cholesterol (Box 3-1).

FATTY ACIDS AND TRIGLYCERIDES

Dietary fats consist mostly of triglycerides—a compound of three fatty acids attached to a glycerol (carbon and

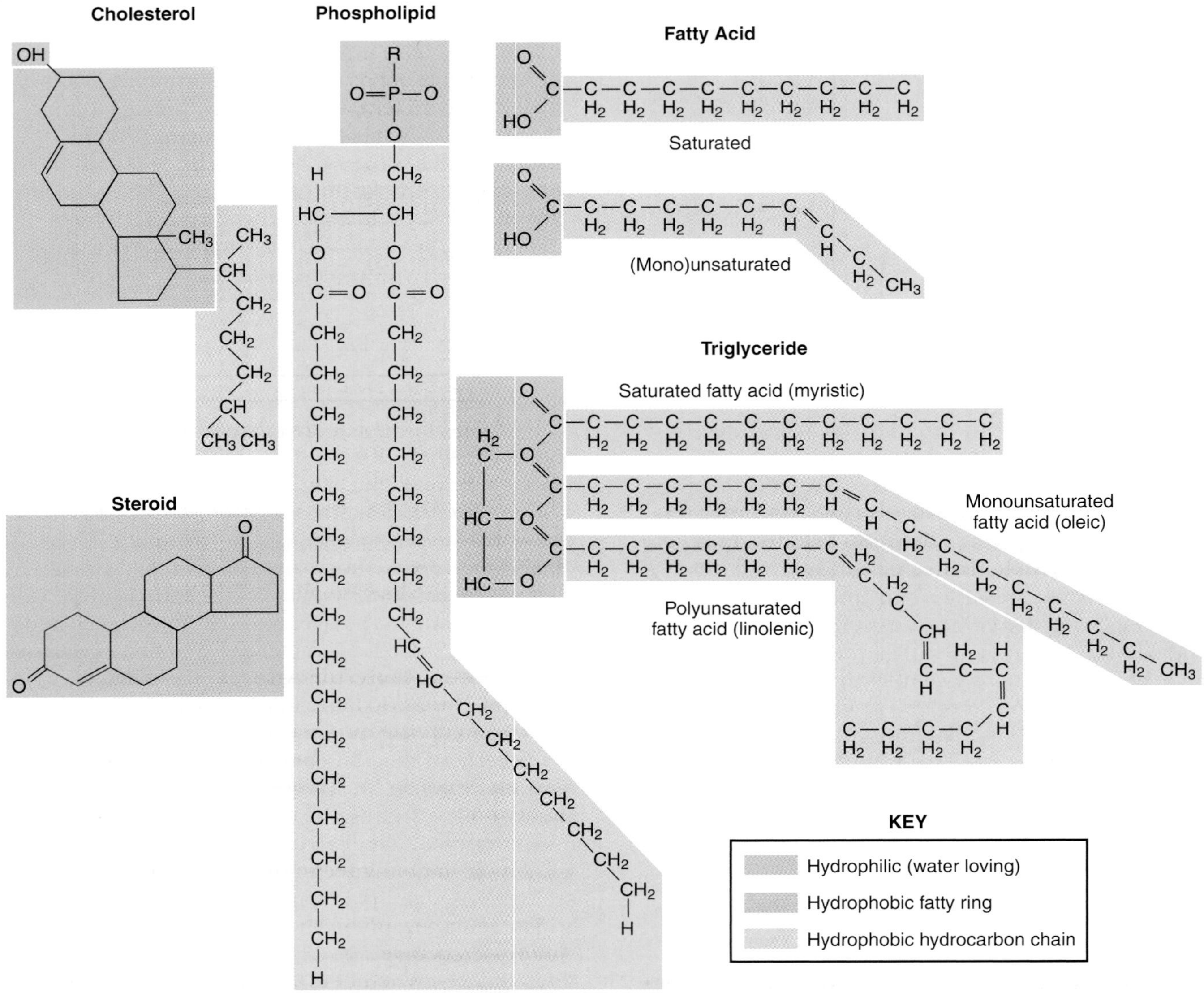

Figure 3-1. Fat structure.

hydrogen structure) backbone. Triglycerides are the chemical form in which most fat exists in food as well as in the body. Fat is stored primarily as triglycerides in **adipose tissue**, providing a ready source of calories and energy in times of energy deprivation or fasting. Triglycerides also provide the body insulation (subcutaneous fat) and protection of vital organs (visceral fat) and bones (fat pads). Once thought to be simply a place for energy storage, adipose tissue is now recognized as a metabolically active endocrine organ that produces hormones including **leptin**, **resistin**, and the cytokine **TNF-alpha**, which functions as part of an immune system response. These hormones have been found to be produced at higher levels in the obese population and have been implicated in inflammatory, atherosclerotic, and insulin resistance processes.[1]

Fatty acids are long hydrocarbon chains with an even number of carbons and varying degrees of saturation with hydrogen. The human body requires fatty acids of differing chain lengths and saturation to meet structural and metabolic needs. The major categories of fatty acids are saturated, monounsaturated, and polyunsaturated.

Saturated Fatty Acids

Saturated fatty acids contain no double bonds between carbon atoms; all carbons are saturated with hydrogens. As a food, saturated fats are typically solid at room temperature and are very stable, which gives them a long shelf life. Saturated fat comes in primarily four forms in the food supply: lauric acid, myristic acid, palmitic acid, and stearic acid. Saturated fats are found

Box 3-1. Are Eggs Good or Bad?

If there is one thing certain about nutrition science, it is that with continuous research and knowledge, nutrition recommendations will change. While this can be extremely frustrating for clients and the general public, it highlights the importance of health professionals staying on top of the latest research and findings.

Historically, one of the most controversial foods has been the egg. Is it healthy or not? It used to be that eggs were well known for their potential health risks given their high cholesterol content (there are 213 mg of cholesterol in one egg yolk—that is 70% of the total daily amount of 300 mg recommended by the 2010 *Dietary Guidelines for Americans*). Then eggs were applauded for their high protein content and, more recently, for the notable amount of heart-healthy DHA omega-3 fatty acid in egg yolk (about 50 mg and up to 400 mg in DHA-enriched eggs). At just about 15 cents each, eggs contain a load of nutrients at a very cheap price, but are they safe and healthy to eat?

A single egg has 70 calories; 6 grams of protein, including all of the essential amino acids; 13 vitamins and minerals; and DHA omega-3 fatty acids. Few other foods could boast such a high nutritional density (Fig. 3-2).

Nutrition Facts
Serving Size 1 egg (50g)

Amount Per Serving	
Calories 70 Calories from Fat 40	
	% Daily Value*
Total Fat 4.5g	**7%**
Sat. Fat 1.5g	**8%**
Trans. Fat 0g	
Cholest. 215mg	**71%**
Sodium 65mg	**3%**
Total Carb. Less than 1g	**0%**
Protein 6g	**10%**

Vitamin A	6%	•	Vitamin C	0%
Calcium	2%	•	Iron	4%

Not a significant source of Dietary Fiber or Sugars.

Figure 3-2. The egg nutrition label.

On the other hand, eggs also contain a high amount of cholesterol. While dietary cholesterol is not very closely associated with elevated cholesterol levels in the body for most people (that has more to do with saturated fat intake), the American Heart Association (AHA) still recommends that people who have elevated cholesterol or increased risk factors for heart disease limit their dietary cholesterol to 200 milligrams per day. That is approximately equivalent to a single egg yolk, thus suggesting that people with heart disease probably should eat eggs only a couple of times per week, or forgo the yolk and just eat the whites. But, notably, the AHA has amended its guidelines and no longer makes a specific recommendation on the number of egg yolks a person should eat per week. Other than their cholesterol amounts, eggs also are a possible source of food-borne illness, though the risk is low. Salmonella infection may be prevented most of the time with good food-handling techniques, including special care to fully cook eggs. Nonetheless, this risk is increased, especially in the elderly and immune-suppressed people.

Ultimately, whether or not clients choose to include eggs in their daily diets will depend on taste preferences and their conclusions regarding the risks versus the benefits, but there is no doubt that eggs are an inexpensive source of a variety of nutrients.

primarily in animal sources like red meat and full-fat dairy products; however, palm and coconut oil are atypical plant sources. Animal sources of saturated fats contain mostly palmitic and stearic acids, while tropical vegetable oils contain largely lauric and myristic acid. The different types of saturated fat induce different effects on cholesterol. When compared to other saturated fats, stearic acid exerts a beneficial effect on cholesterol levels (decreases LDLs and decreases the ratio of total to HDL cholesterol). However, when compared to unsaturated fats, stearic acid increases LDL, decreases HDL, and increases the ratio of total to HDL cholesterol.[2] Lauric acid and myristic acid cause a greater increase in total cholesterol than palmitic acid. Though lauric acid causes an increase in cholesterol, the increase comes mostly from increasing the high-density lipoprotein (HDL), the "good" cholesterol.[3]

Because saturated fat increases low-density lipoprotein (LDL), which is referred to as the "bad" cholesterol for its atherosclerotic properties (see discussion of "cholesterol" below), the American Heart Association and the government's dietary guidelines have long advised consumers to avoid saturated fat. However, a growing body of research seems to suggest that saturated fat in and of itself may not actually lead to increased risk of cardiovascular or cancer death. This news has driven a growing interest in the once-maligned coconut oil (see Box 3-2).

Box 3-2. Coconut Oil, Saturated Fat, and the 'Great [Health] Debate'

Once maligned as a cholesterol-raising, artery-clogging, and waist-widening ingredient to be avoided, coconut oil has made a surprising comeback among health enthusiasts. While the science of nutrition has long been recognized as volatile and fluid (e.g., Eggs healthy or not? Soy good or bad? Margarine or butter?), the rise of coconut oil from a demonized "bad" food to the purported "cure all" for a variety of health ailments is unexpected. The nutritional composition of coconut oil remains the same—namely, about 90% saturated fat—so why the sudden change of heart?

The growing interest in coconut oil is due to at least two factors: (1) the scientific understanding of the effects of saturated fat on heart health has evolved, and (2) a growing number of people who either avoid animal fats or are looking for a new flavor have discovered that coconut oil can transform a bland dish or baked product into a masterpiece, among its other purported benefits.

EVOLVING SCIENCE: SATURATED FAT NO LONGER A VILLAIN

The 2010 *Dietary Guidelines for Americans* and the American Heart Association recommendations for optimal heart health both advise consumers to avoid saturated fats and keep intake to less than 10% of total calories consumed. The Academy of Nutrition and Dietetics recommends an intake of 7% to 10% of total energy.[28] Physicians, nutritionists, and other health experts have long warned patients and clients of the risks of a diet that contains too much saturated fat—primarily, a sharp rise in low-density lipoprotein (LDL), the "bad" cholesterol.

While coconut oil is mostly comprised of lauric acid, a type of saturated fat that raises heart-healthy HDL much more than LDL cholesterol, it also contains other types of saturated fat that raise LDL cholesterol. However, even though saturated fat raises LDL levels, a growing body of scientific evidence suggests that overall saturated fats are not quite as bad as previously believed. A meta-analysis published in 2010 evaluated the findings of 21 studies that looked at the relationship between saturated fat intake and risk of coronary heart disease, stroke, and cardiovascular disease. The researchers found that even at the extremes of very low intake compared to very high intake of saturated fat there was no difference in any of the studied health outcomes.[26] However, a pooled analysis of 11 studies found that when saturated fat is replaced with other types of fat (especially polyunsaturated fatty acids), cardiovascular disease risk decreases significantly.[27] These studies and others like them have provoked discussion and debate in the health and medical communities around the role of fat and health.

A description and summary of the "Great Fat Debate" was published as a series of short articles written by leading nutrition experts in the *Journal of the American Dietetic Association*.[25] Overall, the debate provided these key recommendations and points:

- It is not the amount of fat intake, but rather the type of fat that is important for health. With that said, fat is more calorie-dense than carbohydrates and proteins and consumers should be careful to balance calories consumed with calories expended.
- The evidence against saturated fat is "not as strong as the dietary guidelines may have interpreted," but polyunsaturated (especially) and monounsaturated fats are clearly healthy.
- Saturated fats should *not* be viewed as "good for you," but a healthy, balanced diet can include saturated fats.
- Replacing saturated fat with polyunsaturated fat (like omega-3 and omega-6 fatty acids) is beneficial for overall health and cardiovascular disease risk reduction.
- Trans fats are unhealthy and should be avoided.
- Remember that dietary fats are never purely one type of fat, thus meal planning should focus on a balance of food types, rather than specific nutrients.

So what does this mean in the case for (or against) coconut oil? Virgin coconut oil may exert a modestly beneficial effect on blood lipids (through elevation of HDL cholesterol) and its consumption probably will not lead to harmful cardiovascular health outcomes. However, oils that are high in polyunsaturated fatty acids (e.g., safflower, poppyseed, flaxseed, and grapeseed oils) and monounsaturated fatty acids (almond, avocado, and olive oils) probably provide greater health benefits. Note that partially hydrogenated coconut oil is detrimental to health due to its high trans fatty acid content.

COCONUT OIL AND ITS MANY USES

Of course, coconut oil connoisseurs love the stuff for much more than its health profile. While some mono- and polyunsaturated fats may be healthier, they do not have the same desirable cooking characteristics of coconut oil, such as the stability to withstand high temperatures, the sweet texture, or the rich taste that make it ideal for cooking.

While many of the purported benefits of coconut oil have not been rigorously studied, some people report improvements in weight, chronic fatigue, Crohn's disease, irritable bowel syndrome, thyroid conditions, and skin health. As research evolves, these claims may be substantiated or proven incorrect.

Monounsaturated Fatty Acids

Unsaturated fatty acids contain one (monounsaturated) or more (polyunsaturated) double bonds between carbon atoms, are typically liquid at room temperature, are found primarily in plant sources, and are fairly unstable. Unsaturated fatty acids are more susceptible to oxidative damage and have a shorter shelf life than saturated fatty acids.

Oleic acid is a **monounsaturated fatty acid**. When used in place of saturated fat, oleic acid lowers total and LDL cholesterol. When used in place of carbohydrates, it decreases triglycerides, increases HDL cholesterol, and increases the total-to-HDL cholesterol ratio.[3] Most plant oils, such as olive, canola, and peanut oils, nuts, seeds, and avocado are excellent sources of monounsaturated fat. The Academy of Nutrition and Dietetics recommends that 15% to 20% of caloric intake come from monounsaturated fatty acids.[28]

Polyunsaturated Fatty Acids

Polyunsaturated fats are especially important for optimal health. In fact, a growing body of research suggests that polyunsaturated fats are the healthiest of the fats, and substituting these fats for saturated fats or refined carbohydrates likely contributes to a significant decrease in cardiovascular disease risk.[4] The Academy of Nutrition and Dietetics recommends that intake from polyunsaturated fatty acids comprise 3% to 10% of total caloric intake.[28] Two polyunsaturated fatty acids that are **essential fatty acids** are **omega-3** (α-linolenic acid) and **omega-6** (linoleic acid).

Omega-3 (a-Linolenic Acid)

Alpha-linolenic acid (ALA) is found primarily in plant oils. It can be converted to eicosapentaenoic acid (EPA) and docosahexanoic acid (DHA). DHA and EPA omega-3 fatty acids are naturally found in egg yolks (amounts vary depending on the chicken feed) as well as in cold-water fish and shellfish like tuna, salmon, mackerel, cod, crab, shrimp, and oysters. Overall, omega-3s reduce blood clotting, dilate blood vessels, reduce inflammation, and act to reduce cholesterol and triglyceride levels. They are important for eye and brain development and are especially important for a growing fetus in the late stages of pregnancy. Omega-3s may also help to preserve brain function and reduce the risk of mental illness and attention deficit hyperactivity disorder, though more research is needed to confirm these mental health benefits.[3]

While there is no established **dietary reference intake** (DRI) for the optimal amount of EPA+DHA intake for the general population, the Institute of Medicine (IOM) has established an **adequate intake** (AI) for ALA, the precursor to EPA+DHA. The IOM considers 1.1 grams per day of ALA to be the minimal amount necessary for normal growth and neural development. The IOM suggests that 10% of the needed ALA could come from EPA or DHA, which suggests a daily intake of about 100 milligrams per day.[5] This amount could be obtained by consuming one serving of light, canned tuna. Some expert panels have recommended much higher intakes of 250 and 500 milligrams per day due to the significant health benefits attributed to these fatty acids, and the low risk of complications such as bleeding.[6,28] Notably, most Americans tend not to consume enough omega-3 fatty acids, although this recommendation can be met through the consumption of approximately 8 ounces of a fatty fish per week. Though natural food sources are best, people who do not meet this recommendation or do not like fish may benefit from supplementation or from fortified foods. In fact, the American Heart Association recommends that, under the care of a physician, individuals with elevated triglycerides take a 2 to 4 gram DHA-plus-EPA supplement.[7] Of note, while many products claim to be fortified with omega-3s, it is important for consumers to read the label. If the omega-3s are mostly ALA, they are unlikely to be optimally converted to EPA and DHA and likely have fewer of the health benefits.

Omega-6 (Linoleic Acid)

Linoleic acid, which is generally consumed in abundance, is an essential fatty acid found in flaxseed, canola, and soybean oils, and green leafy vegetables.

Eicosanoids

While both omega-3 and omega-6 fatty acids are used to make **eicosanoids**, eicosanoids made from omega-6 fatty acids tend to contribute to inflammation and increase blood pressure and blood clotting. Eicosanoids made from omega-3 fatty acids have the opposite effect: they reduce blood clotting, dilate blood vessels, and reduce inflammation. The pathways by which these eicosanoids are made compete, therefore it is a balancing act between omega-6 and omega-3 to maintain normal circulation and other biological processes. In the past, scientists hypothesized that reducing consumption of omega-6 fatty acids and increasing consumption of omega-3 fatty acids might lower chronic disease risk, but more recent research has shown that maintaining a high consumption of both omega-3 and omega-6 fatty acids has cardiovascular health benefits.[6] The American Heart Association and the Academy of Nutrition and Dietetics recommend that Americans consume 3-5% to 10% and the Academy of Nutrition and Dietetics of calories as omega-6 polyunsaturated fatty acids; that is, about 12 grams per day for women and 17 grams per day for men.[8,28] On the other hand, the World Health Organization and the Food Agriculture Organization advise a 2% to 3% intake from omega-6 polyunsaturated fatty acids.[29] Table 3-1 shows the fatty acid composition of commonly used vegetable and animal fats and oils.

Hydrogenation

Hydrogenation is the process of converting an unsaturated fatty acid to a saturated fatty acid by replacing the double bonds with hydrogen. The hydrogenation process involves breaking the double bonds of the unsaturated fat and forming an altered unsaturated fat, referred to as a "synthetic" or "industrial" trans fat (transformation from the *cis* formation to a *trans* formation). **Trans fat**, listed as **partially hydrogenated** or hydrogenated oil on a food ingredient list, results mostly from a man-made effort to make an unsaturated fat solid at room temperature and therefore more resistant to oxidation and more shelf stable. Some beef and milk products, though, contain small amounts of natural or "ruminant" trans fat. Once consumed, these fatty acids with trans double bonds are incorporated into phospholipids that form cell and organelle membranes. Therefore, both partial hydrogenation and full hydrogenation cause changes to cell membrane fluidity and negatively affect cell function. The process also interferes with some of the heart-healthy properties of the original unsaturated fat, such as the desaturation and elongation of linoleic acid and ALA to form the heart-healthy EPA and DHA polyunsaturated fatty acids.[9] Synthetic trans fats significantly elevate LDL and are implicated in the development and progression of cardiovascular disease.

Legislation requires food manufacturers to include the amount of trans fat on the nutrition label *if* it is more than 0.5 gram per serving. Food manufacturers now use food processing techniques that do not produce trans fats. Many processed foods that used to be high in trans fat such as chips, crackers, cakes, peanut butter, and margarine are now "trans-fat free." However, as of the time of this writing, many foods still contain notable amounts of trans fat. This is likely to change due to a 2013 Food and Drug Administration preliminary ruling that would ban trans fats.[30] Until final approval and implementation, consumers should check the label to determine if a food contains trans fat. The dietary guidelines recommend that for good health consumers strictly avoid synthetic trans fats[10] (see Communication Strategies).

COMMUNICATION STRATEGIES

Engaging in Science and Policy

The *Dietary Guidelines for Americans* provide evidence-based nutritional guidance to promote health, reduce the risk of chronic diseases, and reduce the prevalence of overweight and obesity through improved nutrition and physical activity. Every 5 years an updated set of dietary guidelines is published which then serves as the cornerstone of nutritional policy in the United States.

In the months to years preceding the release of updated dietary guidelines, the United States Department of Agriculture provides consumers an opportunity for public comment. (For information about the development of the 2015 dietary guidelines and a link to the full 2010 document, visit www.dietaryguidelines.gov.)

Based on your review of the "Fats" section of the 2010 dietary guidelines and your understanding of the role of fat intake in health, compose a letter to the dietary guidelines committee with your comments about the guidelines and/or suggestions for improvement.

SPEED BUMP

1. **List the functions of fat in the body.**
2. **Describe the differences between saturated fat, unsaturated fat, and trans fat.**

PHOSPHOLIPIDS

Phospholipids such as **lecithin** and **sphingomyelin** are structurally similar to triglycerides, but the glycerol backbone is modified so that the molecule is water-soluble at one end and water-insoluble at the other end. Phospholipids play a critical role in maintaining cell-membrane structure and function. Lecithin, a major component of HDL, functions to remove cholesterol from cell membranes. Common food sources of lecithin include liver, egg yolks, soybeans, peanuts, legumes, spinach, wheat germ, and animal products.

FAT DIGESTION AND ABSORPTION

While the majority of dietary fat is consumed as triglycerides and excess fat is stored as triglycerides, dietary fat must still be broken down into its component parts through the process of digestion, transferred to the bloodstream through absorption, and then delivered to the cells to either use for energy or to rebuild into triglycerides and be stored in **adipocytes**.

Fat digestion begins in the mouth with the release of **lingual lipase**, which cleaves short- (fatty acid tail

Table 3-1. **Fatty Acid Composition of Commonly Used Vegetable and Animal Fats and Oils**

OIL LENGTH OF CHAIN: NUMBER OF DOUBLE BONDS[a]	KCAL	TOTAL FA	SFA	LAURIC 12:0	MYRISTIC 14:0	PALMITIC 16:0	STEARIC 18:0	TOTAL MUFA	OLEIC 18:1	TOTAL PUFA	LINOLEIC 18:2(N-6)	LINOLENIC 18:3(N-3)
Almond	120	13.6	1.1	—	—	0.9	0.2	9.5	9.4	2.4	2.4	—
Avocado	124	14	1.6	—	—	1.5	0.1	9.9	9.5	1.9	1.8	0.1
Butter	102	11.5	7.3	0.4	1.1	3.1	1.4	3	2.8	0.4	0.3	0.1
Canola	124	14	1	—	—	0.6	0.3	8.9	8.6	3.9	2.6	1.3
Coconut	117	13.6	11.8	6.1	2.2	1.1	0.4	0.8	0.8	0.3	0.3	—
Corn	120	13.6	1.8	—	—	1.4	0.3	3.8	3.8	7.4	7.2	0.2
Flaxseed	120	13.6	1.2	—	—	0.7	0.5	2.5	2.5	9.2	2	7.2
Grapeseed	120	13.6	1.3	—	—	0.9	0.4	2.2	—	9.5	9.5	—
Hazelnut	120	13.6	1	—	—	0.7	0.3	10.6	10.6	1.4	1.4	—
Lard	115	12.8	5	—	0.2	3	1.7	5.8	5.3	1.4	1.3	0.1
Olive	119	13.5	1.9	—	—	1.5	0.3	9.9	9.6	1.4	1.3	0.1
Palm	120	13.6	6.7	—	0.1	5.9	0.6	5	5	1.3	1.2	—
Peanut	119	13.5	2.3	—	—	1.3	0.3	6.2	6	4.3	4.3	—
Safflower (high oleic)	120	13.6	1	—	—	0.7	0.3	10.2	10.2	1.7	1.7	—
Salmon	123	13.6	2.7	—	0.4	1.3	0.6	3.9	2.3	5.5	0.2	0.1
Sesame	120	13.6	1.9	—	—	1.2	0.7	5.4	5.3	5.7	5.7	—
Soybean	120	13.6	2.1	—	—	1.4	0.6	3.1	3.1	7.9	6.9	0.9
Sunflower (high oleic)	124	14	1.4	—	—	0.5	0.6	11.7	11.6	0.5	0.5	—
Vegetable, palm kernel	117	13.6	11	6.4	2.2	1.1	0.4	1.6	1.6	0.2	0.2	—
Walnut	120	13.6	1.2	—	—	1	0.2	3.1	3	8.6	7.1	1.4

[a]All nutritional values are per 1 tablespoon of oil.
Source: USDA National Nutrient Database for Standard Reference (http://ndb.nal.usda.gov).

with less than 6 carbons) and medium- (fatty acid tail with 6 to 12 carbons) chain fatty acids. After swallowing, fat moves to the stomach, where **gastric lipase** further digests these fats. The mixing and churning of the food in the small intestine helps to increase the surface area for digestion by pancreatic enzymes.

The presence of fat in the small intestine triggers the release of the hormone **cholecystokinin** (CCK). This hormone stimulates the release of **gastric inhibitory peptide**, which decreases gut movement and slows digestion. This explains why high-fat meals increase feelings of fullness compared with lower fat meals. In the small intestine, bile acids **emulsify** the lipids, further increasing surface area so that pancreatic lipases can break the lipids into fatty acids, cholesterol, and lysolecithin. Products of lipid digestion and fat-soluble vitamins are carried by micelles to the absorptive surface of the intestinal cells, where they diffuse across the luminal membrane. Once inside the enterocyte they are converted back into triglycerides, cholesterol, and phospholipids. While medium-chain triglycerides can pass directly into the portal circulation, long-chain triglycerides join an apoprotein to form a chylomicron. These fats and fat-soluble vitamins are transferred into the **lymphatic system**. At the thoracic duct, a large lymphatic vein that drains into the heart, chylomicrons pass into the bloodstream, where they travel to the liver. In the liver, chylomicrons are degraded and the lipids can be repackaged into lipoproteins. The VLDL transports triglycerides to cells for energy or to adipose tissue for storage (see Myths and Misconceptions). Triglycerides that will be broken down to provide energy are sent to the working cells where the enzyme **lipoprotein lipase** cleaves off the fatty acid. These fatty acids can be broken down via the metabolic process of fatty acid (beta) oxidation to produce energy.

Myths and Misconceptions

Eating Fat Makes You 'Fat'

The Myth
Eating fat makes you "fat."

The Logic
Because most dietary fat is triglycerides and fat in the body is stored as triglycerides, it seems logical that they should be one and the same. Further, fat is loaded with calories: 9 calories per 1 gram of fat, compared to 4 calories per 1 gram of carbohydrate or protein.

The Science
The (im)balance of calories consumed versus calories expended determines whether the energy in food (whether it be comprised of carbohydrate, protein, and/or fat) ultimately is stored as fat. Because fat is more filling than carbohydrates, people may tend to eat less of a high-fat product than a high-carbohydrate product. During the low-fat craze of the 1990s, many people replaced higher fat foods with "low-fat" or "fat-free" foods. Unfortunately, "low fat" doesn't always mean low calorie. In fact, some low-fat products are equal to or higher in calorie content than full fat products. How might this trend have contributed to the obesity epidemic?

FAT METABOLISM AND STORAGE

Fat consumed in the diet beyond what is immediately needed as an energy source is stored in adipose tissue. Primarily used as an energy reserve, adipose tissue also functions to provide thermal insulation and serve as a cushion for vital organs. The average 80-kilogram young adult man stores about 12,300 grams of body fat. That translates into about 110,000 calories of fat (12,300 grams × 9 calories/gram), most of which can be mobilized to provide energy to fuel exercise.

Adipose tissue grows in two ways: **hyperplasia** (abnormal increase in the number of fat cells) and hypertrophy (abnormal increase in the size of current fat cells). Genetic predisposition may contribute to the number of fat cells, but excessive energy also plays a role in adipose tissue deposition. When fat cells reach their maximum size, additional fat cells may be created as storage sites.

Parallel to the two types of muscle cells (slow twitch and fast twitch), humans also have two types of fat cells: white fat cells and brown fat cells. White fat cells function primarily to store fat and provide thermal insulation. Brown fat cells, which get their color from the large number of iron-containing mitochondria, are more metabolically active and tend to consume energy. Brown fat cells help to generate body heat, primarily in newborns since newborns are unable to shiver to produce heat. Previously, scientists believed that all brown fat cells were converted to white fat cells as an infant entered childhood and by adulthood all fat was white fat; however, more recent studies suggest that even adults still may have some brown fat. Moreover, there is some emerging evidence that certain types of exercise may help convert the more metabolically inert white fat cells into calorie-burning brown fat cells (see Evaluating the Evidence).

During times of increased energy needs due either to increased energy expenditure or decreased caloric intake, the body mobilizes fat stores to provide energy through fatty acid oxidation (more on this in Chapter 6).

EVALUATING THE EVIDENCE

Does Brown Fat Make You Thin?

The cardiovascular training regimen of one of your lean male clients includes running in very cold temperatures without a shirt, hat, or gloves. When you ask him why he engages in this regimen, he responds simply "brown fat." He goes on to tell you that he has been running in the cold for the last 3 years after he read about brown fat in a newspaper article. He says that he is 100% convinced that his regimen is the reason for his lean physique.

Curious as to the validity of his claim for brown fat, you first search the lay press for a few stories from reputable sources to help you get an overview of the issue. You come across these two stories from the *New York Times*:

1. "Brown fat, triggered by cold or exercise, may yield a key to weight control," by Gina Kolata, January 24, 2012.
2. "Calorie-burning fat? Studies say you have it," by Gina Kolata, April 8, 2009.

Based on your review of these articles and the scientific studies cited within the newspaper articles, answer the following questions:

1. What is the purpose of brown fat? How does it work?
2. Where is brown fat stored in adult humans? When is it activated?
3. What is the difference in amount and activity of brown fat in lean versus obese, men versus women, young versus old participants?
4. How might exercise affect brown fat stores?
5. Why are researchers so excited about the possibility of brown fat and its role in weight control?
6. What are some unanswered questions and limitations to the research?
7. What are some limitations to the way that the research findings are presented in the articles?
8. Are there other more recent scientific studies or articles that provide major updates to the information provided in the two newspaper articles mentioned above?
9. Overall, do you think that your client's conclusion regarding brown fat and his lean physique is warranted?
10. How will this information affect the advice you offer your clients?

SPEED BUMP

3. Outline the process of fat digestion, absorption, and storage.

GENERAL FAT RECOMMENDATIONS

The dietary reference intakes (DRIs) set an acceptable macronutrient distribution range (AMDR) of fat as 20% to 35% of total calories from fat. The average American consumes about 34% of calories from fat, which narrowly fits within the recommended range.

The DRIs do not establish recommended intakes for the types of fat other than the essential fats. The adequate intake (AI) of linolenic acid (omega-3) is 1.6 and 1.1 grams per day for men and women, respectively. The AI for linoleic acid (omega-6) is 17 grams for men and 12 grams for women daily. The 2010 *Dietary Guidelines for Americans* advise the general population to consume fewer than 10% of calories from saturated fat and less than 300 milligrams per day of dietary cholesterol, and to consume more monounsaturated and polyunsaturated fats and less saturated and trans fats. The guidelines introduced the term **solid fats and added sugars** (SoFAS) and recommend avoiding these substances for optimal health. The American College of Sports Medicine and the Academy of Nutrition and Dietetics endorse these guidelines for the general population as well as athletes.

FAT AND HEALTH

Fat intake has long been implicated in the development of **coronary heart disease** (CHD), a leading killer of both men and women in the United States. CHD develops from atherosclerosis, or an accumulation of fat and cholesterol in the lining of the arteries that supply oxygen and nutrients to the heart muscle. Over time, blood flow is reduced and oxygenation to the heart muscle can become limited, leading to **angina** (chest pain) and **myocardial infarction** (heart attack). The risk factors for CHD in children are not significantly different from those for adults, and atherosclerosis can begin to develop in childhood. High blood cholesterol levels—in particular, high levels of low-density lipoprotein (LDL) and its susceptibility to oxidation—are the main culprits in the development of atherosclerosis. Adipocyte dysfunction can be characterized by the inability of the adipocytes to store excess energy consumption, resulting in increased blood glucose and triglyceride levels and cytokine production. The resultant inflammatory reactions may impair the body's ability to regulate satiety and modulate insulin resistance.[11]

Allied health professionals can help clients minimize their **cardiovascular disease** risk by educating them about risk factors and encouraging them to talk with their physicians about their personal risk. The importance of monitoring risk factors such as age, LDL cholesterol, HDL cholesterol, smoking, systolic blood pressure, family history, obesity, and diabetes should be emphasized.[12] Both older adults, who may have already developed one or more risk factors and now must vigorously work to reverse them, or at least prevent their progression, and younger individuals, who appear to be healthy, should be monitored.

Regardless of a person's overall risk, everyone should be encouraged to follow these nutrition recommendations to optimize heart health:

- Replace saturated fat with polyunsaturated fat whenever possible, or otherwise with monounsaturated fat. Polyunsaturated fats lower LDL cholesterol and improve the HDL:total cholesterol ratio, often by increasing the HDL component. Monounsaturated fats have a more neutral effect.
- Choose healthful fats over "low fat" foods that contain refined carbohydrates, as these foods decrease HDL cholesterol, increase triglycerides, and overall worsen the **atherogenic dyslipidemia** associated with obesity and insulin resistance.[4]
- Consume omega-3 fatty acids in the diet at least two times per week.
- Avoid trans fats, as they decrease HDL cholesterol and increase total cholesterol.
- Keep in mind that total fat intake and ratio of omega-3 to omega-6 fatty acids are not predictors of heart health.
- Exercise regularly to decrease LDL levels and prevent reduction in HDL associated with a diet higher than recommended in total fat and saturated fatty acids.[13] The American Heart Association and the American College of Sports Medicine recommend 150 minutes per week of moderate exercise or 75 minutes a week of vigorous exercise. It can be as simple as a total of 30 minutes of brisk walking 5 days a week.

FAT AND WEIGHT MANAGEMENT

The long-held and inaccurate belief that "eating fat makes you fat" has inspired many very low fat diets in the past and a residual disdain for fat-containing foods among consumers trying to lose weight. While fat is more calorically dense than proteins and carbohydrates—225% more calories per gram (9 calories per gram compared to 4 calories per gram)—fat also contributes to increased feelings of satiety and fullness. These feelings of satiety should lead to reduced food intake in people who regulate their intake based on physiological cues of hunger and fullness (rather than emotional or nonphysiologically driven eating).

Several studies investigating the role of dietary fats in weight management have found that as long as caloric intake is equal across diets, the percentage of calories from fat, protein, or carbohydrates does not make a difference in sustained weight loss. In fact, research has consistently played out that higher fat diets are just as good for weight loss and health benefits, if not better in some cases, than a low-fat, high-carbohydrate diet.[14-16]

FAT AND ATHLETIC PERFORMANCE

The effectiveness of various dietary strategies to use fat as an ergogenic aid is inconclusive. According to a position statement of the Academy of Nutrition and Dietetics and the American College of Sports Medicine, to date there is no evidence for performance benefit from a very low-fat diet (< 15% of total calories) or from a high-fat diet.[17] However, there has been interest in **fat loading**, a dietary approach in which an athlete increases consumption of fat in an effort to provide a ready supply of fat as an energy source. Fat loading can be done immediately before exercise or long term by adopting a high-fat, low-carbohydrate diet. The theory is that if a progressively greater percentage of fat is consumed in the diet, fat oxidation will be increased during exercise. Energy can be produced from fat, and therefore, carbohydrate stores can be spared. Typically, carbohydrate stores can only fuel about 3 hours of endurance activity. By using more fat for fuel, the belief is that it will take longer to deplete muscle glycogen stores and the athlete will be able to maintain long-distance activities for a longer period of time at a higher intensity. This is referred to as **fat adaptation**.

Dietary periodization is another strategy that involves consuming a high-fat, low-carbohydrate diet for a designated period while training for an endurance event, followed by a period of glycogen restoration during which a high-carbohydrate, low-fat diet is consumed. While in theory this sounds like it may benefit athletic performance, and some studies that have looked at fat-adaptation strategies have found that whole-body rates of fat oxidation are increased in well-trained athletes, the effects of fat adaptation strategies on endurance performance have been equivocal. Some athletes experience worsened performance, presumably due to factors such as fatigue. Part of the problem is due to reduced muscle glycogen stores from a low-carbohydrate diet (due to high fat).[18]

The role of fat in athletic performance is described in detail in Chapter 7. Overall, similar to the general population, athletes are advised to consume fats within the AMDR of 20% to 35% of total calories.[17]

SPEED BUMP

4. **Describe the effect of various fats on health and disease risk.**
5. **Describe the role of fat in weight management.**

CHOOSING FATS

Clearly, fat serves many essential functions in the body and adequate dietary intake of fats is critical to not only maintain body weight but also for optimal health. In fact, contrary to the dietary teaching of previous decades which advised strict avoidance of fat, certain fats are healthy and consensus among leading nutrition experts is that fats are better for health than the refined sugars that food manufacturers have used to replace fat in the highly processed fat-free crackers, cookies, chips, breads, and ice creams found on grocery store shelves.[19]

Arguably, the most heart-healthy way of eating, the Mediterranean diet, is based on an eating plan that contains significantly more calories from fat (about 35% to 40% of calories) than what the American Heart Association has historically recommended (< 30%). However, this eating plan is also characterized by low intakes of red meat, refined grains, and sweets. Instead, it features fatty fish, nuts, whole grains, fruits, vegetables, and moderate alcohol intake, particularly red wine, with the majority of fat intake coming from monounsaturated fat in olive oil. Research continues to demonstrate that the Mediterranean diet is associated with decreased risk of heart disease, stroke, and several forms of cancer.[20-22] Additional research shows a possible correlation between adherence to a Mediterranean diet and neurological disease, including decreased risk of mild cognitive impairment, dementia, and Alzheimer's disease.[23, 24] As research supporting the beneficial effects of the Mediterranean diet accumulates, more consideration may need to be given to education in this area.

WHAT TO TELL YOUR CLIENTS

A panel of expert contributors to the "Great Fat Debate" in the *Journal of the American Dietetic Association* offer these key practice points to registered dietitians (and Allied Health Professionals) when discussing nutrition with clients:[25]

- Use liquid vegetable oils (a mix of monounsaturated fatty acids and polyunsaturated fatty acids) whenever possible.
- When solid fats are necessary, keep trans fat intake as low as possible.
- Balance calories by limiting refined carbohydrates and not through avoidance of the healthy polyunsaturated and monounsaturated fats.
- While saturated fats are not "good for you," they can fit in an overall healthy eating plan when limited to less than 10% of total fat intake.
- Remember that dietary fats are never purely polyunsaturated, monounsaturated, or saturated fats, but rather a combination of fats.
- Provide education in terms of a food-based (not chemical-based) discussion.
- Promote fruits, vegetables, and whole grains as ideal sources of carbohydrates rather than refined or heavily processed carbohydrates.
- Emphasize that dietary patterns are more important than single dietary components. A healthful eating plan includes fruits, vegetables, unprocessed whole grains, fish, lean meat, low-fat dairy, and vegetable oils.
- Calorie balance should emphasize quality of food selection.

Allied health professionals can empower clients to make informed decisions by helping them learn to read a nutrition label to glean important nutrient information, including fat content. Box 3-3 demonstrates how one might help a client understand the health value of a serving of walnuts.

SPEED BUMP

6. List several principles to share with clients when discussing fat intake.

Box 3-3. Understanding the Food Label

A client requests your help in understanding the food label. A discussion of the relationship between the serving size and percentage of calories from fat follows:

Nutrition Facts

Serving Size 1 ounce (28g)		(A)
Amount Per Serving		
Calories 185	Calories from Fat 154	(B)
	% Daily Value*	
Total Fat 18g	**28%**	(C)
Sat. Fat 2g	**9%**	(D)
Trans. Fat		
Cholest. 0mg	**0%**	
Sodium 1mg	**0%**	
Total Carb. 4g	**1%**	
Protein 4g	**8%**	
Vitamin A 0% • Vitamin C 1%		
Calcium 3% • Iron 5%		

*Percent Daily Values are based on a 2,000 calorie diet. Your daily values may be higher or lower depending on your calorie needs.

1. Serving size. What might be a tool that your client could use to help estimate how much is 1 ounce of walnuts?
2. What is the significance of noting the "calories from fat" on the nutrition label?
3. What does "total fat" on the label mean? How is the percent daily value of fat determined? Is the 28% stated on the food label applicable to your client's fat needs?
4. a. What is the significance of 2 g of saturated fat? Is that an acceptable amount of saturated fat per serving?
   b. You can use the USDA National Nutrient Database (http://ndb.nal.usda.gov/), then click on "full report (all nutrients)" to determine the types of fat contained in the other 16 grams of fat per serving, or the USDA's Supertracker (supertracker.usda.gov), then click "Food-A-Pedia" and "nutrient info" for complete nutrition information. Do you think the types and amounts of fat influences the health value of walnuts?
   c. On the front of the walnut package there is a *qualified health claim* that states: "Supportive but not conclusive research shows that eating 1.5 ounces per day of walnuts, as part of a low saturated fat and low cholesterol diet and not resulting in increased caloric intake, may reduce the risk of coronary heart disease. See nutrition information for fat [and calorie] content." A qualified health claim characterizes a relationship between a substance (specific food component or a specific food) and a disease (e.g., heart disease) or health-related condition (e.g., high blood pressure), and is supported by scientific evidence, but there is not significant scientific agreement (which is required for a health claim), thus the claim must be "accompanied by a disclaimer or otherwise qualified." Qualified health claims were initially authorized to help consumers make healthier nutrition choices even though claims may be accompanied by inconclusive evidence. Do you think qualified health claims help or hinder consumers from making well-informed nutrition choices? Why?

KEY POINTS SUMMARY

1. Fats serve many important critical functions in the body including energy storage, insulation, protection, transport of fat-soluble vitamins, precursor to hormones, and cell membrane structure.
2. Triglycerides consist of three fatty acids joined to a glycerol backbone. Both dietary fats and stored fats consist mostly of triglycerides.
3. Fat cells are called adipocytes. They are stored in the body as adipose tissue. Adipose tissue is a metabolically active endocrine organ that produces hormones that have been implicated in contributing to the obesity and diabetes epidemics.
4. The major categories of fatty acids include saturated fatty acids, monounsaturated fatty acids, and polyunsaturated fatty acids. Polyunsaturated fats (especially omega-3 fatty acids) are the most heart-healthy fats, followed by monounsaturated fats. An emerging body of research suggests that saturated fats are not as bad for health as previously thought, though they are clearly inferior to the polyunsaturated and monounsaturated fats. Polyunsaturated fatty acids that have trans fats are harmful to human health and should be avoided.

5. Dietary fat is digested and absorbed in the gastrointestinal system. The digestion of triglycerides with short- and medium-chain fatty acids begins in the mouth and stomach, whereas the digestion of long-chain fatty acids does not begin until the food has reached the small intestine. Fat digestion finishes in the small intestine, where lipid droplets are carried as micelles to the absorptive surface of the small intestine. Once the lipids are absorbed into the mucosal surface of the small intestine, they are reconfigured as triglycerides, phospholipids, and cholesterol. The lipids with short- and medium-chain fatty acids (the minority of dietary fats) can pass directly to the portal circulation and to the liver. The lipids with long-chain fatty acids are carried as chylomicrons to the lymphatic system. The chylomicrons are carried to the liver, where triglycerides are repackaged into lipoproteins and transported primarily to the adipose tissue for metabolism and storage.
6. Fat is stored in large amounts in the human body. White fat cells serve as a reservoir of calories and energy, while brown fat cells—which are typically activated by cold—expend energy. Some researchers speculate that exercise may stimulate brown fat cells and may also act to convert some white fat cells into brown fat cells.
7. The AMDR for fat is 20% to 35% of calories. The 2010 *Dietary Guidelines for Americans* recommend that less than 10% of total calories come from saturated fat and that Americans consume less than 300 milligrams per day of cholesterol. The guidelines also advise Americans to avoid solid fats and added sugars (SoFAS).
8. To optimize heart health, health professionals should advise consumers to replace saturated fat with polyunsaturated (preferably) or monounsaturated fat, whenever possible. Replacing saturated fat with refined carbohydrates does not benefit health. Trans fats negatively affect health and should be avoided. Research suggests that adopting a low-fat diet does not improve health or facilitate weight loss when compared to a higher fat diet of equal calories.
9. Health professionals must be knowledgeable of the latest advances in nutritional science as well as the latest trends among consumers to provide reliable nutrition information to consumers.

PRACTICAL APPLICATIONS

1. Which of the following substances, when oxidized, distributes cholesterol to the inner linings or walls of arteries and may form a plaque and ultimately cause atherosclerosis?
   A. Chylomicrons
   B. Phospholipids
   C. Intermediate-density lipoproteins (IDLs)
   D. Low-density lipoproteins (LDLs)
2. Olives, nuts, seeds, and avocados are excellent sources of which type of fat?
   A. Monounsaturated fat
   B. Polyunsaturated fat
   C. Saturated fat
   D. Hydrogenated fat
3. Clients at risk for heart disease can be challenged by the health professional to eat fewer than 200 milligrams each day of:
   A. Sodium
   B. Total fat
   C. Cholesterol
   D. Sugar
4. Which of the following statements is true regarding the latest research on dietary fat?
   A. A healthy, balanced diet should not include saturated fats.
   B. The evidence against saturated fat is not as strong as originally interpreted.
   C. Trans fats can be included in small amounts in a balanced diet.
   D. It is not the type of fat intake, but rather the amount of fat that is important for health.
5. Which of the following hormones is responsible for the increased feelings of satiety after a high-fat meal?
   A. Ghrelin
   B. Insulin
   C. Glucocorticoid
   D. Cholecystokinin
6. Which of the following anatomical structures is typically activated by cold and functions to expend energy?
   A. Muscle tissue
   B. Brown fat
   C. White fat
   D. Collagen

7. According to the *Dietary Guidelines for Americans*, less than what percentage of daily calories should come from saturated fat?
   A. 3%
   B. 5%
   C. 10%
   D. 15%
8. Sanjay is an ultra-marathoner who believes that he can increase performance if he increases his consumption of fat in an effort to provide a ready supply of fat as an energy source. This dietary approach is known as:
   A. Fat loading
   B. Carbohydrate loading
   C. Carbohydrate sparing
   D. Protein sparing
9. Which of the following diet plans recommends the least amount of daily calories from fat?
   A. Zone diet
   B. Paleo diet
   C. Mediterranean diet
   D. American Heart Association diet
10. To optimize heart health, allied health professionals should advise consumers to replace saturated fat with:
   A. Polyunsaturated fat
   B. Monounsaturated fat
   C. Trans fat
   D. Refined carbohydrates

Case 1 Susan, the Middle-Aged Overweight Hiker

Susan is a 55-year-old overweight teacher who has struggled with her weight since childhood. After her best friend suffered a debilitating heart attack, she decided to change her lifestyle and achieve a healthier weight. As part of her fitness program, she is training to hike the Grand Canyon with her 17-year-old daughter and a guide. She is 5′2″ and 180 pounds (BMI 32.9 kg/m2). According to the USDA's Supertracker, Susan needs about 2,000 calories per day to *maintain* her weight.

1. What is the AMDR for fat intake?
2. What range of calories per day should Susan get from fats to maintain her weight?
3. Susan tells you that she is confused as to whether fat in her diet matters or not. She says that the last she remembers, the recommendation was to eat a "low-fat" diet but then she heard that the Mediterranean diet, which is high in olive oil and fatty fish, is very healthy, and now she has read a lot of information that says "saturated fat is good." She asks you to please clarify which fats are "good," which are "bad," and what she should be eating.

Case 2 Scott, the Professional Triathlete

Scott is a 29-year-old professional triathlete. It is the off-season and his current training regimen is of relatively low intensity. He is 6′2″ and 170 pounds (BMI 21.8 kg/m2). He needs about 3,200 calories per day to maintain his weight.

1. What is the AMDR for fat for athletes?
2. a. What range of calories from fat should Scott get each day?
   b. How might Scott's fat needs within this range change over the course of the year?
3. Scott has experimented with several dietary manipulations during the off-season in an effort to identify a regimen that will give him the competitive edge during the training and competitive seasons. He has recently started a *fat loading* diet with the following regimen:

DAY 1	DAY 2	DAY 3	DAY 4	DAY 5	DAY 6	DAY 7
High-fat diet (70% of calories from fat, 15% CHO, 15% protein)					High carbohydrate (70% calories from CHO, 15% fat, 15% protein) and rest	"Brick" (45 min swim, 2 hr ride, 1.5 hr run)
Run for 20 min at 70% VO_2 max + interval training	3-4 hr ride	2 hr run	3-4 hr ride	1.5 hr swim		

a. Describe the rationale behind "fat loading." Include a discussion of "fat adaptation."
b. What are the pros and cons of the dietary plan (called "dietary periodization") that Scott is following?
c. What advice do you have for Scott as he experiments with this diet/training regimen?

TRAIN YOURSELF

1. What is the recommended AMDR for fat for you?
2. Using supertracker.usda.gov, estimate your daily caloric needs. Based on that estimate, what range of calories from fat should you get each day?
3. Record your food intake for a 24-hour period using supertracker.usda.gov. Then, answer the following questions:
   a. What is the percentage of calories from fat? How does this compare to the AMDR?
   b. How many grams of saturated fat did you eat? What percentage of total calories came from saturated fat?
   c. How many empty calories did you eat?
   d. List several of the fatty foods that you ate. Using the USDA National Nutrient Database (http://ndb.nal.usda.gov/) or the Supertracker food analysis tool, determine the amount of the various types of fat in each of the foods. Rank saturated fat, polyunsaturated fat, and monounsaturated fat from "most eaten" to "least eaten."

RESOURCES

USDA National Nutrient Database (http://ndb.nal.usda.gov) provides detailed nutrition information for thousands of foods.

REFERENCES

1. Vendrell J, Broch M, Vilarrasa N, et al. Resistin, adiponectin, ghrelin, leptin, and proinflammatory cytokines: relationships in obesity. *Obes Res*. 2004;12:962–971. doi: 10.1038/oby.2004.118.
2. Hunter JE, Zhang J, Kris-Etherton PM. Cardiovascular disease risk of dietary stearic acid compared with trans, other saturated, and unsaturated fatty acids: a systematic review. *Am J Clin Nutr.* January 2010;91(1):46-63.
3. Kris-Etherton PM, Innis S, American Dietetic A, Dietitians of C. Position of the American Dietetic Association and Dietitians of Canada: dietary fatty acids. *J Am Diet Assoc.* September 2007;107(9):1599-1611.
4. Siri-Tarino PW, Sun Q, Hu FB, Krauss RM. Saturated fat, carbohydrate, and cardiovascular disease. *Am J Clin Nutr.* March 2010;91(3):502-509.
5. Institute of Medicine, National Academy of Sciences. *Dietary reference intakes for energy, carbohydrate, fiber, fat, fatty acids, cholesterol, protein, and amino acids*. Washington, DC: National Academies Press; 2005.
6. Harris W. Omega-6 and omega-3 fatty acids: partners in prevention. *Curr Opin Clin Nutr Metab care.* March 2010; 13(2):125-129.
7. Miller M, Stone NJ, Ballantyne C, et al. Triglycerides and cardiovascular disease: a scientific statement from the American Heart Association. *Circulation.* May 24 2011; 123(20):2292-2333.
8. Harris WS, Mozaffarian D, Rimm E, et al. Omega-6 fatty acids and risk for cardiovascular disease: a science advisory from the American Heart Association Nutrition Subcommittee of the Council on Nutrition, Physical Activity, and Metabolism; Council on Cardiovascular Nursing; and Council on Epidemiology and Prevention. *Circulation.* February 17 2009;119(6):902-907.
9. Kummerow FA, Mohfouz MM, Zhou Q. Trans fatty acids in partially hydrogenated soybean oil inhibit prostacyclin release by endothelial cells in presence of high level of linoleic acid. *Prostaglandins Other Lipid Mediat.* 2007;84:138-153.
10. U.S. Dept. of Agriculture. 2010 Dietary Guidelines for Americans backgrounder, history and process. Washington, DC: U.S. Dept. of Agriculture; 2010. Available at: http://purl.fdlp.gov/GPO/gpo4085.
11. Balagopal P, de Ferranti SD, Cook S, et al. Nontraditional risk factors and biomarkers for cardiovascular disease: mechanistic, research, and clinical considerations for youth: a scientific statement from the American Heart Association. *Circulation.* 2011;123:2749-2769. doi:10.1161/CIR.0b013e31821c7c64.
12. Greenland P, Alpert JS, Beller GA, et al. 2010 ACCF/AHA guideline for assessment of cardiovascular risk in asymptomatic adults. Executive summary: a report of the American College of Cardiology Foundation/American Heart Association Task Force on Practice Guidelines. *Circulation.* 2010; 122:2748-2764.
13. Thompson PD, Lim V. Physical activity in the prevention of atherosclerotic coronary heart disease. *Curr Treat Options Cardiovasc Med.* 2003;5:279-285.
14. Foster GD, Wyatt HR, Hill JO, et al. A randomized trial of a low-carbohydrate diet for obesity. *N Engl J Med.* May 22 2003;348(21):2082-2090.
15. Gardner CD, Kiazand A, Alhassan S, et al. Comparison of the Atkins, Zone, Ornish, and LEARN diets for change in weight and related risk factors among overweight premenopausal women: the A TO Z Weight Loss Study: a randomized trial. *JAMA.* March 7 2007;297(9):969-977.
16. Dansinger ML, Gleason JA, Griffith JL, Selker HP, Schaefer EJ. Comparison of the Atkins, Ornish, Weight Watchers, and Zone diets for weight loss and heart disease risk reduction: a randomized trial. *JAMA.* January 5 2005; 293(1):43-53.
17. Rodriguez NR, DiMarco NM, Langley S. Position of the American Dietetic Association, Dietitians of Canada, and the American College of Sports Medicine: nutrition and athletic performance. *J Am Diet Assoc.* March 2009; 109(3):509-527.
18. Yeo WK, Carey AL, Burke L, et al. Fat adaptation in well-trained athletes: effects on cell metabolism. *Appl Physiol Nutr Metab.* 2011;36:12-22.
19. WGBH Educational Foundation. Did the low-fat era make us fat? *Frontline.* April 8, 2004. www.pbs.org/wgbh/pages/frontline/shows/diet/themes/lowfat.html. Accessed April 19, 2013.

20. Fung TT, Rexrode KM, Mantzoros CS, et al. Mediterranean diet and incidence of and mortality from coronary heart disease and stroke in women. *Circulation.* 2009;119(8), 1093-1100.
21. Estruch R, Ros E, Salas-Salvado J, et al. Primary prevention of cardiovascular disease with a Mediterranean diet. *N Engl J Med.* 2013. doi: 10.1056/NEJMoa1200303.
22. Buckland G, Agudo A, Luján L, et al. (2010). Adherence to a Mediterranean diet and risk of gastric adenocarcinoma within the European Prospective Investigation into Cancer and Nutrition (EPIC) cohort study. *Am J Clin Nutr*. 2010; 91(2):381-390.
23. Scarmeas N, Stern Y, Mayeux R, et al. Mediterranean diet and mild cognitive impairment. *Arch Neurol.* 2009; 66(2):216-225. doi:10.1001/archneurol.2008.536.
24. Féart C, Samieri C, Rondeau V, et al. Adherence to a Mediterranean diet, cognitive decline, and risk of dementia. *JAMA*. 2009;302(6):638-648. doi:10.1001/jama.2009.1146.
25. Zelman K. The great fat debate: a closer look at the controversy-questioning the validity of age-old dietary guidance. *J Am Diet Assoc.* May 2011;111(5):655-658.
26. Siri-Tarino PW, Sun Q, Hu FB, Krauss RM. Meta-analysis of prospective cohort studies evaluating the association of saturated fat with cardiovascular disease. *Am J Clin Nutr.* March 2010;91(3):535-546.
27. Jakobsen MU, O'Reilly EJ, Heitmann BL, et al. Major types of dietary fat and risk of coronary heart disease: a pooled analysis of 11 cohort studies. *Am J Clin Nutr.* May 2009; 89(5):1425-1432.
28. Vannice, G & Rasmussen, H. Position of the Academy of Nutrition and Dietetics: Dietary fatty acids for healthy adults. *J Acad Nutr Diet* 2014;114:136-153.
29. World Health Organization/Food Agriculture Organization. Fats and fatty acids in human nutrition. Report of an expert consultation. *FAO Food Nutr Pap*. 2010; 91: 1-166.
30. Food and Drug Administration. FDA takes step to further reduce *trans* fats in processed foods. FDA News Release, November 7, 2013. Available at: www.fda.gov/newsevents/newsroom/pressannouncements/ucm373939.htm. Retrieved January 19, 2014.

CHAPTER 4

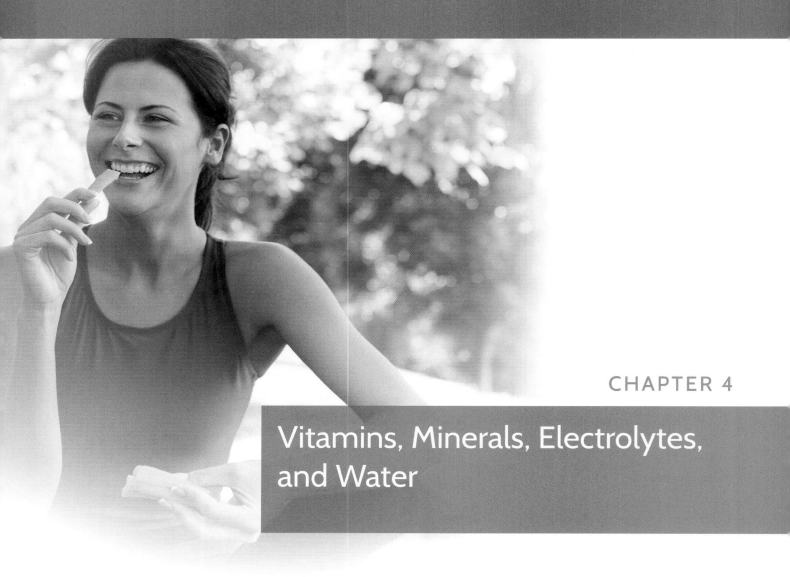

Vitamins, Minerals, Electrolytes, and Water

CHAPTER OUTLINE

CHAPTER OUTLINE–cont'd

LEARNING OBJECTIVES

After studying this chapter, the reader should be able to:

4.1 Define the term *micronutrient* and explain the different categories of micronutrients.
4.2 Describe the role of electrolytes in athletic performance.
4.3 List the micronutrients most commonly deficient in athletes.
4.4 Describe the benefit or lack of benefit of vitamin and mineral supplementation.
4.5 Explain the importance of water for health and athletic performance.

KEY TERMS

active transport The passage of a particle from an area of low concentration to an area of high concentration made possible through the use of adenosine triphosphate (ATP).
anion A negatively charged molecule.
antioxidant A substance that prevents or repairs oxidative damage; includes vitamins C and E, some carotenoids, selenium, quinones, and bioflavonoids.
cation A positively charged molecule.
chelation compounds A compound that consists of a molecule bonded to a single atom, usually a metal, which allows the metal to be more efficiently absorbed by the body.
cofactor A substance that needs to be present in addition to an enzyme in order for a chemical reaction to occur.
colonic bacteria Benign bacteria that colonize the large intestine (the colon) of the human gut.
dehydration A state of decreased total body fluid, which is categorized as mild (< 2% loss of body weight), moderate (2% to 7%), and severe (> 7%).
duodenum The approximately 1-foot long first portion of the small intestine where the majority of chemical digestion of food occurs.
electrolytes Minerals that exist as charged ions in the body and are extremely important for normal cellular function.
enriched food A food to which specific nutrients, such as B vitamins and iron, are added to replace nutrients lost during processing.
facilitated diffusion The passage of a particle from an area of high concentration to an area of low concentration with a protein carrier.
fat-soluble vitamins Vitamins that are stored in and absorbed by fat; vitamins A, D, E, and K.
female athlete triad A syndrome characterized by an eating disorder (or low energy availability), amenorrhea, and decreased bone mineral density.
ferritin The storage form of iron.
fortified food A food to which specific nutrients not inherently available in that food are added, such as vitamin D in milk.

functional anemia Low iron ferritin levels in the context of normal hemoglobin concentration.
glycogenolysis The process of breaking down glycogen into glucose molecules.
heat stroke A severe heat-related illness with extreme increase in core body temperature resulting from prolonged exposure to heat without adequate replacement of fluids and electrolytes; symptoms include lack of sweating, strong and rapid pulse, disorientation, and loss of consciousness; often fatal without rapid treatment.
heme iron Iron bound within the iron-carrying proteins of hemoglobin and myoglobin complex found in meat, fish, and poultry.
hemoglobin An iron-rich protein of red blood cells that carries oxygen to working cells.
hyponatremia An abnormally low concentration of blood sodium (less than 135 millimoles per liter (mmol/L)) which, when severe, can lead to brain swelling and death.
ileum The final portion of the small intestine, which is approximately 12 feet in length, where absorption of vitamin B_{12}, bile salts, and digestive products not already absorbed in the jejunum occurs.
iron deficiency anemia A condition resulting from too little iron in the body, which decreases hemoglobin concentration and thus impairs oxygen delivery to cells.
jejunum The middle portion of the small intestine, which is approximately 8 feet in length; where much of food absorption occurs.
micronutrient A nutrient that is needed in small quantities for normal growth and development; includes vitamins and minerals.
myoglobin An oxygen- and iron-binding protein found in muscle and cardiac tissue which delivers oxygen to the working muscle cells.
osteopenia A condition in which bone density is lower than normal; a precursor to osteoporosis.
osteoporosis Weakening of the bones due to chronic calcium deficiency, which can lead to fracture of the hip, spine, and other skeletal sites.
oxidation The process of binding oxygen to a molecule.
passive diffusion See *simple diffusion.*
phytochemicals Substances in plants that are not necessarily required for normal functioning, but improve health and reduce the risk of disease.
prohormone A precursor to a hormone.
provitamin Inactive vitamin that can be converted to an active vitamin with enzyme activation.
quasi-vitamins Similar to vitamins in having important roles in the normal functioning and health of the body, but currently there are no known human requirements.
simple diffusion When a substance moves from an area of high concentration to an area of low concentration without the need for a carrier protein.
sports anemia A pseudo-anemia characterized by low hemoglobin concentration due to increased plasma volume in response to exercise; the actual total hemoglobin content is normal and the athlete does not have true anemia.
transferrin The protein that binds and transports iron.
vegan A pure vegetarian who excludes all animal-derived foods from the diet.
vitamins Organic substances obtained from plant and animal foods that are essential in small quantities for normal growth and activity of the body.
water-soluble vitamins Vitamins that are readily dissolved in water and thus are not effectively stored in the human body.

INTRODUCTION

On the heels of a research study warning of the possible increased risk of mortality from red meat consumption,[1] a top running magazine published an article proclaiming the benefits of red meat for athletes. The long list of cited benefits included: a "great source" of zinc and iron; the high B vitamins "help convert carbohydrates into the fuel needed to make it through a training run"; vitamin B_6, which "can increase your metabolism"; the salt-heavy turkey pastrami is a "great source of electrolytes"; and athletes lose enough salt through sweat so the sodium content is unimportant.[2] In the article, several sports dietitians were quoted endorsing red meat's benefits (see Communication Strategies). But does the relatively higher vitamin and mineral composition described above for red meat really make it a superior protein source for athletes? How do micronutrient needs for athletes differ compared with the general population? What are the best food sources to optimize micronutrient intake?

As their name implies, **micronutrients,** including vitamins and minerals, are only needed in small amounts. The World Health Organization (WHO) refers to these nutrients as the "magic wands that enable the body to produce enzymes, hormones, and other substances that are essential for proper growth and development."[3] When the body is deprived of or excessively overloaded with micronutrients, the consequences are severe. But when the micronutrients are consumed in the right amounts through a varied, balanced, and nutrient-rich diet, vitamins and minerals contribute to optimal health, function, and well-being.

COMMUNICATION STRATEGIES

Working With The Media

Working with the media is an effective way to share health and nutrition information with the general population while at the same time enhancing your credibility and reputation as a professional. With that being said, health experts need to be thoughtful when working with the media. Prior to responding to a query from a reporter, consider investigating that reporter's past work; understand the purpose of the piece and if you agree with it; and remember that everything is "on the record." Then make yourself a valuable resource by responding promptly and honestly with well-informed and simple statements.

Practice with this sample query:

A reporter contacts you for information on an article that she is writing about the benefits for athletes of what she considers to be unfairly maligned red meat. She believes that red meat is necessary for athletes to compete at their best. She asks you the following questions:

1. What are the vitamin and mineral benefits of red meat for athletes?
2. Do you recommend that your clients eat red meat? If so, what kind and why?
3. What tips do you have for shoppers on how to select the best protein source for optimal athletic performance?

Answer the questions with the understanding that she may publish a summary of your comments or quote you directly for the article.

Now, think about the topic and review the answers that you wrote when answering the following questions:

1. Do you agree with the writer's premise that red meat is especially beneficial for athletes?
2. Did you use any scientific research or studies to back up your point? If so, which ones? If not, try to find a scientific study or report that supports your statements. If you cannot find one, reconsider your statements.
3. Could the writer take any quotes from your responses that, by themselves, might not accurately reflect your opinion on the benefits of red meat for athletes?

VITAMIN FUNCTIONS, NEEDS, AND FOOD SOURCES

Vitamins are organic (carbon containing), noncaloric micronutrients that are essential for normal physiological function. Vitamins must be consumed through foods, with the following exceptions: vitamin K and biotin, which can be produced by normal intestinal flora (bacteria that live in the intestines and are critical for normal gastrointestinal function); vitamin D, which can be self-produced with sun exposure; and niacin and vitamin A, which can be synthesized from tryptophan and beta-carotene, respectively. No "perfect" food contains all the vitamins in just the right amount. Instead, a variety of nutrient-dense foods must be consumed to ensure adequate vitamin intake. Many foods, such as breads and cereals, are **enriched** or **fortified** with some nutrients to reduce the risk of vitamin deficiency. Some foods contain inactive vitamins, which are called **provitamins**. The human body contains enzymes to convert these inactive vitamins into active vitamins.

Humans need 13 different vitamins, which are divided into two categories: water-soluble vitamins (the B vitamins and vitamin C) and fat-soluble vitamins (vitamins A, D, E, and K). Some B vitamin derivatives, known as **quasi-vitamins**, also have important roles in the normal functioning and health of the body; however, their human requirements are not yet known. Inositol, choline, and para-aminobenzoic acid (PABA) are examples of quasi-vitamins. Choline, which plays a crucial role in neurotransmitter and platelet functions, may help prevent Alzheimer's[4] and fatty liver disease,[5] and is essential for normal fetal brain development.[6] Inositol has been linked to improving metabolic syndrome (a combination of risk factors such as obesity, high blood pressure, high blood sugar, and high cholesterol that increase the risk for conditions such as heart disease and stroke) in postmenopausal women.[7]

The human body needs vitamins to varying degrees. Dietary reference intake (DRI) is a collective term used to refer to three types of reference values:

- **Recommended dietary allowances (RDAs):** the daily dietary intake of a nutrient known to meet the nutritional needs of 97% of healthy persons in age- and gender-specific groups. The Food and Nutrition Board, an entity of the Institute of Medicine, establishes RDAs.

- **Estimated average requirement (EAR):** an amount of nutrient known to be adequate to meet nutritional needs in 50% of an age- and gender-specific group.
- **Tolerable upper intake level (UL):** the maximum intake that is unlikely to pose risk of adverse health effects to almost all individuals in an age- and gender-specific group.

If an RDA cannot be based on an EAR, then the adequate intake (AI), the amount of intake that is believed to cover the needs of all healthy individuals in the groups, is used. The recommended intake for each of the vitamins is included in Table 4-1. Table 4-2 summarizes the vitamin functions, signs of deficiency and toxicity, and food sources.

Water-Soluble Vitamins

Thiamin, riboflavin, niacin, pantothenic acid, folate, vitamin B_6, vitamin B_{12}, biotin, and vitamin C are referred to as the **water-soluble vitamins**. Their ability to dissolve in water (which gives them similar absorption and distribution in the body) and their roles as **cofactors** of enzymes involved in metabolism (i.e., without them, the enzyme will not work) are common traits. With the exception of vitamins B_6 and B_{12}, water-soluble vitamins cannot be stored in the body and, in general, are readily excreted in urine. This decreases the risk of toxicity from overconsumption and makes their regular intake a necessity.

Though generally the body does not store the water-soluble vitamins, the effects of a period of inadequate dietary consumption of the water-soluble vitamins vary considerably. For example, clinical signs of niacin deficiency can present as early as a couple of weeks, vitamin C deficiency from 1 to 6 months, and signs of vitamin B_{12} deficiency may result only after years of insufficient intake.

The water-soluble vitamins play many important roles in the human body. Some B vitamins—thiamin (vitamin B_1), riboflavin (vitamin B_2), niacin (vitamin B_3), and pantothenic acid (vitamin B_5)—are cofactors in energy metabolism. In other words, these vitamins are necessary to unlock the energy in food. One of the major roles of vitamin C is in the production of collagen, a fibrous protein, which is an essential component of skin, bone, and other connective structures.

Thiamin

Thiamin (vitamin B_1) is essential for carbohydrate metabolism and plays a role in nerve function. Signs of thiamin deficiency include decreased appetite, weight loss, and cardiac and neurological irregularities that progress to beriberi—a constellation of symptoms that includes mental confusion, muscular wasting, swelling, decreased sensation in the feet and hands, a fast heart rate, and an enlarged heart. Thiamin deficiency is rare in the United States because of enrichment in rice and cereal products. Other food sources of thiamin include nuts and seeds, lean and organ meats, legumes, and whole grains. Deficiency occasionally manifests in alcoholics, who have impaired thiamin absorption.

Riboflavin

Riboflavin (vitamin B_2) assists in carbohydrate, amino acid, and lipid metabolism. It also helps with **antioxidant** protection through its role in reduction-oxidation (redox) reactions. Consumption of meat, dairy products, and green leafy vegetables helps prevent riboflavin deficiency (known as ariboflavinosis), which causes eye problems, including sensitivity to light; excessive tearing, burning, and itching; and loss of vision, as well as soreness and burning of the mouth, tongue, and lips.

Niacin

Niacin (vitamin B_3) acts as a cofactor for more than 200 enzymes involved in carbohydrate, amino acid, and fatty-acid metabolism. Lean meats, poultry, fish, peanuts, and yeast contain ample amounts of niacin. Muscular weakness, anorexia, indigestion, and skin abnormalities are early signs of niacin deficiency and can cause the disease pellagra, which is characterized by the "four Ds": dermatitis (eczema), dementia, diarrhea, and eventually death.

Vitamin B_6

Vitamin B_6 (pyridoxine) plays an important role in many bodily functions, including protein metabolism, red blood cell production, **glycogenolysis** (in which glycogen is broken down to glucose), conversion of the amino acid tryptophan to niacin, neurotransmitter formation, and immune-system function. Meats, whole-grain products, vegetables, and nuts contain high concentrations of vitamin B_6, though bioavailability of the nutrient is highest in animal products. Deficiency leads to decreased neurological and dermatological function and weakened immunity.

Folate

Folate (also known as folic acid in its supplement form) is named for its abundance in plant foliage such as green leafy vegetables. Folate plays a crucial role in the production of deoxyribonucleic acid (DNA), formation of red and white blood cells, formation of neurotransmitters, and metabolism of amino acids. Deficiency is relatively common because folate is easily lost during cooking and food preparation. Perhaps more importantly, most people do not eat enough green leafy vegetables in sufficient quantities. Folate deficiency in early pregnancy can be devastating for a developing embryo and can lead to neural tube defects such as spina bifida. For this reason, the Centers for Disease Control and Prevention recommends that all women of childbearing age take a daily folate supplement. Deficiency also causes megaloblastic anemia, skin lesions, and poor growth. Notably, excessive consumption of folate can mask a vitamin B_{12} deficiency.[8]

Table 4-1. **Dietary Reference Intakes: Recommended Dietary Allowances and Adequate Intakes, Vitamins**

Life Stage Group	Vitamin A (μg/d)[a]	Vitamin C (mg/d)	Vitamin D (μg/d)[b,c]	Vitamin E (mg/d)[d]	Vitamin K (μg/d)	Thiamin (mg/d)	Riboflavin (mg/d)	Niacin (mg/d)[e]	Vitamin B_6 (mg/d)	Folate (μg/d)[f]	Vitamin B_{12} (μg/d)	Pantothenic Acid (mg/d)	Biotin (μg/d)	Choline (mg/d)[g]
Infants														
0 to 6 mo	400*	40*	10	4*	2.0*	0.2*	0.3*	2*	0.1*	65*	0.4*	1.7*	5*	125*
6 to 12 mo	500*	50*	10	5*	2.5*	0.3*	0.4*	4*	0.3*	80*	0.5*	1.8*	6*	150*
Children														
1–3 y	**300**	**15**	**15**	**6**	30*	**0.5**	**0.5**	**6**	**0.5**	**150**	**0.9**	2*	8*	200*
4–8 y	**400**	**25**	**15**	**7**	55*	**0.6**	**0.6**	**8**	**0.6**	**200**	**1.2**	3*	12*	250*
Males														
9–13 y	**600**	**45**	**15**	**11**	60*	**0.9**	**0.9**	**12**	**1.0**	**300**	**1.8**	4*	20*	375*
14–18 y	**900**	**75**	**15**	**15**	75*	**1.2**	**1.3**	**16**	**1.3**	**400**	**2.4**	5*	25*	550*
19–30 y	**900**	**90**	**15**	**15**	120*	**1.2**	**1.3**	**16**	**1.3**	**400**	**2.4**	5*	30*	550*
31–50 y	**900**	**90**	**15**	**15**	120*	**1.2**	**1.3**	**16**	**1.3**	**400**	**2.4**	5*	30*	550*
51–70 y	**900**	**90**	**15**	**15**	120*	**1.2**	**1.3**	**16**	**1.7**	**400**	**2.4*h***	5*	30*	550*
> 70 y	**900**	**90**	**20**	**15**	120*	**1.2**	**1.3**	**16**	**1.7**	**400**	**2.4*h***	5*	30*	550*
Females														
9–13 y	**600**	**45**	**15**	**11**	60*	**0.9**	**0.9**	**12**	**1.0**	**300**	**1.8**	4*	20*	375*
14–18 y	**700**	**65**	**15**	**15**	75*	**1.0**	**1.0**	**14**	**1.2**	**400*i***	**2.4**	5*	25*	400*
19–30 y	**700**	**75**	**15**	**15**	90*	**1.1**	**1.1**	**14**	**1.3**	**400*i***	**2.4**	5*	30*	425*
31–50 y	**700**	**75**	**15**	**15**	90*	**1.1**	**1.1**	**14**	**1.3**	**400*i***	**2.4**	5*	30*	425*
51–70 y	**700**	**75**	**15**	**15**	90*	**1.1**	**1.1**	**14**	**1.5**	**400**	**2.4*h***	5*	30*	425*
> 70 y	**700**	**75**	**20**	**15**	90*	**1.1**	**1.1**	**14**	**1.5**	**400**	**2.4*h***	5*	30*	425*

Continued

Table 4-1. Dietary Reference Intakes: Recommended Dietary Allowances and Adequate Intakes, Vitamins–cont'd

Life Stage Group	Vitamin A (μg/d)[a]	Vitamin C (mg/d)	Vitamin D (μg/d)[b,c]	Vitamin E (mg/d)[d]	Vitamin K (μg/d)	Thiamin (mg/d)	Riboflavin (mg/d)	Niacin (mg/d)[e]	Vitamin B_6 (mg/d)	Folate (μg/d)[f]	Vitamin B_{12} (μg/d)	Pantothenic Acid (mg/d)	Biotin (μg/d)	Choline (mg/d)[g]
Pregnancy														
14–18 y	**750**	**80**	**15**	**15**	75*	**1.4**	**1.4**	**18**	**1.9**	**600*j***	**2.6**	6*	30*	450*
19–30 y	**770**	**85**	**15**	**15**	90*	**1.4**	**1.4**	**18**	**1.9**	**600*j***	**2.6**	6*	30*	450*
31–50 y	**770**	**85**	**15**	**15**	90*	**1.4**	**1.4**	**18**	**1.9**	**600*j***	**2.6**	6*	30*	450*
Lactation														
14–18 y	**1,200**	**115**	**15**	**19**	75*	**1.4**	**1.6**	**17**	**2.0**	**500**	**2.8**	7*	35*	550*
19–30 y	**1,300**	**120**	**15**	**19**	90*	**1.4**	**1.6**	**17**	**2.0**	**500**	**2.8**	7*	35*	550*
31–50 y	**1,300**	**120**	**15**	**19**	90*	**1.4**	**1.6**	**17**	**2.0**	**500**	**2.8**	7*	35*	550*

Source: Food and Nutrition Board, Institute of Medicine, National Academies

NOTE: This table (taken from the DRI reports, see www.nap.edu) presents recommended dietary allowances (RDAs) in **bold type** and adequate intakes (AIs) in ordinary type followed by an asterisk (*). An RDA is the average daily dietary intake level sufficient to meet the nutrient requirements of nearly all (97% to 98%) healthy individuals in a group. It is calculated from an estimated average requirement (EAR). If sufficient scientific evidence is not available to establish an EAR, and thus calculate an RDA, an AI is usually developed. For healthy breastfed infants, an AI is the mean intake. The AI for other life stage and gender groups is believed to cover the needs of all healthy individuals in the groups, but lack of data or uncertainty in the data prevent being able to specify with confidence the percentage of individuals covered by this intake.

a. As retinol activity equivalents (RAEs). 1 RAE = 1 g retinol, 12 g carotene, 24 g carotene, or 24 g cryptoxanthin. The RAE for dietary provitamin A carotenoids is two-fold greater than retinol equivalents (RE), whereas the RAE for preformed vitamin A is the same as RE.

b. As cholecalciferol. 1 μg cholecalciferol = 40 IU vitamin D.

c. Under the assumption of minimal sunlight.

d. As -tocopherol. -Tocopherol includes *RRR-* -tocopherol, the only form of -tocopherol that occurs naturally in foods, and the *2R*-stereoisomeric forms of -tocopherol (*RRR-*, *RSR-*, *RRS-*, and *RSS-* -tocopherol) that occur in fortified foods and supplements. It does not include the *2S*-stereoisomeric forms of -tocopherol (*SRR-*, *SSR-*, *SRS-*, and *SSS-* -tocopherol), also found in fortified foods and supplements.

e. As niacin equivalents (NE). 1 mg of niacin = 60 mg of tryptophan; 0–6 months = preformed niacin (not NE).

f. As dietary folate equivalents (DFE). 1 DFE = 1 μg food folate = 0.6 μg of folic acid from fortified food or as a supplement consumed with food = 0.5 μg of a supplement taken on an empty stomach.

g. Although AIs have been set for choline, there are few data to assess whether a dietary supply of choline is needed at all stages of the life cycle, and it may be that the choline requirement can be met by endogenous synthesis at some of these stages.

h. Because 10% to 30% of older people may malabsorb food-bound B_{12}, it is advisable for those older than 50 years to meet their RDA mainly by consuming foods fortified with B_{12} or a supplement containing B_{12}.

i. In view of evidence linking folate intake with neural tube defects in the fetus, it is recommended that all women capable of becoming pregnant consume 400 μg from supplements or fortified foods in addition to intake of food folate from a varied diet.

Table 4-2. **Vitamins**

VITAMIN	FUNCTION	SOLUBILITY	DEFICIENCY DISEASE	TOLERABLE UPPER INTAKE LEVEL (UL)/DAY	OVERDOSE DISEASE	MAJOR FOOD SOURCES
Thiamin (B_1)	Coenzyme in carbohydrate and branched-chain amino acid metabolism and neural function	Water	Early sign anorexia and weight loss; Beriberi (mental confusion, muscle wasting, swelling, neuropathy — "wet form" from high carbohydrate intake + strenuous activity); Wernicke-Korsakoff (alcoholic encephalopathy); apathy, decrease in short-term memory, confusion, and irritability; muscle weakness; and cardiovascular effects such as an enlarged heart	Insufficient data to set	No reports of adverse effects	Enriched, fortified, or whole-grain products; mixed foods whose main ingredient is grain; and ready-to-eat cereals
Riboflavin (B_2)	Coenzyme in numerous redox reactions and carbohydrate, amino acid, and lipid metabolism; component of *flavin adenine dinucleotide (FAD)* in aerobic/anaerobic metabolism	Water	"Ariboflavinosis" sore throat; redness and swelling of the oral mucous membranes; cracking of lips and mouth; glossitis (magenta tongue); seborrheic dermatitis ("cradle cap"); and normochromic, normocytic anemia	Insufficient data to set	No reports of adverse effects	Milk and milk drinks; bread products and fortified cereals; green leafy vegetables
Niacin (B_3)	Coenzyme for over 200 enzymes involved in carbohydrate, fatty acid, and	Water	Initial signs include weakness, anorexia, indigestion; later leads to pellagra (the "4 Ds": dermatitis [colored rash	35 mg May be lower for individuals with hepatic dysfunction or a history of liver disease,	Flushing; adverse effects such as nausea, vomiting, and signs and	Meat, fish, poultry; enriched and whole-grain breads and bread products; and fortified ready-to-eat cereals

Continued

Table 4-2. Vitamins–cont'd

VITAMIN	FUNCTION	SOLUBILITY	DEFICIENCY DISEASE	TOLERABLE UPPER INTAKE LEVEL (UL)/DAY	OVERDOSE DISEASE	MAJOR FOOD SOURCES
	amino acid metabolism; this is part of the *nicotinamide adenine dinucleotide (NAD)* which is transferred to ATP in aerobic and anaerobic metabolism		that develops symmetrically in areas exposed to sun], dementia, diarrhea, and death)	diabetes mellitus, active peptic ulcer disease, gout, cardiac arrhythmias, inflammatory bowel disease, migraine headaches, and alcoholism	symptoms of liver toxicity have been observed at nicotinamide intakes of 3,000 mg/day	
Pyridoxine (B_6)	Coenzyme in the metabolism of amino acids, glycogen, and sphingoid bases; several ongoing randomized trials are addressing whether supplementation will decrease risks of CHD	Water	Rash, microcytic anemia, seizures and depression and confusion	100 mg	Sensory neuropathy and dermatological lesions	Meats; fortified, ready-to-eat cereals; white potatoes and other starchy vegetables; and noncitrus fruits
Folate	Coenzyme in single-carbon transfers in the metabolism of nucleic and amino acids; important for red and white blood cell formation	Water	Rise in homocysteine concentration, and megaloblastic changes in the bone marrow and other tissues with rapidly dividing cells and subsequent megaloblastic anemia; neural tube defects in developing fetus of deficient mother	1,000 μg	May impair zinc absorption	Green, leafy vegetables (especially spinach, asparagus, and broccoli); lean beef; potatoes; whole wheat bread

Cobalamin (B_{12})	Coenzyme in amino acid and other metabolism, especially important for gastrointestinal tract, bone marrow, and nervous system	Water	Pernicious anemia (may take several years of inadequate intake to develop signs)	Insufficient data to determine		Liver and kidney, milk, eggs, fish, cheese, muscle meats
Biotin	Important for gluconeogenesis, fatty acid synthesis, and amino acid metabolism	Water	Rash, hair loss, and paralysis	Insufficient data to determine		Milk, liver, egg yolk
Pantothenic acid	Important for fatty acid, amino acid, and carbohydrate metabolism (component of acetyl CoA)	Water	Skin, liver, adrenal and nervous system dysfunction	Insufficient data to determine	Massive doses may cause mild intestinal distress and diarrhea	Meat, mushrooms, avocados, broccoli, egg yolk, skim milk, sweet potatoes
Vitamin C	Antioxidant, enzyme cofactor, promotes resistance to infection	Water	Scurvy (generally after 45 to 80 days of deprivation) characterized by impaired wound healing; swelling; bleeding; and weakness of bones, teeth, and connective tissue	2,000 mg	GI distress and diarrhea	Citric fruits and vegetables, organ meats
Vitamin A	Important roles in vision, growth, immune function, reproduction, and maintenance of epithelial tissue	Fat	Blindness, increased susceptibility to infection	3,000 μg	Hypervitaminosis (dry lips, scaling and peeling of skin, hair loss, nail fragility); liver disease; high levels toxic to developing embryo	Liver, milk, eggs, cod and halibut, carrots, spinach, sweet potatoes, cantaloupe

Continued

Table 4-2. **Vitamins–cont'd**

VITAMIN	FUNCTION	SOLUBILITY	DEFICIENCY DISEASE	TOLERABLE UPPER INTAKE LEVEL (UL)/DAY	OVERDOSE DISEASE	MAJOR FOOD SOURCES
Vitamin D	Maintenance of calcium and phosphorus homeostasis; may have many other important systemic functions	Fat	Rickets (impaired mineralization of growing bones) in children and osteomalacia (decreased bone density) in adults	2,000 IU/day	High calcium and phosphorus levels leading to calcification of soft tissues such as kidney, heart, lungs, and inner ear	Fish liver oils, fortified milk, sun
Vitamin E	Antioxidant	Fat	May take 5 to 10 years to develop; loss of deep tendon reflexes, impaired position sensation, and visual disturbances	1,000 mg	Can interfere with utilization of other fat-soluble vitamins	Oils
Vitamin K	Blood clotting	Fat	Bleeding	Insufficient data to determine	Massive dose could potentially cause hemolytic anemia	Green, leafy vegetables (especially broccoli, cabbage, turnip greens, dark lettuces)

Source: Dietary Reference Intakes (various volumes). Copyright 1997, 1998, 2000, 2001, 2010 by the National Academy of Sciences.

Vitamin B_{12}

Vitamin B_{12} (cobalamin) is important for the normal function of cells of the gastrointestinal tract, bone marrow, and nervous tissue. Uniquely, vitamin B_{12} can be stored in the liver and requires a protein carrier called intrinsic factor for absorption. The richest sources of vitamin B_{12} include clams and oysters, milk, eggs, cheese, muscle meats, fish, liver, and kidney. Long-time **vegans** are at risk for deficiency, as are the elderly, who tend to have a decreased ability to absorb the nutrient due to decreased food intake or decreased intrinsic factor. Deficiency leads to megaloblastic anemia and neurological dysfunction, in which neurons become demyelinated. This causes numbness, tingling, and burning of the feet, as well as stiffness and generalized weakness of the legs.

Biotin

Biotin (vitamin B_7) is the ultimate "helper vitamin." Typically bound to protein, it carries a carboxyl (-COOH) group, which it lends to any of four different enzymes that are important in various metabolic functions. Ultimately, biotin plays an important role in the metabolic functions of pantothenic acid, folic acid, and vitamin B_{12}. The most important sources of biotin include milk, liver, and egg yolk. Deficiency is uncommon.

Pantothenic Acid

Pantothenic acid, which is present in all plant and animal tissues, forms an integral component of coenzyme A and acyl-carrier protein. These proteins are essential for metabolism of fatty acids, amino acids, and carbohydrates, as well as for normal protein function. Deficiency is rare due to pantothenic acid's availability in many foods.

Vitamin C

Vitamin C plays an important role as an antioxidant. Vitamin C is also necessary to make collagen, a fibrous protein that is part of skin, bones, teeth, ligaments, and other connective structures. Deficiency can result in scurvy (a disease that can cause dark purplish spots on the skin and spongy or bleeding gums). Vitamin C improves iron absorption, promotes resistance to infection, and helps with steroid, neurotransmitter, and hormone production. Citrus fruits and green leafy vegetables are excellent sources of vitamin C. Signs of deficiency include impaired wound healing, swelling, bleeding, and weakness in bones, cartilage, teeth, and connective tissues.

Fat-Soluble Vitamins

Vitamins A, D, E, and K are the **fat-soluble vitamins** and are often found in fat-containing foods. They are stored in the liver or adipose tissue until needed, and therefore are closely associated with fat. If fat absorption is impaired, so is fat-soluble-vitamin absorption. Unlike water-soluble vitamins, fat-soluble vitamins can be stored in the body for extended periods of time and eventually are excreted in feces. This storage capacity increases the risk of toxicity from overconsumption, but also decreases the risk of deficiency.

Vitamin A

Vitamin A and its provitamin beta-carotene are important for vision, growth, and development; the development and maintenance of epithelial tissue, including bones and teeth; immune function; and reproduction. Animal products, including liver, milk, and eggs, are rich in preformed vitamin A. Dark green leafy vegetables, and yellow-orange vegetables and fruit contain lots of provitamin A carotenoids. (A good rule of thumb: The deeper the color, the higher the level of carotenoids.) Deficiency of vitamin A is the most common cause of preventable blindness in the developing world. It begins with night blindness and progresses to poor growth and increased susceptibility to infection. Excess consumption, which overwhelms the capacity of the liver to store the vitamin (generally resulting from overconsumption of supplements or therapeutic retinoids), leads to dryness and cracking of the skin and mucous membranes, headache, nausea and vomiting, and liver disease.[9]

Vitamin D

The effects of vitamin D on bone, namely its role in calcium and phosphorus absorption and homeostasis, are well studied. The effects of vitamin D on the rest of the body—including its role in athletic performance—are less certain but a source of intense interest among researchers.

Vitamin D is obtained in the body through two major mechanisms. Vitamin D is referred to as the "sunshine vitamin," because small amounts of sunlight exposure (about 10 to 15 minutes twice a week, depending on latitude and skin pigmentation) induce the body to make sufficient vitamin D from cholesterol. (The fact that the body can produce vitamin D makes it technically a **prohormone** rather than a vitamin). The second source of vitamin D comes from food and supplement intake. Fish liver oils provide an abundance of vitamin D. Smaller amounts are found in butter, cream, egg yolk, and liver. Typically, Americans get the majority of their dietary vitamin D intake from fortified milk, which is poorly absorbed.

Vitamin D comes in two forms: vitamin D_3, or cholecalciferol, from sunlight, animal products, and certain supplements; and vitamin D_2, or ergocalciferol, from plant sources and certain supplements. Structurally and functionally both forms are very similar. Both vitamin D_3 and vitamin D_2 must be modified in order to become activated in the body.

This process of modification and activation is outlined in Figure 4-1. Essentially, the inactive compounds vitamin D_2 and vitamin D_3 are converted in the liver to another inactive compound, 25-hydroxy vitamin D

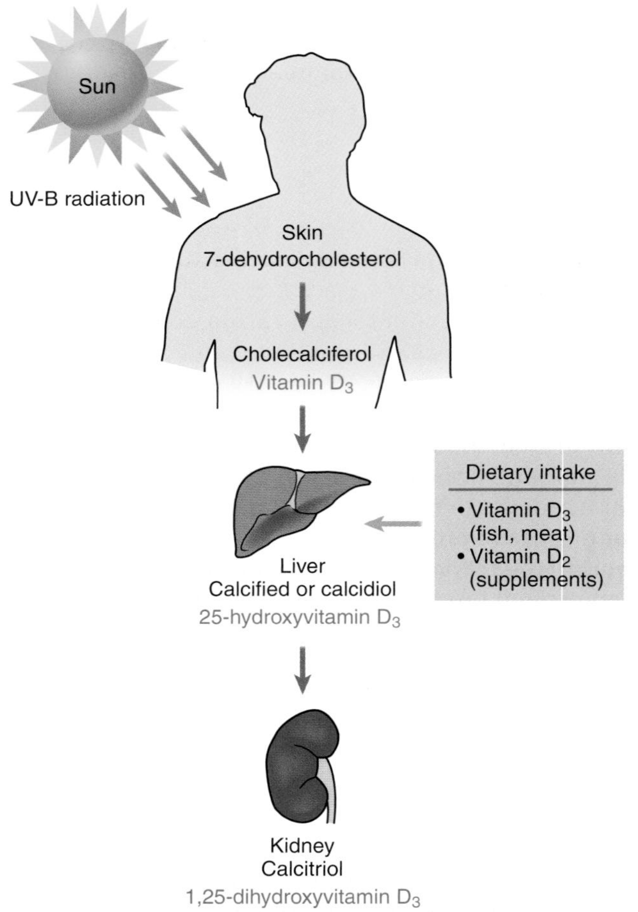

Figure 4-1. **Overview of vitamin D synthesis, intake, and activation.** *From Overview of vitamin D synthesis, intake, and activation in* Dietary Reference Intakes for Calcium and Vitamin D, *by A.C. Ross, C.L. Taylor, A.L. Yaktine, & H.B. Del Valle, Eds; National Academies Press, 2011.*

(25-OHD), the main circulating form of vitamin D. In the kidney, vitamin D (25-OHD) is converted to the active form 1,25-dihydroxy vitamin D (1,25-$(OH)_2$D), also known as calcitriol. Calcitriol is responsible for vitamin D's biological effects.

Calcitriol acts at the level of the kidney, intestines, bone, immune cells, brain, heart, skin, gonads, breast, and skeletal and smooth muscle by binding to the vitamin D receptor. Once calcitriol binds to the vitamin D receptor, a cascade of reactions ensues. The ultimate effect of vitamin D binding its receptor in bone is increased calcium deposition in bones. If too little vitamin D is available in the body, adults can develop osteomalacia, a condition in which the bones become weak, leading to muscular weakness and bone tenderness. This condition can also lead to pseudofractures, which are calluses on the bone, and can increase the risk of fracture, in particular of the wrist and pelvis. Low vitamin D intake may also play a role in the development of osteoporosis in postmenopausal women. Without vitamin D, children whose bones have not yet fully developed will experience impaired mineralization, which can lead to rickets and bowing of the weight-bearing large bones. On the other hand, too much vitamin D causes elevated calcium and phosphorus levels and may lead to headache, nausea, and eventually calcification of the kidney, heart, lungs, and the tympanic membrane of the ear, leading to deafness.

Vitamin D also has a significant role in immune function and physical performance related to muscle health, which are only now being investigated due to a vitamin D deficiency epidemic affecting 1 billion people worldwide. Vitamin D deficiency is especially problematic for athletes who may be at risk for such problems as stress fractures, respiratory infections, and muscle injuries.[10] As previously noted, investigating the non-bone effects of vitamin D—including whether vitamin D helps improve athletic performance—is an area of intense scientific research (see Evaluating the Evidence). However, despite a growing body of evidence suggesting that vitamin D may be a highly health-promoting vitamin and that the majority of people do not get enough of this vitamin, the Institute of Medicine released a report that concluded that the currently available data does not provide compelling evidence that vitamin D provides benefits beyond bone health, or that intakes higher than the DRIs provide any additional benefit.[11]

EVALUATING THE EVIDENCE

Vitamin D and Athletic Performance

The prospect of a potential ergogenic effect of vitamin D has provided intrigue and speculation among researchers, coaches, athletes, sports nutritionists, allied health professionals, and others highly invested in optimizing athletic performance. In fact, it was the topic of a "Phys Ed" column in the *New York Times*, inspiring over 100 comments from readers. In that article, the columnist summarized several studies that suggest there may be a role for vitamin D in performance.[30]

She mentions an early study of sprinters that was conducted in Russia several decades ago. Athletes trained for a 100-meter dash after half were exposed to artificial ultraviolet light and the other half were not. The researchers found that during the test run, the control group improved their time by almost 2%, while the runners who got the light therapy beat their old times by over 7%. The finding suggests that the light therapy activated intrinsic vitamin D production, which enhanced muscular power.

In another study mentioned in the piece, researchers tested the vertical jump of a small group of adolescent athletes. As a whole, the athletes

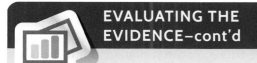

EVALUATING THE EVIDENCE–cont'd

with the lowest levels of vitamin D performed worse. The researchers speculated that too little vitamin D impaired muscular strength.

The column author also notes that a series of studies have shown that year-round athletes who exercise outside tend to have higher maximal oxygen intake in the late summer and are fittest in August. She notes that ultraviolet radiation is at its peak during this time. Then, unexpectedly, with the onset of fall, maximal oxygen consumption and performance falters, just as ultraviolet radiation lessens.

The columnist then wonders: Could athletes with vitamin D deficiency boost performance with normalized levels? Should athletes routinely undergo vitamin D screenings? Should they spend more time in the sun, sunscreen-free? Should athletes routinely take vitamin D supplements?

1. Conceptualize and describe a research study design that would convince you of the role of vitamin D in athletic performance.
2. What is your response to the rhetorical questions posed by the columnist, namely, should athletes routinely undergo vitamin D screenings? Should they spend more time in the sun, sunscreen-free? Should athletes routinely take vitamin D supplements?
3. What would you say to athletes who ask you about the role of vitamin D in athletic performance?

Vitamin E

Vitamin E exists in eight different forms: alpha-, beta-, gamma-, and delta-tocopherol; and alpha-, beta-, gamma-, and delta-tocotrienol. Vitamin E is sometimes referred to as alpha-tocopherol because that is the most active form in humans. Vitamin E plays a fundamental role in the metabolism of all cells. It may help protect against conditions related to oxidative stress including aging, air pollution, arthritis, cancer, cardiovascular disease, cataracts, diabetes, and infection, though research remains contradictory and inconclusive. (A more detailed discussion of the role of antioxidants is presented later in this chapter.) Vitamin E is synthesized by plants. The richest sources of vitamin E are polyunsaturated plant oils, wheat germ, whole grains, green leafy vegetables, nuts, and seeds. Vitamin E is easily destroyed by heat and oxygen, therefore, its richest source, oils, should be stored in a cool, dark location. Although vitamin E deficiency is rare in humans, it results in a hemolytic anemia (lysing, or destruction, of the red blood cells), and tends to occur only in cases of fat malabsorption and transport problems. Toxicity is uncommon, though when present may decrease the absorption of other fat-soluble vitamins, impair bone mineralization, and lead to prolonged clotting times. This is especially relevant for individuals on anticlotting medication such as warfarin (Coumadin).

Vitamin K

Vitamin K, which is produced by bacteria in the colon and present in large amounts in green, leafy vegetables (especially broccoli, cabbage, turnip greens, and dark lettuce), is important for blood clotting and maintenance of strong bones. Due to vitamin K's critical role in blood clotting, individuals on blood-thinning medications that interfere with vitamin K absorption need to carefully titrate their vitamin K intake through diet under the supervision of a physician. Insufficient vitamin K intake can lead to hemorrhage and potentially fatal anemia. Fortunately, vitamin K deficiency is rare and usually found only in association with lipid malabsorption, destruction of intestinal flora (often due to chronic antibiotic therapy), and liver disease. Newborns are at risk for vitamin K deficiency, as the vitamin does not cross the placenta and is negligible in breast milk. For this reason, newborn infants routinely receive a vitamin K shot after birth to prevent (or slow) a rare problem of bleeding into the brain weeks after birth. Toxicity of vitamin K only occurs with excessive intake of the synthetic form, which is called menadione. At doses of about 1,000 times the RDA, vitamin K can cause severe jaundice in infants and hemolytic anemia.

MINERAL FUNCTIONS, NEEDS, AND FOOD SOURCES

Minerals serve many critical roles in the human body, such as regulating enzyme activity, maintaining acid–base balance, assisting with muscle contraction, and helping with growth. The body's ability to use minerals is dependent on their bioavailability, or the degree to which the mineral can be absorbed by the body. Nearly all minerals, with the exception of iron, are absorbed in their free form; that is, in their ionic state unbound to organic molecules and complexes. When bound to a complex, the mineral is not bioavailable and will be excreted in feces. Typically, minerals with high bioavailability (> 40%) include sodium, potassium, chloride, iodide, and fluoride. Minerals with low bioavailability (1% to 10% absorption) include iron, zinc, chromium, and manganese. (Bioavailability is 20% to 30% for **heme iron**, which is the iron bound within the iron-carrying proteins of hemoglobin and myoglobin complex found in meat, fish, and poultry). All other minerals, including calcium and magnesium, are of medium bioavailability (30% to 40% absorption).

An important consideration when consuming minerals, and particularly when taking mineral supplements, is the possibility of mineral–mineral interactions. Some minerals can interfere with the absorption of other minerals. For example, zinc absorption may be decreased through iron supplementation. Similarly, zinc excesses can decrease copper absorption. Too much calcium limits the absorption of manganese, zinc, and iron. When a mineral is not absorbed properly, a deficiency may develop.

Minerals are typically categorized as macrominerals (major elements) and microminerals (trace elements). Macrominerals are elements the body requires in amounts of 100 milligrams or more per day. These include calcium, phosphorus, magnesium, sulfur, sodium, chloride, and potassium. Microminerals are minerals the body requires in amounts less than 20 milligrams per day. These include iron, iodine, selenium, zinc, chromium, copper, and various other minerals that do not have an established DRI and will not be discussed in this chapter. The recommended mineral intakes are included in Table 4-3. Table 4-4 summarizes the mineral functions, signs of deficiency and toxicity, and food sources.

Macrominerals

By definition, macrominerals are essential for adults in amounts of 100 milligrams per day or more. The elements calcium, phosphorus, magnesium, and sulfur are described below.

Calcium

Calcium is the most abundant mineral in the human body and serves various functions including mineralization of the bones and teeth, muscle contraction, blood clotting, blood-pressure control, immunity, and possibly colon-cancer prevention.[12] Calcium homeostasis is an excellent example of how the body maintains adequate calcium levels. Calcium is absorbed in different parts of the intestine depending on whether the body level is high or low. The kidney is involved in excreting and reabsorbing calcium to maintain proper calcium levels. Finally, the bones store 99% of the body's calcium. If calcium levels get low, calcium is released from the bones.

Significant sources of calcium include milk products, small fish with bones, green leafy vegetables, and legumes. Most people in the United States do not consume the recommended amounts of calcium from food sources. To help counter this problem, calcium supplements are often used to increase intake. Calcium carbonate is inexpensive, does not cause discomfort, and is a good source of calcium. Calcium citrate supplements are preferred for people who do not produce enough stomach acid or take medications that inhibit acid production.[13] Calcium supplements with other minerals, such as magnesium, are not necessary, although those with vitamin D can provide added benefits because the vitamin is required for calcium absorption. No more than 500 milligrams of calcium should be taken at one time because that is the maximum amount the body can absorb at once. Calcium carbonate should be taken with food to help with absorption; calcium citrate can be taken with or without food.[13]

Calcium deficiency in childhood and adolescence can contribute to decreased peak bone mass and suboptimal bone strength. Calcium deficiency in adulthood, particularly in postmenopausal women, can lead to **osteopenia** and **osteoporosis**. Calcium toxicity, particularly when combined with vitamin D toxicity, can lead to hypercalcemia and calcification of soft tissues, particularly of the kidneys. High calcium intake also interferes with the absorption of other minerals, including iron, zinc, and manganese. Relatively common effects of excessive calcium intake include constipation and renal stones.

Phosphorus

Phosphorus is the second most abundant mineral in the body.[14] Like calcium, phosphorus plays a role in mineralization of bones and teeth. Phosphorous also helps filter out waste in the kidneys and contributes to energy production in the body by participating in the breakdown of carbohydrates, protein, and fats. Phosphorus is needed for the growth, maintenance, and repair of all tissues and cells, and for the production of the genetic building blocks DNA and RNA. Phosphorus is also needed to balance and metabolize other vitamins and minerals including vitamin D, calcium, iodine, magnesium, and zinc. Animal products such as meat, fish, poultry, eggs, and milk are excellent sources of phosphorus. As a general rule, any food high in protein is also high in phosphorus. The outer coating of many grains contains phosphorus, but in the form of phytic acid, a bound form of phosphorus that is not bioavailable. The leavening process unbinds the phosphorus, making leavened breads a good source of the mineral. Phosphorus is also present in sodas. Deficiency of phosphorus is practically unheard of in the United States. In fact, most individuals consume much more than the DRIs. People taking phosphate-binding medications may be at risk of deficiency, which can present with neuromuscular, skeletal, hematological, and renal abnormalities and may be deadly. Too much phosphorus intake interferes with calcium absorption and may lead to decreased bone mass and density.

Magnesium

Magnesium, which is present primarily in bone, muscle, soft tissue, and body fluids, is important for bone mineralization, protein production, muscle contraction, nerve conduction, enzyme function, and healthy teeth. Excellent food sources include nuts, legumes, whole grains, dark green leafy vegetables, and milk. In general, a diet high in vegetables and unrefined grains will include more than adequate amounts of magnesium. Unfortunately, most Americans eat a diet high in refined foods and meat and do not meet recommended

Table 4-3. **Dietary Reference Intakes (DRIs): Recommended Dietary Allowances and Adequate Intakes, Elements**

Life Stage Group	Calcium (mg/d)	Chromium (μg/d)	Copper (μg/d)	Fluoride (mg/d)	Iodine (μg/d)	Iron (mg/d)	Magnesium (mg/d)	Manganese (mg/d)	Molybdenum (μg/d)	Phosphorus (mg/d)	Selenium (μg/d)	Zinc (mg/d)	Potassium (g/d)	Sodium (g/d)	Chloride (g/d)
Infants															
0 to 6 mo	200*	0.2*	200*	0.01*	110*	0.27*	30*	0.003*	2*	100*	15*	2*	0.4*	0.12*	0.18*
6 to 12 mo	260*	5.5*	220*	0.5*	130*	**11**	75*	0.6*	3*	275*	20*	**3**	0.7*	0.37*	0.57*
Children															
1–3 y	**700**	11*	**340**	0.7*	**90**	**7**	**80**	1.2*	**17**	**460**	**20**	**3**	3.0*	1.0*	1.5*
4–8 y	**1,000**	15*	**440**	1*	**90**	**10**	**130**	1.5*	**22**	**500**	**30**	**5**	3.8*	1.2*	1.9*
Males															
9–13 y	**1,300**	25*	**700**	2*	**120**	**8**	**240**	1.9*	**34**	**1,250**	**40**	**8**	4.5*	1.5*	2.3*
14–18 y	**1,300**	35*	**890**	3*	**150**	**11**	**410**	2.2*	**43**	**1,250**	**55**	**11**	4.7*	1.5*	2.3*
19–30 y	**1,000**	35*	**900**	4*	**150**	**8**	**400**	2.3*	**45**	**700**	**55**	**11**	4.7*	1.5*	2.3*
31–50 y	**1,000**	35*	**900**	4*	**150**	**8**	**420**	2.3*	**45**	**700**	**55**	**11**	4.7*	1.5*	2.3*
51–70 y	**1,000**	30*	**900**	4*	**150**	**8**	**420**	2.3*	**45**	**700**	**55**	**11**	4.7*	1.3*	2.0*
> 70 y	**1,200**	30*	**900**	4*	**150**	**8**	**420**	2.3*	**45**	**700**	**55**	**11**	4.7*	1.2*	1.8*
Females															
9–13 y	**1,300**	21*	**700**	2*	**120**	**8**	**240**	1.6*	**34**	**1,250**	**40**	**8**	4.5*	1.5*	2.3*
14–18 y	**1,300**	24*	**890**	3*	**150**	**15**	**360**	1.6*	**43**	**1,250**	**55**	**9**	4.7*	1.5*	2.3*
19–30 y	**1,000**	25*	**900**	3*	**150**	**18**	**310**	1.8*	**45**	**700**	**55**	**8**	4.7*	1.5*	2.3*
31–50 y	**1,000**	25*	**900**	3*	**150**	**18**	**320**	1.8*	**45**	**700**	**55**	**8**	4.7*	1.5*	2.3*
51–70 y	**1,200**	20*	**900**	3*	**150**	**8**	**320**	1.8*	**45**	**700**	**55**	**8**	4.7*	1.3*	2.0*
> 70 y	**1,200**	20*	**900**	3*	**150**	**8**	**320**	1.8*	**45**	**700**	**55**	**8**	4.7*	1.2*	1.8*

Continued

Table 4-3. Dietary Reference Intakes (DRIs): Recommended Dietary Allowances and Adequate Intakes, Elements–cont'd

Life Stage Group	Calcium (mg/d)	Chromium (μg/d)	Copper (μg/d)	Fluoride (mg/d)	Iodine (μg/d)	Iron (mg/d)	Magnesium (mg/d)	Manganese (mg/d)	Molybdenum (μg/d)	Phosphorus (mg/d)	Selenium (μg/d)	Zinc (mg/d)	Potassium (g/d)	Sodium (g/d)	Chloride (g/d)
Pregnancy															
14–18 y	**1,300**	29*	**1,000**	3*	**220**	**27**	**400**	2.0*	**50**	**1,250**	**60**	**12**	4.7*	1.5*	2.3*
19–30 y	**1,000**	30*	**1,000**	3*	**220**	**27**	**350**	2.0*	**50**	**700**	**60**	**11**	4.7*	1.5*	2.3*
31–50 y	**1,000**	30*	**1,000**	3*	**220**	**27**	**360**	2.0*	**50**	**700**	**60**	**11**	4.7*	1.5*	2.3*
Lactation															
14–18 y	**1,300**	44*	**1,300**	3*	**290**	**10**	**360**	2.6*	**50**	**1,250**	**70**	**13**	5.1*	1.5*	2.3*
19–30 y	**1,000**	45*	**1,300**	3*	**290**	**9**	**310**	2.6*	**50**	**700**	**70**	**12**	5.1*	1.5*	2.3*
31–50 y	**1,000**	45*	**1,300**	3*	**290**	**9**	**320**	2.6*	**50**	**700**	**70**	**12**	5.1*	1.5*	2.3*

Source: Food and Nutrition Board, Institute of Medicine, National Academies. Dietary Reference Intakes for Calcium, Phosphorous, Magnesium, Vitamin D, and Fluoride (1997); Dietary Reference Intakes for Thiamin, Riboflavin, Niacin, Vitamin B_6, Folate, Vitamin B_{12}, Pantothenic Acid, Biotin, and Choline (1998); Dietary Reference Intakes for Vitamin C, Vitamin E, Selenium, and Carotenoids (2000); Dietary Reference Intakes for Vitamin A, Vitamin K, Arsenic, Boron, Chromium, Copper, Iodine, Iron, Manganese, Molybdenum, Nickel, Silicon, Vanadium, and Zinc (2001); Dietary Reference Intakes for Water, Potassium, Sodium, Chloride, and Sulfate (2005); and Dietary Reference Intakes for Calcium and Vitamin D (2011). These reports may be accessed via www.nap.edu

NOTE: This table (taken from the DRI reports, see www.nap.edu) presents recommended dietary allowances (RDAs) in bold type and adequate intakes (AIs) in ordinary type followed by an asterisk (*). An RDA is the average daily dietary intake level sufficient to meet the nutrient requirements of nearly all (97% to 98%) healthy individuals in a group. It is calculated from an Estimated Average Requirement (EAR). If sufficient scientific evidence is not available to establish an EAR, and thus calculate an RDA, an AI is usually developed. For healthy breastfed infants, an AI is the mean intake. The AI for other life stage and gender groups is believed to cover the needs of all healthy individuals in the groups, but lack of data or uncertainty in the data prevent being able to specify with confidence the percentage of individuals covered by this intake.

Table 4-4. Minerals

NAME	ELEMENTAL SYMBOL	FUNCTION	BIO-AVAILABILITY	DEFICIENCY DISEASE	TOLERABLE UPPER INTAKE LEVEL (UL)	OVERDOSE DISEASE	MINERAL-MINERAL INTERACTIONS RELEVANT TO NUTRIENT REQUIREMENTS	FOOD SOURCES
Calcium	Ca^{2+}	Development of peak bone mass and maintenance of bone strength	Moderate	Osteomalacia-osteoporosis	2,500 mg	Hypercalcemia and calcification of soft tissues such as the kidneys, constipation, renal stones	High levels may interfere with other *divalent cations* (iron, zinc, manganese)	Dark green leafy vegetables (such as kale, collards, turnips, mustard greens, broccoli), sardines, clams, oysters, soybeans
Phosphorus	P^{3-}	Bone development; important in protein, fat, and carbohydrate utilization	Moderate	Widespread negative effects leading to death	4 g	Decreased bone mass and potentially fractures	High intakes can decrease calcium balance	Meat, poultry, fish, eggs
Magnesium	Mg^{2+}	Stabilize the structure of ATP in ATP-dependent enzyme reactions	Moderate	Tremor, muscle spasm, personality changes, anorexia, vomiting	350 mg (as medication, not in food or supplement)	May inhibit bone calcification	High intake of calcium increases magnesium requirements	Seeds, nuts, legumes, unmilled cereal grains, dark green vegetables, milk
Sulfur	S^{-}	Constituent of 2 amino acids, DNA, heparin	Moderate	Very rare	Insufficient data to determine	Metabolic byproducts decrease reabsorption of calcium	High levels can contribute to low calcium levels	Meat, poultry, fish, eggs, dried beans, broccoli, cauliflower
Iron	Fe^{2+}	Hemoglobin formation, improves blood quality, increases resistance to stress and disease	Low	Most common nutritional deficiency; anemia	45 mg	Increased oxidation of LDL, excessive accumulation of free radicals; increased risk of heart disease and cancer	High levels decrease zinc absorption; high levels of manganese, zinc, magnesium, and phosphorus decrease iron absorption; high levels of copper increase iron absorption. Iron absorption increased with vitamin C consumption	Liver, oysters, seafood, lean meat, poultry, fish, dried beans and vegetables

Continued

Table 4-4. **Minerals–cont'd**

NAME	ELEMENTAL SYMBOL	FUNCTION	BIO-AVAILABILITY	DEFICIENCY DISEASE	TOLERABLE UPPER INTAKE LEVEL (UL)	OVERDOSE DISEASE	MINERAL-MINERAL INTERACTIONS RELEVANT TO NUTRIENT REQUIREMENTS	FOOD SOURCES
Iodine	I^-	Growth and metabolism	High	Goiter	1,100 µg	Goiter, thyroid disease		Iodized salt, seafood
Selenium	Se^-	Protects body tissues against oxidative damage from radiation, pollution, and normal metabolic processing	Moderate	Exceedingly rare	400 µg	*Selenosis* — skin and nail changes, decay of teeth, and neurological abnormalities		Brazil nuts, fish, clams, oysters, sunflower seeds
Zinc	Zn^{2+}	Involved in digestion and metabolism; important in development of reproductive system; aids in healing	Low	Growth retardation, delayed wound healing, skin lesions, immune deficiencies, behavioral disturbances	40 mg	Anemia, fever, central nervous system disturbances; excess intake may decrease HDL level	Excess intake interferes with copper and iron absorption	Lean meats, liver, eggs, seafood, whole grains
Chromium	$Cr^{3+,\,6+}$	Increase effects of insulin, restore glucose tolerance	Low	Very rare	Insufficient to determine	No serious adverse effects		Corn oil, clams, whole-grain cereals, brewer's yeast

magnesium intakes. High intakes of calcium, protein, vitamin D, and alcohol increase the body's magnesium requirements. Magnesium deficiency is very rare; however, the elderly may experience a magnesium deficit due to depletion as well as insufficient intake. Depletion is based on the aging process including common pathologies, such as insulin dependent diabetes, and use of treatments such as hypermagnesuric diuretics. Magnesium depletion may contribute to many chronic illnesses and is associated with heart arrhythmias and myocardial infarction (heart attack). Magnesium toxicity may prevent bone calcification, but toxicity is also very rare, even in cases of supplement overuse.

Sulfur

Sulfur is an important component of many important body compounds, including two amino acids (cystine and methionine); three vitamins (thiamin, biotin, and pantothenic acid); and heparin, an anticoagulant found in the liver and other tissues. Meat, poultry, fish, eggs, dried beans, broccoli, and cauliflower are good food sources of the mineral. Sulfur deficiency is relatively uncommon and does not appear to cause any symptoms. Excess sulfur intake may lead to decreased bone mineralization, though sulfur toxicity is very rare. No AI, RDA, or UL has been established for sulfur.

Microminerals

Microminerals (trace elements) are found in minute amounts (less than 20 mg per day) in the body. Despite the need for minimal amounts of these minerals, they are critical for optimal growth, health, and development. Six of the major trace elements are described below: iron, iodine, selenium, zinc, chromium, and copper.

Iron

Iron plays an essential role in normal human function. It regulates cell growth and differentiation. Iron is also essential for the production of **hemoglobin**, the protein that carries inhaled oxygen from the lungs to the tissues; **myoglobin**, the protein responsible for making oxygen available for muscle contraction; and helps produce energy.

Iron can be stored in the body for future use as the protein complex **ferritin**. This stored iron provides a reserve during times of inadequate dietary intake of iron. Iron absorbed from food; stored as ferritin in the liver, spleen, and bone marrow; and released from the breakdown of red blood cells is transferred to working cells via a carrier protein called **transferrin**.

Sufficient iron intake is essential for optimal health as well as optimal athletic performance. When iron intake is low, the body makes less hemoglobin, and consequently, less oxygen can be delivered to the working cells. Signs of iron deficiency include fatigue, poor work performance, and decreased immunity.

Many foods are rich in iron (Table 4-5), but the absorption and bioavailability of iron varies based on

Table 4-5. Iron-Rich Food Sources

FOOD, STANDARD AMOUNT	IRON (mg)
Clams, canned, drained, 3 oz	23.8
*Fortified dry cereals (various), about 1 oz	1.8 to 21.1
Cooked oysters, 3 oz	10.2
Organ meats (liver, giblets), cooked, 3 oz	5.2 to 9.9
*Fortified instant cooked cereals (various), 1 packet	4.9 to 8.1
*Soybeans, mature, cooked, ½ cup	4.4
*Pumpkin and squash seed kernels, roasted, 1 oz	4.2
*White beans, canned, ½ cup	3.9
*Blackstrap molasses, 1 Tbsp	3.5
*Lentils, cooked, ½ cup	3.3
*Spinach, cooked from fresh, ½ cup	3.2
Beef, chuck, blade roast, cooked, 3 oz	3.1
Beef, bottom round, cooked, 3 oz	2.8
*Kidney beans, cooked, ½ cup	2.6
Sardines, canned in oil, drained, 3 oz	2.5
Beef, rib, cooked, 3 oz	2.4
*Chickpeas, cooked, ½ cup	2.4
Duck, meat only, roasted, 3 oz	2.3
Lamb, shoulder, cooked, 3 oz	2.3
*Prune juice, ¾ cup	2.3
Shrimp, canned, 3 oz	2.3
*Cowpeas, cooked, ½ cup	2.2
Ground beef, 15% fat, cooked, 3 oz	2.2
*Tomato puree, ½ cup	2.2
*Lima beans, cooked, ½ cup	2.2
*Soybeans, green, cooked, ½ cup	2.2
*Navy beans, cooked, ½ cup	2.1
*Refried beans, ½ cup	2.1
Beef, top sirloin, cooked, 3 oz	2.0

Food sources are ranked by milligrams of iron per standard amount. (All amounts listed provide 10% or more of the RDA for teenage and adult females, which is 18 mg/day.)
*These are nonheme iron sources. To improve absorption, eat these with a vitamin-C rich food.
Source: www.healthierus.gov/dietaryguidelines (2005).

whether the iron source is *heme iron* or *nonheme elemental iron* . Heme iron is the iron obtained from animal sources; bioavailability is 10% to 35%. Nonheme elemental iron is the iron obtained from plant sources; bioavailability is about 2% to 10%. Iron absorption can be increased by combining an iron-rich food with a vitamin C-rich food, while absorption is decreased when combined with coffee or tea, excessive amounts of certain minerals (zinc, magnesium, or calcium), or high amounts of phytic acid from dietary fiber. Figure 4-2 provides an overview of iron absorption and metabolism.

Many people who do not obtain adequate amounts of iron in their diets rely on iron supplementation to treat or avoid **iron deficiency anemia**, the most common micronutrient deficiency in the world. Young children, teenagers, and premenopausal women are at highest risk of iron deficiency.

Athletes who experience small amounts of exercise-induced blood loss in urine, gastrointestinal bleeding, high sweat rates, or large amounts of mechanical trauma (such as from runners' feet hitting the pavement) experience increased red blood cell destruction and loss of iron. However, rarely are these iron losses large enough to cause iron-deficiency anemia. Rather, these athletes may be at risk for exercise-induced pseudoanemia or **sports anemia**. For these athletes, if a blood test was done to measure hemoglobin levels the level would be low, officially meeting criteria for "anemia." However, the actual iron levels in the body would be normal. This results from the increase in plasma volume in response to physical training; the *total hemoglobin* is unchanged, but the *hemoglobin concentration* (total hemoglobin divided by total volume) is decreased.

A client with suspected iron-deficiency anemia or a client who is at risk for iron deficiency may benefit from a visit with the primary care provider to test for iron deficiency. The doctor can order a laboratory panel to evaluate for iron deficiency (Table 4-6). Clients with confirmed iron-deficiency anemia will likely be advised to take an iron supplement for 3 to 6 months to replenish iron stores. Some clients may not meet criteria for iron deficiency but may suffer from **functional anemia** or iron insufficiency (also referred to as *iron depletion without anemia*). This occurs when a person has depleted iron stores (characterized by a low ferritin level) but a low-normal hemoglobin level. For example, one study of female rowers found that rowers with functional anemia (depleted iron stores) trained 10 minutes less per day and had 0.3 L/min lower VO_2 max than the nondepleted rowers.[14] In these cases, boosting iron stores through increased consumption of high-iron foods or an iron supplement may increase exercise performance.

While iron supplementation is beneficial for athletes with iron insufficiency or deficiency, athletes with normal hemoglobin and ferritin levels do not benefit from, and may be harmed by, iron supplementation. Potential side effects of iron supplements include nausea, vomiting, constipation, diarrhea, dark-colored stools, and abdominal pain. Excessive iron intake can cause severe weakness and fatigue, unexplained joint and abdominal pain, diabetes, change in skin color, liver toxicity, and sometimes even death.

Iodine

Iodine, a mineral stored in the thyroid gland and essential for normal growth and metabolism, is found naturally in seafood, though the most common source

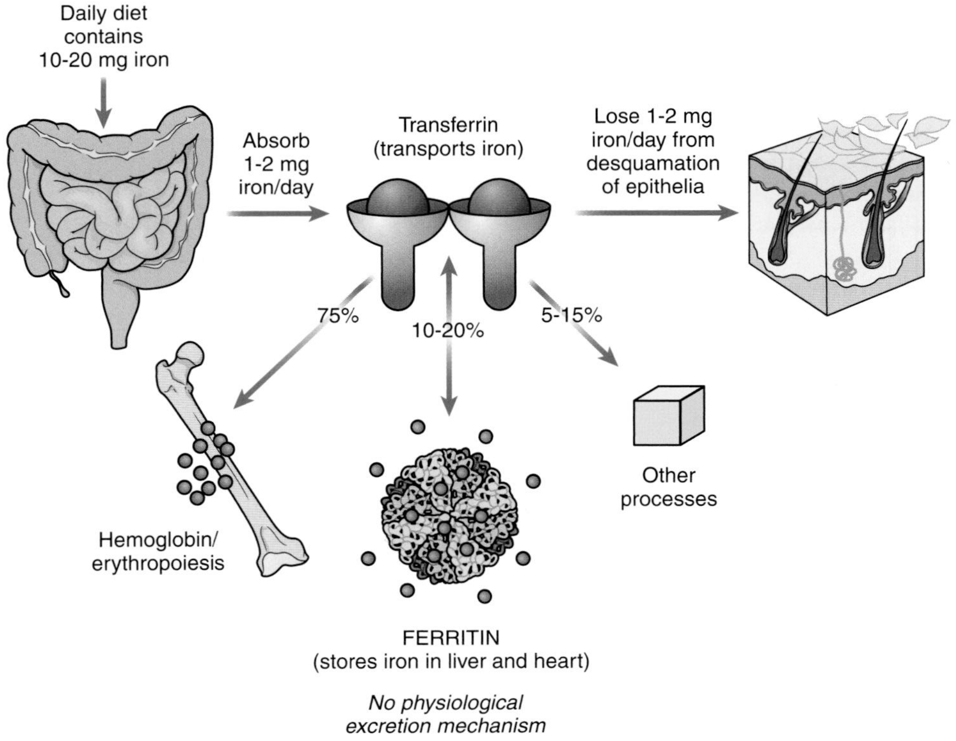

Figure 4-2. Iron absorption and metabolism.

Table 4-6. The Iron Deficiency Workup: What Is the Doctor Testing and What Does It Mean?

TEST	EXPLANATION	IRON DEFICIENCY
Hemoglobin 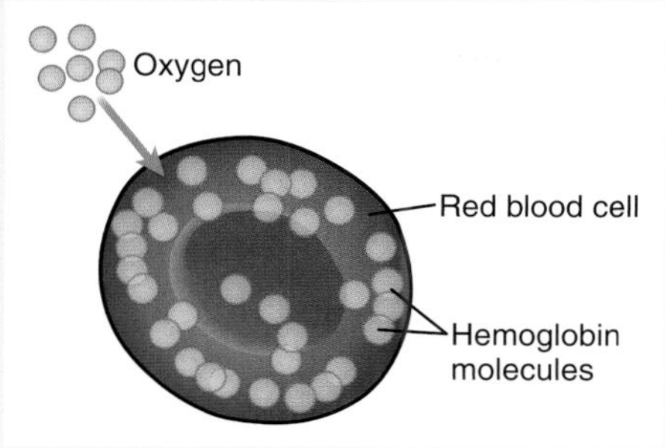	An iron-containing oxygen-carrying compound	Low
Hematocrit 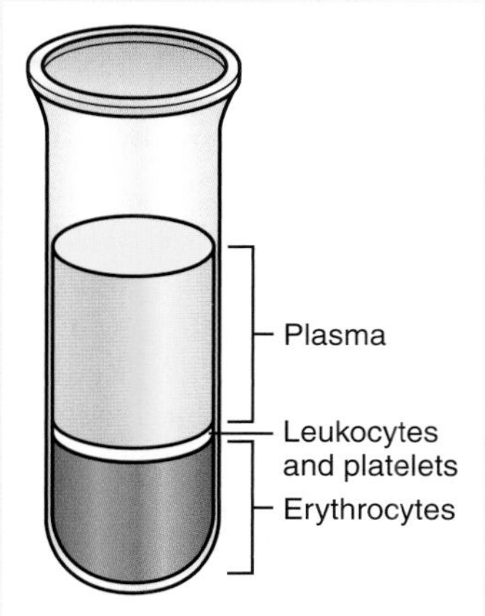	Proportion of total blood made up of red blood cells	Low
Ferritin 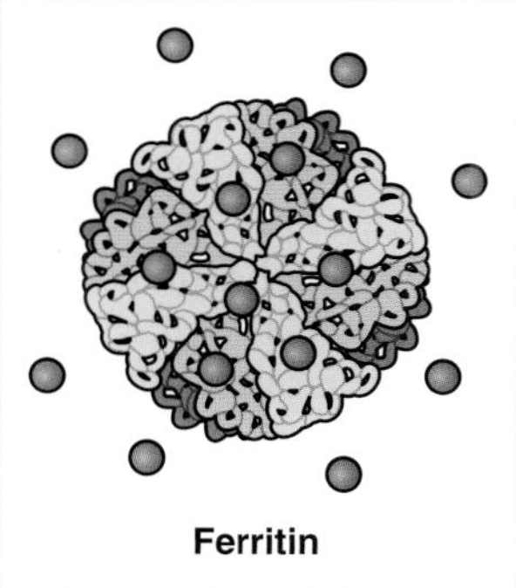	Measure of iron stores in liver and heart	Low
Iron 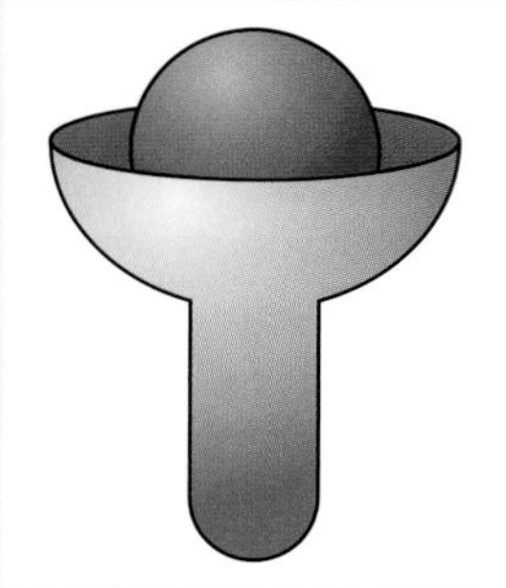	The amount of iron carried in blood by transferrin	Low

Continued

Table 4-6. The Iron Deficiency Workup: What Is the Doctor Testing and What Does It Mean?—cont'd

TEST	EXPLANATION	IRON DEFICIENCY
Total iron binding capacity 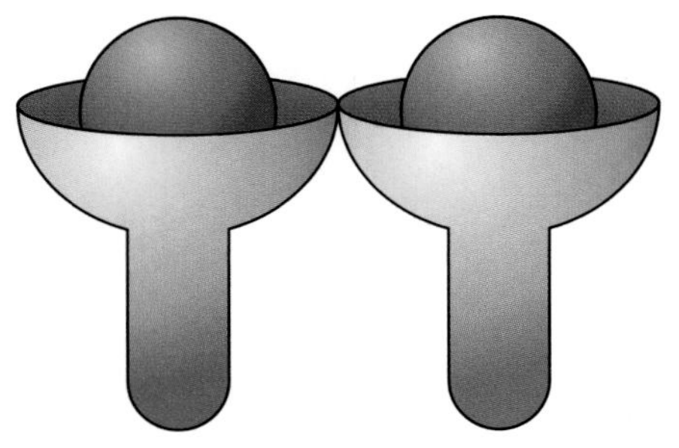	A measure of available iron binding sites on transferrin (in this case 50% since only half of transferrin has iron)	High
Reticulocyte count 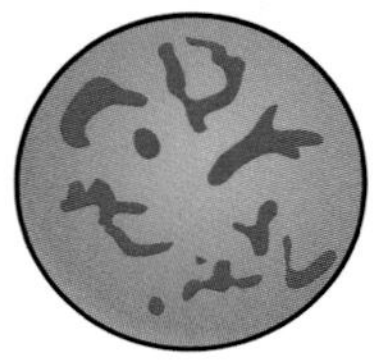 Reticulocyte	Immature red blood cells; levels are low in iron deficiency anemia due to lack of available iron to make red blood cells	Low

of iodine in the United States is iodized salt. Thanks to this fortification, iodine deficiency is rare in developed countries. However, in some developing countries, deficiency can cause goiter (enlargement of the thyroid gland) and cretinism (severely short stature and severe mental retardation) in children of mothers who were iodine-deficient during pregnancy. Excessive iodine can potentially lead to goiter or thyroid disease,[15] such as hypothyroidism.

Selenium

Selenium, an important antioxidant found mostly in plant foods grown in selenium-rich soil, is needed only in small amounts for optimal function. A lack of this mineral may lead to heart disease, hypothyroidism, and a weakened immune system. Too much selenium can lead to a condition called selonosis, which is manifested as gastrointestinal distress, hair loss, white blotchy nails, garlic breath odor, fatigue, irritability, and nerve damage.

Zinc

Zinc is found in almost every cell and is the second most abundant trace element after iron. It stimulates the activity of enzymes, supports a healthy immune system, assists with wound healing, strengthens the senses (especially taste and smell), supports normal growth and development, and helps with DNA synthesis. Foods rich in zinc include meat, fish, poultry, milk products, and seafood such as oysters and other shellfish. Zinc deficiency causes delayed wound healing and immune-system dysfunction. Toxicity is rare in otherwise healthy individuals, although too much zinc as a result of overzealous supplementation can decrease healthy HDL cholesterol, interfere with copper absorption, and alter iron function

Chromium

Chromium is a trace mineral that helps to increase the effectiveness of insulin and aids in glucose metabolism. Many researchers have an increased interest in chromium supplementation as a possible treatment to help improve the symptoms of type 2 diabetes, although studies to date have not proven that it is an effective treatment.[16,17] Food sources rich in chromium include corn oil, clams, whole-grain cereals, and brewer's yeast. Both chromium deficiency and chromium toxicity are very rare.

Copper

Copper, which is found throughout the body, helps make red blood cells and keeps nerve cells and the immune system healthy. It helps in the formation of collagen and cellular energy production. Copper may also act as an antioxidant by eliminating free radicals, which can damage cells. Copper helps in the absorption of iron and is found in oysters, liver, organ meats, and dried legumes.

It is rare for a person to be truly deficient in copper. Signs of possible copper deficiency include anemia, low body temperature, bone fractures, and osteoporosis.

Electrolytes

Known as **electrolytes**, sodium, potassium, and chloride are macrominerals that exist as ions in the body and are extremely important for normal cellular function. All three of these electrolytes play at least four essential roles in the body: water balance and distribution, osmotic equilibrium (i.e., assuring that the negative ions (**anions**) balance with positive ions (**cations**) when electrolytes move in and out of cells), acid–base balance, and intracellular/extracellular differentials (i.e., assuring that the sodium and chloride stay mostly outside the cell while potassium stays mostly inside the cell).

Serious consequences may occur when electrolytes are imbalanced, as when there is a high concentration of electrolytes, which can happen with **dehydration**, or when there is not enough sodium circulating in the body, known as **hyponatremia**. Symptoms of dehydration include nausea, vomiting, dizziness, disorientation, weakness, irritability, headache, cramps, chills, and decreased performance. Symptoms of hyponatremia include nausea, vomiting, extreme fatigue, respiratory distress, dizziness, confusion, disorientation, coma, and seizures. In severe cases, both conditions can result in death.

Electrolytes are excreted in urine, feces, and sweat. Generally, overt electrolyte deficiencies do not occur. In fact, sodium excess (and consequently, for certain genetically susceptible people, hypertension) is increasingly common given the typical American diet of highly processed and salty foods. Sodium excess may also contribute to osteoporosis, as high sodium increases calcium excretion. Potassium tends to be underconsumed, because most people do not consume enough fruits and vegetables. Insufficient potassium intake is linked to hypertension and osteoporosis. Table 4-7 summarizes the recommended intakes and roles of the electrolytes and water. See Chapter 8 for more information.

SPEED BUMP

1. **Define the term *micronutrient* and explain the different categories of micronutrients.**
2. **Describe the role of electrolytes in athletic performance.**

Table 4-7. Dietary Reference Intakes (DRIs): Recommended Dietary Allowances and Adequate Intakes, Electrolytes and Water

NUTRIENT	FUNCTION	LIFE STAGE GROUP	AI	UL[a]	SELECTED FOOD SOURCES	ADVERSE EFFECTS OF EXCESSIVE CONSUMPTION	SPECIAL CONSIDERATIONS
Sodium	Maintains fluid volume outside of cells and thus normal cell function.	Infants	(g/d)	(g/d)	Processed foods to which sodium chloride (salt)/benzoate/phosphate have been added; salted meats, nuts, cold cuts; margarine; butter; salt added to foods in cooking or at the table. Salt is ~ 40% sodium by weight.	Hypertension; increased risk of cardiovascular disease and stroke.	The AI is set based on being able to obtain a nutritionally adequate diet for other nutrients and to meet the needs for sweat losses for individuals engaged in recommended levels of physical activity. Individuals engaged in activity at higher levels or in humid climates resulting in excessive sweat may need more than the AI. The UL applies to apparently healthy individuals without hypertension; it thus may be too high for individuals who already have hypertension or who are under the care of a health-care professional.
		0–6 mo	0.12	ND[b]			
		7–12 mo	0.37	ND[b]			
		Children	1.0	1.5			
		1–3 y	1.2	1.9			
		4–8 y	1.5	2.2			
		Males	1.5	2.3			
		9–13 y	1.5	2.3			
		14–18 y	1.5	2.3			
		19–30 y	1.3	2.3			
		31–50 y	1.2	2.3			
		50–70 y	1.5	2.2			
		> 70 y	1.5	2.3			
		Females	1.5	2.3			
		9–13 y	1.5	2.3			
		14–18 y	1.3	2.3			
		19–30 y	1.2	2.3			
		31–50 y	1.5	2.3			
		50–70 y	1.5	2.3			
		> 70 y	1.5	2.3			
		Pregnancy	1.5	2.3			
		14–18 y					
		19–50 y					
		Lactation					
		14–18 y					
		19–50 y					

Continued

Table 4-7. Dietary Reference Intakes (DRIs): Recommended Dietary Allowances and Adequate Intakes, Electrolytes and Water–cont'd

NUTRIENT	FUNCTION	LIFE STAGE GROUP	AI	UL[a]	SELECTED FOOD SOURCES	ADVERSE EFFECTS OF EXCESSIVE CONSUMPTION	SPECIAL CONSIDERATIONS
Chloride	With sodium, maintains fluid volume outside of cells and thus normal cell function.	Infants 0–6 mo 7–12 mo Children 1–3 y 4–8 y Males 9–13 y 14–18 y 19–30 y 31–50 y 50–70 y > 70 y Females 9–13 y 14–18 y 19–30 y 31--50 y 50–70 y > 70 y Pregnancy 14–18 y 19–50 y Lactation 14–18 y 19–50 y	(g/d) 0.18 0.57 1.5 1.9 2.3 2.3 2.3 2.3 2.0 1.8 2.3 2.3 2.3 2.3 2.0 1.8 2.3 2.3 2.3 2.3	(g/d) ND[b] ND[b] 2.3 2.9 3.4 3.6 3.6 3.6 3.6 3.6 3.4 3.6 3.6 3.6 3.6 3.6 3.6 3.6 3.6 3.6	See above; about 60% by weight of salt.	In concert with sodium, results in hypertension.	Chloride is lost usually with sodium in sweat, as well as in vomiting and diarrhea. The AI and UL are equimolar in amount to sodium since most of sodium in diet comes as sodium chloride (salt).
Potassium	Maintains fluid volume inside/outside of cells and thus normal cell function; acts to blunt the rise of blood pressure in response to excess sodium intake, and decrease markers of bone turnover and recurrence of kidney stones.	Infants 0–6 mo 7–12 mo Children 1–3 y 4–8 y Males 9–13 y 14–18 y 19–30 y 31–50 y 50–70 y > 70 y Females 9–13 y 14–18 y 19–30 y 31–50 y 50–70 y > 70 y Pregnancy 14–18 y 19–50 y Lactation 14–18 y 19–50 y	(g/d) 0.4 0.7 3.0 3.8 4.5 4.7 4.7 4.7 4.7 4.7 4.5 4.7 4.7 4.7 4.7 4.7 4.7 4.7 5.1 5.1	No UL.	Fruits and vegetables; dried peas; dairy products; meats; and nuts.	None documented from food alone; however, potassium from supplements or salt substitutes can result in hyperkalemia and possibly sudden death if excess is consumed by individuals with chronic renal insufficiency (kidney disease) or diabetes.	Individuals taking drugs for cardiovascular disease such as ACE inhibitors, ARBs (Angiotensin Receptor Blockers), or potassium sparing diuretics should be careful to not consume supplements containing potassium and may need to consume less than the AI for potassium.

Table 4-7. Dietary Reference Intakes (DRIs): Recommended Dietary Allowances and Adequate Intakes, Electrolytes and Water–cont'd

NUTRIENT	FUNCTION	LIFE STAGE GROUP	AI	UL[a]	SELECTED FOOD SOURCES	ADVERSE EFFECTS OF EXCESSIVE CONSUMPTION	SPECIAL CONSIDERATIONS
Water	Maintains homeostasis in the body and allows for transport of nutrients to cells and removal and excretion of waste products of metabolism.	Infants 0–6 mo 7–12 mo Children 1–3 y 4–8 y Males 9–13 y 14–18 y 19–30 y 31–50 y 50–70 y > 70 y Females 9–13 y 14–18 y 19–30 y 31–50 y 50–70 y > 70 y Pregnancy 14–18 y 19–50 y Lactation 14–18 y 19–50 y	(L/d) 0.7 0.8 1.3 1.7 2.4 3.3 3.7 3.7 3.7 3.7 2.1 2.3 2.7 2.7 2.7 2.7 3.0 3.0 3.8 3.8	No UL.	All beverages, including water, as well as moisture in foods (high moisture foods include watermelon, meats, soups, etc.).	No UL because normally functioning kidneys can handle more than 0.7 L (24 oz) of fluid per hour; symptoms of water intoxication include hyponatremia, which can result in heart failure and rhabdomyolosis (skeletal muscle tissue injury) which can lead to kidney failure.	Recommended intakes for water are based on median intakes of generally healthy individuals who are adequately hydrated; individuals can be adequately hydrated at levels below as well as above the AIs provided. The AIs provided are for total water in temperate climates. All sources can contribute to total water needs: beverages (including tea, coffee, juices, sodas, and drinking water) and moisture found in foods. Moisture in food accounts for about 20% of total water intake. Thirst and consumption of beverages at meals are adequate to maintain hydration.

NOTE: The table is adapted from the DRI reports. See www.nap.edu. Adequate intakes (AIs) may be used as a goal for individual intake. For healthy breastfed infants, the AI is the mean intake. The AI for other life stage and gender groups is believed to cover the needs of all individuals in the group, but lack of data prevent being able to specify with confidence the percentage of individuals covered by this intake; therefore, no recommended dietary allowance was set.

a. UL = The maximum level of daily nutrient intake that is likely to pose no risk of adverse effects. Unless otherwise specified, the UL represents total intake from food, water, and supplements. Due to lack of suitable data, ULs could not be established for potassium, water, and inorganic sulfate. In the absence of ULs, extra caution may be warranted in consuming levels above recommended intakes.

b. ND = Not determinable due to lack of data of adverse effects in this age group and concern with regard to lack of ability to handle excess amounts.

Source of intake should be from food only to prevent high levels of intake.

Source: Dietary Reference Intakes for Water, Potassium, Sodium, Chloride, and Sulfate. These reports may be accessed via www.nap.edu.

MICRONUTRIENT DIGESTION AND ABSORPTION

While vitamin and mineral absorption varies by nutrient, the majority of vitamin and mineral digestion and absorption occurs in the small intestine. Figure 4-3 provides an overview of micronutrient digestion, absorption, and distribution to tissues.

Vitamin Digestion and Absorption

By the time the vitamins pass to the small intestine, most of the vitamins have been separated from the

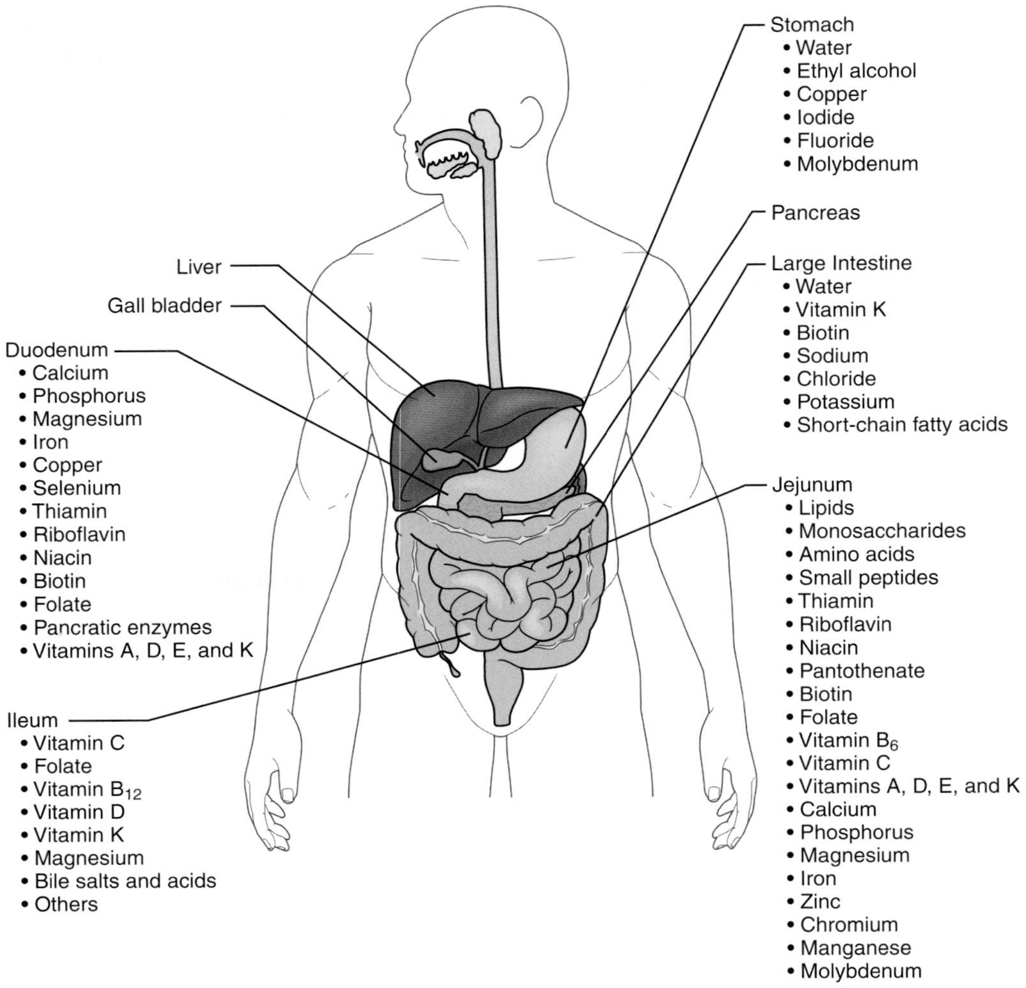

Figure 4-3. Micronutrient digestion, absorption, and distribution.

other food components. The vitamins pass unchanged primarily from the middle and lower portions of the small intestine (the **jejunum** and **ileum**) into the blood by **passive** or **simple diffusion**, movement from an area of high concentration to one of low concentration without the need for a carrier protein. For the most part, water-soluble vitamins are absorbed in the jejunum and the fat-soluble vitamins in the ileum. Fat-soluble vitamins are then incorporated into chylomicrons and other blood lipoproteins and delivered throughout the body. Fat-soluble vitamins are stored in adipose tissue and the liver.

Vitamin K, vitamin B_{12}, thiamin, and riboflavin can also be produced by **colonic bacteria** in the large intestine; from there they are absorbed into the bloodstream.

Mineral Digestion and Absorption

Mineral digestion and absorption is considerably more complex than vitamin digestion and absorption. In the stomach, the digestive enzymes and stomach acids already have separated minerals from the other food components. The cations, or positively charged minerals (such as calcium, iron, zinc, and magnesium), dissolve into the acidic stomach chyme. As the dissolved minerals pass into the less acidic solution in the small intestine, the minerals form insoluble compounds with hydroxide molecules and protein carriers. These compounds are known as **chelation compounds**. For the most part, this phase of mineral digestion, referred to as the *intraluminal stage,* occurs in the uppermost portion of the small intestine, the **duodenum**. The small anions, or negatively charged minerals, are unaffected by pH and are easily digested and absorbed.

The negatively charged minerals pass across the border of the small intestine for absorption through simple diffusion. The positively charged minerals, formed into the chelation compounds, cross the small intestinal border through **facilitated diffusion**, from high concentration to low concentration, with a protein carrier that they are attached to in order to cross the small intestinal border, and/or **active transport**, from low concentration to high concentration, made possible through the use of ATP. The method of transport depends on the concentration of the mineral on either side of the small intestinal border. This stage of absorption is referred to as the *translocation stage*.

Finally, once the mineral complex has crossed the small intestinal border it arrives into the portal blood circulation, which will deliver it to the liver for processing and then distribution to the rest of the body. This is the *mobilization stage*. Some of the mineral complexes may not ultimately pass across the small intestinal border and instead may be sequestered within the absorptive cell for later use.

The bioavailability of the minerals depends on many factors. One factor is the presence or absence of other minerals. This is in large part due to the nonspecific nature of the carrier proteins required for facilitated diffusion and active transport. For example, high levels of iron and zinc may inhibit copper absorption, while high levels of copper may decrease iron and molybdenum absorption. Cobalt and iron compete with and inhibit each other's absorption. Another factor includes the availability of the protein that binds with the mineral to form the chelation complex. For example, iron requires transferrin for absorption while many other minerals require the nonspecific albumin protein carrier. In most cases, these protein carriers are undersaturated. However, if the mineral is consumed in excessive amounts, the mineral can overwhelm the carrier sites and lead to toxicity. Mineral absorption also can be impaired if minerals bind to free fatty acids in the intestinal lumen or if a mineral is present in very high concentrations, forming a nonabsorbable precipitate.

While most minerals are digested and absorbed in the small intestine, sodium and potassium are absorbed in the large intestine.

Antioxidants and Phytochemicals

Many of the vitamins and minerals already discussed, including vitamin C, beta-carotene, vitamin E, and selenium, function as antioxidants. Just as metal rusts over time when exposed to water and oxygen, cells are damaged from chronic oxygen exposure. This damage-causing process is called **oxidation** and can set in motion various chemical reactions that at best cause aging and at worst cause cancer. Antioxidants function to prevent or repair oxidative damage. In the past, antioxidants were considered potent disease fighters. Subsequent research suggests that the agents not only fail to protect against disease, but that in excess some of them may act to increase the risk of cancer, heart disease, and mortality in some individuals.[18,19] Their true role in disease pathology has yet to be determined.

What remains undisputed is that a diet high in fruits and vegetables is associated with a lower risk of developing chronic disease, such as heart disease, cancer, and possibly Alzheimer's disease. Their beneficial effects could be due to antioxidants, fiber, agents that stimulate the immune system to combat free radicals, monounsaturated fatty acids, B vitamins, folic acid, or various other potential **phytochemicals**—substances in plants that are not necessarily required for normal functioning, but improve health and reduce the risk of such diseases as cancer, diabetes, and cardiovascular disease.

Vitamin and Mineral Supplements

Clearly vitamins and minerals consumed at recommended levels are essential for optimal health. What is less clear is whether vitamins taken in pill form as a sort of "insurance" in the case of potential inadequate intake from whole foods provide any benefit. Physicians, scientists, dietitians, and other health professionals have long touted the importance of getting enough of these nutrient powerhouses—and consumers have been listening. About one-half of U.S. adults use a supplement with about one-third of all adults taking a multivitamin.[20] This adds up to about $11 billion per year in multivitamin and mineral supplements,[21] not counting the huge market for heavily fortified nutrition bars, which tend to contain similar levels of vitamins and minerals as a multivitamin (Box 4-1).

Box 4-1. A Closer Look at Nutrition Bars

Sarah is a college water polo player who constantly finds herself rushing in the morning to get to practice on time before she sits through a day of lectures. To make sure that she still gets a quick and balanced breakfast despite the time crunch, she starts each day with a nutrition bar advertised as having 100% of the RDA for 12 vitamins and minerals. She never questioned this routine until she had a conversation with a friend who adopted a 60-day "processed-free food" pledge. This got her wondering—should she change her breakfast routine to include only "real" foods and not the heavily fortified nutrition bar?

A variety of nutrition and energy bars are readily available, not only for athletes looking for a boost in performance, but also for busy individuals looking for a prepackaged "balanced" meal or snack. Similar to the bar that Sarah relies on, many nutrition bars provide much of the recommended daily allowance of many vitamins and minerals, serve as quick and easy snacks, and if chosen carefully, can be a welcome component of a busy person's eating plan. But consumers must be cautious.

Because most of the bars are vitamin-fortified, consumers should be careful not to overconsume vitamins and minerals by eating too many bars, or

Continued

Box 4-1. A Closer Look at Nutrition Bars–cont'd

eating them in addition to taking a multivitamin or other supplement. While it is very rare to develop signs of vitamin or mineral toxicity from eating too much of a food, it can occur with consumption of too many fortified food products or supplements.

Many nutrition bars are high-calorie foods so people who are underactive or who are trying to lose weight should use them as a meal replacement and not as a snack. Of course, many nutrition bars contain more calories than their food counterparts, are not that filling, and do not contain disease-fighting nutrients found in fruits and vegetables. While an occasional nutrition bar is unlikely to do any harm and may be helpful for some individuals who otherwise would not consume a balanced diet, nutrition bars should not serve as a food substitute altogether. In the best case, athletes and consumers in general would get a plentiful mix of a variety of nutrients through a balanced and varied mix of whole foods.

The latest research results from studies evaluating the health benefits of vitamins 'supplements' so it is clear that we are referring to vitamin supplements have largely been disappointing. A study of 161,000 older women enrolled in the Women's Health Initiative concluded that calcium supplements with or without vitamin D increased the risk of cardiovascular events, particularly myocardial infarction.[22] A study of 84,000 physicians from the Physician's Health Study found no difference in heart disease in men taking vitamins E, C, or a multivitamin compared to those not taking supplements.[23] Other studies have found that not only do vitamin E and selenium not decrease the risk of prostate cancer[24] as once thought, but vitamin E supplementation may actually increase risk.[25] Overall, most studies have shown no significant association between vitamin supplements and improved health,[21] with some notable exceptions, especially folic acid supplementation in pregnant women[26] and physician-directed treatment of disorders such as iron-deficiency anemia and osteoporosis. While, in general, the interest among researchers in studying the effect of vitamins on health has waned with the growing evidence of minimal benefit, there has been a surge in evaluation of the effects of vitamin D deficiency on health and the role that supplementation might play in warding off a variety of health conditions (and possibly improving athletic performance), but so far the data is lacking.[11] More information on supplements can be found in Chapter 10.

Vitamins, Minerals, and Athletic Performance

Micronutrients play important roles in energy production, red blood cell formation, bone strength, immune function, muscle repair, and protection from oxidative damage—all critical functions to help set the stage for optimal athletic performance. Because exercise increases demands on the micronutrient-requiring metabolic processes, athletes probably have increased vitamin and mineral needs compared to the sedentary or less active population, though the published DRIs are the same for active individuals as the sedentary population (see Myths and Misconceptions). The exception is vitamin C, which extreme athletes such as professional triathletes do require in larger amounts.

Myths and Misconceptions

Vitamins Provide Energy

The Myth
Vitamins provide energy.

The Logic
If the supplement, bar, and drink manufacturers say it's so, it must be true. Plus, physiologically, vitamins are necessary to unlock the energy from carbohydrates, fat, and protein.

The Science
Vitamins contain no calories. Scientifically, the term *energy* is equivalent to *calories*. Therefore, vitamins do not provide energy. However, it is true that in the absence of vitamins—in particular, the B vitamins—energy from food cannot be unlocked and used by the working cells. But intake of a vitamin beyond the RDA or AI provides no additional benefit or "energy" boost.

Most athletes do not suffer from vitamin and mineral deficiencies despite potential increased needs. Due to the generally higher food intake of athletes, they are able to meet their nutritional needs. However, an athlete who severely restricts intake of specific food groups or does not consume a generally balanced and wholesome diet may suffer from a nutritional deficiency. Athletes are at highest risk for low levels of the B vitamins, vitamins C and E, beta-carotene, calcium and vitamin D, selenium iron, zinc, and magnesium.[27]

The B vitamins have at least two essential roles during exercise: supporting energy production (thiamin, riboflavin, niacin, pyridoxine (B_6), pantothenic acid, and biotin) and supporting the formation of oxygen-containing red blood cells (folate and cobalamin (B_{12})). While necessary in recommended amounts for optimal athletic performance, taking "extra" B vitamins does not benefit athletic performance. At the same time, a short-term dietary lapse leading to marginally deficient B vitamins probably will not negatively affect exercise performance. However, vitamin B_{12} deficiency, which often takes months to years to develop, or folate deficiency, can contribute to anemia, which reduces the oxygen-carrying capacity of the red blood cells and may subsequently negatively affect cardiorespiratory performance. Female athletes, especially vegetarians and those with disordered eating habits, are most likely to suffer B vitamin deficiency.

The antioxidant vitamins C and E, beta-carotene, and selenium protect the body from oxidative damage resulting from exercise. Without sufficient dietary intake of the antioxidants, high levels of physical activity could deplete the body's reserves. However, most athletes consume adequate amounts of the antioxidants from their diet. Athletes on a calorically restricted, low-fat diet with minimal fruits, vegetables, and whole grains are at increased risk of deficiency, which in some cases could affect performance. There is some evidence that, in the case of deficiency, restored vitamin E and vitamin C levels could enhance exercise performance and recovery.[28] There is also evidence that supplementation with vitamins E and C can reduce the risk of upper respiratory infections, especially in men.[29]

Calcium and vitamin D play important roles in maintaining and optimizing bone health. Female athletes tend to be at highest risk for negative effects from low calcium and vitamin D consumption, especially female athletes who engage in weight-sensitive sports like gymnastics, running, and cycling. Women who meet criteria for or show signs of the **female athlete triad**, which is characterized by disordered eating, amenorrhea, and osteoporosis (discussed in detail in Chapter 16), must pay extra attention to vitamin D and calcium intakes in order to preserve bone mass and decrease the risk for fracture. Vitamin D may be essential for more than bone health, and, in fact, vitamin D status could predict athletic performance.[10]

In addition to being at increased risk for low calcium intake, female athletes also have high rates of iron-deficiency anemia. Iron carries oxygen in the blood to all cells in the body, and levels within normal limits are essential for endurance activities. Many adolescent females have low iron levels due to inadequate intake combined with menstrual and exercise losses. If a female athlete feels abnormally fatigued with diminished performance relative to training and effort or otherwise is concerned about possible iron-deficiency, the allied health professional should encourage her to make an appointment with her primary care physician to evaluate iron levels and the need, if any, for iron supplementation. While male athletes can also suffer iron deficiency, it is rare.

Some athletes, usually females, also consume less-than-recommended amounts of zinc and magnesium. Low zinc levels can negatively affect athletic performance by decreasing cardiorespiratory endurance and muscle strength. Wrestlers, dancers, gymnasts, and tennis players, who may restrict their energy intake to maintain a specific weight, are at highest risk for low magnesium intake. Magnesium deficiency worsens endurance performance through increased oxygen requirements at any given submaximal intensity.[27]

Vitamins, Minerals, and Weight Management

Though vitamins and minerals are calorie-free (and thus are not a source of energy), they are essential for optimal health. Given the body's demands for vitamins and minerals and the relative caloric-restriction many clients may follow in an effort to lose weight, it is especially important for clients who are attempting to lose weight to adopt a nutrient-dense, low-calorie eating plan. Not only should clients limit "empty calories" from nutrient-poor foods, but they should also pay special care to eat a balanced diet that includes all of the major food groups so as to ensure sufficient vitamin and mineral intake. Certain clients who restrict whole food groups or who have adopted a very restrictive eating plan should discuss the necessity of a daily multivitamin with their physician.

SPEED BUMP

3. **List the micronutrients most commonly deficient in athletes.**
4. **Describe the benefit or lack of benefit of vitamin and mineral supplementation.**

WATER

When people think of nutrition, they often forget to think about water. Loss of only 20% of total body water could cause death. A 10% loss causes severe disorders (Fig. 4-4). In general, adults can survive up to 10 days without water, while children can survive for up to 5 days.[12]

Water Absorption

Consumed water passes through the digestive system to the large intestine where it is absorbed by passive diffusion (osmosis). Approximately one-half to a full liter of water contained within chyme passes to the large intestine each day. The majority of this water is absorbed into the portal circulation. About 50 to 200 milliliters is not absorbed and passes into stool.

Water Functions

Water is the single largest component of the human body, making up approximately 50% to 70% of body weight. In other words, about 85 to 119 pounds (39 to 54 kg) of a 170-pound (77-kg) man is water weight. Physiologically, water has many important functions, including regulating body temperature, protecting vital

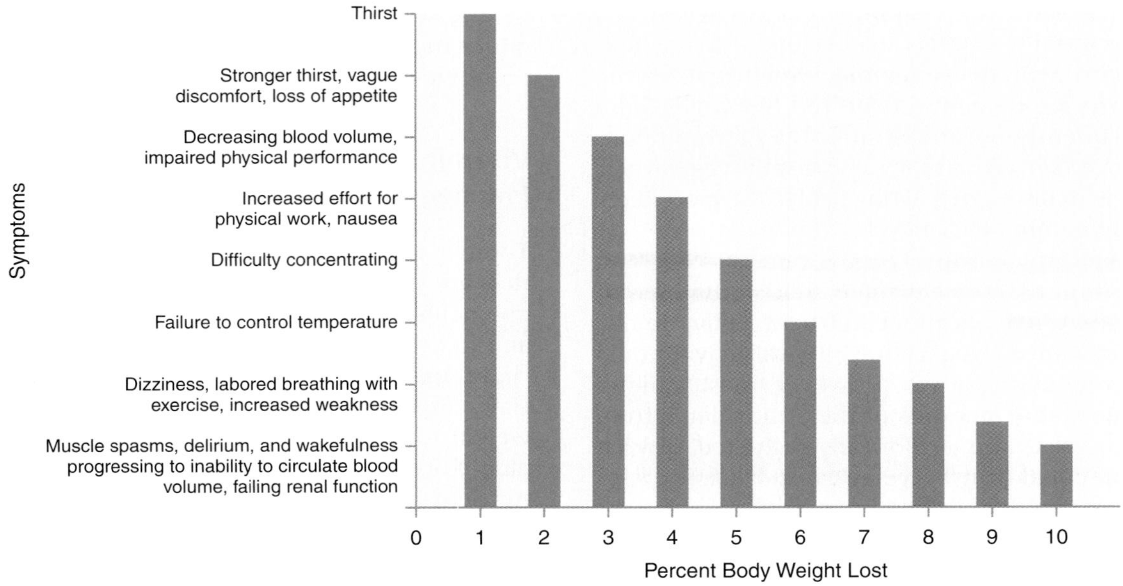

Figure 4-4. Effects of dehydration.

organs, providing a driving force for nutrient absorption, serving as a medium for all biochemical reactions, and maintaining a high blood volume for optimal athletic performance. In fact, total body water weight is higher in athletes compared to nonathletes and tends to decrease with age due to diminishing muscle mass.

Water volume can be influenced by a variety of factors, such as food and drink intake; sweat, urine, and feces excretion; metabolic production of small amounts of water; and losses of water that occur with breathing. These factors play an especially important role during exercise when metabolism is increased. The generated body heat causes a person to sweat, which is a solution of water, sodium, and other electrolytes.

Risks of Water Imbalance

If fluid intake is not increased to replenish the lost fluid, the body attempts to compensate by retaining more water and excreting more concentrated urine. Under these conditions, the person is said to be dehydrated. Severe dehydration can lead to **heat stroke**. On the other hand, if people ingest excessive amounts of fluid to compensate for minimal amounts of water lost in sweat they may become overloaded with fluid, a condition called hyponatremia. When the blood's water-to-sodium ratio is severely elevated, excess water can leak into brain tissue, leading to encephalopathy, or brain swelling.

Fortunately, the human body is well-equipped to withstand dramatic variations in fluid intake during exercise and at rest with little or no detrimental health effects. Individuals at highest risk of negative consequences due to fluid imbalance include infants and young children, vigorously exercising athletes, hospitalized patients, and the sick and elderly, who may have diminished thirst sensation.

SPEED BUMP

5. Explain the importance of water for health and athletic performance.

CHAPTER SUMMARY

There is broad consumer interest in the roles of vitamins and minerals in optimizing health and athletic performance. Magazines, talk shows, friends, celebrities, cited experts, and professional athletes all influence the questions and actions of the recreational athlete who is interested in the latest food or supplement with promises to improve fitness and well-being. While the research on the precise roles of each nutrient in optimizing human health and performance is constantly evolving, a basic understanding of the functions and food sources of each nutrient prepares the allied health professional to logically evaluate the latest trends and claims.

KEY POINTS SUMMARY

1. The dietary reference intakes (DRIs) provide recommended intakes of the vitamins and minerals depending on gender and age. While athletes may have higher micronutrient needs compared to the sedentary population, there are no separate DRIs for athletes. This does not pose a problem for most athletes, as athletes tend to consume more calories and thus have

more opportunities to obtain high levels of vitamins and minerals.

2. Vitamins are classified as water-soluble and fat-soluble. Water-soluble vitamins include all of the B vitamins and vitamin C. Fat-soluble vitamins include vitamins A, D, E, and K. Water-soluble vitamins have limited capacity for storage in the human body, with deficiency resulting from months to rarely years (in the case of vitamin B_{12}) of inadequate intake. Due to this decreased storage capacity, water-soluble vitamins must be taken in very large amounts to cause toxicity, as the body typically excretes excessive vitamins in urine. Fat-soluble vitamins require fat for absorption and are readily stored in fat tissue in the body—which is helpful for individuals at risk of vitamin deficiency but potentially harmful for individuals who consume very large amounts of the vitamin, as fat-soluble vitamins are not readily excreted.
3. Minerals are classified as macrominerals and microminerals. The macrominerals are needed in larger amounts and include calcium, phosphorus, magnesium, sulfur, sodium, chloride, and potassium. Microminerals are needed only in small amounts and include iron, iodine, selenium, zinc, chromium, and others.
4. The electrolytes sodium, potassium, and chloride are macrominerals that play an important role in maintaining normal cellular function. All three electrolytes play at least four essential roles in the body: water balance and distribution, osmotic pressure, acid–base balance, and intracellular/extracellular differentials. An imbalance of electrolytes can cause severe disability or death.
5. The majority of vitamin and mineral digestion and absorption occurs in the small intestine. While vitamins are well absorbed and utilized by the body, the bioavailability of minerals is much less. Minerals with high bioavailability (> 40%) include sodium, potassium, chloride, iodide, and fluoride. Minerals with low bioavailability (1% to 10% absorption) include iron, zinc, chromium, and manganese. (Bioavailability is 20% to 30% for heme iron.) All other minerals, including calcium and magnesium, are of medium bioavailability (30% to 40% absorption). Many factors affect a mineral's bioavailability, including the effects of mineral-mineral interactions
6. Antioxidants include vitamin C, beta-carotene, vitamin E, and selenium. Antioxidants function to prevent or repair oxidative damage. In the past, antioxidants were considered potent disease fighters. However, subsequent research suggests the agents may not protect against disease and in excess (generally from supplements) some of them may act to increase the risk of cancer, heart disease, and mortality in some individuals.
7. A diet high in fruits and vegetables is associated with a lower risk of developing chronic disease, such as heart disease, cancer, and possibly Alzheimer's disease. Their beneficial effects could be due to antioxidants, fiber, agents that stimulate the immune system, monounsaturated fatty acids, B vitamins, folic acid, or various other potential phytochemicals.
8. While nearly half of the adult population takes a multivitamin, there is no evidence that taking a multivitamin leads to improved health outcomes. Generally, vitamin and mineral supplements are not warranted. Notable exceptions include folic acid supplementation in pregnant women and physician-directed treatment of disorders such as iron-deficiency anemia or iron insufficiency (in athletes) and osteoporosis or osteopenia. There is also emerging evidence that many people could benefit from vitamin D supplementation.
9. Athletes are at highest risk for low levels of the B vitamins, vitamins C and E, beta-carotene, calcium and vitamin D, selenium, iron, zinc, and magnesium.
10. Clients on very-low-calorie or restrictive diets need to be aware of micronutrient intakes to avoid deficiency.
11. Water makes up 50% to 70% of body weight. Its balance is essential for optimal health and performance. Water has many important functions, including regulating body temperature, protecting vital organs, providing a driving force for nutrient absorption, serving as a medium for all biochemical reactions, and maintaining a high blood volume for optimal athletic performance.
12. Water volume can be influenced by a variety of factors, such as food and drink intake; sweat, urine, and feces excretion; metabolic production of small amounts of water; and losses of water that occur with breathing. These factors play an especially important role during exercise when metabolism is increased. The generated body heat is released through sweat, which is a solution of water, sodium, and other electrolytes.
13. Athletes need to consume sufficient—but not too much—water before, during, and after exercise to maintain fluid balance.

PRACTICAL APPLICATIONS

1. Which of the following statements about vitamins is true?
   A. Vitamins are essential nutrients.
   B. Vitamins are inorganic compounds.
   C. Large amounts of vitamins are needed for overall good health.
   D. There are 10 vitamins in all.

2. Which of the following nutrients can be stored in the body for extended periods of time?
   A. Vitamin C
   B. Biotin
   C. Thiamin
   D. Vitamin D
3. What is an important function of vitamin A?
   A. Vision
   B. Lowering of LDL cholesterol
   C. Absorption of calcium and phosphorus
   D. Cell membrane protection
4. Plant oils are excellent sources of __________ and liver is an excellent source of __________.
   A. vitamin K; vitamin A
   B. vitamin E; vitamin D
   C. vitamin E; vitamin A
   D. vitamin D; vitamin K
5. Which of the following nutrients plays an integral role in the development of the bones and teeth, muscle contraction, and blood-pressure control?
   A. Amino acids
   B. Calcium
   C. Triglycerides
   D. Phosphorous
6. A lack of which of the following substances is known to be the cause of the most common micronutrient deficiency in the world?
   A. Folate
   B. Iron
   C. Niacin
   D. Biotin
7. Which of the following nutrients provide the body with necessary electrolytes?
   A. Vitamins
   B. Proteins
   C. Minerals
   D. Fats
8. Symptoms of dehydration during exercise include all of the following except:
   A. An increase in appetite
   B. Disorientation
   C. Chills
   D. A decrease in performance
9. Where does the majority of vitamin and mineral digestion and absorption take place?
   A. Small intestine
   B. Mouth
   C. Large intestine
   D. Stomach
10. Approximately what percentage of total body weight is made up of water?
    A. 30% to 50%
    B. 50% to 70%
    C. 45% to 65%
    D. 65% to 85%

Case 1 Adele, the Active Octogenarian

Adele is an 85-year-old woman who is relatively new to physical activity. After her husband died last year she committed to a fitness program to help her maintain her independence. She participates in water fitness classes 5 days per week, weight trains with a personal trainer 2 hours per week, and attends yoga for 1 hour 2 days per week.

1. Adele tells you that her doctor told her that she is at risk for calcium and vitamin D deficiency and that she should make sure to get recommended amounts of the nutrients.
   a. Explain the importance of calcium and vitamin D for older adults.
   b. What are the recommended calcium and vitamin D intakes for Adele? Make a list of foods that she could consume to meet these daily needs.
   c. Adele could meet her vitamin D needs through food intake, sunlight, or supplementation. What are the risks and benefits of each of these options?
   d. How would Adele know if she has a calcium or vitamin D deficiency?
2. Adele also shares with you that most of her friends get vitamin B_{12} shots to prevent or treat vitamin B_{12} deficiency. She tells you that she prefers not to take a supplement but she is concerned about getting enough of the vitamin because she heard that low levels are "bad news."
   a. What are the symptoms of vitamin B_{12} deficiency? How long does it take for these symptoms to develop?
   b. What is the recommended level of vitamin B_{12} intake for Adele?
   c. What is the rationale behind vitamin B_{12} shots for older adults?
   d. Make a list of foods that are high in vitamin B_{12}.

Case 2 Brian, the High School Basketball Player

Brian is a 15-year-old high school basketball player. He is 6′2″ and 180 pounds. He tells you that his mom has been telling him that he needs to eat better.

Appreciating that teens do not always consume a balanced diet, you decide to look up what is considered to be the "typical" teenage diet. You learn that the typical teen diet is characterized by an abundance of sweetened beverages, French fries, pizza, and fast food. It typically lacks adequate fruits, vegetables, low-fat dairy products, whole grains, lean meats, and fish. This makes for a diet very high in fat, saturated fat, trans fat, and added sugar and too low in calcium; iron; zinc; potassium; vitamins A, D, and C; and folic acid.

You are not surprised to find that Brian is no exception. When you ask him what kinds of foods he typically eats he tells you that he knows that he has an overall lousy diet but that he is motivated to eat better because he knows it will help to improve his basketball game.

You are especially concerned about Brian's micronutrient intake.

1. Fill in the following table. What "superfoods" are good sources of more than one of the micronutrients?

Nutrient	Recommended Intake for Brian	Good Food Sources Appropriate for Client
Calcium		
Iron		
Zinc		
Potassium		
Vitamin A		
Vitamin D		
Vitamin C		
Folic acid		

2. Brian asks you how eating a more balanced diet with sufficient amounts of the nutrients listed in the table might affect his athletic performance.

   For each of the nutrients listed in the table below, briefly summarize the nutrient's importance as it relates to exercise.

Nutrient	Role in Exercise
Calcium	
Iron	
Zinc	
Potassium	
Vitamin A	
Vitamin D	
Vitamin C	
Folic acid	

TRAIN YOURSELF

1. Meeting Nutritional Needs
   a. Based on your gender, age, activity level, and dietary habits, for which micronutrients do you think that you may not meet recommended intakes?
   b. For the nutrients you listed above, what are the recommended daily intakes for you?
   c. Plan a 1-day menu for yourself that would include the recommended amounts of the nutrients you listed above.
   d. On a scale of 1 (highly unlikely) to 10 (extremely likely), what is the likelihood that you will follow this plan? Explain why.
2. Cooking for Optimal Nutrition
   a. Consider how you select, store, and prepare fruits and vegetables. How could you select, store, and prepare fruits and vegetables differently to optimize the amount of micronutrients you consume?

REFERENCES

1. Pan A, Sun Q, Bernstein AM, et al. Red meat consumption and mortality: results from 2 prospective cohort studies. *Arch Intern Med.* April 9 2012;172(7):555-563.
2. Girdwain J. Meaty issues. *Runners World.* www.runnersworld.com/article/0,7120,s6-242-300—14241-0,00.html April 2012.
3. World Health Organization. Nutrition: Micronutrients. *WHO.* www.who.int/nutrition/topics/micronutrients/en/.
4. McDaniel MA, Maier SF, Einstein GO. "Brain-specific" nutrients: a memory cure? *Nutrition.* November-December 2003;19(11-12):957-975.
5. Fischer LM, da Costa KA, Kwock L, Galanko J, Zeisel SH. Dietary choline requirements of women: effects of estrogen and genetic variation. *Am J Clin Nutr.* November 2010; 92(5):1113-1119.
6. Zeisel SH, Niculescu MD. Perinatal choline influences brain structure and function. *Nutr Rev.* April 2006;64(4):197-203.
7. Santamaria A, Giordano D, Corroado F, et al. One-year effects of myo-inositol supplementation in postmenopausal women with metabolic syndrome. *Climacteric.* 2012;15(5): 490-495.
8. Centers for Disease Control and Prevention. Folic acid. www.cdc.gov/ncbddd/folicacid/recommendations.html. Accessed April 21, 2013.
9. National Institutes of Health. Dietary supplement fact sheet: vitamin A. http://ods.od.nih.gov/factsheets/VitaminA-HealthProfessional/#disc. Accessed April 21, 2013.
10. Angeline ME, Gee AO, Shindle M, et al. The effects of vitamin D deficiency in athletes. *Am J Sports Med.* 2013 February;41(2):461-464.
11. Slomski A. IOM endorses vitamin D, calcium only for bone health, dispels deficiency claims. *JAMA.* February 2 2011;305(5):453-454, 456.
12. Mahan LK, Escott-Stump S. *Krause's Food Nutrition and Diet Therapy* (13th ed.). Philadelphia: W.B. Saunders Company; 2011.
13. National Institutes of Health. Dietary supplement fact sheet: calcium. http://ods.od.nih.gov/factsheets/Calcium-HealthProfessional/. Accessed April 21, 2013.
14. Della Valle DM, Haas JR. Iron status is associated with endurance performance and training in female rowers. *Med Sci Sports Exerc.* 2012; Epub ahead of print February 2012.
15. Teng W, Shan Z, Teng X, et al. Effect of iodine intake on thyroid diseases in China. *N Engl J Med.* 2006 June 29; 354(26):2783-2793.
16. Cefalu WT, Rood J, Pinsonat P, et al. Characterization of the metabolic and physiologic response to chromium supplementation in subjects with type 2 diabetes mellitus. *Metabolism.* 2010 May;59(5):755-762.
17. Ali ND, Ma Y, Reynolds J, et al. Chromium effects on glucose tolerance and insulin sensitivity in persons at risk for diabetes mellitus. *Endocr Pract.* 2011 January-February;17(1): 16-25. doi: 10.4158/EP10131.OR.
18. Bjelakovic G, Nikolova D, Gluud LL, Simonetti RG, Gluud C. Mortality in randomized trials of antioxidant supplements for primary and secondary prevention: systematic review and meta-analysis. *JAMA.* February 28 2007;297(8): 842-857.
19. Halliwell B. Dietary polyphenols: good, bad, or indifferent for your health? *Cardiovasc Res.* January 15 2007;73(2): 341-347.
20. Bailey RL, Gahche JJ, Lentino CV, et al. Dietary supplement use in the United States, 2003-2006. *J Nutr.* February 2011;141(2):261-266.
21. Kamangar F, Emadi A. Vitamin and mineral supplements: do we really need them? *Int J Prev Med.* March 2012;3(3): 221-226.
22. Bolland MJ, Grey A, Avenell A, Gamble GD, Reid IR. Calcium supplements with or without vitamin D and risk of cardiovascular events: reanalysis of the Women's Health Initiative limited access dataset and meta-analysis. *BMJ.* 2011;342:d2040.
23. Muntwyler J, Hennekens CH, Manson JE, Buring JE, Gaziano JM. Vitamin supplement use in a low-risk population of US male physicians and subsequent cardiovascular mortality. *Arch Intern Med.* July 8 2002;162(13):1472-1476.
24. Lippman SM, Klein EA, Goodman PJ, et al. Effect of selenium and vitamin E on risk of prostate cancer and other cancers: the Selenium and Vitamin E Cancer Prevention Trial (SELECT). *JAMA.* January 7 2009;301(1):39-51.
25. Klein EA, Thompson IM, Jr., Tangen CM, et al. Vitamin E and the risk of prostate cancer: the Selenium and Vitamin E Cancer Prevention Trial (SELECT). *JAMA.* October 12 2011; 306(14):1549-1556.
26. Blencowe H, Cousens S, Modell B, Lawn J. Folic acid to reduce neonatal mortality from neural tube disorders. *Int J Epidemiol.* April 2010;39 Suppl 1:i110-121.
27. Rodriguez NR, Di Marco NM, Langley S. American College of Sports Medicine position stand. Nutrition and athletic performance. *Med Sci Sports Exerc.* March 2009;41(3):709-731.
28. Rodriguez NR, DiMarco NM, Langley S. Position of the American Dietetic Association, Dietitians of Canada, and the American College of Sports Medicine: nutrition and athletic performance. *J Am Diet Assoc.* March 2009;109 (3):509-527.
29. Fondell, E, Bälter O, Rothman KJ, et al. Dietary intake and supplement use of vitamins C and E and upper respiratory tract infection. *J Am Coll Nutr.* 2011 August;30(4):248-258.
30. Reynolds G. Phys Ed: can vitamin D improve your athletic performance? *New York Times* .

CHAPTER 5

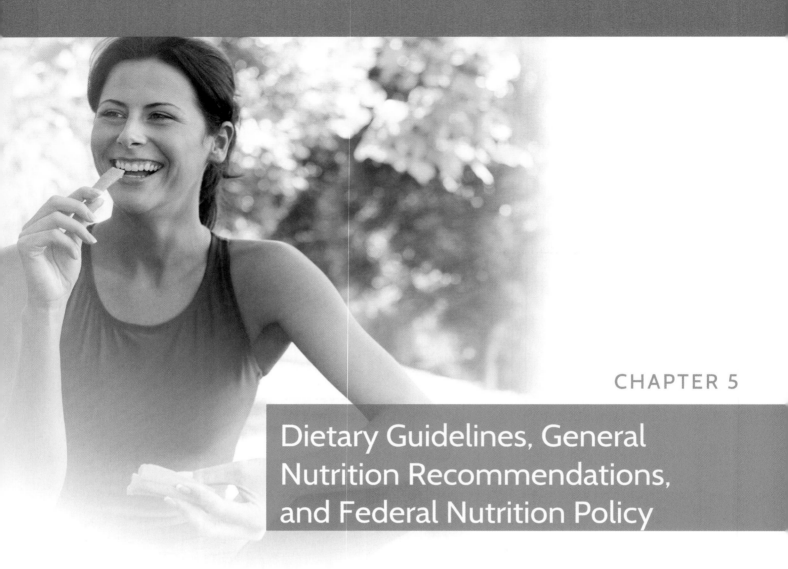

Dietary Guidelines, General Nutrition Recommendations, and Federal Nutrition Policy

CHAPTER OUTLINE

LEARNING OBJECTIVES

After studying this chapter, the reader should be able to:

5.1 Summarize the major recommendations from the 2010 *Dietary Guidelines for Americans*.

5.2 Describe the major features of MyPlate.

5.3 Define the Dietary Reference Intakes, including RDA, EAR, UL, and AI.

5.4 Dissect a nutrition label to determine the total number of calories; calories from fat, protein, and carbohydrates; and overall nutritional value of a product.

5.5 List several important food safety principles when selecting, storing, and preparing food.

5.6 Describe four ways that allied health professionals can get involved to shape policy and advocate for healthier lifestyles.

KEY TERMS

Centers for Disease Control and Prevention (CDC) An agency of the federal government whose mission is to work with other health agencies to optimally promote health, prevent disease, reduce injury and disability, and prepare for and respond to health threats.

daily value (DV) The recommended level of intake for a nutrient.

Dietary Guidelines for Americans Federally released guidelines that provide evidence-based nutrition information and advice for people age 2 and older, and serve as the basis for federal food and nutrition education programs.

Federal Trade Commission The government agency tasked with the job of preventing unfair methods of competition and enforcement of "unfair and deceptive acts or practices," such as misleading advertisements.

Food and Drug Administration (FDA) An agency within the Department of Health and Human Services which, among other functions, monitors food and drug safety, oversees nutrition labeling, regulates tobacco products, and provides the public with credible health information.

food frequency questionnaire A method used to identify typical eating habits, which is composed of a checklist of foods and beverages with a section for the client to mark how often each of the listed foods are eaten.

percent daily value The percentage of recommendations for key nutrients based on a 2,000-calorie diet.

qualified health claims A health claim on a packaged food that is supported by scientific research that attests a relationship between a substance and its ability to reduce the risk of a disease or health-related condition.

recommended dietary allowance (RDA) The amount of nutrient known to be adequate to meet the nutritional needs of nearly all healthy persons.

social-ecological model A model for health behavior change that emphasizes the development of coordinated partnerships, programs, and policies to support healthy eating and active living.

structure-function claims A health claim on a packaged food that describes the effect that a substance has on the structure or function of the body. An example is "calcium builds strong bones." Structure-function claims must be truthful and not misleading and are not pre-reviewed or authorized by the FDA.

tolerable upper intake level The maximum intake that is unlikely to pose risk of adverse health effects to almost all individuals in an age- and gender-specific group.

U.S. Department of Agriculture (USDA) An agency of the federal government responsible for developing and implementing policy on food and dietary recommendations, farming, and agriculture.

CALCULATIONS

Carbohydrate = 4 Calories/gram

Protein = 4 Calories/gram

Fat = 9 Calories/gram

INTRODUCTION

During her first term in the White House, First Lady Michelle Obama launched the ambitious Let's Move campaign with the goal of eliminating childhood obesity within a generation. During that same time period, the federal government replaced the MyPyramid dietary tool with a simpler icon—a dinner plate. The goal was to translate the federal government's nutrition recommendations for the general population into an easy-to-understand-and-implement symbol.

The push toward personalizing nutrition and activity advice offers an opportunity to reach more people and perhaps begin to make a dent in the epidemic of poor eating habits and physical inactivity. Athletes require a balanced diet of carbohydrates, protein, and fat to ensure they are amply fueled for activity. Getting the proper amount of nutrients from all the food groups is one of the best ways to prevent deficiencies as well as fuel the body. In order to meet nutrient needs, athletes must focus on a variety of foods. But which foods are best? The federal government's dietary guidelines provide a starting point.

DIETARY GUIDELINES

Published every 5 years by the **U.S. Department of Agriculture (USDA)** and the Department of Health and Human Services, the ***Dietary Guidelines for Americans*** is the government's best advice on how to eat to promote health. The dietary guidelines offer a foundation from which to develop an eating plan for most Americans. The guidelines include 23 recommendations for the general population and 6 additional recommendations for specific groups, which are grouped into four categories:[1]

1. **Balance calories to achieve and maintain a healthy weight.** The guidelines encourage Americans to prevent or reduce overweight by eating better and exercising more. This includes eating fewer calories for people who are overweight or obese, increasing physical activity, and decreasing time spent in sedentary behaviors like watching television or browsing the Internet. Table 5-1 shows estimated calorie needs per day according to age, gender, and physical activity level.
2. **Foods and food components to reduce.** The dietary guidelines advise Americans to: reduce sodium intake to less than 2,300 mg per day for the general population and to less than 1,500 mg for higher risk populations such as older adults, African Americans, and people with hypertension, diabetes, or chronic kidney disease; consume fewer than 10% of calories from saturated fat and instead consume monounsaturated and polyunsaturated fats; consume less than 300 mg per day of dietary cholesterol; minimize consumption of trans fatty acids; reduce caloric intake from sugar and solid fats; and consume alcohol in moderation (one drink per day for women and two drinks per day for men).
3. **Foods and nutrients to increase.** The dietary guidelines advise Americans to eat more fruits and vegetables, especially dark-green and red

Table 5-1. Estimated Calorie Needs Per Day by Age, Gender, and Physical Activity Level[a]

Estimated amounts of calories needed to maintain calorie balance for various gender and age groups at three different levels of physical activity. The estimates are rounded to the nearest 200 calories. An individual's calorie needs may be higher or lower than these average estimates.

GENDER	AGE (YEARS)	PHYSICAL ACTIVITY LEVEL[b]		
		Sedentary	**Moderately Active**	**Active**
Child (female and male)	2–3	1,000–1,200	1,000–1,400[c]	1,000–1,400[c]
Female[d]	4–8	1,200–1,400	1,400–1,600	1,400–1,800
	9–13	1,400–1,600	1,600–2,000	1,800–2,200
	14–18	1,800	2,000	2,400
	19–30	1,800–2,000	2,000–2,200	2,400
	31–50	1,800	2,000	2,200
	51+	1,600	1,800	2,000–2,200
Male	4–8	1,200–1,400	1,400–1,600	1,600–2,200
	9–13	1,600–2,000	1,800–2,200	2,000–2,600

Table 5-1. Estimated Calorie Needs Per Day by Age, Gender, and Physical Activity Level[a]—cont'd

GENDER	AGE (YEARS)	PHYSICAL ACTIVITY LEVEL[b]		
		Sedentary	**Moderately Active**	**Active**
	14–18	2,000–2,400	2,400–2,800	2,800–3,200
	19–30	2,400–2,600	2,600–2,800	3,000
	31–50	2,200–2,400	2,400–2,600	2,800–3,000
	51+	2,000–2,200	2,200–2,400	2,400–2,800

a. Based on Estimated Energy Requirements (EER) equations, using reference heights (average) and reference weights (healthy) for each age/gender group. For children and adolescents, reference height and weight vary. For adults, the reference man is 5 feet 10 inches tall and weighs 154 pounds. The reference woman is 5 feet 4 inches tall and weighs 126 pounds. EER equations are from the Institute of Medicine. Dietary Reference Intakes for Energy, Carbohydrate, Fiber, Fat, Fatty Acids, Cholesterol, Protein, and Amino Acids. Washington (DC): The National Academic Press; 2002.

b. Sedentary means a lifestyle that includes only the light physical activity associated with typical day-to-day life. Moderately active means a lifestyle that includes physical activity equivalent to walking about 1.5 to 3 miles per day at 3 to 4 miles per hour, in addition to the light physical activity associated with typical day-to-day life. Active means a lifestyle that includes physical activity equivalent to walking more than 3 miles per day at 3 to 4 miles per hour, in addition to the light physical activity associated with typical day-to-day life.

c. The calorie ranges shown are to accommodate needs of different ages within the group. For children and adolescents, more calories are needed at older ages. For adults, fewer calories are needed at older ages.

d. Estimates for females do not include women who are pregnant or breastfeeding.

Source: www.cnpp.usda.gov/Publication/DietaryGuidelines/20120/Policy Doc.pdf

and orange vegetables; consume at least half of all grains as whole grains; increase intake of fat-free or low-fat milk products; choose lean proteins and especially try to increase the amount of seafood eaten (Box 5-1); replace high-fat proteins with leaner proteins; use oil instead of solid fat; and try to consume more potassium, fiber, calcium, and vitamin D. Sources of these nutrients include fruits, vegetables, whole grains, milk, and milk products. Athletes also need increased amounts of certain nutrients such as iron to prevent anemia and the resulting feelings of exhaustion and fatigue.

4. **Building healthy eating patterns.** A healthy eating pattern meets nutrient needs through consumption of nutrient-dense foods while staying within calorie limits. Some examples of well-known and effective healthy eating

Box 5-1. Selecting and Preparing Fish

The *Dietary Guidelines for Americans* emphasize that Americans should eat more seafood, which contains omega-3 fats and many other nutrients, for optimal health. However, the average American may not be accustomed to eating the recommended two or more servings of seafood per week. Some tips from the FDA for safely selecting and preparing seafood are:

- Buy your seafood from a retailer that follows proper food-handling techniques and from a clean-looking and clean-smelling facility.
- Fresh fish should smell fresh and mild. Whole fish and fillets should have firm, shiny flesh that springs back when pressed. Make sure there is no darkening or drying around the edges and that the eyes are clear, not cloudy.
- Don't buy frozen fish that is positioned above the "frost line" or top of the freezer case in the store's freezer. Also, avoid fish in packages that are open, torn, or crushed around the edges. Look for signs of frost or ice crystals, an indication that the fish has been stored for too long.
- Put seafood in the refrigerator if you will eat it within 2 days, otherwise store it in the freezer.
- Take the same food safety precautions you would when preparing raw beef or chicken. Avoid cross-contamination and defrost in the refrigerator.
- Cook fish to an internal temperature of 145°F. Properly cooked fish flesh should be opaque and separate easily.
- Never leave raw or cooked seafood out of the refrigerator for more than 2 hours.
- Pregnant women, young children, older adults, immunocompromised persons, and those with decreased stomach acidity are at increased risk of foodborne illness and should not eat raw or partially cooked fish or shellfish. Shark, swordfish, king mackerel, and tilefish contain high amounts of mercury, which can harm an unborn child's developing nervous system. Pregnant women should instead eat up to 12 ounces per week of fish that is low in mercury such as shrimp, canned light tuna, salmon, pollock, and catfish.

Table 5-2. DASH Eating Plan: Serving Sizes, Examples, and Significance

The following eating plan is based on 2,000 calories per day. The number of daily and weekly servings varies according to calorie requirements.

FOOD GROUP	DAILY SERVINGS	SERVING SIZES	EXAMPLES AND NOTES	SIGNIFICANCE OF EACH FOOD GROUP TO THE DASH EATING PLAN
Grains[a]	6–8	1 slice bread 1 oz dry cereal[b] ½ cup cooked rice, pasta, or cereal[b]	Whole-wheat bread and rolls, whole-wheat pasta, English muffin, pita bread, bagel, cereals, grits, oatmeal, brown rice, unsalted pretzels and popcorn	Major sources of energy and fiber
Vegetables	4–5	1 cup raw leafy vegetable ½ cup cut-up raw or cooked vegetable ½ cup vegetable juice	Broccoli, carrots, collards, green beans, green peas, kale, lima beans, potatoes, spinach, squash, sweet potatoes, tomatoes	Rich sources of potassium, magnesium, and fiber
Fruits	4–5	1 medium fruit ¼ cup dried fruit ½ cup fresh, frozen, or canned fruit ½ cup fruit juice	Apples, apricots, bananas, dates, grapes, oranges, grapefruit, grapefruit juice, mangoes, melons, peaches, pineapples, raisins, strawberries, tangerines	Important sources of potassium, magnesium, and fiber
Fat-free or low-fat dairy products[c]	2–3	1 cup milk or yogurt 1½ oz cheese	Fat-free milk or buttermilk; fat-free, low-fat, or reduced-fat cheese; fat-free/low-fat regular or frozen yogurt	Major sources of calcium and protein
Lean meats, poultry, and fish	6 or less	1 oz cooked meats, poultry, or fish 1 egg[d]	Select only lean; trim away visible fats; broil, roast, or poach; remove skin from poultry	Rich sources of protein and magnesium
Nuts, seeds, and legumes	4–5 per week	⅓ cup or 1½ oz nuts 2 Tbsp peanut butter 2 Tbsp or ½ oz seeds ½ cup cooked legumes (dried beans, peas)	Almonds, filberts, mixed nuts, peanuts, walnuts, sunflower seeds, peanut butter, kidney beans, lentils, split peas	Rich sources of energy, magnesium, protein, and fiber
Fats and oils[e]	2–3	1 tsp soft margarine 1 tsp vegetable oil 1 Tbsp mayonnaise 2 Tbsp salad dressing	Soft margarine, vegetable oil (canola, corn, olive, safflower), low-fat mayonnaise, light salad dressing	The DASH study had 27% of calories as fat, including fat in or added to foods
Sweets and added sugars	5 or less per week	1 Tbsp sugar 1 Tbsp jelly or jam ½ cup sorbet, gelatin dessert 1 cup lemonade	Fruit-flavored gelatin, fruit punch, hard candy, jelly, maple syrup, sorbet and ices, sugar	Sweets should be low in fat

a. Whole grains are recommended for most grain servings as a good source of fiber and nutrients.

b. Serving sizes vary between ½ cup and 1¼ cups, depending on cereal type. Check the product's Nutrition Facts label.

c. For lactose intolerance, try either lactase enzyme pills with dairy products or lactose-free or lactose-reduced milk.

d. Because eggs are high in cholesterol, limit egg yolk intake to no more than four per week; two egg whites have the same protein content as 1 oz of meat.

e. Fat content changes the serving amount for fats and oils. For example, 1 Tbsp regular salad dressing = one serving; 1 Tbsp low-fat dressing = one-half serving; 1 Tbsp fat-free dressing = zero servings.

Source: National Heart, Lung, and Blood Institute, National Institutes of Health. Following the DASH eating plan. Available at www.nhlbi.nih.gov/health/health-topics/topics/dash/followdash.html#footnotea. Accessed April 22, 2013.

patterns include the Dietary Approaches to Stop Hypertension (DASH) diet (Table 5-2), the Mediterranean diet (see Evaluating the Evidence), and a well-planned vegetarian diet. It is a common misconception that athletes who follow vegetarian diets cannot meet their nutrient needs. A diet rich in plant-based protein and nutrients of concern (typically iron, zinc, vitamins B_{12}, vitamin D, and omega-3 fats) can certainly be achieved with proper dietary instruction.

EVALUATING THE EVIDENCE

Does Adherence to a Mediterranean Diet Increase Longevity?

The Greek island of Crete is famous for more than its stunning scenery and ancient roots. More than 50 years ago, American scientist Ancel Keys, who himself lived to 100, attributed the exceptional longevity and miniscule rates of cardiovascular disease and cancer on the island to the "Cretan" Mediterranean diet–a diet rich in fruits, vegetables, legumes, whole grains, fish, and olive oil, and moderate in red wine. Since then, a large body of research on the Mediterranean diet has been accumulated, suggesting that adhering to a Mediterranean diet offers numerous benefits such as enhanced weight loss, heart health, and mental health, and reduced Alzheimer's disease, cancer, and Parkinson disease.[14] But is there enough evidence to support the assertion that adopting a Mediterranean diet may add years to your life?

WHAT DOES THE EVIDENCE SAY?

Greek researchers from the University of Athens medical school set out to rigorously evaluate the assertion that adherence to a Mediterranean diet may improve longevity.[15] They enrolled 22,043 adults in Greece who completed a comprehensive survey that included a **food frequency questionnaire** aimed to evaluate how closely the diet resembled the traditional Mediterranean diet. The researchers rated adherence to the Mediterranean diet on a nine-point scale that incorporated the major features of the Mediterranean diet. They then checked up on the study participants 44 months later, after which 275 participants had died. A higher degree of adherence to the Mediterranean diet was associated with a lower likelihood of death from any cause as well as death from cardiovascular disease or cancer. Interestingly, associations between individual food groups within the Mediterranean diet and mortality were not significant. The authors concluded that adherence to the traditional Mediterranean diet is associated with a significant reduction in mortality and that greater adherence to a Mediterranean diet may be related to the increased longevity.

1. Based on this study, is it fair to conclude that a Mediterranean diet increases longevity? Why or why not?
2. What are three important limitations to this study?
3. This study was published in the ***New England Journal of Medicine***, among the most prestigious and rigorous medical journals. Why do you think the journal may have selected this article for publication?
4. The authors evaluated adherence to a Mediterranean diet with a scale very similar to the one below.[13] Based on this scale, how closely does your typical diet resemble the Mediterranean diet? Give yourself one point for each "yes." If you score 6 or higher, you're eating like you live in the Mediterranean.

	Yes	No
Vegetables (other than potatoes), 4 or more servings per day		
Fruits, 4 or more servings per day		
Whole grains, 2 or more servings per day		
Beans (legumes), 2 or more servings per week		
Nuts, 2 or more servings per week		
Fish, 2 or more servings per week		
Red and processed meat, 1 or fewer servings per day		
Dairy foods, 1 or fewer servings per day		
Alcohol, ½ to 1 drink per day for women, 1 to 2 for men		

This chapter's Evaluating the Evidence is based on the following article: Trichopoulou A, Costacou T, Bamia C, Trichopoulos D. Adherence to a Mediterranean diet and survival in a Greek population. *N Engl J Med* 2003;348:2599-608.

The guidelines advise Americans to follow food safety recommendations when preparing and eating foods so as to reduce the risk of foodborne illness (discussed in more detail later in this chapter).

The dietary guidelines strive to help Americans to eat the variety and amount of foods necessary to optimize nutrition while avoiding excessive caloric intake. Athletes benefit as much as the general public in adopting these guidelines, even in the case of prolonged endurance sessions when overall calorie and carbohydrate needs increase. Though athletes may have increased caloric needs, including consumption of rapidly digestible carbohydrates, it is preferred to obtain energy from healthful natural sugar sources rather than highly processed alternatives.

Help Americans Make Healthy Choices

The guidelines charge all sectors of society to play an active role in the movement to make the United States healthier by developing coordinated partnerships, programs, and policies to support healthy eating. Food and activity behaviors should be viewed in the context of a **social-ecological model**. The guidelines describe this model as an approach that emphasizes the development of coordinated partnerships, programs, and policies to support healthy eating and active living. In this framework, interventions should extend well beyond providing traditional education to individuals and families about healthy choices, and should help build skills, reshape the environment, and reestablish social norms to facilitate individuals' healthy choices. The social-ecological model takes into consideration *individual factors* such as age, gender, socioeconomic status, and knowledge; *environmental settings* including homes, schools, workplaces, and other community venues; *sectors of influence* such as government, marketing and media, and industry; and *social and cultural norms and values* including belief systems, religion, lifestyle, and body image (see Communication Strategies).

Health professionals play an important role in responding to the dietary guidelines' call to action to: (1) ensure that all Americans have access to nutritious foods and opportunities for physical activity; (2) facilitate individual behavior change through environmental strategies; and (3) set the stage for lifelong healthy eating, physical activity, and weight management behaviors.

MYPLATE

Based on the *Dietary Guidelines for Americans,* MyPlate is a symbol of healthy eating designed to replace the MyPyramid icon (Fig. 5-1). MyPlate simplifies the government's nutrition messages into an easily understood and implemented graphic—a dinner plate divided into four sections: fruits, vegetables, protein, and grains accompanied by a glass of 1% or non-fat milk or dairy alternative like soy milk. The goal of this icon is to

COMMUNICATION STRATEGIES

Putting the Social-Ecological Model to Use

You are working with a 21-year-old recreational college athlete who wants to improve her soccer game. She is a committed athlete and pushes herself in soccer practice and at games. She recognizes that her dietary habits are poor. She believes that eating at the college dorms is impeding her ability to choose a healthy diet.

The dietary guidelines recommend using the social-ecological model as a framework to understand the context in which people make nutrition and activity decisions.[13] It is a useful model to keep in mind when advising clients on how to make healthful lifestyle changes. During the initial interview when a client is making nutrition and activity goals, it is important for the health professional to consider the client's current nutrition and activity behaviors, environmental and social supports and barriers, and self-efficacy and readiness to change among the other factors contained within the social-ecological model.

CLASS ACTIVITY

Working in pairs, assign one partner to be the client and the other to be the health professional.

The client should play the part of this recreational soccer player who wants to improve her soccer game but is struggling to adopt a healthy diet. Take 10 minutes to make a list of potential individual factors, environmental settings, sectors of influence, and social and cultural values and norms that may be affecting her nutrition choices. (Remember, you are role playing this client so feel free to take liberties in developing her story, perhaps drawing upon some of your own experiences and challenges).

The health professional should aim to gather information about the factors that are interfering with the client's ability to eat a healthy diet. Once you've gathered this information, think of potential strategies you might use to help overcome one barrier in each of the domains (individual factors, environmental settings, sectors of influence, and social and cultural values and norms).

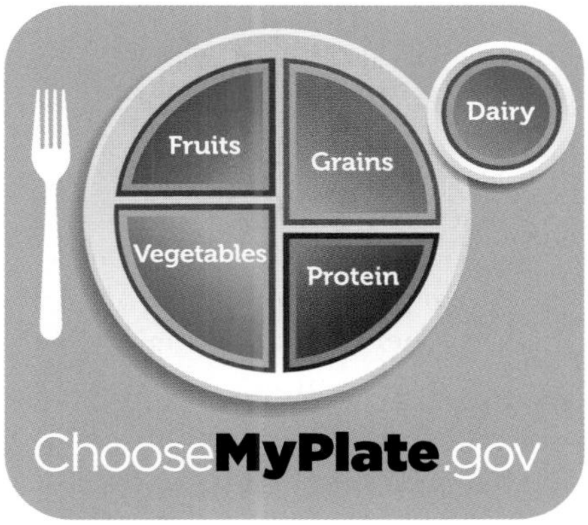

Figure 5-1. MyPlate.

create a better visual of a balanced diet that is about 50% fruits and vegetables, with remaining portions being made up of lean protein, grains, and dairy.

On the MyPlate website (www.choosemyplate.gov), consumers can input their age, gender, height, weight, and physical activity level into the SuperTracker tool and receive an individualized eating plan to meet caloric needs. The program calculates estimated energy expenditure based on this demographic information. Within seconds, users are categorized into one of 12 different energy levels (anywhere from 1,000 to 3,200 calories) and are given the recommended number of servings—measured in cups and ounces—to eat from each of the five food groups (vegetables, fruit, protein, grains, dairy). A set number of discretionary calories (i.e., the leftover calories available for sugar or additional fats or an extra serving from any of the food groups) are also allocated for that individual. By following these recommendations, users are presented with a diet plan for disease prevention and weight maintenance based on their personalized needs. The SuperTracker tool is a beneficial starting point for recreational athletes as well as the general population. Competitive athletes often have higher caloric requirements.

Overall, the tools available at choosemyplate.gov encourage people to:

1. Balance calorie intake with calories expended through physical activity.
2. Enjoy food, but make sure portions are appropriate. Eat slowly to truly enjoy the food (and key in to the body's internal cues of hunger and fullness) and try to minimize distractions like television and cell phones.
3. Avoid oversized portions. MyPlate recommends smaller plates, smaller serving sizes, and more mindful eating.
4. Eat more vegetables, fruits, whole grains, and fat-free or low-fat dairy products (or dairy-free alternatives) for adequate potassium, calcium, vitamin D, and fiber.
5. Make half your plate fruits and vegetables. Most Americans need nine servings of fruits and vegetables per day for optimal health. According to 2013 CDC data, though, the average adult in the United States consumes fruit about 1.1 times per day and vegetables about 1.6 times per day[2] (see Myths and Misconceptions).
6. Switch to fat-free or low-fat (1%) milk or a dairy alternative such as soy milk. Full-fat dairy products provide excess calories and saturated fat in exchange for no nutritional benefit over fat-free and low-fat versions.
7. Make half your grains whole grains (ideally even more than that). This will help to ensure adequate fiber intake and decrease intake of highly processed foods.
8. Eat fewer foods high in solid (typically saturated and trans) fat, added sugars, and salt.
9. Compare sodium in foods and then choose the lower sodium versions.
10. Drink water instead of sugary drinks to help cut sugar and unnecessary calories.

The plan is for each of these messages to be emphasized during a multi-year campaign by Let's Move and the USDA to promote better nutrition. Online tools and how-to strategies are available.

DIETARY REFERENCE INTAKES

From 1941 to 1995, health professionals and the public used the recommended dietary allowance (RDA) values to guide nutrition choices. In 1995, the Food and Nutrition Board of the Institute of Medicine published the dietary reference intakes (DRIs), a more comprehensive approach for recommending nutrients that addresses higher intakes of certain nutrients needed to promote health, the use of dietary supplements and fortified foods, and individual, rather than group, needs. DRIs encompass the following reference values used to plan and assess nutrient recommendations for healthy individuals:

- RDA is the sufficient average intake for most healthy individuals. RDA values may vary based on age and gender.
- Estimated average requirement (EAR) is an adequate intake (AI) in 50% of an age- and gender-specific group.
- Tolerable upper intake level (UL), the maximum intake of a nutrient that is unlikely to pose risk of adverse health effects to almost all individuals in an age- and gender-specific group.
- AI is used when a RDA cannot be determined. AI is a recommended nutrient intake level that is based on research and is sufficient for healthy individuals.

DRIs have been established for calcium, vitamin D, phosphorus, magnesium, and fluoride; folate and other B vitamins; antioxidants (vitamins C and E, selenium); macronutrients (protein, carbohydrates, and fat); trace elements (iron, zinc); and electrolytes and water. Many of the dietary guidelines and advice contained within MyPlate are based on the DRIs. The complete set of DRIs is available at www.iom.edu. Refer to Chapter 4 for the DRIs for various micronutrients.

Myths and Misconceptions

It is Impossible to Eat Healthy on a Tight Budget

One of the most commonly cited reasons people give for not eating healthy is that healthy food "costs too much." With the average consumer spending only about $7 per day on food according to the U.S. Department of Labor Statistics,[3] it may seem near impossible to get the recommended five to nine servings of fruits and vegetables per day on such a tight budget. But that's not necessarily the case. With a little bit of planning, a family of four can get by on about $28 per day ($7 each) including a wholesome breakfast, lunch, and dinner and even a few snacks along the way (see sample recipes below).

Clients can put every food dollar to excellent use by adopting some of the following cost-cutting tips whenever possible.

- Eat at home more often. Not only does it cost less, but you also have better control over portion sizes and can freeze any leftovers for another day when you don't have time to cook.
- Don't go to the grocery store on a whim. Rather, check what you already have in your refrigerator and pantry and have your shopping list in hand. This will help you avoid overbuying. The Let's Move initiative offers an easy-to-use grocery list template that will help boost the nutritional value of your purchases. It's available at www.letsmove.gov/sites/letsmove.gov/files/Grocery_List.pdf.
- It seems obvious, but buy only food that you're actually going to eat, and then actually eat it. If time gets away from you and you have overripe fruits and vegetables in the refrigerator, think of creative ways to use them. How about tomatoes to make a marinara sauce, leftover meat and vegetables in a soup, or ripe fruit for muffins or a smoothie?
- At the store, check packages and perishable items for expiration dates and try to pick the latest one possible.
- Learn the value of a food budget. Use price, need, nutritional value, and portion size to determine buying decisions.

Following is a day's worth of breakfast, lunch, dinner, and snacks that can feed a family of four for approximately $28. The recipes are set up so that you can save money and optimize nutritional value by substituting vegetables and meats based on what is in season or on sale. Pantry items such as salt, pepper, and olive oil are listed at the end of the ingredient lists and are not factored into the price.

Breakfast:

"Banana bread" oatmeal ($1.50)

2 cups uncooked oats
3 cups of water
2 tablespoons brown sugar
2 ripe bananas

Cook basic oatmeal as instructed. Add 2 tablespoons of brown sugar to basic oatmeal recipe. Peel 2 ripe bananas into a bowl and mash with a fork. Finally, add bananas to oatmeal and cook for another 5 minutes.

Lunch:

Grilled Chicken Pita Wraps with Creamy Bean Spread ($8.00)

1 can (15 ounces) cannellini beans
2 skinless chicken breasts
2 whole wheat pitas, separated into 4 pieces
2 cups of baby spinach, washed and dried
2 medium carrots, shredded
½ medium cucumber, sliced
Pantry items: salt, pepper, olive oil

To prepare bean spread: Place 1 can of cannellini beans (including liquid in can) in a blender. Add salt and pepper to taste.

To prepare chicken: Cut each chicken breast in half widthwise (so each chicken breast is thinner). Heat pan on stove at medium heat. Sprinkle each side of the chicken breasts with salt and pepper. Place 2 tablespoons of olive oil in pan. Put two pieces of chicken in pan and cook for 6 to 7 minutes. Flip chicken and cook for another 6 to 7 minutes, until well cooked. Repeat with remaining two pieces of chicken. When chicken is finished cooking, lay flat on cutting board and cut into half-inch strips.

To prepare wraps: Spread 2 tablespoons of bean dip on pita bread. Next, top with one-half cup of spinach, followed by carrots and cucumber, then chicken. Roll up, cut in half, and serve.

Dinner:

Pork and Vegetable Whole Wheat Chow Mein ($12.00)

1 pack of whole wheat spaghetti, cooked according to package directions
2 boneless pork chops
½ medium onion, sliced
1 inch piece of fresh ginger, grated
3–4 cloves of garlic, finely chopped
2 medium carrots, cut into quarter-inch slices
2 large broccoli crowns, cut into small florets
1 large red pepper, cut into thin strips
1 cup of green onions, chopped

Myths and Misconceptions–cont'd

¼ cup of reduced sodium soy sauce
½ cup of water
Pantry items: olive oil
To prepare the meat: Slice the pork into thin slices, approximately ¼ inch in width. Place 2 tablespoons of olive oil in a pan over medium heat. Place onions, ginger, and garlic in pan and cook for 3 to 4 minutes, stirring occasionally. Add sliced meat to pan and cook for 3 to 4 minutes or until meat is almost cooked. Add carrots, broccoli, and red pepper to the pan, followed by soy sauce and water. Cook for approximately 2 minutes. Lastly, add cooked noodles to pan and mix all ingredients well. Cook for another 2 to 3 minutes and serve.

Snacks:

Creamy Garlic Bean Spread with Baked Pita Chips ($3.00)

1 can of white beans (also known as cannellini beans)
2 tablespoons of olive oil
2 tablespoons of water
3 garlic cloves
Place all ingredients in a blender and blend until smooth. Serve with baked pita chips, vegetables, or as an alternative to mayo on sandwiches.

Baked Pita Chips

4 whole wheat pitas
Pantry items: olive oil, salt and pepper
Preheat oven to 400 degrees. Cut each whole wheat pita into eight wedges. Place in bowl and toss with 2 tablespoons of olive oil. Sprinkle with salt and pepper. Place pita wedges on a baking tray evenly and put into oven. Bake for 15 minutes, or until pita chips are crispy.

Strawberry-Banana Yogurt Smoothies ($3.00)

2 ripe bananas
1 cup of plain low-fat yogurt
1 orange, peeled
½ cup of frozen strawberries
Place all ingredients in a blender and blend until smooth. Divide into 4 glasses and serve.

SPEED BUMP

1. **Summarize the major recommendations from the 2010 *Dietary Guidelines for Americans.***
2. **Describe the major features of MyPlate.**
3. **Define DRI and its components: RDA, EAR, UL, and AI.**

FOOD LABELS

Understanding what nutrients contribute to a healthy diet and which foods contain those nutrients contribute to healthy nutrition decisions. The food label, or nutrition facts panel, a required component of nearly all packaged foods, provides knowledge that can inform healthy food choices (Fig. 5-2).

Dissect the food label by starting from the top with the serving size and the number of servings per container. In general, serving sizes are standardized so that consumers can compare similar products. All of the nutrient amounts listed on the food label are for one serving. Thus, it is important to determine how many servings an individual actually consumes to accurately assess nutrient intake. Next, look at the calories, which indicate how much energy a person gets from a particular food. This part of the nutrition label is the most important factor for weight control. In general, 40 calories per serving is considered low, 100 is moderate, and 400 or more is high.[4] The next two sections of the label note the nutrient content of the food product. Values are based on a 2,000-calorie per day diet for adults and children older than age 4, though many athletes require more, and more sedentary individuals require less. Clients should try to minimize intake of the first three nutrients listed:

- Fat (in particular saturated and trans fat): Clients on a 2,000 calorie per day diet should aim for a total per day of ≤ 65 g of total fat and ≤ 20 g of saturated fat
- Cholesterol: Goal of ≤ 300 mg
- Sodium: Goal of ≤ 2,300 mg

Clients should aim to consume adequate amounts of protein (50 g), total carbohydrate (300 g), fiber (goal of ≥ 25 g), vitamin A (goal of ≥ 5,000 IU), vitamin C (goal of ≥ 60 mg), calcium (goal of ≥ 1,000 mg), and iron (goal of ≥ 18 mg for women ages 19 to 50 who are not pregnant or lactating; goals are less for males and younger and older females). Amounts will vary based on the client's calorie needs (see Box 5-2). Additional considerations should be made for athletes. For example, many athletes may require more than 2,300 mg of sodium because they lose more from sweat.

The **daily values** (DVs) are recommended levels of intake for nutrients. The DVs shown in the footnote on the label are for a 2,000- or 2,500-calorie diet. The **percent daily values** (PDVs) listed on the label are percentages based on a 2,000-calorie diet of the recommended intake for key nutrients. In general, 5% daily value or less is considered low, while 20% daily value or more

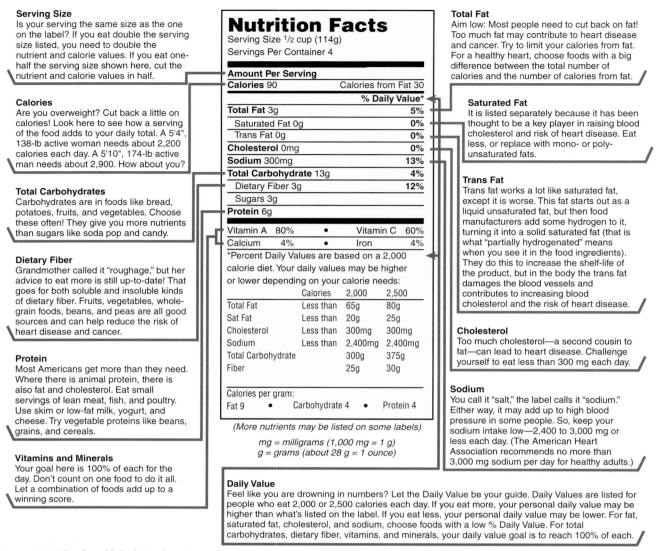

Serving Size
Is your serving the same size as the one on the label? If you eat double the serving size listed, you need to double the nutrient and calorie values. If you eat one-half the serving size shown here, cut the nutrient and calorie values in half.

Calories
Are you overweight? Cut back a little on calories! Look here to see how a serving of the food adds to your daily total. A 5'4", 138-lb active woman needs about 2,200 calories each day. A 5'10", 174-lb active man needs about 2,900. How about you?

Total Carbohydrates
Carbohydrates are in foods like bread, potatoes, fruits, and vegetables. Choose these often! They give you more nutrients than sugars like soda pop and candy.

Dietary Fiber
Grandmother called it "roughage," but her advice to eat more is still up-to-date! That goes for both soluble and insoluble kinds of dietary fiber. Fruits, vegetables, whole-grain foods, beans, and peas are all good sources and can help reduce the risk of heart disease and cancer.

Protein
Most Americans get more than they need. Where there is animal protein, there is also fat and cholesterol. Eat small servings of lean meat, fish, and poultry. Use skim or low-fat milk, yogurt, and cheese. Try vegetable proteins like beans, grains, and cereals.

Vitamins and Minerals
Your goal here is 100% of each for the day. Don't count on one food to do it all. Let a combination of foods add up to a winning score.

Nutrition Facts
Serving Size 1/2 cup (114g)
Servings Per Container 4

Amount Per Serving	
Calories 90	Calories from Fat 30
	% Daily Value*
Total Fat 3g	**5%**
Saturated Fat 0g	**0%**
Trans Fat 0g	**0%**
Cholesterol 0mg	**0%**
Sodium 300mg	**13%**
Total Carbohydrate 13g	**4%**
Dietary Fiber 3g	**12%**
Sugars 3g	
Protein 6g	

Vitamin A	80%	Vitamin C	60%
Calcium	4%	Iron	4%

*Percent Daily Values are based on a 2,000 calorie diet. Your daily values may be higher or lower depending on your calorie needs:

	Calories	2,000	2,500
Total Fat	Less than	65g	80g
Sat Fat	Less than	20g	25g
Cholesterol	Less than	300mg	300mg
Sodium	Less than	2,400mg	2,400mg
Total Carbohydrate		300g	375g
Fiber		25g	30g

Calories per gram:
Fat 9 • Carbohydrate 4 • Protein 4

(More nutrients may be listed on some labels)

mg = milligrams (1,000 mg = 1 g)
g = grams (about 28 g = 1 ounce)

Total Fat
Aim low: Most people need to cut back on fat! Too much fat may contribute to heart disease and cancer. Try to limit your calories from fat. For a healthy heart, choose foods with a big difference between the total number of calories and the number of calories from fat.

Saturated Fat
It is listed separately because it has been thought to be a key player in raising blood cholesterol and risk of heart disease. Eat less, or replace with mono- or poly-unsaturated fats.

Trans Fat
Trans fat works a lot like saturated fat, except it is worse. This fat starts out as a liquid unsaturated fat, but then food manufacturers add some hydrogen to it, turning it into a solid saturated fat (that is what "partially hydrogenated" means when you see it in the food ingredients). They do this to increase the shelf-life of the product, but in the body the trans fat damages the blood vessels and contributes to increasing blood cholesterol and the risk of heart disease.

Cholesterol
Too much cholesterol—a second cousin to fat—can lead to heart disease. Challenge yourself to eat less than 300 mg each day.

Sodium
You call it "salt," the label calls it "sodium." Either way, it may add up to high blood pressure in some people. So, keep your sodium intake low—2,400 to 3,000 mg or less each day. (The American Heart Association recommends no more than 3,000 mg sodium per day for healthy adults.)

Daily Value
Feel like you are drowning in numbers? Let the Daily Value be your guide. Daily Values are listed for people who eat 2,000 or 2,500 calories each day. If you eat more, your personal daily value may be higher than what's listed on the label. If you eat less, your personal daily value may be lower. For fat, saturated fat, cholesterol, and sodium, choose foods with a low % Daily Value. For total carbohydrates, dietary fiber, vitamins, and minerals, your daily value goal is to reach 100% of each.

Figure 5-2. The food label. At the time of publication of this text, the FDA is revising the food label to make it more useful for consumers. For information on the changes, go to www.fda.gov and search "nutrition facts label."

Box 5-2. Calculating Caloric Value

Each of the three macronutrients has a per gram caloric value:
Carbohydrate = 4 Calories/gram
Protein = 4 Calories/gram
Fat = 9 Calories/gram

These values can be used to calculate the caloric value of a specific amount of food. For example, a 5-gram portion of sugar (the approximate amount in 1 teaspoon) contains 20 calories (5 multiplied by 4). A teaspoon of oil contains about 5 grams of fat, or 45 calories (5 multiplied by 9). These calculations can also be used when reading a food label. If a food label reads that there are 10 grams of protein per serving, there are 40 calories from protein.

These values can also be used to calculate the percent macronutrient content. For example, if a serving of food contains 250 calories per serving, with 10 grams of total carbohydrates, it can be determined that there are 40 calories from carbohydrate (10 multiplied by 4). By then dividing this value by the total calorie value (40 divided by 250), this serving of food is 16% carbohydrate.

is considered high for all nutrients.[4] PDVs are listed for key nutrients to facilitate product comparisons (just make sure that the serving sizes are similar), nutrient content claims (does a reduced sugar cereal contain less carbohydrates than the original cereal?), and dietary tradeoffs (balance consumption of a high-fat product for lunch with lower fat products throughout the rest of the day).

Individuals who need more or less calories than those shown on the label should adjust recommendations accordingly. For example, 3 grams of fat provides 5% of the recommended amount for someone on a 2,000-calorie diet and 7% for someone on a 1,500-calorie diet. The footnote also includes daily values for nutrients to limit (total fat, saturated fat, trans fat, cholesterol, sodium), recommended carbohydrate intake for a 2,000-calorie diet (60% of calories), and minimal fiber recommendations for 2,000- and 2,500-calorie diets.

Legislation requires food manufacturers to list all potential food allergens on food packaging. The most common food allergens are fish, shellfish, soybean, wheat, egg, milk, peanuts, and tree nuts. This information usually is included near the list of ingredients on the package. Note that the ingredient list is in decreasing order of substance weight in the product. That is, the ingredients that are listed first are the most abundant ingredients in the product. Try to avoid foods with sugar, high fructose corn syrup, bleached flour, or partially hydrogenated oils near the top of the list.

While the food label is found on the side or the back of products, myriad health and nutrition claims are visibly displayed on the front of the box. The FDA closely regulates these claims, which must meet strict criteria.

SPEED BUMP

4. Locate a food with a nutrition label. Dissect the label to determine the total number of calories; calories from fat, protein, and carbohydrates; and overall nutritional value of a product based on the nutritional information, including percent daily values and ingredient list.

FOOD SAFETY AND SELECTION

Though the federal government plays a prominent role in protecting consumers from food-related illness, the system is not without fail. Foodborne illnesses strike 76 million unsuspecting Americans each year, causing 325,000 hospitalizations and 5,000 deaths.[5] While some infections result from consumer errors in storage and preparation, outbreaks expose holes in the U.S. food safety system.

In the United States, food safety oversight is divided primarily among three agencies: the USDA regulates meat, poultry, and eggs; the **Food and Drug Administration** oversees produce and seafood; and the **Centers for Disease Control and Prevention** gathers statistics to monitor the progression of outbreaks. The CDC also publishes educational materials to help prevent future outbreaks. In January 2013, President Obama signed the Food Safety Modernization Act, the first revision to some national food safety standards in over 70 years. Many of the new laws in this act implement standards for the produce industry. Due to limitations in the government's authority to mandate recalls and force changes, and limitations in government resources and personnel, contaminated food frequently makes it into the food supply. For these reasons, consumers need to be educated and take proper precautions with food selection and preparation.

Foodborne Illnesses

The health consequences from exposure to contaminated food range from asymptomatic to deadly. In general, signs and symptoms of foodborne illness may include abdominal pain, nausea, vomiting, diarrhea, and dehydration. In some cases, symptoms can become severe, requiring hospitalization. Treatment methods for foodborne infections can also vary, but one of the most important treatments is rehydration to replace fluid loss. Special populations most at-risk include pregnant women, infants and young children, older adults, and people who are immunocompromised. Table 5-3 describes the most common foodborne illnesses, their symptoms, and how they are usually treated.

Reducing Exposure to Foodborne Illnesses

While no consumer can fully protect his or her family from exposure to foodborne illness, several precautions help to reduce risk. From choosing wisely at the grocery store to safe food preparation and storage, consumers can exert some control in stamping out foodborne contamination. Following are a few tips for consumers to keep in mind when selecting foods:

- Check produce for bruises and punctures, either may allow for contamination.
- Look for a sell-by date for breads and baked goods, a use-by date on some packaged foods, an expiration date on yeast and baking powder, and a pack date on canned and some packaged foods. While some foods are good for a few days after the sell-by or expiration date, play it safe by choosing the product with the latest date. Use the product well before its marked expiration.
- Make sure packaged goods are not torn, and cans are not dented, cracked, or bulging. Dented cans may indicate the presence of botulism. Bulging cans may indicate the food is contaminated.
- Separate fish and poultry from other purchases by wrapping them separately in plastic bags. Once home, prevent leakage and cross contamination. Store these foods away from produce and other ready to eat foods. Even though these products will later be cooked to a safe temperature to kill bacteria, other uncooked contaminated foods can harbor the infection.
- When shopping, choose refrigerated and frozen foods last. Try to make sure all perishable items are refrigerated within 1 hour of purchase. Microorganisms stop or greatly reduce the rate of growth at freezing or cold temperatures. However, once the products start to warm, the bacteria rapidly multiply.

Consumers may also want to note where the product was processed and packaged. All beef, lamb, pork, fish, shellfish, perishable agricultural commodities,

Table 5-3. **Common Foodborne Illnesses (From Most to Least Common)**

PATHOGEN	FOOD SOURCE	SYMPTOMS	TREATMENT	PREVENTION
Salmonella	Raw poultry, eggs, beef, unwashed fruit and vegetables	Fever, diarrhea, abdominal cramps, and headache lasting 4–7 days.	None needed usually.	Avoid raw eggs, beef, and poultry. Wash produce before eating.
Campylobacter	Raw poultry, fresh produce, unpasteurized milk products	Crampy abdominal pain, watery diarrhea, fever 2–4 days after exposure.	Replace electrolytes and fluids.	Cook foods well and practice good hygiene.
Shigella	Fecal-oral route (food, toys, restroom surfaces)	Abdominal pain and cramping; watery diarrhea with blood or mucus; fever; nausea, vomiting.	Replace electrolytes and fluids.	Good hand hygiene.
Cryptosporidium	Contaminated water	Diarrhea (may last for up to a month).	Replace electrolytes and fluids.	Good hand hygiene.
E. Coli 0157:H7	Undercooked beef, bean sprouts, fresh leafy vegetables	Severe bloody diarrhea and abdominal cramps 3–4 days after exposure. Can cause hemolytic uremic syndrome in kids.[a]	Do not use antibiotics; hospitalization may be necessary. Can be fatal.	Change in slaughter operations for cattle.
E. Coli non-0157:H7	Contaminated water, salad, raw seafood, undercooked meat	Profuse watery diarrhea, abdominal cramping.	Replace electrolytes and fluids.	Avoid potentially contaminated foods when traveling abroad.
Yersinia	Raw or undercooked pork	Most common in young children: fever, abdominal pain, and bloody diarrhea 4–7 days after exposure.	Antibiotics in severe cases.	Avoid undercooked pork; practice good hygiene.
Vibrio	Oysters	Watery diarrhea with cramping, nausea, vomiting, fever, chills.	Replace electrolytes and fluids.	Cook seafood thoroughly.
Listeria	Meat, cheese, milk, poultry, seafood	None in healthy individuals including pregnant women; meningitis in immune-deficient and neonates.	Antibiotics	Avoid unpasteurized products. Heat until steaming. Wash produce. Avoid rare meat and seafood.
Cyclospora	Contaminated water or food	Watery, explosive diarrhea.	Antibiotics	Avoid contaminated water.
Staph Aureus[b]	Desserts, salads, baked goods, products with mayonnaise	Quick onset nausea, vomiting, diarrhea, and bloating.	Replacement of fluids and electrolytes.	Frequent handwashing. Refrigerate leftovers within 2 hours.

Table 5-3. Common Foodborne Illnesses (From Most to Least Common)—cont'd

PATHOGEN	FOOD SOURCE	SYMPTOMS	TREATMENT	PREVENTION
Botulism[b]	Canned food; honey in children < 1yr	Double vision, blurred vision, drooping eyelids, slurred speech, difficulty swallowing, dry mouth, and muscle weakness.	Antitoxin; hospitalization. Can be fatal.	Avoid home canning. Avoid food in dented or bulging cans.

a. Hemolytic-uremic syndrome is a potentially life-threatening condition that is usually treated in an intensive care unit. Blood transfusions and kidney dialysis are often required. Per CDC data, with intensive care, the death rate for hemolytic uremic syndrome is 3% to 5%.
b. Staph Aureus and Botulism incidence data were not collected by the CDC FoodNet.
Source: Centers for Disease Control and Prevention. FoodNet Surveillance; www.cdc.gov/foodnet/surveillance.htm. Accessed July 16, 2011.

including fresh and frozen fruits and vegetables, and peanuts and other nuts, must be labeled with their country of origin. The information can be printed on a food label or displayed on a placard in the grocery store. Processed and cooked foods are exempt from country of origin labeling (COOL), thus restaurants and other food service establishments are not required to label their foods.

The 2010 *Dietary Guidelines for Americans* include an appendix devoted to food safety. The guidelines offer several simple steps to safe food handling that are critical to reduce exposure to foodborne illness. Additional information can be found at www.fightbac.org.

- Wash hands often with warm water and soap for at least 20 seconds. This is the single most important defense to reduce risk of microbial infection.
- Clean hands, food contact surfaces, and fruits and vegetables. To prevent cross contamination, meat and poultry should *not* be washed or rinsed.
- Separate raw, cooked, and ready-to-eat foods while shopping, preparing, or storing foods.
- Cook foods to a safe temperature to kill microorganisms (bacteria grow most rapidly between the temperatures of 40°F and 140°F). Pregnant women and people over age 65 should only eat deli meats that have been reheated to steaming hot to reduce risk of infection. Frankfurters must be cooked to a safe internal temperature (typically 160°F).
- Refrigerate perishable food within 2 hours (on a hot day over 90°F within 1 hour) and defrost foods properly. Eat refrigerated leftovers within 3 to 4 days. Remember, when in doubt, throw it out.
- Avoid raw (unpasteurized) milk or any products made from unpasteurized milk, soft cheeses, raw or partially cooked eggs or foods containing raw eggs, raw or undercooked meat and poultry, raw fish, unpasteurized juice, and raw sprouts. This is especially important for infants and young children, pregnant women, older adults, and those who are immunocompromised.

While food safety lapses higher in the production scale may allow a contaminated food product into the marketplace, adhering to these recommendations makes it less likely that the microbe will have the opportunity to cause an infection.

SPEED BUMP

5. List several important food safety principles when selecting, storing, and preparing food.

NUTRITION POLICY

Food safety regulations are just one area where federal government food policy can significantly affect health outcomes. Nutrition policy from the dietary guidelines and MyPlate, to ordinances and regulations that shape food choices and sales, may also play an important role in setting the stage for Americans to adopt a healthier lifestyle.

As Americans have continued to eat more and become more sedentary, countless health professionals, including nutrition and fitness experts, have focused on inspiring healthful change one individual at a time. Unfortunately, adherence to healthful eating habits and regular physical activity programs has been poor. This is not necessarily due to a lack of willpower and motivation, but more to an environment that discourages many health-promoting behaviors. Consider the following: there are 3,800 calories available in the food supply for each person daily (the average American needs only 2,350 calories); most Americans eat at least one-third of their calories away from home; and 90% of Saturday morning cartoon food ads—watched by highly impressionable youngsters—are for sugar- and fat-laden junk food.[6] Modern conveniences such as remote controls, elevators, car washes, washing machines, leaf blowers, and drive-through windows rob us of expending about 8,800 calories per month; that adds up to about 2.5 pounds of fat.[7]

A commentary published in the *Journal of the American Medical Association* (*JAMA*) outlined several policy strategies that may be effective in helping to increase nutrition and physical activity habits on a population-level and, hopefully, reduce obesity rates and improve health:[8]

- **Taxation.** *Imposing higher taxes on calorie-dense and nutrient-poor foods might lower consumption of unhealthy foods and generate revenue to subsidize healthful foods.* Politicians have long debated whether adding an "obesity tax" on non-diet sodas and other sugar-sweetened beverages might generate tax revenue and decrease unhealthy habits.
- **Food prohibitions.** *Removing harmful ingredients from the food supply eliminates their health risk.* New York City was the first U.S. city to impose a trans-fat ban in all restaurants; soon after, other cities and states followed suit. In 2013, the FDA recommended complete elimination of trans fats in the food supply.
- **Regulation of food marketing to children and adolescents.** *Restricting food advertising during children's programs, counter-advertising to promote good nutrition and physical activity, limiting use of cartoon characters, and other regulations may help protect children who are unable to critically evaluate advertisements.* The role of food advertisements in the epidemic of childhood obesity has been well studied. The charge to eliminate unhealthy food ads in children's programming has been a source of ongoing debate.
- **School policies.** *Many school districts already have removed vending machines, provided healthier menus, and offered more physical activity opportunities for school children. However, much work remains to be done.* Over the past few years, several policies have helped make the school environment healthier. The task of aligning the school nutrition and activity environment with the government recommendations for optimal nutrition and health is underway. All public schools are required to have a school wellness committee and adhere to a school wellness policy. Many school programs are incorporating more nutrition education into curriculums. Efforts are also being made to establish school gardens and farm-to-school programs to help increase fruit and vegetable consumption.
- **The "built" environment.** *Zoning laws to limit the number of fast-food restaurants, expand recreational facilities, and encourage healthier lifestyles would increase the ability for people to live and play healthfully, especially in poor neighborhoods where access to parks and healthy foods is severely limited.* As zoning and development are under the jurisdiction of local governments, individual community members and leaders must step up to help change from an environment that fosters poor diet and inactivity to one that fosters a healthy lifestyle and sense of community.
- **Disclosure.** *Restaurants and manufacturers could be required to disclose nutritional content and health warnings so that consumers may make more informed decisions.* An increasing number of states and jurisdictions require chain restaurants to provide calorie counts and nutritional information on restaurant menus and menu boards.
- **Tort liability.** *Lawsuits against companies such as fast-food giants for selling "unreasonably hazardous" products might force companies to offer healthier alternatives and provide accurate information.* Legal and financial repercussions may also inspire some large food giants to be more discriminating in their health claims. Since 2002, the FDA has allowed **qualified health claims** (claims linking a food substance to prevention of a disease) on food labels for products that have a basis of scientific evidence to support the claim. While many food companies push the limits, several have received sanctioning letters from the FDA. For example, POM Wonderful, a pomegranate juice company, received a violation letter for claiming that the juice will treat, prevent, or cure disease such as diabetes, hypertension, and cancer. These types of claims are not allowed on food products. Spectrum Organic Products was sanctioned for making nutrient claims such as "cholesterol free" and "less saturated fat than butter" without meeting the legal requirements for those claims.[9]

  Companies also inappropriately use **structure-function claims** in promoting a food's benefits. Structure-function claims describe a way in which the food purportedly affects a body structure or function (such as "calcium builds strong bones"). For example, the **Federal Trade Commission** sanctioned Kellogg's for claiming that Frosted Mini-Wheats was "clinically shown to improve kids' attentiveness by 20%" and then later for claiming that Rice Krispies cereal "now helps support your child's immunity."[9]
- **Surveillance.** *Similar to how health departments monitor infectious disease, states could monitor chronic diseases such as diabetes.* New York City has led the way in adopting surveillance measures to monitor the health and nutrition status of its residents. The New York City Health and Nutrition Examination Survey randomly sampled residents to undergo a physical examination, clinical and laboratory tests, and interview.[10] Results revealed that the prevalence of diabetes and pre-diabetes is higher than expected, with more than one-third of New Yorkers with abnormal glucose levels.[10] In an effort to further improve surveillance and management of diabetes, the New York City A1C Registry was started. The registry collects hemoglobin A1C results (a measure of blood sugar control) from city laboratories; sends quarterly reports of patients' A1C level to their providers; and reminds patients to follow up with their providers.

- **"Training" Communities.** A commentary published in *JAMA* offers three strategies to improve the health of communities: (1) consider individuals within the larger social, economic, and cultural context; (2) form partnerships; and (3) influence larger political and policy debates.[11] Interventions that focus on changing physical activity behavior through building, strengthening, and maintaining social networks are highly effective in increasing physical activity and overall physical fitness.[12]

Health professionals are ideally positioned to inspire lasting improvements in health. Efforts that extend beyond working with individuals to incorporate social, community, environmental, and political change will go a long way in helping to make a physically active lifestyle the norm (Box 5-3).

SPEED BUMP

6. Describe four ways that allied health professionals can get involved to shape policy and advocate for healthier lifestyles.

Box 5-3. Shaping Policy: A Primer for Health Professionals

Health professionals are in a position to advocate for local, state, and federal initiatives and policies that encourage increased physical activity and health. By working with schools, advocacy agencies, the media, and elected officials, you can reach "clients" far beyond the confines of an office, gym, or playing field. Here are a few ways you can get started:

- Join an advocacy organization such as the National Coalition for the Promotion of Physical Activity (ncppa.org) or Action for Healthy Kids (afhk.org). These organizations will keep you up to date with the latest relevant legislation and make it easy for you to voice your concerns to your local legislators.
- Start or join a local obesity prevention or physical activity coalition. Work together with other interested stakeholders to influence activity-promoting changes in your local community.
- Complete advocacy training to learn how to become optimally effective in sharing your message and inspiring change.
- Learn about resources in your community that promote, encourage, or inspire physical activity.
- Become a resource in your community. Coach a local team, offer a few sessions of pro bono exercise training to low-income clients, or work with your local parks and recreation organization to secure resources to build a walking trail in an underserved community.
- Speak up. Lobby your local, state, and federal representatives to pass bills that will promote physically active lifestyles, or oppose bills that will cut funding or support for healthy nutrition and optimal fitness and recreation.
- Write a letter to the editor in support of local efforts to improve physical activity.
- Write articles for newsletters or magazines that provide information and education about physical activity.
- Live it. Be physically active every day and share your passion for healthy eating and exercise and activity with anyone who will listen.

CHAPTER SUMMARY

The federal government plays a large role in researching and understanding the major components of an optimal diet, promoting an optimal eating plan, developing food policy agendas, regulating the safety and quality of the food supply, and funding nutritional programs. While athletes may have specific nutritional needs compared to the general population, a thorough understanding of federal dietary recommendations gives health professionals a basis from which to make general nutrition recommendations while staying within one's professional scope of practice.

KEY POINTS SUMMARY

1. The 2010 *Dietary Guidelines for Americans* emphasize balancing calories to maintain a healthy weight; decrease intake of solid fats (saturated and trans fats), cholesterol, sugar, and to consume alcohol in moderation; increase fruits and vegetables, whole grains, low-fat dairy, lean protein and seafood; adopt an overall healthy eating plan; and help to create a healthier environment that supports optimal nutrition and physical activity.
2. Overall, MyPlate encourages Americans to balance caloric intake and control portion sizes; make half of their plate fruits and vegetables; make the other half of their plate protein and grains (preferably whole grains); choose 1% or fat-free milk; choose foods low in salt and saturated and trans fat; and drink water instead of sugary drinks.
3. Recommended nutrient intake is based upon reference values known as Dietary Reference Intakes. The most commonly used DRI is the RDA, which is the amount of nutrient known to be adequate to meet the nutritional needs of nearly all healthy persons.

4. The Nutrition Facts Panel provides consumers important information to help make healthy nutrition decisions. Understanding how to interpret and evaluate the food label is a critical skill that health professionals should not only master but also be able to teach to clients.
5. When evaluating a food label, remember that there are 4 calories per gram of protein and carbohydrate and 9 calories per gram of fat. A food with a percent of daily value greater than 20% for any given nutrient is considered to be an "excellent source" of that nutrient.
6. Vigilance in choosing, storing, and preparing foods in a safe manner is essential to help prevent foodborne illness. Try to refrigerate foods within 1 hour of purchase and store leftovers within 2 hours of preparation. Keep leftovers in the refrigerator no longer than 4 days.
7. Consider potential social, community, environmental, and political changes when considering ways in which to help facilitate increased nutrition habits and physical activity.

PRACTICAL APPLICATIONS

1. The 2010 *Dietary Guidelines for Americans* emphasize balancing caloric intake with caloric expenditure to maintain a healthy weight. If your 22-year-old female client (5′4″ and 125 pounds) burns 500 calories per workout and exercises 5 days per week, about how many calories does she need each day to maintain her weight?
   A. 1,800
   B. 2,000
   C. 2,200
   D. 2,400
2. Dave is a 20-year-old lacrosse player who recently underwent a comprehensive nutrition evaluation. He says the evaluation helped him realize that he goes out to eat too frequently. If he is like the typical American, which nutrients is Dave most likely to consume in insufficient amounts?
   A. Sodium, potassium, iron, and vitamin C
   B. Calcium, fiber, protein, and vitamin D
   C. Protein, fiber, essential fatty acids, and calcium
   D. Potassium, fiber, calcium, and vitamin D
3. Based on a 2,000-calorie diet, how many servings of fruits and vegetable should Americans eat according to MyPlate?
   A. 3 to 5 servings per day (1.5 to 2.5 cups)
   B. At least 5 servings per day (2.5 cups)
   C. 9 servings per day (4.5 cups)
   D. 11 servings per day (5.5 cups)
4. Which of the following dinner plates most resembles the MyPlate ideal?
   A. Mixed vegetable primavera with whole grain pasta, an orange, sliced grilled chicken breast, and a glass of skim milk
   B. Beef tacos with shredded lettuce, tomato, and cheese, a glass of water, and fruit Jello
   C. Cheese pizza, a small dinner salad, and a glass of skim milk
   D. Baked salmon, brown rice, black beans, steamed broccoli, and a glass of water
5. You are working with a 45-year-old avid surfer. He asks you about how much vitamin B_6 he should eat to meet his nutritional needs. You look up the Dietary Reference Intakes for vitamin B_6. Which one of the DRIs should you tell him?
   A. Recommended Dietary Allowance
   B. Estimated Average Requirement
   C. Tolerable Upper Intake Level
   D. Adequate Intake
6. You are teaching a client to read the nutrition label. Together you are looking at the following label from a sports nutrition bar. As you analyze the contents you notice a few discrepancies in the reported nutrient composition and the nutrient composition based on the calculations you have been taught to use. Assuming that the number of grams of fat, carbohydrates, and protein on the label are accurate, what is the total calories and percentage of calories from fat, carbohydrates, and protein in the total package based on the calculations you learned?

Nutrition Facts	Amount/Serving	% DV*	Amount/Serving	% DV*	Amount/Serving	% DV*
Serv. Size 1 Bar (68g)	**Total Fat** 6g	9%	**Sodium** 180mg	8%	Insoluble Fiber 2g	
Calories 240	Sat. Fat 2.5g	13%	**Potassium** 180mg	5%	Sugars 22g	
Calories from Fat 50	Trans. Fat 0g		**Total Cab.** 43g	14%	Other Carb. 16g	
*Percent Daily Values (DV) are based on a 2,000 calorie diet.	**Cholest.** 0mg	0%	Dietary Fiber 5g	20%	**Protein** 10g	20%
	Vit. A 10%, Vit. C 50%, Calcium 25%, Iron 25%, Vit. D 10%, Vit. E 50%, Vit. K 25%, Thiamin (B1) 10%, Riboflavin (B2) 15%, Niacin (B3) 15%, Vit. B6 20%, Folate 20%, Vit. B12 15%, Biotin 10%, Pantothenic Acid 20%, Phosphorus 10%, Iodine 10%, Magnesium 10%, Zinc 10%, Selenium 10%, Copper 15%, Manganese 10%, Chromium 4%					

A. Total calories: 240, percentage of calories from fat: 20; percentage of calories from protein: 16; percentage of calories from carbohydrates: 70
B. Total calories: 265, percentage of calories from fat: 20, percentage of calories from protein: 15; percentage of calories from carbohydrates: 65
C. Total calories: 265, percentage of calories from fat: 20; percentage of calories from protein: 16; percentage of calories from carbohydrates: 70
D. Total calories: 240, percentage of calories from fat: 20; percentage of calories from protein 15; percentage of calories from carbohydrates: 65

7. Based on the nutrition label shown in question 6, this sports bar is an excellent source of which nutrients?
A. Calcium, iron, dietary fiber
B. Fat, carbohydrate, potassium
C. Calcium, iron, zinc
D. Vitamin C, vitamin E, and vitamin A

8. How long can you leave leftovers out of the refrigerator before microorganism growth may become high enough to cause infection?
A. 2 hours
B. 3 hours
C. 4 hours
D. 5 hours

9. What is the best treatment for most foodborne illnesses that cause multiple bouts of diarrhea and/or vomiting?
A. Antibiotics
B. Rest
C. Rehydration
D. Over-the-counter medicine

10. You are the coach of a little league baseball team. The local ice cream shop is your team sponsor. As a perk they offer free ice cream cones for the whole team for every game that your team wins. While you are grateful for their support, you wish that the kids weren't rewarded with unhealthy food and wish instead that healthy snacks were provided for the team. After talking with several of the other coaches, you learn that their team sponsors are mostly fast-food restaurants that provide free meal coupons for the kids. What should you do to help the children to have healthier snacks and reduce incentives to eat unhealthy foods?
A. Tell the ice cream shop to stop providing the free ice cream cones because it is contributing to the childhood obesity epidemic.
B. Ask the little league leadership to ban food rewards and incentives effective immediately, as these practices promote an unhealthy relationship with food.
C. Ask the little league leadership to stop accepting sponsorship from food companies, as it unduly influences eating preferences in kids.
D. Ask other coaches, parents, and little league leadership to join a coalition whose goal is to explore the best ways to promote healthy nutrition for the players.

Case 1: Brian, the High School Basketball Player

Brian is a 15-year-old high school basketball player. He is 6′2″ and 180 pounds. His mom feels that he needs to eat a better diet. She goes to the choosemyplate.gov website and prints out his ideal eating plan:

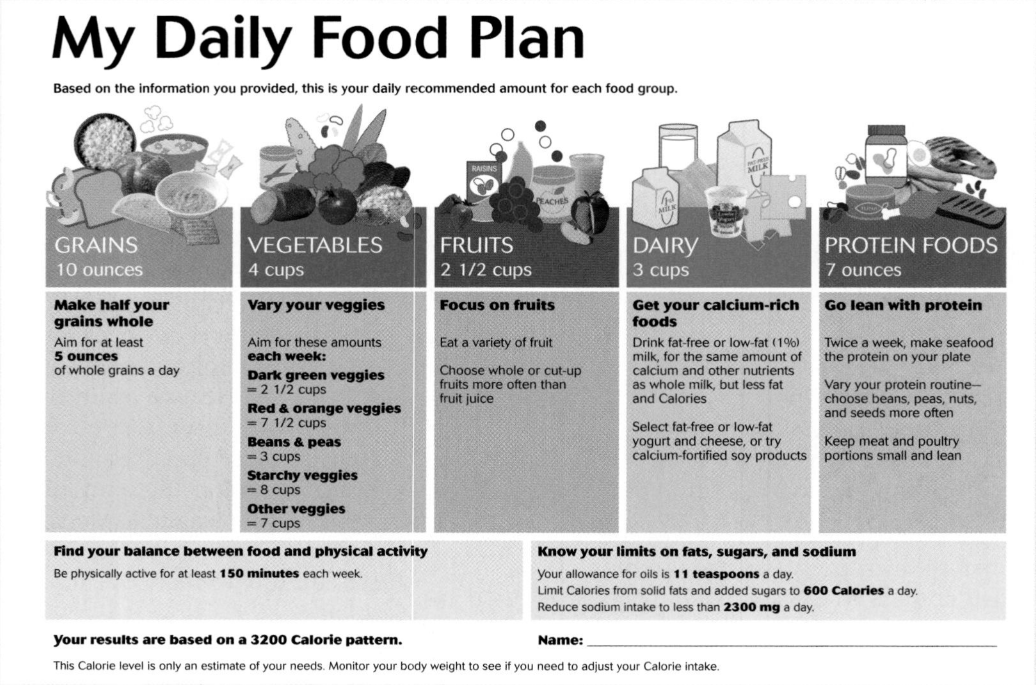

My Daily Food Plan

Based on the information you provided, this is your daily recommended amount for each food group.

GRAINS 10 ounces	VEGETABLES 4 cups	FRUITS 2 1/2 cups	DAIRY 3 cups	PROTEIN FOODS 7 ounces
Make half your grains whole Aim for at least **5 ounces** of whole grains a day	**Vary your veggies** Aim for these amounts **each week:** **Dark green veggies** = 2 1/2 cups **Red & orange veggies** = 7 1/2 cups **Beans & peas** = 3 cups **Starchy veggies** = 8 cups **Other veggies** = 7 cups	**Focus on fruits** Eat a variety of fruit Choose whole or cut-up fruits more often than fruit juice	**Get your calcium-rich foods** Drink fat-free or low-fat (1%) milk, for the same amount of calcium and other nutrients as whole milk, but less fat and Calories Select fat-free or low-fat yogurt and cheese, or try calcium-fortified soy products	**Go lean with protein** Twice a week, make seafood the protein on your plate Vary your protein routine—choose beans, peas, nuts, and seeds more often Keep meat and poultry portions small and lean

Find your balance between food and physical activity
Be physically active for at least **150 minutes** each week.

Know your limits on fats, sugars, and sodium
Your allowance for oils is **11 teaspoons** a day.
Limit Calories from solid fats and added sugars to **600 Calories** a day.
Reduce sodium intake to less than **2300 mg** a day.

Your results are based on a 3200 Calorie pattern.

Name: ____________________

This Calorie level is only an estimate of your needs. Monitor your body weight to see if you need to adjust your Calorie intake.

Brian's mom has asked you to help them figure out how to convert this recommendation into a reasonable eating plan.*

1. Put together a potential 1-day eating plan for Brian that fulfills the nutritional needs described above. Include breakfast, lunch, dinner, and two snacks. (Note: You can divide the Daily Food Plan into food groups and don't necessarily have to list specific food items. For example, breakfast might be 2 ounces of grains, 1 cup of fruit, and 1 cup of dairy.)

   Breakfast:

   Snack:

   Lunch:

   Snack:

   Dinner:

   What was the most difficult component to developing Brian's eating plan? What special considerations would you need to keep in mind in helping to develop an eating plan for a competitive athlete?

2. Brian's mom reports to you that she is having a difficult time getting Brian to cut out the fast foods and eat an overall healthier and more balanced diet. What strategies might you suggest to help her?
3. Apply the social-ecological model to describe a potential large-scale environmental change that could make it easier for Brian to eat healthier.

*Note: This activity is intended to explore concepts from the chapter. Meal planning is outside the scope of practice of a non-registered dietitian or licensed nutritionist.

Case 2: Adele, the Active Octogenarian

Adele is an 85-year-old woman who is relatively new to physical activity. After her husband died last year she committed to a fitness program to help her maintain her independence. She participates in water fitness classes 5 days per week, weight trains with a personal trainer 2 hours per week, and attends yoga for 1 hour 2 days per week. Her doctor recently diagnosed her with hypertension and told her that she needs to eat a DASH diet.

1. Put together a potential 1-day eating plan for Adele based on the DASH diet described in Table 5-2. More detailed information about the DASH diet can be found at www.nhlbi.nih.gov/health/health-topics/topics/dash/followdash.html#footnotea and www.nhlbi.nih.gov/health/public/heart/hbp/dash/new_dash.pdf.
   Breakfast:
   Snack:
   Lunch:
   Snack:
   Dinner:

The eating plan shown in Table 5-2 is based on a 2,000-calorie diet. Adele tells you that she thinks that this will be far too much food for her. How might you advise her to modify the plan? Refer to Table 5-1.

2. How is the DASH Diet similar to the MyPlate eating plan? How is it different?
3. Adele tells you that she sometimes has a difficult time eating all of the leftovers before they go bad. She asks you how long she can keep leftovers in the refrigerator. In addition to answering this question, you decide to discuss overall food safety with her. What do you tell her? (Cover the highlights as if you are having a conversation with Adele; i.e., use lay terms and more simple terms.)

TRAIN YOURSELF

1. Go to supertracker.usda.gov and input your demographic information to receive an individualized meal plan based on the *Dietary Guidelines for Americans*. Develop an ideal 1-day meal plan divided among your typical meals and snacks.
2. Keep a record of all of the food and drink you consume for a 24-hour period on a typical day. Then, input this information into Supertracker for a summary of how your diet compares to your ideal diet.
3. How is your ideal MyPlate plan different from your typical eating habits? What are some barriers you experience in trying to eat according to the MyPlate guidelines? What are some strategies you could try to improve your eating habits? What are some large-scale policy strategies that, if implemented, would make it easier for you to eat healthier?

REFERENCES

1. U.S. Dept. of Agriculture. 2010 Dietary Guidelines for Americans backgrounder, history and process. Washington, DC: U.S. Dept. of Agriculture; 2010: http://purl.fdlp.gov/GPO/gpo4085.
2. Centers for Disease Control and Prevention. State Indicator Report on Fruits and Vegetables 2013.www.cdc.gov/nutrition/downloads/State-Indicator-Report-Fruits-Vegetables-2013.pdfAccessed January 19, 2014.
3. U.S. Department of Labor. Consumer expenditures in 2008. 2010; www.bls.gov/cex/csxann08.pdf. Accessed July 12, 2011.
4. U.S. Food and Drug Administration. How to use and understand the nutrition facts label. 2013. Available at www.fda.gov/food/resourcesforyou/consumers/nflpm/ucm274593.htm.
5. Mead PS, Slutsker L, Griffin PM, Tauxe RV. Food-related illness and death in the United States reply to Dr. Hedberg. *Emerg Infect Dis.* November 1999;5(6):841-842.
6. Center for Science in the Public Interest. Why it's hard to eat well and be active in America today. 2009; cspinet.org/nutritionpolicy/food_advertising.html. Accessed July 10, 2011.
7. Blair SN, Nichaman MZ. The public health problem of increasing prevalence rates of obesity and what should be done about it. *Mayo Clin Proc.* February 2002;77(2):109-113.
8. Gostin LO. Law as a tool to facilitate healthier lifestyles and prevent obesity. *JAMA.* January 3, 2007;297(1):87-90.
9. Government Accountability Office. *FDA Needs to Reassess Its Approach to Protecting Consumers from False or Misleading Claims;* 2011.
10. Thorpe LE, Upadhyay UD, Chamany S, et al. Prevalence and control of diabetes and impaired fasting glucose in New York City. *Diabetes Care.* January 2009;32(1):57-62.
11. Shortell SM, Swartzberg J. The physician as public health professional in the 21st century. *JAMA.* December 24 2008; 300(24):2916-2918.
12. Recommendations to increase physical activity in communities. *Am J Prev Med.* May 2002;22(4 Suppl):67-72.
13. U.S. Dept. of Agriculture. *Dietary Guidelines for Americans.* Available at: www.cnpp.usda.gov/DGAs2010-Policy Document.htm
14. Sofi F, Cesari F, Abbate R, Gensini GF, Casini A. Adherence to Mediterranean diet and health status: meta-analysis. *BMJ.* 2008;337:a1344.
15. Trichopoulou A, Costacou T, Bamia C, Trichopoulos D. Adherence to a Mediterranean diet and survival in a Greek population. *N Engl J Med.* Jun 26 2003;348(26):2599-2608.

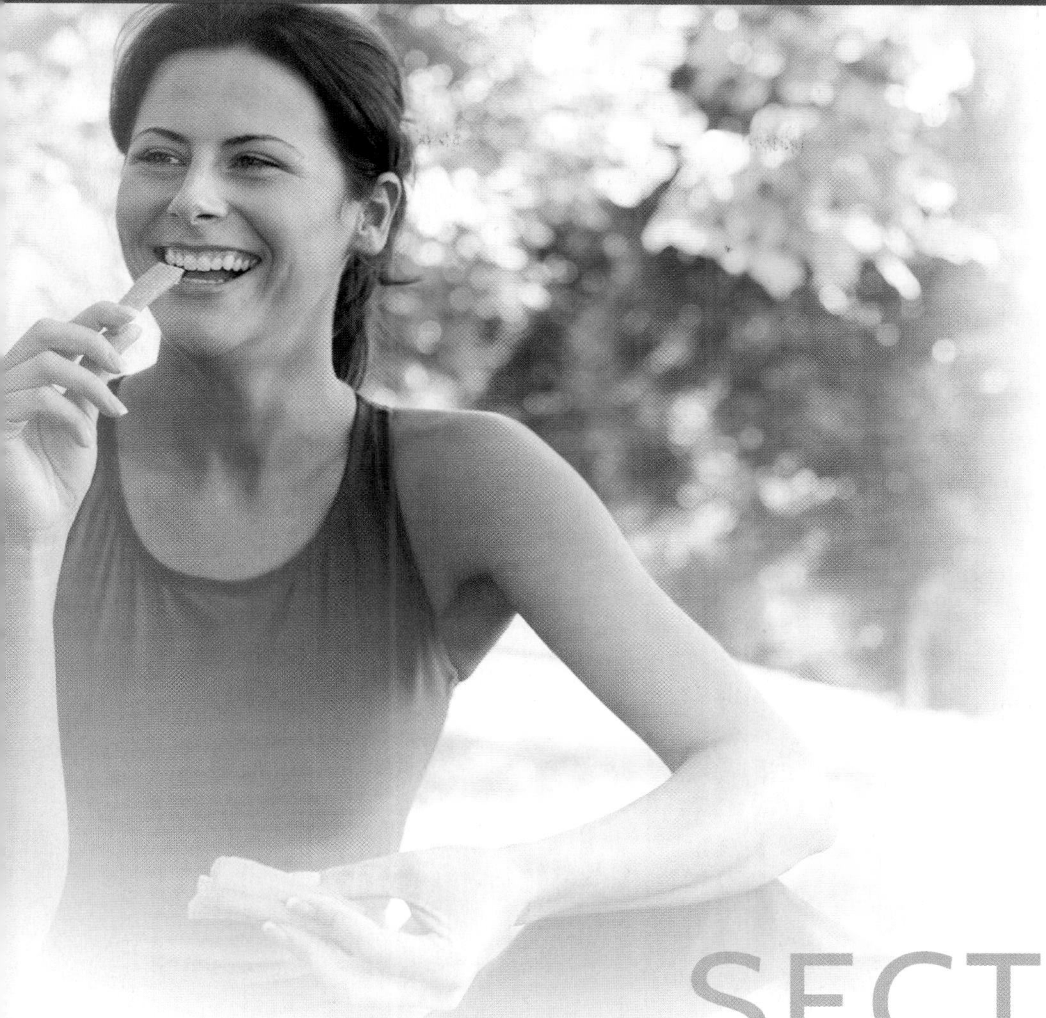

SECTION 2

Optimizing Sports Performance

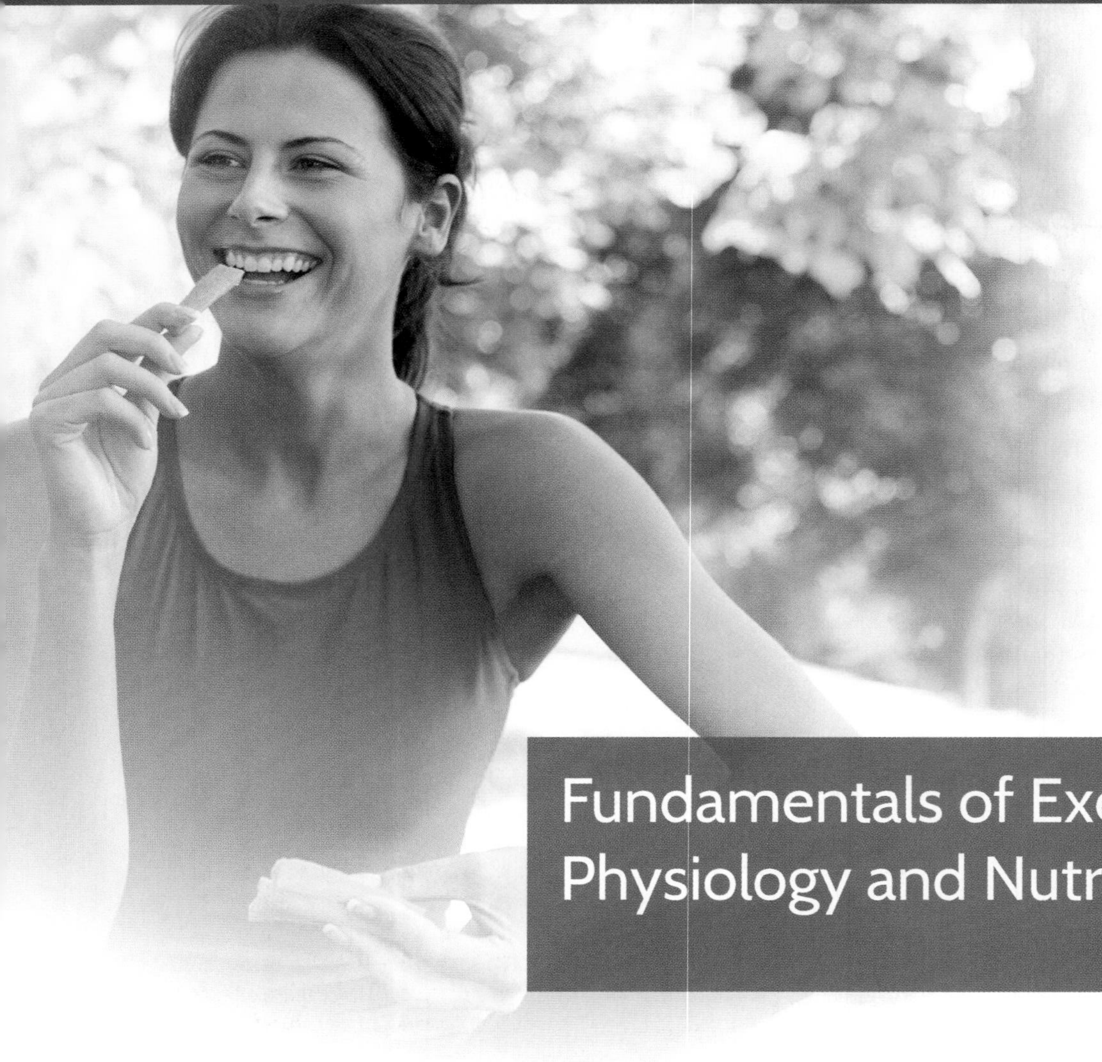

CHAPTER 6

Fundamentals of Exercise Physiology and Nutrition

CHAPTER OUTLINE

LEARNING OBJECTIVES

After studying this chapter, the reader should be able to:

6.1 Trace the pathway of a food starting with consumption and ending with usable energy.

6.2 Outline the metabolic pathways including the phosphagen system, anaerobic glycolysis, aerobic glycolysis, and fatty acid oxidation as they relate to exercise performance.

6.3 Explain how energy is stored in the skeletal muscles and other tissues, and how other nutrients are delivered via the digestion and absorption system.

6.4 Apply energy metabolism to design of nutrition strategies for active individuals and populations.

KEY TERMS

aerobic respiration The 10-step metabolic process of breaking glucose down to intermediate pyruvate, which is converted to acetyl-CoA and enters the citric acid cycle. Occurs in the mitochondria and cytoplasm in the presence of oxygen; produces a net 36 ATP.

anaerobic respiration The 10-step metabolic process of breaking glucose down to intermediate pyruvate and then lactic acid; occurs in the cytoplasm of cells; produces a net 2 ATP.

anaerobic threshold Point in exercise when lactate accumulation begins. Also known as *lactate threshold* or *ventilatory threshold*.

beta oxidation The process in which carbon fragments are removed from the fatty acid. These carbon molecules produce acetyl CoA, which enters the citric acid cycle and electron transport chain.

bioenergetics The process of studying the capture, conversion, and use of energy from ATP.

cardiac output (Q) The volume of blood pumped through the heart per minute (mL blood/min); calculated as stroke volume (mL blood/beat) × heart rate (beat/min).

citric acid cycle A metabolic pathway involved in the chemical conversion of carbohydrates, fats, and proteins into carbon dioxide and water to generate a form of usable energy. Also known as *Krebs cycle* and *tricarboxylic acid cycle*.

creatine phosphate An important source of stored energy; its breakdown to creatine plus a high-energy phosphate can rapidly fuel the first 5 to 10 seconds of exercise.

cross-bridge cycle The process whereby a series of molecular actions cause myosin and actin to interact and produce muscle contraction.

electron-transport chain The process of stripping NADH and FADH of their hydrogen molecules through a series of chemical reduction-oxidation reactions, which ultimately powers the conversion of ADP plus Pi to ATP and provides energy to the working cell.

excess post-exercise oxygen consumption (EPOC) The elevated oxygen consumption after high-intensity exercise has stopped.

flavin adenine dinucleotide (FADH) A hydrogen-carrying molecule that enters the electron transport chain to produce 2 ATPs per molecule of FADH.

gluconeogenesis The production of glucose from precursors in the liver.

glycolysis The process through which glucose is converted to pyruvate.

Krebs cycle See *citric acid cycle*.

lactate A salt of lactic acid produced in the body.

lactate threshold Point in exercise when lactate accumulation begins. Also known as *anaerobic threshold* or *ventilatory threshold*.

lactic acid A metabolic byproduct of anaerobic glucose metabolism.

lipogenesis The production of fat from excess carbohydrate, protein, or fat that is consumed beyond what the body immediately can use for energy, structural support, or glycogen storage.

mitochondria Organelles known as the "power plant" of the body's cells; the location where most ATP production occurs.

nicotinamide adenine dinucleotide (NADH) A hydrogen-carrying molecule that enters the electron transport chain to produce 3 ATPs per molecule of NADH.

oxidative phosphorylation Process in which energy from electrons passed through the electron transport chain is captured and stored to produce ATP.

oxygen-carrying capacity The body's ability to get the oxygen that is breathed in from the environment into the lungs and bloodstream; affected by two main factors: (1) the ability to adequately ventilate the alveoli in the lungs, and (2) hemoglobin concentration in the blood.

oxygen deficit Oxygen shortage in cells that occurs with anaerobic activity.

oxygen delivery The ability of the body to transport oxygen from the lungs to the mitochondria of the working cells; the amount delivered is a function of cardiac output.

oxygen extraction The ability to transfer oxygen from the blood to the working muscle cells.

pharynx The portion of the respiratory system extending from the base of the skull to the tip of the larynx and esophagus (the throat).

phosphagen system The energy system used when there is an immediate energy need, generally within the first 5 to 10 seconds of exercise. Utilizes creatine phosphate to produce ATP.

CALCULATIONS

Cardiac output (Q) = heart rate (HR) × stroke volume (SV)

VO_2 = cardiac output × avO_2 difference

VO_2 max = Q (CaO_2 (arterial oxygen content) 2 CvO_2 (venous oxygen content))

respiratory quotient (RQ) The amount of carbon dioxide, the end product of metabolism, produced by the body divided by the amount of oxygen consumed. Also called *respiratory exchange ratio*.

SAID principle Stands for "specific adaptation to imposed demands"; a training principle which describes that when the body is placed under stress it starts to make adaptations to improve the body's functioning in the future when it experiences that same stress.

stroke volume The amount of blood pumped out of the heart with each heart beat.

triacylglycerols Stored triglycerides (fats); compound consisting of three fatty acids and one glycerol molecule.

tricarboxylic acid cycle See *citric acid cycle*.

urea cycle A complex metabolic system that removes nitrogen from organic compounds and prepares the remaining nitrogenous structure (urea) for excretion in urine.

ventilatory threshold Point in exercise when lactate accumulation begins. Also known as *anaerobic threshold* or *lactate threshold*.

VO_2 max A measure of maximal oxygen uptake; liters of O_2 consumed per kilogram of body weight per minute.

INTRODUCTION

Kate is a 22-year-old recreational athlete. Marathon season is underway and Kate is intensifying her training in hopes of qualifying for the Boston Marathon. Kate has finished three marathons, but despite her best efforts she has yet to finish in the Boston-qualifying time of 3 hours 35 minutes. Her current personal record is 4 hours. With her prior training she focused exclusively on physical training and made no changes to her diet or eating habits. This time around, Kate wonders if application of basic sports nutrition principles might help shave 25 minutes off of her marathon time and give her the energy she needs to train for peak performance. In anticipation of a major dietary overhaul, she sets out to understand the relationship between sports nutrition and peak performance.

Most people understand eating a healthful diet is good for their bodies. However, what may be harder to comprehend is why certain foods are considered healthier than others or how different food groups work differently in the body. For instance, how does protein help build muscles, or why are carbohydrates the best energy source for endurance training?

By understanding the basics of nutrition, digestion, and absorption, the health professional will be better able to explain nutrition recommendations and suggestions, and answer questions clearly and with certainty for active individuals. This chapter focuses on nutrient digestion and absorption, and how consumption of food ultimately results in usable energy for the body. Further, metabolic systems such as the phosphagen system, anaerobic and aerobic glycolysis, and fatty acid oxidation as it relates to exercise performance, are explained. The foundation of biology, chemistry, biochemistry, and physiology will help the health professional to develop nutrition strategies for active individuals and populations.

THE DIGESTIVE SYSTEM

In addition to oxygen, which enters the body through the lungs and is transported to the cells of the body, the cells need a constant supply of nutrients to provide energy and perform metabolic functions. This energy can be obtained either from stored nutrients (e.g., stored fat, calcium from bones, glycogen) or from the breakdown of food through the digestive system. As discussed in earlier chapters, the gastrointestinal tract forms a long hollow tube from mouth to anus where digestion and absorption occur. It is made up of the mouth, esophagus, stomach, small intestine, large intestine, liver, gallbladder, and pancreas (see Fig. 1-1). With the first bite of food, the saliva and its digestive enzymes begin to digest and moisten the food. With swallowing, the food passes through the **pharynx** to enter the esophagus (the epiglottis prevents food from entering the trachea). Muscles in the esophagus push food to the stomach through a wave-like motion called peristalsis. The stomach mixes up the food, liquids, and its digestive juices to break food down into absorbable nutrients and energy. Next, the stomach empties its contents into the small intestine. The amount of time it takes for gastric emptying depends on the type of food (carbohydrates are emptied the fastest, followed by protein and then fat), amount of muscle action of the stomach and the receiving small intestine, and such factors as the amount of liquid versus solids (liquids empty rapidly, while solids stay longer in the stomach) and the gastric volume (increased food volume increases gastric emptying). In general, for the typical adult 10% of food will pass from the stomach to the small intestine in 1 hour, 40% in 2 hours, and 90% by 4 hours.

The small intestine, specifically the duodenum (the almost foot-long first portion of the small intestine), is the site of the majority of food digestion. Pancreatic digestive juices and bile produced in the liver and stored in the gallbladder help the duodenum digest the food into chyme, which then passes to the jejunum and ileum, the second and third portions of the small intestine, respectively, that comprise about 20 feet of small intestine. This is where most of the nutrients from the food are absorbed. The nutrients cross the intestinal brush border, a membrane ideal for absorbing large amounts of nutrients due to its numerous tiny finger-like projections (villi), and are absorbed into the bloodstream. This blood gets fast-tracked directly to the liver (known as portal circulation) for processing and distribution of nutrients to the rest of the body. Food spends about 1 to 4 hours in the small intestine.

The waste and indigestibles (such as fiber) leftover in the small intestine are passed through the ileocecal valve to the 5-foot long large intestine. Here a few minerals and a lot of water are reabsorbed into the blood. As more water gets reabsorbed, the waste passing through the colon portion of the large intestine becomes firmer until it is finally excreted as solid waste from the rectum and anus. Food can stay in the large intestine from hours to days. Total transit time from mouth to anus usually takes anywhere from 18 to 72 hours, thus what's considered to be a "normal" frequency of bowel movements can range from three times daily to once every 3 days or more.

SPEED BUMP

1. Outline the basic anatomy of the digestive system.

FUNDAMENTALS OF THE NUTRITIONAL BIOCHEMISTRY OF EXERCISE

A foundational understanding of nutritional biochemistry helps to make sense of the body's response to exercise and how to best fuel the body for peak athletic performance.

Fuel Utilization During Exercise

The basic principle is simple: food gives us energy to exercise. Glucose is the preferred energy source, which is delivered by the blood to the working cells. These cells break down the glucose to carbon dioxide and water, releasing usable energy—adenosine triphosphate (ATP)—which biochemically is an adenosine molecule joined with three phosphate molecules. The energy produced from the breakdown of ATP fuels metabolism, muscle contraction, heart pumping, and the myriad other demands required to maintain exercise performance. The process of studying the capture, conversion, and use of energy is known as **bioenergetics**.

ATP and Creatine Phosphate

ATP is used for all processes that require energy, including fueling muscle contraction. Muscle cells are made up of many proteins, including two contractile proteins, actin and myosin. Together these proteins allow for the muscle shortening and force that occurs with a muscle contraction. The following steps occur when a muscle contracts:

Step 1: Neuron action potential arrives at the end of the motor neuron. This stimulates release of acetylcholine (ACh), a neurotransmitter.

Step 2: ACh binds to receptors on the motor end plate, which creates an action potential.

Step 3: Calcium is released from the sarcoplasmic reticulum.

Step 4: Calcium binds to troponin.

Step 5: Troponin changes shape and tropomyosin shifts to expose binding sites of actin.

Step 6: During the **cross-bridge cycle**, ATP binds to myosin and is hydrolyzed to adenosine-*di*phosphate (ADP) and inorganic phosphate (Pi). The activated myosin head binds to actin, creating a cross bridge, and Pi is released (Fig. 6-1).

Step 7: ADP is released and the myosin head pivots, pulling the actin toward the center; the muscle is contracting.

Step 8: ATP molecules bind to the myosin head, detaching it from the actin, and the cross bridge is broken.

There is only a limited amount of stored ATP to fuel muscle contraction, approximately 3 seconds' worth. Shortly after the onset of vigorous exercise as the stored ATP is depleted, the ADP byproduct of ATP catabolism combines with **creatine phosphate** (CP), a high-energy phosphate compound, to produce more ATP (Fig. 6-2). This one-step reaction does not require oxygen, making the **phosphagen system** a source of immediate energy. The concentration of creatine phosphate stored in the muscle is five times that of stored ATP. Energy from stored ATP and stored creatine phosphate is enough to fuel about 5 to 10 seconds of an intense athletic effort, such as sprinting for 100 meters.

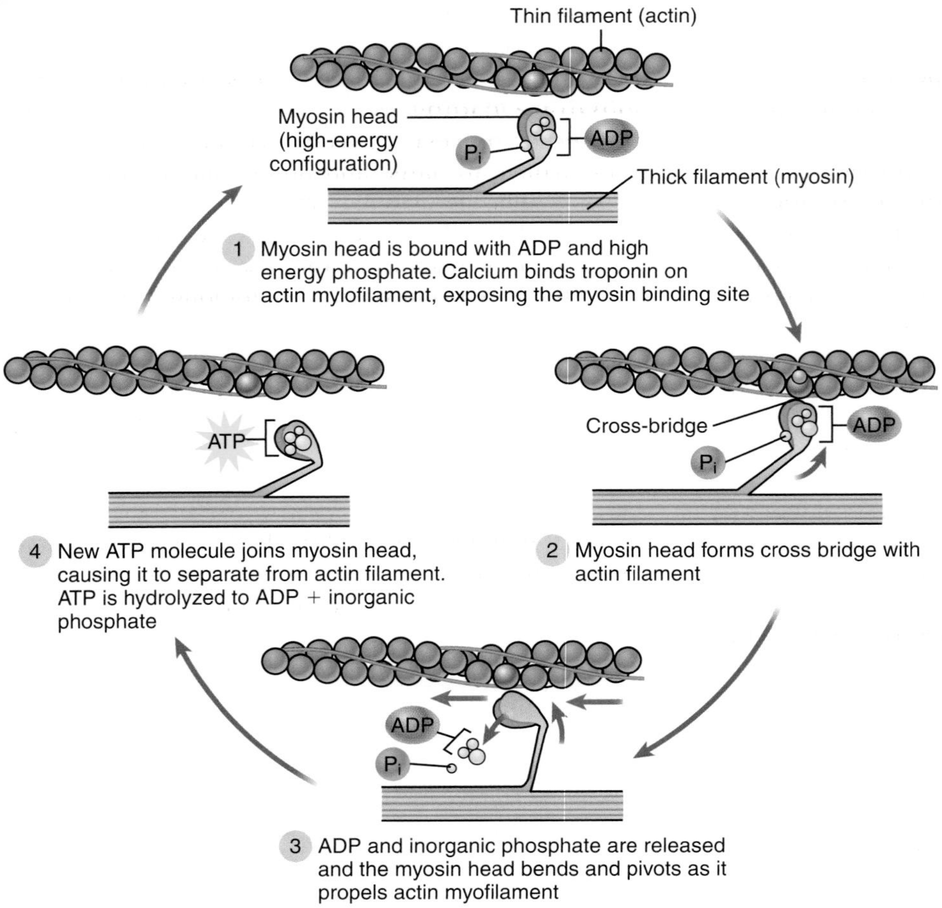

Figure 6-1. Muscle contraction and ATP.

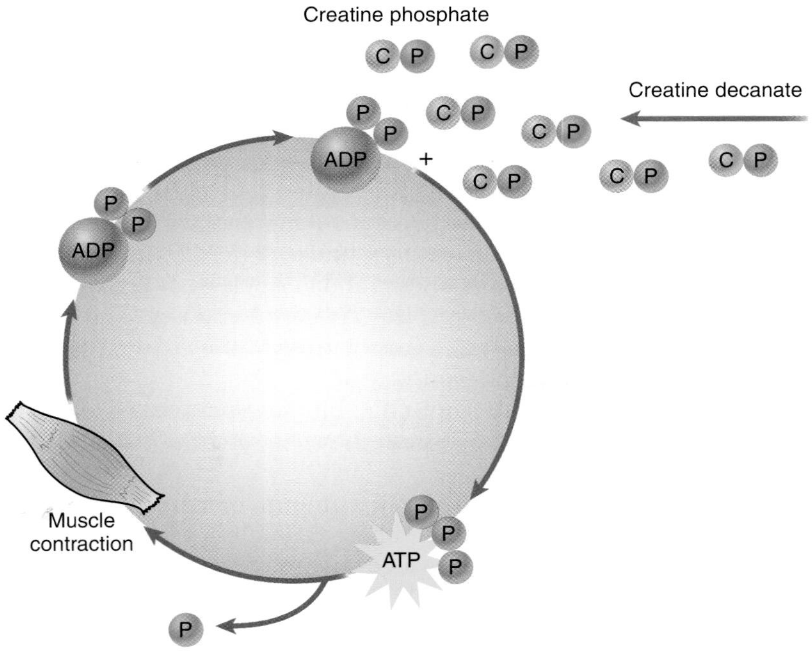

Figure 6-2. The phosphagen system. CP donates its phosphate molecule to ADP in the presence of an enzyme called creatine phosphokinase (CPK) or creatine kinase (CK) to form ATP.

Glycolysis System

While the body can fuel 5 to 10 seconds of exercise with stored ATP and creatine phosphate, these energy sources are just temporary supplies while the metabolic machinery revs up to metabolize glucose readily available in the bloodstream and make more glucose available through the breakdown of glycogen, a long chain of glucose molecules.

Through glycogenolysis, glycogen is broken down into single glucose molecules. The glucose is converted to pyruvate during **glycolysis**, then the cell uses

anaerobic respiration, which involves a 10-step process to convert pyruvate to ATP and lactic acid (Fig. 6-3). The muscles release **lactate**, the salt of **lactic acid** found in the body, into the bloodstream, and it is oxidized to produce more energy.

Glycolysis produces 4 ATPs and 2 hydrogen-carrying molecules, **nicotinamide adenine dinucleotide (NADH)**; however, 2 ATPs are used during the glycolysis process, resulting in a net of 2 ATP and 2 NADH for each glucose molecule. The process of glycolysis does not require oxygen and is the predominant energy-producing system for intense exercises lasting about 1 to 3 minutes. For example, glycolysis would provide energy for someone swimming 400 meters between 1 and 3 minutes (for more on this, see the discussion of VO_2 max later in the chapter).

Glucose is the body's preferred energy source, thus athletes are well-served to have a continual and ready supply of glucose available to fuel exercise. One key way to do this is through optimization of glycogen stores. Approximately 90 grams, or 360 calories, can be stored in the liver and 150 grams, or 600 calories, can be accumulated in the muscles. However, with physical training muscle glycogen storage can increase by fivefold. **Carbohydrate loading** also increases glycogen stores (see Chapter 7); however, glycogen contains water molecules, which are large and bulky, making long-term boosts in glycogen storage impossible. What happens then if a person continues to consume more carbohydrates than the body can either use or store? The body converts the extra glucose into fat for long-term storage.

Aerobic Respiration

For those who are exercising longer than several minutes, the body must rely on the breakdown of carbohydrates, fat, and sometimes protein to supply a continued source of ATP. Exercise triggers a cascade of reactions that direct each of the body's systems to help optimize nutrient and oxygen delivery to the working muscle cells. The heart beats faster and pushes out more blood with each beat to deliver more oxygen and

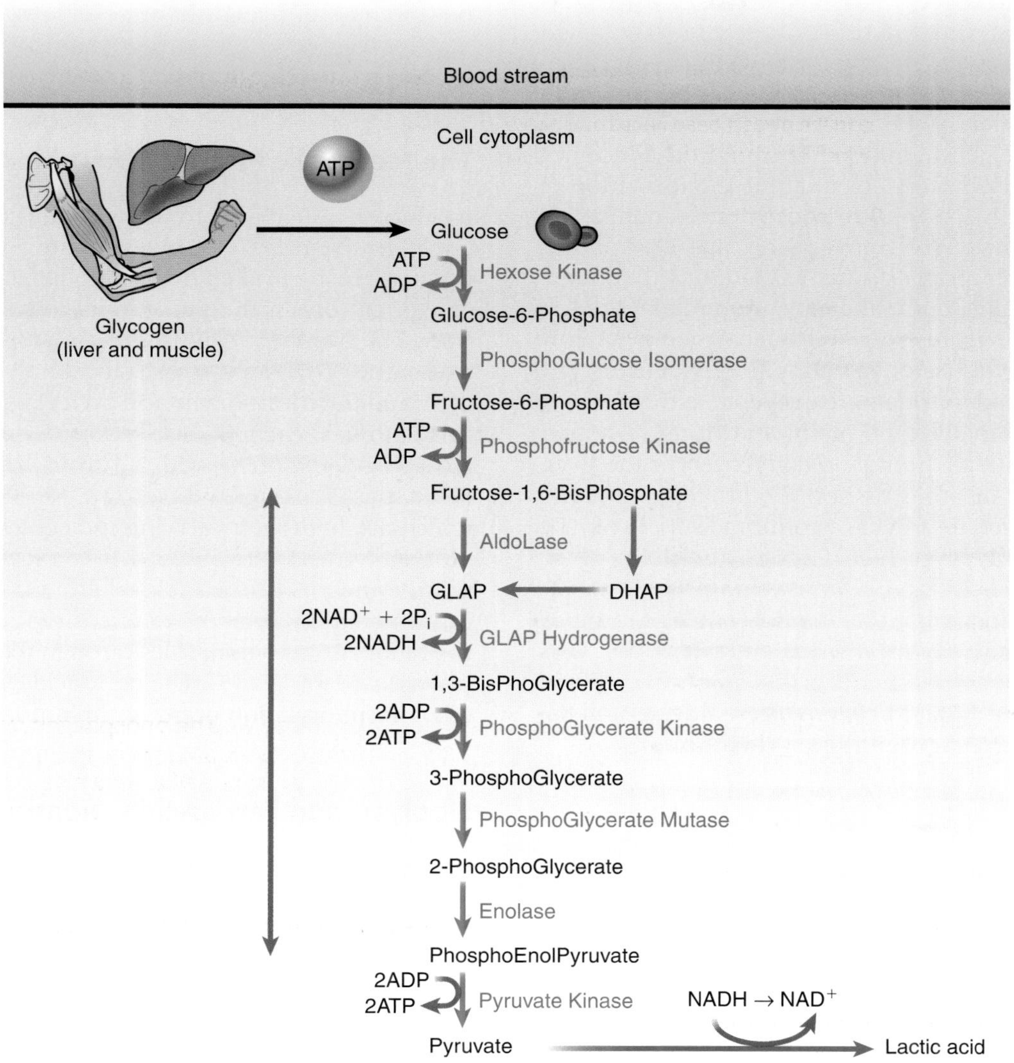

Figure 6-3. Glycogenolysis and glycolysis.

nutrients to working cells. Respiratory rate increases to ensure optimal amounts of oxygen are available. The digestive system slows in an effort to help divert blood flow to working muscles. The endocrine system releases more epinephrine, norepinephrine, and cortisol as part of the nervous system's activation of the sympathetic system. Metabolic activity increases in the working muscles.

The increased metabolic activity in the muscle cells ensures the nutrients are broken down into ATP through the process of **aerobic respiration**, which occurs in the **mitochondria** in the presence of oxygen. Glucose is broken down into pyruvate, which in turn is converted to acetyl CoA and enters the citric acid cycle.

Oxygen and Nutrient Delivery

Oxygen-rich and nutrient-rich blood must be delivered to the working cells to fuel ongoing activity. How well the body is able to deliver these essential ingredients (oxygen and nutrients) is a major determinant of exercise performance. The body's ability to obtain oxygen from the air inhaled into the lungs and transported to the bloodstream is known as **oxygen-carrying capacity**. Oxygen-carrying capacity is affected by two main factors: (1) the ability to adequately ventilate the alveoli in the lungs, and (2) hemoglobin concentration in the blood. Athletes who consume a diet with inadequate amounts of iron may suffer from iron-deficiency anemia. Because iron is essential for the formation of hemoglobin, athletes with iron-deficiency anemia will suffer from reduced oxygen-carrying capacity and thus decreased endurance performance. On the other hand, athletes who have optimal dietary iron intake are less likely to suffer from iron deficiency anemia or low hemoglobin levels (see Evaluating the Evidence).

As oxygen and nutrients are delivered to the working cells, the carbohydrates, protein, and/or fat (whether from food intake or from stored glycogen in the liver, adipose tissue, or other tissues) are broken down and oxygen is utilized to provide a continual supply of ATP.

Oxygen delivery, which describes the ability of the body to transport oxygen from the lungs to the working cells, is a function of the quantity of blood pumped through the heart per minute (**cardiac output**). Cardiac output is determined by the amount of blood pumped with each heartbeat (**stroke volume**) and the number of heartbeats per minute (heart rate).

$$\text{Cardiac output (Q)} = \text{stroke volume (SV)} \times \text{heart rate (HR)}$$

Cardiac output increases due to increases in both SV and HR. HR typically increases with increased exercise intensity in a linear fashion up to maximal levels. SV increases with increased exercise intensity up until a point (about 40% to 50% of VO_2 max—more on this concept later in this chapter) and then plateaus. Thus, with increasing exercise intensity, more oxygen (and nutrients) are delivered to the working cells to provide continuous replenishment of the ingredients necessary to produce ATP.

VO_2 max, maximal oxygen uptake, is an indicator of a person's potential for aerobic endurance during high-intensity exercise. It refers to the maximum amount of oxygen an individual can use during intense or maximal exercise. VO_2 max is expressed as a number that reflects how many millimeters of oxygen are used in 1 minute per kilogram of body weight or ml/kg/min.

$$VO_2 \text{ max} = Q\ (CaO_2 \text{ (arterial oxygen content)} - CvO_2 \text{ (venous oxygen content))}$$

VO_2 max is generally considered the best indicator of a person's cardiovascular fitness and aerobic endurance. The theory is the more oxygen used during intense exercise the more ATP (energy) is produced. Typically, elite endurance athletes have very high VO_2 max levels. Numerous studies have shown VO_2 max can be increased by working out at an intensity that raises the heart rate to between 65% and 85% of its maximum for at least 20 minutes, three to five times a week.[1]

VO_2 should not be confused with **lactate threshold** (or **anaerobic threshold** or **ventilatory threshold**), which refers to the intense, exhaustive exercise that causes lactate to accumulate in the muscles.

The Metabolic Pathway (Aerobic Glycolysis)

As glucose is delivered to the working cell, it is broken down into pyruvate. However, now instead of the pyruvate being broken down into lactic acid, as in the case of glycolysis, the pyruvate is converted to acetyl-CoA. The acetyl-CoA passes to the mitochondria and enters the **citric acid cycle** (also known as the Krebs cycle and the tricarboxylic acid cycle; Fig. 6-4). Through this pathway, each glucose molecule produces 2 ATP along with 8 NADH and 2 **flavin adenine dinucleotide** (FADH), and 6 CO_2. NADH and FADH, which are hydrogen-carrying molecules, go on to the **electron-transport chain**, where they are stripped of their hydrogen and pass through a series of reactions until the energy from electrons is captured and stored to produce 28 ATP molecules through **oxidative phosphorylation** (Fig. 6-5). The citric acid cycle and oxidative phosphorylation occur in the mitochondria.

Lipolysis and Fatty Acid Oxidation

When exercise continues for more than 20 minutes, fat becomes the predominant fuel. To get energy from fat, **triacylglycerols** (stored triglycerides) must first be broken down through the process of lipolysis into glycerol plus three fatty acids. The fatty acids are then carried by albumin through the bloodstream to the working cells. Fatty acids enter the mitochondria where they are

EVALUATING THE EVIDENCE

What Variables Predict Endurance Performance?

Endurance performance depends upon the interplay between oxygen-carrying capacity, oxygen delivery, and oxygen extraction. But to what extent does each variable predict endurance performance? The following study of 16 competitive cyclists (1 female, 15 males, ages 29 years ± 6 years) sought to answer that question by isolating the most important physiological determinants of endurance performance in highly trained endurance athletes. This is the study abstract:

> Human endurance performance can be predicted from maximal oxygen consumption (VO(2max)), lactate threshold, and exercise efficiency. These physiological parameters, however, are not wholly exclusive from one another and their interplay is complex. Accordingly, we sought to identify more specific measurements explaining the range of performance among athletes. Out of 150 separate variables we identified 10 principal factors responsible for hematological, cardiovascular, respiratory, musculoskeletal, and neurological variation in 16 highly trained cyclists. These principal factors were then correlated with a 26-kilometer time trial and test of maximal incremental power output. Average power output during the 26-kilometer time trial was attributed to, in order of importance, oxidative phosphorylation capacity of the m. vastus lateralis ($p = 0.0005$), steady state submaximal blood lactate concentrations ($p = 0.0017$), and maximal leg oxygenation (O(2LEG)) ($p = 0.0295$), accounting for 78% of the variation in time trial performance. Variability in maximal power output, on the other hand, was attributed to total body hemoglobin mass (Hb(mass); $p = 0.0038$), VO(2max) ($p = 0.0213$), and O(2LEG) ($p = 0.0463$). In conclusion: (1) skeletal muscle oxidative capacity is the primary predictor of time trial performance in highly trained cyclists; (2) the strongest predictor for maximal incremental power output is Hb(mass); and (3) overall exercise performance (time trial performance + maximal incremental power output) correlates most strongly to measures regarding the capability for oxygen transport, high VO(2max) and Hb(mass), in addition to measures of oxygen utilization, maximal oxidative phosphorylation, and electron transport system capacities in the skeletal muscle.[2]

1. Describe the concepts of *VO_2 max, lactate threshold,* and *exercise efficiency* in terms of oxygen-carrying capacity, oxygen delivery, and oxygen extraction.
2. A client asks you what factors are most important in determining endurance performance. Having just read this article, you are excited to share the findings with your client. Summarize in lay terms the objective, design, results, and conclusions of this study.
3. Following are a list of several athletes. For each athlete, state whether or not the findings from this study are directly applicable and why or why not:
   a. A 22-year-old female lacrosse player
   b. A 33-year-old male endurance cyclist
   c. A 19-year-old male power lifter
   d. A 50-year-old triathlete
4. In what ways might (or might not) the results of this study influence your approach to working with clients?
5. Based on the findings of this study, what nutritional strategies do you think might help boost athletic performance?

broken down to acetyl CoA and hydrogen through **beta oxidation**. The process of beta oxidation produces NADH and $FADH_2$ which enter the electron transport chain to make more ATP. The acetyl-CoA enters into the citric acid cycle to form carbon dioxide and ATP. Note that carbohydrate availability is essential to support lipolysis as glycolysis serves to "drive" the citric acid cycle, the metabolic process largely responsible for the conversion of fat to ATP. Depending on the size of the fatty acid, a fatty acid molecule can produce up to 147 ATP. For example, palmitic acid has 16 carbons and can produce 130 ATP (Fig. 6-6).

Fatty acid oxidation provides a nearly limitless supply of ATP. Stored fat contains anywhere from 50,000 to 100,000 calories of potential energy stored in adipocytes and 3,000 calories stored as intramuscular triacylglycerols. This process takes upward of 20 minutes to mobilize the fatty acids and break them down.

Importantly, fats can provide energy for the working muscle cells, but they are not a useful source of energy for the brain or red blood cells, which rely exclusively on glucose for energy. Fat cannot be converted to glucose and cannot be metabolized unless some carbohydrate and oxygen is available. Thus, muscle glycogen and blood glucose availability are limiting factors in athletic performance, regardless of intensity or duration (Table 6-1).

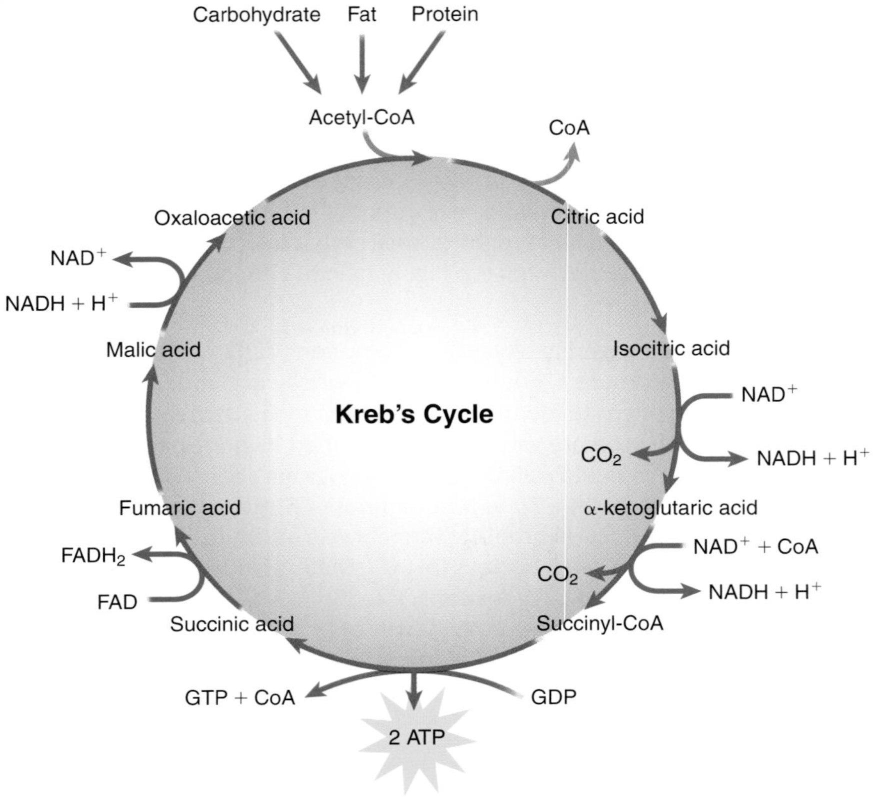

Figure 6-4. The citric acid, or Krebs, cycle.

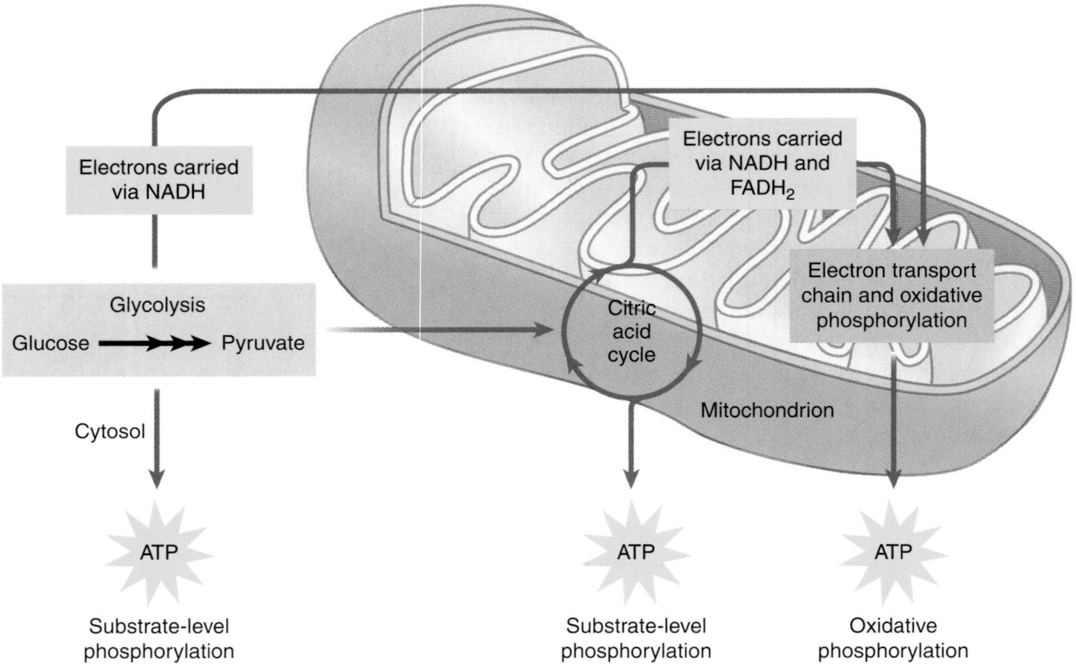

Figure 6-5. Oxidative phosphorylation.

Deamination and Protein as Energy

When endurance exercise or heavy training lasts longer than 1 hour, and no carbohydrates have been ingested, blood glucose levels begin to dwindle. After 1 to 3 hours of continuous moderate-intensity exercise muscle glycogen stores may become depleted. When this happens, protein can be broken down to produce energy. The amino acids undergo deamination (nitrogen removal) through the **urea cycle** in the liver. The *glucogenic* amino acids may then either be converted to glucose through **gluconeogenesis** or may enter the citric acid cycle to form ATP (Fig. 6-7). *Ketogenic* amino acids cannot be used

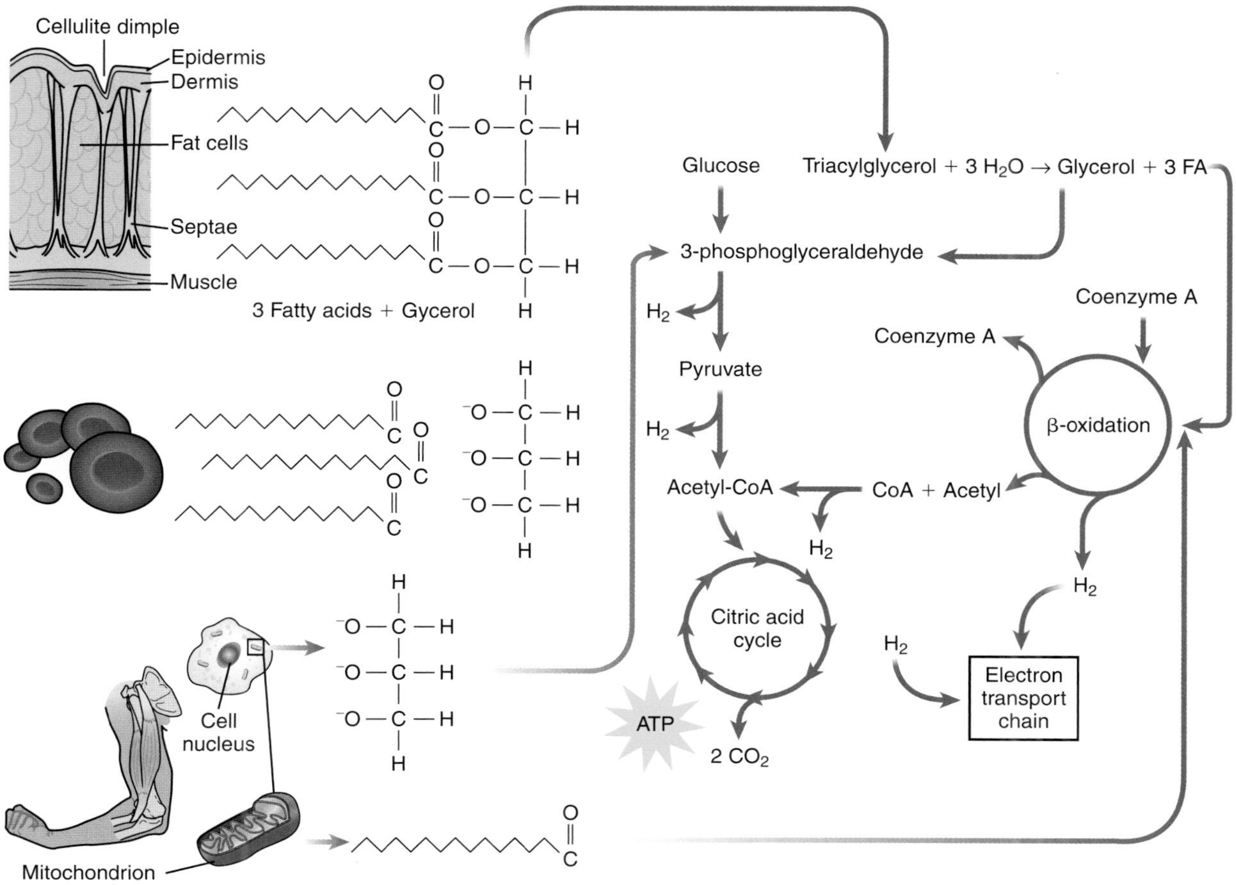

Figure 6-6. Lipolysis and fatty acid oxidation.

Table 6-1. The Energy Systems

ENERGY SYSTEM	SUBSTRATE	LIMITATION TO PRODUCE ATP	PRIMARY USE
Anaerobic			
Phosphagen	Creatine phosphate (CP) and stored ATP	Muscle stores very little CP and ATP	High-intensity, short-duration activities; less than 10 seconds to fatigue
Anaerobic glycolysis	Glucose and glycogen	Lactic acid forms and disassociates into lactate, which can be used as fuel by muscles, and hydrogen	High-intensity, short-duration activities; 1 to 3 minutes to fatigue
Aerobic			
Aerobic glycolysis	Glucose and glycogen	Depletion of muscle glycogen	Long-duration, subanaerobic threshold activities; longer than 3 minutes to fatigue
Fatty acid oxidation	Fatty acids	Depletion of muscle glycogen and blood glucose	Long-duration, lower intensity activities; longer than 20 minutes to fatigue

to make glucose but can be converted to acetyl-CoA and enter the citric acid cycle or be converted to fat.

While protein can be used for energy or to produce glucose, this situation is not ideal, as the majority of the amino acids come from the breakdown of muscle. To avoid muscle wasting, athletes need to ensure adequate carbohydrate intake to fuel exercise and assure a continual glucose energy supply (Fig. 6-8 and Communication Strategies).

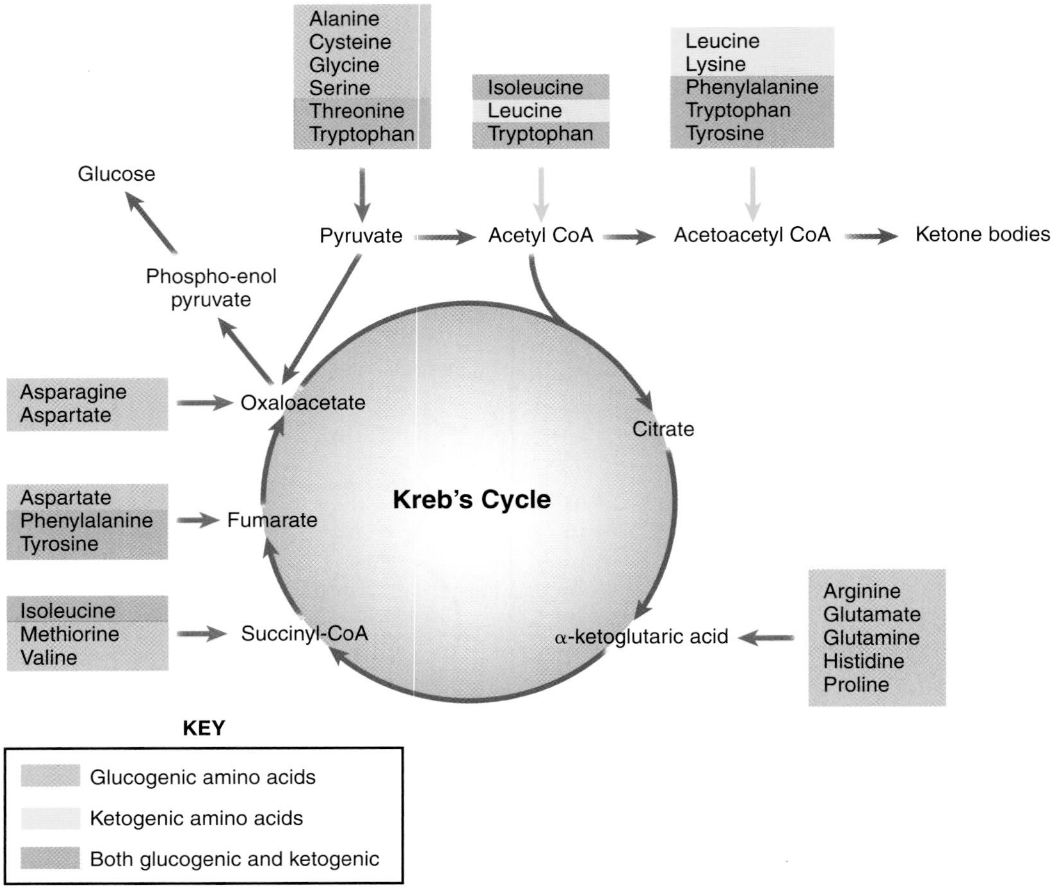

Figure 6-7. Gluconeogenesis and protein as energy.

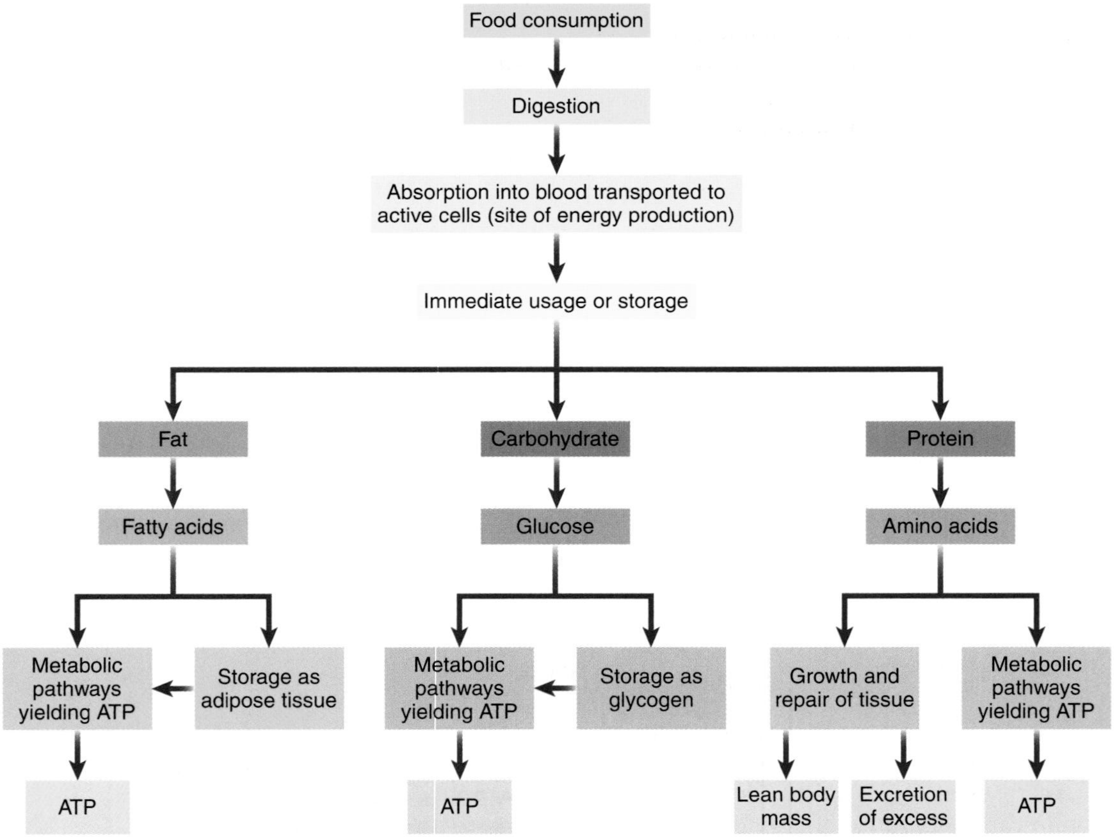

Figure 6-8. The pathways from food to energy. *From* ACE Personal Trainer Manual: The Ultimate Resource for Fitness Professionals. *4th ed. Monterey, CA: Coaches Choice; 2010. Reprinted with permission.*

COMMUNICATION STRATEGIES

Adult Learning Theory

Your instructor has asked you to give a 10-minute presentation to your sports nutrition classmates choosing one of the following three prompts (or she says that you can come up with one of your own, based on the chapter's content):

1. Outline the pathway of a nutrition bar that is consumed 30 minutes prior to a 10-mile endurance run.
2. Describe the energy systems in use during the beginning, middle, and end of a 4-hour bike ride.
3. Describe what happens to a high-carbohydrate meal eaten 30 minutes after a strenuous endurance workout. What happens if the athlete keeps eating? Outline the metabolic pathways in use.

While preparing your presentation, you run into a friend who is working on a doctorate in education. She suggests that you familiarize yourself with "adult learning theory" in order for your presentation to be most useful for your classmates. In doing so, you learn that this theory is based on the following six premises:[3]

- Adults prefer to be independent and self-directed in learning experiences
- Adults prefer to learn in terms of practical applications to day-to-day life
- Adults prefer active learning
- Adult education should be appropriate to the adult learner's readiness to learn and their need to know the information
- Adult learning should be oriented toward performing tasks and solving problems
- Adults need to know *why* they are learning the material

Class Activity

Working in groups of two, prepare a 10-minute learning session using one of the prompts above. Be sure to integrate adult learning theory into your approach.

Lipogenesis

Any excess carbohydrate, protein, or fat that is consumed beyond what the body can immediately use for energy, structural support, or glycogen storage is converted to fat and stored in adipocytes through **lipogenesis** (Fig. 6-9). In this process, the pancreas releases insulin, which induces an increased transport of glucose into adipose cells. Here the glucose is converted to glycerol, which joins with three free fatty acids to form triacylglycerols for storage. The fatty acids are delivered to the adipose cell by way of very low density lipoprotein (VLDL) from the liver and chylomicrons from the bloodstream. Fatty acids also may be produced from glucose by way of acetyl CoA, a compound produced during aerobic glycolysis and the main substrate for fatty acid synthesis.

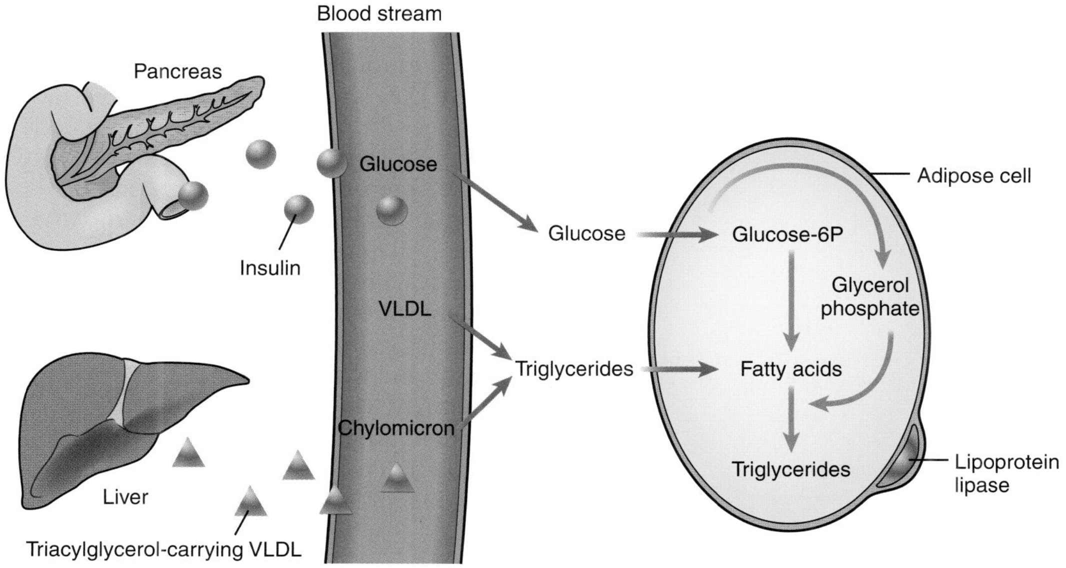

Figure 6-9. Lipogenesis

SPEED BUMP

2. **Describe the pathway of a food starting with consumption and digestion and ending with usable energy.**
3. **Describe the metabolic pathways including the phosphagen system, anaerobic glycolysis, aerobic glycolysis, and fatty acid oxidation.**

A CASE EXAMPLE

Perhaps the easiest way to understand the nutritional biochemistry of exercise is with an example. For purposes of this chapter, the example is of a marathon training program that incorporates long runs and sprints. However, the principles apply to other sports. The same energy systems that predominate during long runs predominate during prolonged biking, swimming, or hiking. Likewise, the main energy systems used during a sprint are also used for weight lifting, speed training, and plyometrics. Also, while exercise intensity and duration determine which energy system predominates, *at no time does any single energy system provide 100% of energy*.

As described in the introduction, Kate is a 22-year-old recreational athlete training for what she hopes will be a Boston-qualifying marathon. Kate's marathon training program consists mostly of long runs, but twice per week she incorporates sprints into her program. Depending on her workout, her body relies on several pathways to varying degrees. The pathways include the phosphagen system, in which creatine is the energy source; anaerobic glycolysis and aerobic glycolysis, where glucose provides energy; and fatty acid oxidation, in which energy comes from the breakdown of fat. Approximately 10% of protein will be burned as a result of these long runs.

Kate's sprinting program consists of several rounds of 400-yard sprints twice per week. Let's start by tracing her body's energy use through one of these sprints:

1. Seconds 0 to 8. Upon starting an all-out physical effort, stored ATP in the muscle is rapidly broken down, releasing ADP, an inorganic phosphate (P_i), and energy:

$$\text{ATP} \xrightarrow{\textit{Myosin ATPase}} \text{ADP} + P_i + \text{Energy}$$

ADP combines with a high-energy phosphate from stored creatine phosphate to produce more ATP and more energy:

$$\text{ADP} + \text{Creatine phosphate} \xrightarrow{\textit{Creatine kinase}} \text{ATP} + \text{Creatine}$$

This rapid energy allows for a high-intensity (> 85% of VO_2 max) effort. By seconds 8 to 10 the stored ATP and creatine phosphate are depleted.

2. Seconds 8 to 120. Glycolysis is at full throttle. The body is working on transporting as much glucose as possible to working muscles. The most readily available is glucose floating around in the bloodstream from recently digested carbohydrate and from glycogen stored in the muscle. Glucose is rapidly broken down to produce 2 ATP molecules per glucose molecule. Kate's sprint is over. Glycolysis:

$$\text{Glucose} \xrightarrow{\text{Glycolysis}} \text{Pyruvate} \longrightarrow \text{Lactic Acid} \quad \text{2 ATP}$$

3. Recovery. Kate is breathing heavily in an involuntary effort to replenish her **oxygen deficit**, the energy supplied to muscles anaerobically at the beginning of exercise. Oxygen consumption slowly declines, but remains elevated above resting level in what is known as **excess post-exercise oxygen consumption (EPOC)** (Fig. 6-10).

As Kate nears the peak of her training program, her long runs get longer. This one is 18 miles. Unlike the sprint sessions, at the beginning of this workout she starts at a moderate intensity. As soon as aerobic exercise begins, increased amounts of ATP are required. To meet this demand, Kate's sympathetic nervous system takes over and stimulates an increase in cardiac output and the release of epinephrine and norepinephrine, which prepare the body for increased metabolic demands. Her initial fuel sources are stored ATP, creatine phosphate, and glucose through anaerobic glycolysis, but these are only primary energy sources for the first 1 to 3 minutes until the aerobic glycolysis system is fully functional. Aerobic glycolysis takes longer to provide ATP because it requires adequate oxygen and multiple systems are working together to produce ATP.

As Kate breathes in, the oxygen passes from nasal passages to lungs to blood to the muscle cells. It takes about 2 to 4 minutes until Kate's body is able to reverse the oxygen deficit and meet the increased metabolic oxygen demands. During this time, the anaerobic energy systems fuel the workout. However, once the aerobic system is able to provide energy, a new level of steady-state oxygen consumption is achieved. Aerobic glycolysis breaks pyruvate down to carbon dioxide, water, and NADH and FADH2. The hydrogen molecules from NADH and FADH2 enter the electron transport chain to produce energy through oxidative phosphorylation. Eventually, one molecule of glucose produces a net total of 36 molecules of ATP.

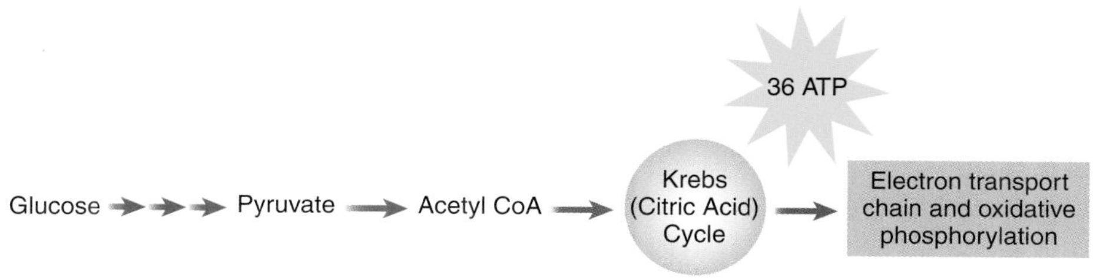

After approximately 20 minutes of moderate-intensity aerobic exercise, fat becomes the predominant energy source through fatty acid oxidation. Glycolysis continues to break down carbohydrates, including glucose, fructose, or galactose, to "drive" the Krebs cycle. Triglycerides are broken down to three fatty acids. Each fatty acid is broken down further to acetyl CoA, which enters the Krebs, or citric acid, cycle directly; NADH and FADH, the hydrogen atom byproducts, are carried into the electron transport chain to produce more ATP. A single fatty acid produces 147 ATP; therefore each triglyceride (three fatty acids) produces 441 ATP from fatty acid oxidation plus an additional 22 ATP from the breakdown of the glycerol backbone of the triglyceride for a total of 463 ATP. The increased ATP comes at a price—a marked increase in the amount of oxygen required per molecule of ATP produced.

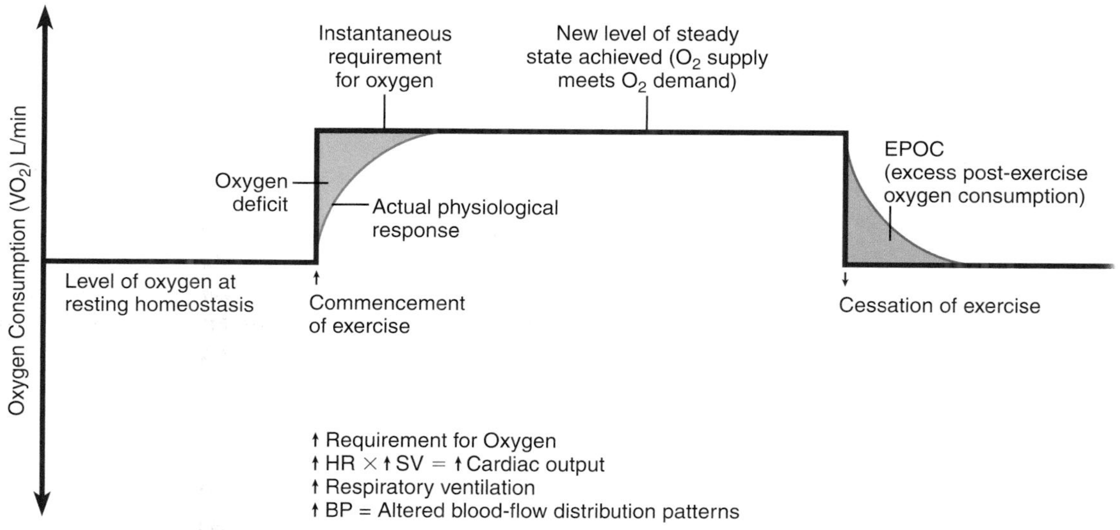

Note: HR = Heart rate; SV = Stroke volume; BP = Blood pressure

Figure 6-10. **Oxygen consumption and exercise.** *From* ACE Personal Trainer Manual: The Ultimate Resource for Fitness Professionals. *4th ed. Monterey, CA: Coaches Choice; 2010. Reprinted with permission.*

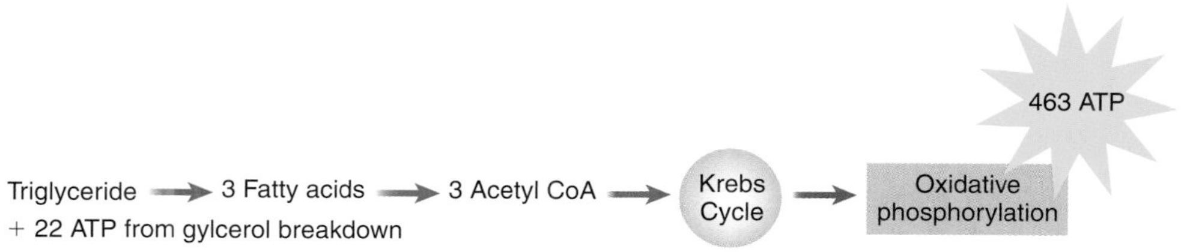

As the endurance run continues, both glucose and fatty acids provide fuel for exercise. The proportion depends on the intensity and duration of exercise and the athlete's fitness level. In general, the lower the intensity, the longer the exercise, and the more fit the athlete, the more the body develops a preference for fat as a fuel. However, importantly, fat cannot be metabolized unless carbohydrate is available. This illustrates the point that while exercise intensity and duration determine which energy system predominates, *at no time does any single energy system provide 100% of energy*. Table 6-1 highlights the capacity of each system at varying exercise intensities and duration.

If Kate wants to achieve her goal of qualifying for the Boston Marathon she will have to integrate high-intensity

Myths and **Misconceptions**

Low-Intensity Exercise Is Best for Weight and Fat Loss

The Myth

You'll lose more weight and body fat if you work out in the lower intensity "fat-burning zone." Thus, you should work out at a lower intensity if you're trying to get rid of excess body fat.

The Logic

Fat supplies a greater percentage of calories than carbohydrate to fuel low-intensity exercise.

The Science

While it is true that a larger *percentage* of calories come from fat during low-intensity exercise, the total energy burned from fat is about the same whether a client works out at 25% of VO_2 max or 85% of VO_2 max.[4] The only difference, of course, is that the client burns more total calories at higher intensity exercise. Those calories just come from carbohydrate rather than fat. But, ultimately, in order to lose weight it comes down to total calories—it doesn't matter whether they come from carbohydrate or fat, the client needs to expend more calories than are consumed.

interval sessions into her aerobic workouts to help boost her overall cardiovascular fitness. When she does sprints she increases intensity beyond the capacity of the aerobic system to supply more energy. Because the aerobic system is already working at full capacity, she has to activate the anaerobic system to provide additional ATP.

Once exercise has stopped, cardiac output, blood pressure, and ventilation return to resting levels. Oxygen consumption slowly declines, but remains elevated above resting level. During this time, phosphagen stores are replenished, remaining H+ is removed from the blood, and the metabolic rate decreases.

Carbohydrate consumption after a strenuous workout helps to replenish depleted glycogen stores. The ingested carbohydrate is broken down into glucose. This blood glucose is transported to liver and muscle cells where it is converted to glycogen (blue arrows in Fig. 6-11). Any leftover lactate in the muscle or bloodstream can also be converted to glycogen. It first is transported to the liver then is used as a substrate for gluconeogenesis (green arrows in Fig. 6-11). This glucose is then converted to glycogen through glycogenesis.

SPEED BUMP

4. **Explain how energy is stored in the skeletal muscles and other tissues.**
5. **Describe oxygen transport in exercise and training (the respiratory and cardiovascular response to exercise).**

EFFECT OF TRAINING

Both recreational and competitive athletes recognize that the beginning of training is the most difficult, but with persistence and patience the same run, amount of weight, or training regimen becomes easier. This is because the body effectively adapts to stresses placed upon it in what is known as the **SAID principle** (specific adaptation to imposed demands). For example, with regular endurance training the same aerobic activity becomes easier. This is in part a result of increased cardiac output efficiency. Stroke volume increases while exercising heart rate decreases. As a

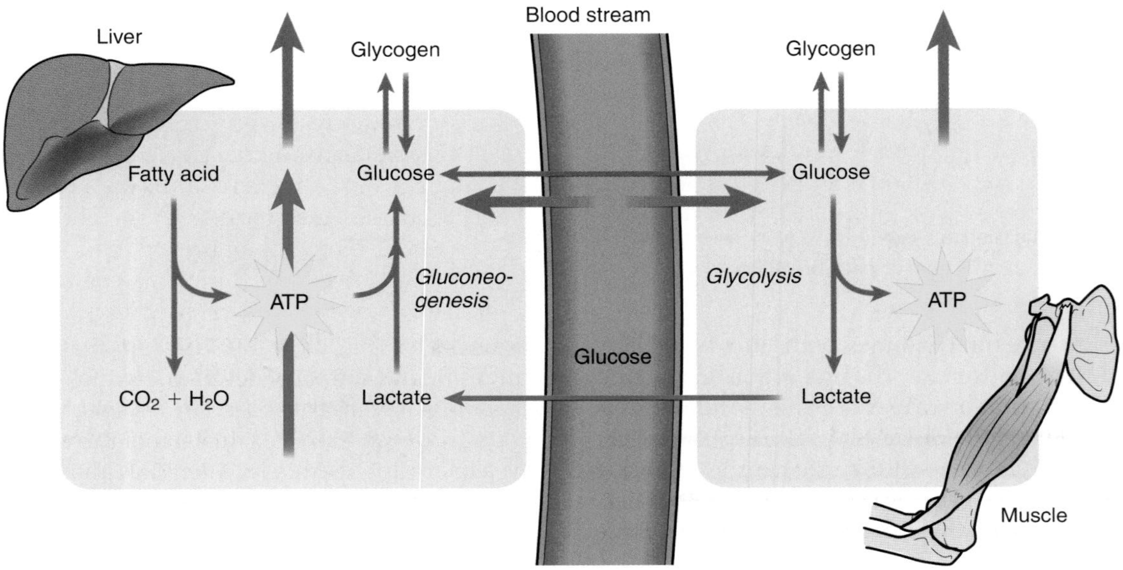

Figure 6-11. Glycogenesis.

result, in order to pump the same amount of blood to the working tissues, the heart pumps harder but with less frequency due to the increased left ventricle size. Increased vascularity around muscle tissues increases the ability to deliver oxygen to the tissues. **Oxygen extraction** also increases as the number of oxidative enzymes and mitochondria increase in the muscle cells, thus increasing the capacity for carbohydrate and fatty acid metabolism. Moreover, the respiratory capacity improves as the body improves its ability through many factors such as enzymes, vasodilation, and increased stroke volume to deliver O_2 to tissues. **Respiratory quotient (RQ)**, or respiratory exchange ratio, is the measurement between oxygen inhaled and carbon dioxide eliminated. The formula is RQ = CO_2 eliminated/O_2 absorbed and is measured during a VO_2 max test. The RQ helps determine the type of fuel being used for energy. As the intensity of the test increases, more carbohydrates (glycogen) are burned for fuel. The RQ estimates how much of the energy came from carbohydrates and how much from fat.

THE INTERRELATIONSHIP OF EXERCISE PHYSIOLOGY AND NUTRITION

The nutritional choices an athlete makes play a large role in athletic performance and overall fitness level. At the cellular level, the available nutrients and oxygen enter biochemical cycles to produce ATP, the body's usable energy source. At the systems level, an athlete who would like to optimize endurance performance would do well to eat a carefully planned high-carbohydrate diet to enhance muscle glycogen stores and the body's ability to maintain a ready supply of glucose for aerobic glycolysis. A strength athlete needs to consume the right type of carbohydrates and protein to optimize creatine stores and muscle rebuilding and hypertrophy. Ultimately, exercise physiology and deep understanding of human sports nutrition empower athletes to accomplish their personal best. *(Keeping this in mind, track Kate's progress in achieving her Boston Marathon goal in the Practical Applications.)*

KEY POINTS SUMMARY

1. Glucose is the body's preferred energy source. It is delivered to the working cells from either the breakdown in the muscle or liver through glycogenolysis or production from protein through gluconeogenesis or from food. The exogenous sources must first pass through the gastrointestinal system, be absorbed in the small intestine, pass through the portal circulation to the liver, and then pass into the systemic bloodstream and track to the working muscles.
2. ATP is the body's usable energy. It is stored in miniscule quantities in the body's muscle cells and must otherwise be produced through the phosphagen system, anaerobic glycolysis, aerobic glycolysis, or fatty acid oxidation.
3. The phosphagen system fuels high-intensity activity lasting 5 to 10 seconds. The energy comes from the breakdown of stored muscle creatine phosphate and ATP.
4. Anaerobic glycolysis relies on breakdown of glucose immediately available from the bloodstream or muscle glycogen. The byproduct pyruvate gets converted to lactic acid. This system, which occurs in the cell cytoplasm without the presence of oxygen, provides the predominant source of ATP for activities lasting 1 to 3 minutes.
5. Aerobic glycolysis relies on the complete breakdown of glucose. Pyruvate is further broken down to acetyl-coA, which then enters the citric acid cycle. Aerobic glycolysis serves as the primary energy system for activities lasting 3 to 20 minutes.
6. Fatty acid oxidation requires oxygen, but also produces large amounts of ATP. Fatty acids are oxidized to acetyl-CoA, which enters the citric acid cycle. Fatty acid oxidation is the primary energy source for low-intensity activities and those lasting longer than about 20 minutes. Importantly, for fatty acid oxidation to continue, glucose is necessary. Thus, if muscle glycogen stores are depleted, athletic performance will falter.
7. Protein is an energy source of last resort. In times of starvation or when there is low glucose availability, ketogenic amino acids can be converted to acetyl-CoA to enter the citric acid cycle while the glucogenic amino acids can be used to produce glucose. Athletes should strive to avoid the situation when protein is used as fuel since the majority of the amino acids can come from muscle tissue. This reinforces the concept of ensuring there is adequate carbohydrate intake so carbohydrates are the main source of energy.
8. At the onset of anaerobic exercise the body produces ATP. It takes the body about 2 to 4 minutes to supply adequate oxygen to meet the metabolic demands. This absence of oxygen at the onset of exercise (oxygen deficit) leads to increased respiration at the end of exercise (EPOC) as the body tries to make up for the oxygen that wasn't initially available.
9. The point at which exercise intensity increases beyond the body's capacity to use oxygen for energy is known as the VO_2 max. To increase VO_2 max, an athlete needs to increase the capacity for oxidation, such as through increased oxygen delivery and extraction. Each of these changes occurs with continued aerobic exercise, especially exercise that pushes the limits of ventilatory capacity. This is the reason why it is important to integrate sprints and other high-intensity exercise into an endurance training program.

10. Any excess carbohydrate, protein, or fat consumed beyond what the body can immediately use for energy, muscle building, or glycogen storage will be converted to and stored as fat.
11. Understanding and application of sports nutrition enables an athlete to set the stage for optimal athletic performance and accomplishment of new personal bests.

PRACTICAL APPLICATIONS

1. What is the path oxygen follows to get from the air to the working cells?
   A. Right atrium, right ventricle, pulmonary artery, alveoli, pulmonary vein, capillaries, cell
   B. Pulmonary artery, left atrium, left ventricle, aorta, alveoli, capillaries, cell
   C. Alveoli, right atrium, left atrium, left ventricle, vena cava, capillaries, cell
   D. Alveoli, pulmonary vein, left atrium, left ventricle, aorta, capillaries, cell

Choose from the following answer choices for questions 2 to 4.

a. Stomach
b. Small intestine
c. Liver
d. Large intestine

2. Where does the majority of digestion occur?
3. Where does the majority of absorption occur?
4. Where does protein get converted to glucose?
5. Jane ate an egg 4 hours prior to beginning a 7-mile run. The amino acids absorbed from the egg have just passed into the bloodstream. What is the most likely pathway for the ketogenic amino acids?
   A. Delivery to muscle for storage
   B. Delivery to fat for storage
   C. Conversion to glucose for energy
   D. Entry into an oxidative pathway for energy

Choose from the answer choices below in response to questions 6 to 8.

a. Phosphagen system
b. Anaerobic glycolysis
c. Aerobic glycolysis
d. Fatty acid oxidation
e. Amino acid deamination

6. What is the primary energy system to fuel a plyometric jump squat?
7. What is the primary energy system to fuel cycling at 70% of VO_2 max for 15 minutes?
8. What is the primary energy system to fuel a sprint at 90% of VO_2 max for 60 seconds?
9. Your client is training for a 10K race. During training he generally runs between 30 and 45 minutes at 65% maximal VO_2, but he sprints the last 200 meters of his workout. What are the main energy substrates used by your client during the sprint?
   A. Amino acids, glucose, and glycogen
   B. Creatine phosphate, amino acids, and fatty acids
   C. Glucose, glycogen, and fatty acids
   D. Fatty acids, amino acids, and glucose
10. The capacity of which energy system is most enhanced in response to a regular endurance training program?
    A. Phosphagen system
    B. Aerobic glycolysis
    C. Anaerobic glycolysis
    D. Fatty acid oxidation

Case 1 Kate the Marathon Runner

Kate is an experienced 22-year-old marathon runner who is trying to qualify for the Boston Marathon. She is 5′6″ and 116 pounds. To qualify, she needs to shave 25 minutes off of her personal record (PR). She asks you to help her develop a nutrition program that will help her achieve her goal. The marathon is in 1 month.

Initial Assessment

1. What are some specific questions you could ask Kate to increase your understanding of each of the following objectives? How would her answers help you in developing a nutrition program?
   a. To determine the healthiness of her diet as well as if she is consuming adequate calories to fuel her workout
   b. To understand what she eats before, during, and after her runs
   c. To assess whether she has an understanding of basic sports nutrition
   d. To get a sense of how much she is working out

Areas for Improvement

2. As you work with Kate, you identify several potential areas of improvement. How would you help her in each of these areas?
   a. Kate routinely skips lunch. Most of her workouts are in the early evening.
   b. During Kate's long runs (90 minutes or more) she only drinks water.
   c. In previous races Kate did not change her nutritional habits in the weeks preceding the marathons.

Applying the Physiology

3. Why would skipping lunch negatively affect Kate's exercise performance?
4. How might a strategic fueling plan during prolonged exercise sessions improve Kate's speed?
5. What performance benefit could Kate get from carbohydrate loading in the week leading up to the marathon?

Follow Up

Kate completes the marathon in 3:34:50. She thanks you profusely for helping her to achieve her goal.

6. What do you think are three important physiological changes that enabled her to achieve this success?

Case 2 Eric the Recreational Bodybuilder

Eric is a 31-year-old competitive bodybuilder. He participates in bodybuilding competitions in the fall and trains the rest of the year. He is 5′11″ and weighs 184 pounds. He currently is in summer training. He asks you to review his current exercise and nutrition plan and see if you can identify any areas for improvement.

Initial Assessment

On your initial intake you learn that Eric follows a well-balanced periodized lifting program. He spends about 2 hours lifting weights 4 days per week. He also spends about 45 minutes 3 days per week running. You also learn that Eric eats a diet that is 40% carbohydrates, 30% protein, and 30% fat.

1. Using the Internet or other reference materials, look up the rationale behind why some athletes follow the 40-30-30 diet.
   a. Describe the rationale here.
   b. Based on your understanding of the physiology of sports nutrition, explain the problems or inaccuracies with this rationale.
   c. Identify a peer-reviewed journal article that addresses this topic. Summarize its findings.
2. How might you go about explaining to Eric your findings in a way that he might understand and be receptive to hearing?

Areas for Improvement

3. What are three changes Eric could make to his eating plan to improve his athletic performance?

Applying the Physiology

Eric reveals to you that he has been taking creatine supplementation to help build his body mass.

4. How might this supplement increase his muscular strength? What are some potential limitations? What do you say when he asks you if you think he should keep taking it?

Eric also shares that he drinks four 8-ounce glasses of whey protein powder per day.

5. Do you think that this is helping, hurting, or not affecting his muscular strength? Why?

Follow Up

You run into Eric in the midst of his competition season and you notice that his muscle mass has drastically increased.

6. What are several possible explanations for how Eric so significantly increased his muscle mass? Briefly describe the physiology behind how each of the explanations would occur.

TRAIN YOURSELF

Use the basic principles of exercise physiology and sports nutrition to your advantage to improve your overall fitness and athletic performance.

Initial Assessment

Identify your current patterns with a 7-day physical activity and sports nutrition log.

1. List the physical activities, time of day, approximate intensity (low, moderate, high), duration of activity, and primary energy system used.
2. Record any meals or snacks you had in the 4 hours preceding the exercise up until 4 hours after exercise.

Areas for Improvement

3. Based on review of your activity log, what are three changes you could make to your current exercise plan to improve your overall fitness and athletic performance?
4. Based on your identified areas of improvement and your current motivation, set a SMART (specific, measurable, attainable, relevant, and time-bound) goal.

Applying the Physiology

5. What energy systems did you use for your physical activities? Was one represented more than the others?
6. What benefits might you gain from incorporating other energy systems?

7. What are some specific exercises or activities you could incorporate into your training regimen to utilize these systems?

Follow Up

8. Based on your understanding of exercise physiology and sports nutrition, and using the SMART goal that you set above as your guide, draft an e-mail to your "future self" outlining a fitness goal you hope to accomplish in the next 3 months. Then, set up your e-mail program to automatically send you that e-mail 3 months from today. Then, when you're least expecting, you'll get a reminder of what you had hoped to accomplish.

RESOURCES

Mahan LK, Raymond JL, and Escott-Stump S. *Krause's food, nutrition, & diet therapy*. 13th ed. Philadelphia: W.B. Saunders; 2011.

REFERENCES

1. French J, Long, M. How to improve your VO_2max. *Athletics Weekly*. November 8 2012; 53.
2. Jacobs RA, Rasmussen P, Siebenmann C, et al. Determinants of time trial performance and maximal incremental exercise in highly trained endurance athletes. *J Appl Physiol*. September 1, 2011.
3. Knowles MS, Holton EF, Swanson RA. *The adult learner: the definitive classic in adult education and human resource development*. 7th ed. Amsterdam: Elsevier; 2011.
4. Romijn JA, Coyle EF, Sidossis LS, et al. Regulation of endogenous fat and carbohydrate metabolism in relation to exercise intensity and duration. *Am J Physiol*. September 1993;265(3 Pt 1):E380-391.

CHAPTER 7

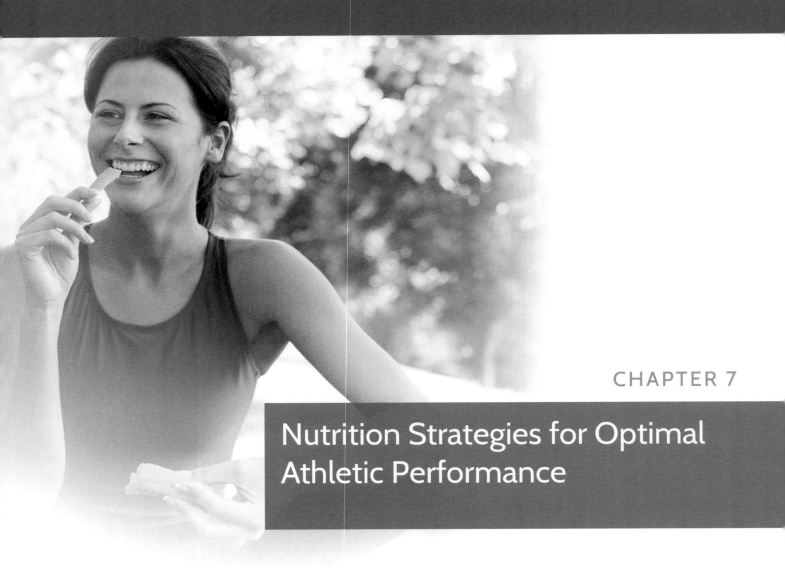

Nutrition Strategies for Optimal Athletic Performance

CHAPTER OUTLINE

LEARNING OBJECTIVES

After studying this chapter, the reader should be able to:

7.1 Describe the pathway of glucose from food to fuel.

7.2 Explain the rationale and effectiveness of carbohydrate loading.

7.3 List the roles of protein in endurance and resistance training.

7.4 Explain the rationale behind "fat loading" and why the method is not recommended.

7.5 Recognize the major goals of pre-exercise, exercise, and post-exercise nutritional strategies.

7.6 List several strategies to optimize pre-exercise, during exercise, and post-exercise nutrition.

KEY TERMS

carbohydrate loading Eating pattern that consists of increasing the amount of carbohydrates consumed in the days leading up to an athletic endurance event to maximize muscle and liver glycogen stores. Typically, activity levels are decreased during this time as well.

fat loading A strategy of progressively increasing percentage of fat intake to increase fatty acid oxidation and thus preserve glycogen stores for prolonged exercise.

gluconeogenesis The production of glucose from precursors such as proteins or fats in the liver.

glycemic index A measurement of the amount of increase in blood sugar after eating particular foods.

glycogen A polysaccharide that is a highly branched chain of glucose molecules. The chief carbohydrate storage material in animals formed and stored in the liver and muscle.

hyperglycemia An abnormally high level of glucose (sugar) in the blood (>100 mg/dL fasting).

hyperinsulinemia An abnormally high level of insulin in the blood.

portal circulation Circulatory system that takes nutrients directly from the stomach, small intestine, colon, and spleen to the liver.

triacylglycerols Compound consisting of three fatty acids and one glycerol molecule.

INTRODUCTION

Dennis Kimetto of Kenya holds the record for the fastest recorded marathon with a 2 hour, 2 minute, and 57 second finish at the 2014 Berlin Marathon—that's about 4 minutes and 42 seconds per mile, or 12.8 miles per hour. These days, it's not just elite runners who are triumphantly finishing 26.2-mile runs. Recreational athletes from teenagers to the elderly (the oldest finisher to date was 100 years old) repeatedly accomplish the feat. But the human body may not have been designed to run such long distances. Legend has it that the first marathoner was the Greek soldier Pheidippides, who ran 25 miles to carry a message from the Battle of Marathon to Athens. He reportedly collapsed and died shortly after reaching his destination. While this story may be part myth, the point is important—without adequate preparation, including regular physical training and good nutrition and hydration, the body is susceptible to overheating and breaking down.

On the other hand, with appropriate training and nutrition, the body can be trained to perform at high levels under highly stressful conditions. For example, in 2010 a Belgian man ran a marathon for every day of the year—365 marathons in as many days. Regardless of whether an athlete is preparing for a 10K run, a century (100-mile) bike ride, or an Ironman distance triathlon (2.4-mile swim, 112-mile bike ride, and a marathon run), or something in between, what he or she eats before, during, and after exercise plays an important role in determining exercise comfort and athletic performance.

THE ANATOMY AND PHYSIOLOGY OF EATING AND EXERCISE

Clients commonly ask what to eat before, during, or after exercise. An avid early morning Spin class attendee may want to know what to eat, if anything, before heading to the gym. A distance runner prone to stomach cramping during long, strenuous runs may ask for recommendations for less cramp-provoking snacks. Or a triathlete who struggles to excel at his evening swim on days when he did a morning training bike ride may ask for guidance with his post-ride recovery snack.

To provide sound information to these clients, it helps to have a good understanding of how digestion and nutrient absorption work, especially as it relates to exercise and the process of transforming food into energy to fuel exercise.

Digestion and Absorption Review

From the moment a person even begins to think about food, the body starts to release enzymes to help break it down into its component parts: carbohydrates, protein, fat, water, vitamins, and minerals. The goal is to free up the usable nutrients and energy for use by the body and to get rid of the waste. The breakdown of the macronutrients, including carbohydrates, protein, and fat, provides the body with the energy to fuel exercise. Foods that are high in carbohydrates are most rapidly digested and absorbed. Foods that are high in fat take much more time to digest and absorb, and the time required for high-protein-containing food lies somewhere in the middle.

Carbohydrates are a source of quick energy due to their rapid transit time through the gastrointestinal tract. It usually takes carbohydrates 1 to 4 hours to be digested, absorbed, and stored as glycogen in muscle or the liver. Once a carbohydrate is consumed, it passes into the stomach and then the small intestine. Carbohydrates can be ingested at a fairly high rate of about 3 grams per minute before causing gastrointestinal upset.[1] The rate-limiting factor in the process of transferring glucose contained in food to usable energy to fuel exercise is the rate of absorption of carbohydrate from the small intestine into the **portal circulation**, a special circulation in which blood passes directly from the small intestine to the liver through the portal vein. The maximal rate of carbohydrate absorption is 1.2 to 1.7 grams per minute.[1] Carbohydrates that pass into the liver may be stored as glycogen or passed into the systemic circulation to provide energy to working muscles and cells, depending on the body's current metabolic needs.

Macronutrient Storage

In addition to the energy available from the breakdown of foods consumed shortly before and during exercise, the body also relies on stored energy to help fuel exercise. Carbohydrates and fat are stored in the body so they can be readily available when needed. When metabolic demands increase, glucose-releasing enzymes free up stored glucose (**glycogen**) from muscle and the liver. In the liver, glucose broken down from the carbohydrates in food can join a pool with the body's stored glucose to pass from the liver into the systemic circulation at a maximum of 1 gram per minute. The glucose can then be taken up by muscle at a similar rate (1 g/min) to be converted to adenosine triphosphate (ATP) to supply energy to fuel exercise (also occurring at a rate of about 1 g/min) (Fig. 7-1).[1]

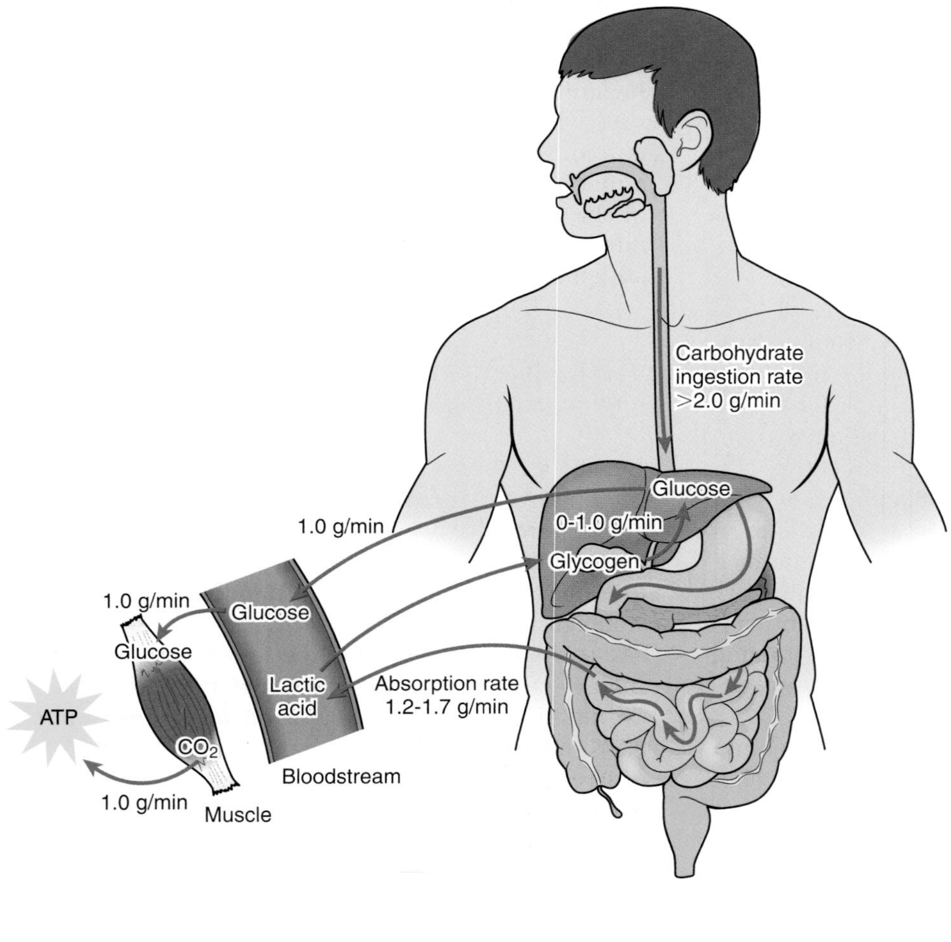

Figure 7-1. The pathway of glucose from food to fuel.

When necessary, stored triglycerides (**triacylglycerols**) in adipose tissue are released as energy-rich fatty acids that can be broken down to make ATP through beta oxidation (see Chapter 6 for more detailed information). While protein that is not immediately used by the body is either excreted or converted to and stored as fat, the carbon skeleton of some amino acids—whether in the blood from a recent meal or being used by the body in muscle or other tissue—can be used to produce glucose for energy through **gluconeogenesis**, the production of glucose from nonsugar substrates such as amino acids. Depending on the duration and intensity of exercise, these stored macronutrients are broken down to regenerate ATP to fuel exercise.

SPEED BUMP

1. Describe the pathway of glucose from food to fuel.

ENERGY INTAKE AND ATHLETIC PERFORMANCE

For optimal performance the working muscles need a constant supply of glucose. When exercise lasts longer than 1 hour and no carbohydrates have been ingested, blood glucose levels begin to dwindle. After 1 to 3 hours of continuous moderate-intensity exercise, muscle glycogen stores may become depleted. If no glucose is consumed, the blood glucose levels drop, resulting in further depletion of liver and muscle glycogen. When this happens, regardless of the athlete's internal toughness or desire to maintain intensity, performance falters (Fig. 7-2).[2]

On the other hand, an optimal eating plan combined with well-planned physical training and rest can set the stage for peak athletic performance. Compared to the general population, endurance athletes require increased fluid to replace sweat losses and increased energy to fuel exercise.

Carbohydrates

Carbohydrates are the body's preferred energy source because they are rapidly digested and absorbed, which provides an immediate energy source. The increased caloric demands of strenuous exercise are best met with an increase in carbohydrate consumption. Consumption of carbohydrates that contain two or three different saccharides (or sugars) such as glucose, fructose, and sucrose, may increase carbohydrate absorption because they use different transport mechanisms from the small intestine to the bloodstream and so decrease competition for transport.[3] For example, glucose uses a transporter called sodium dependent glucose transporter 1 (SGLT 1), whereas fructose is transported by glucose transporter 5 (GLUT5).[3] Increased carbohydrate absorption may lead to increased athletic performance by making more fuel available for exercise more quickly. Not only can consuming foods and drinks that contain more than one kind of carbohydrate enhance athletic performance, but it might also decrease gastrointestinal distress during exercise. By using different transporters for absorption, less carbohydrate remains in the gastrointestinal tract. Less carbohydrate in the gut means less bloating, nausea, and discomfort.[3] Most sports drinks companies understand this well, with almost all brands of sports drink comprising multiple types of sugar. For example, Gatorade is a combination of sucrose, glucose, and fructose.

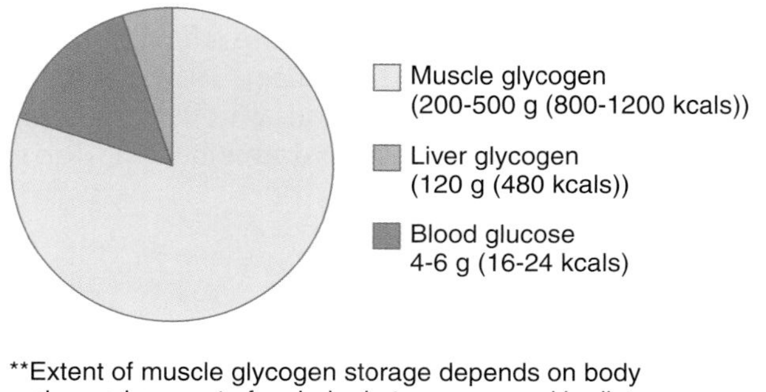

Figure 7-2. Carbohydrate distribution in the body.

Carbohydrate Loading for Endurance Athletes

Individuals training for long-distance endurance events lasting more than 90 minutes, such as a marathon or triathlon, may benefit from **carbohydrate loading** in the days or weeks prior to competition. Consuming more carbohydrates prepares the muscles and liver to store more carbohydrates as glycogen. This increased stored glycogen means the athlete has more fuel to burn before the glycogen becomes depleted. The Academy of Nutrition and Dietetics (formerly called the American Dietetic Association) and the American College of Sports Medicine[4] reviewed 23 studies that have looked at rates and amounts of macronutrient consumption during the training period before an athletic competition. Nine of the studies found that consumption of a high-carbohydrate diet (>60% of energy) in the training period and the week prior to competition resulted in increased muscle glycogen concentrations and/or improvement in performance. Nine studies found no difference. Two found no additional benefit beyond eating 6 grams of carbohydrates per kilogram body weight. Two found gender differences indicating that women may be less able to increase muscle glycogen concentrations through increased carbohydrate consumption. The last study found that performance increased when a high-fat diet for 10 days was followed by a high-carbohydrate diet for 10 days (see Reference 4 for a description of the studies and full reference list).

The assumption behind carbohydrate loading is that eating more carbohydrates helps muscles store more carbohydrates in the form of glycogen. If more glycogen is stored, it will take longer to deplete the body's preferred energy source during a prolonged workout. During carbohydrate loading, clients should taper their workout intensity and/or duration as they near an event so that muscle glycogen stores are not depleted prior to the competition. Carbohydrate loading may contribute to water-based weight gain because carbohydrates require sizeable amounts of water for storage. Various carbohydrate-loading regimens exist, including 7-day, 6-day, 3-day, and 1-day protocols that typically involve two stages:

- Glycogen depletion stage: moderate-to-high intensity exercise to deplete glycogen stores, coupled with low-to-moderate carbohydrate intakes (<55% of total kcal)
- Glycogen loading stage: tapered exercise (low-intensity, short-duration), coupled with high carbohydrate intakes (>70% of total kcal)

There are two basic methods of carbohydrate loading that follow this regimen: classical and modified. In the 1960s, Scandinavian researchers found endurance athletes could double glycogen stores by:[5]

- Two sessions of intense exercise to exhaustion to deplete glycogen
- Two days of less than 10% carbohydrates to "starve" muscle
- Three days of rest while taking in 90% or more carbohydrates

This classical version of carbohydrate loading has serious side effects. The 10% carbohydrate sessions can cause irritability and dizziness, and therefore loss of productive training.

Current research has proven runners can implement a modified version of carbohydrate loading, which increases glycogen stores (between 20% to 40%) but avoids adverse effects. An example of a modified 1-week plan follows:

Days 1 to 3: Moderate carbohydrate diet (50% of calories).

Days 4 to 6: High carbohydrate diet (80% of calories). The recommendation is for about 4.5 grams of carbohydrate per pound of body weight. For example, a 170-lb man would consume 765 grams, or 3,000 calories, from carbohydrates per day.

Day 7: Competitive event. Pre-event meal (typically dinner the night before the event) with carbohydrates (>80% of calories from carbohydrates).

While carbohydrate loading may benefit athletic performance during a prolonged endurance session, it is not without drawbacks. Mental and physical fatigue, irritability, mood disturbances, poor recovery, and increased risk of injury can occur during glycogen depletion stages. Bloating, gastrointestinal distress, weight gain, lethargy, and frustration associated with altered training schedules frequently occur during carbohydrate loading stages.[6] Also, it is worth noting that carbohydrate loading may not always contribute to increased athletic performance. Multiple variables including the loading strategy, type of carbohydrate consumed (low- vs. high-glycemic), timing, gender, and exercise characteristics (endurance, sprint, etc.) affect performance.[6] Carbohydrate loading is most effective for long-distance endurance athletes. Athletes whose sports events span less than 90 minutes (e.g., sprinters) will probably experience adverse effects of carbohydrate loading, such as weight gain. Those clients serious about optimizing sports performance may consider a consultation with a sports dietitian to help them adopt the most appropriate dietary plan and carbohydrate loading regimen. Devising a carbohydrate loading regimen is outside the scope of practice for most health professionals.

Glycemic Index

The role of **glycemic index** and exercise performance has been a source of ongoing research for the past two decades. Initial studies suggested a low glycemic index diet prior to exercise can facilitate increased glycogen availability and improved performance. Research participants who consumed a low glycemic index meal prior to exercise, such as oatmeal with strawberries, had a decreased level of postprandial **hyperglycemia** and **hyperinsulinemia**. As a result, there was an increase in free fatty acid oxidation and thus more carbohydrate available during exercise.[7] Other studies support that low glycemic index foods interact with fatty acid oxidation, which may contribute to increased performance.[8,9] While this still seems to be true, further research found this benefit is negated as soon as a carbohydrate-containing sports drink, gel, or bar is consumed during an exercise session.[7] It is worth noting that some low glycemic index foods, such as dried fruits, are high in fiber, which can cause gastrointestinal distress like gas, abdominal cramps, and diarrhea.

It seems logical that foods with a high glycemic index, such as white bread, bananas, and pancakes, would be effective at replenishing glycogen stores after exercise. After all, carbohydrates with a high glycemic index are rapidly absorbed and quickly release sugar into the bloodstream. Thus, they should be more effective at replenishing energy stores than low glycemic index foods, which are broken down more slowly and take longer to release sugar into the bloodstream. While an early body of research supported this supposition, some more recent studies have found that low glycemic index foods interact with fatty acid oxidation, which may contribute to increased performance in future events.[8,9] Overall, despite years of research on glycemic and endurance performance, there is still no agreement about how glycemic index affects performance (see Evaluating the Evidence). Athletes should follow standard recommendations and personal experience when choosing carbohydrates before, during, and after exercise.[10]

Fat

A 1995 article touted **fat loading** as the "next magic bullet" to improve athletic performance.[11] The idea was that if a progressively greater percentage of fat was

EVALUATING THE EVIDENCE

Do High Glycemic Index Foods Optimize Glycogen Replenishment?[9]

It had long been thought that consumption of high glycemic index foods immediately following a strenuous endurance workout would boost glycogen stores more than consumption of a low glycemic index diet. Then, a few studies such as the one described below were published. These studies suggested that glycemic index of a post-exercise snack does not affect muscle or liver glycogen replenishment, but that a low glycemic index diet would help to increase fatty acid oxidation and thus indirectly salvage glycogen stores. Here is the study abstract:

The glycemic index of dietary carbohydrates influences glycogen storage in skeletal muscle and circulating nonesterified fatty acid (NEFA) concentrations. We hypothesized that diets differing only in glycemic index would alter intramuscular lipid oxidation and glycogen usage in skeletal muscle and the liver during subsequent exercise. Endurance-trained individuals (n = 9) cycled for 90 minutes at 70% Vo(2peak) and then consumed either high- or low-glycemic index meals over the following 12 hours. The following day after an overnight fast, the 90-minute cycle was repeated. (1)H and (13)C magnetic resonance spectroscopy was used before and after exercise to assess intramuscular lipid and glycogen content of the vastus muscle group and liver. Blood and expired air samples were collected at 15-minute intervals throughout exercise. NEFA availability was reduced during exercise in the high-glycemic index compared with the low-glycemic index trial (area under curve 44.5 +/- 6.0 vs. 38.4 +/- 7.30 mM/h, P <0.05). Exercise elicited an approximately 55% greater reduction in intramyocellular triglyceride (IMCL) in the high- versus low-glycemic index trial (1.6 +/- 0.2 vs. 1.0 +/- 0.3 mmol/kg wet wt, P <0.05). There was no difference in the exercise-induced reduction of the glycogen pool in skeletal muscle (76 +/- 8 vs. 68 +/- 5 mM) or in the liver (65 +/- 8 vs. 71 +/- 4 mM) between the low- and high-glycemic index trials, respectively. High-glycemic index recovery diets reduce NEFA availability and increase reliance on IMCL during moderate-intensity exercise. Skeletal muscle and liver glycogen storage or usage are not affected by the glycemic index of an acute recovery diet.

1. Do you have any knowledge gaps that need to be addressed before fully understanding this abstract? What are they and how would you close them?
2. Do you feel like you have enough information from the abstract or would you prefer to read the whole article? Why or why not? What extra information would the full article contain that might be helpful?
3. In lay terms, how would you summarize the results of this study for a client?
4. Do the results of this study have clinical relevance to you and your job? That is, will this study change the way you practice your profession?
5. As a practicing professional, how might you stay on top of the latest research and advances in your profession while at the same time running a busy clinical practice?

consumed in the diet, then fat oxidation would be increased during exercise. Energy would be produced from fat and, therefore, carbohydrate stores could be spared. Typically, carbohydrate stores can only fuel about 3 hours of endurance activity. The thinking was that by shifting to using more fat for fuel it would take longer to deplete muscle glycogen stores and long-distance activities could be maintained for a longer period of time at a higher intensity.

Many studies have been done to test both the short-term and long-term effects of fat loading on endurance performance. Short-term exposure to a high-fat (>60% of calories from fat), low-carbohydrate diet is clearly detrimental: fat utilization during exercise is unchanged and muscle glycogen stores are decreased.[12] However, adoption of a high-fat, low-carbohydrate diet for several days may offer some limited benefits. With longer-term fat adaptation, fat utilization during exercise likely is increased with perhaps some sparing of glycogen stores, but there may also be a decreased total amount of glycogen available. Although studies suggest high levels of physical performance can be maintained across varying levels of fat consumption, it has also been found that a much greater mental effort is required to perform when on a high-fat diet.[13] To summarize, it seems performance is optimized when glycogen stores are maintained by efforts to enhance carbohydrate availability, like carbohydrate loading and eating carbohydrates before and during a prolonged session, and not fat loading.

Protein

Protein plays important roles in endurance and resistance training exercise. Both modes of exercise stimulate muscle protein synthesis[14] which is further enhanced with consumption of protein around the time of exercise.[15] Consumption of protein immediately post-exercise helps in the repair and synthesis of muscle proteins.[16] Protein intake during exercise has not been shown to offer any additional performance benefit if sufficient amounts of carbohydrates—the body's preferred energy source—are consumed.[16] However, for endurance athletes who may struggle to consume adequate calories to fuel extended training sessions, or for the average exerciser striving to lose weight, research suggests that protein helps to preserve lean muscle mass and assure that the majority of weight lost comes from fat rather than lean tissue.[14] While these may seem like great reasons to boost protein intake, it is worth noting that most people habitually consume more than even the most liberal protein intake recommendations.[17] For women and men between the ages of 19 to 70+ the RDA for protein is 46 grams and 56 grams, respectively.[18] Protein consumption beyond these amounts is unlikely to result in further muscle gains because the body has a limited capacity to utilize amino acids to build muscle.[17]

SPEED BUMP

2. **Explain the rationale and effectiveness of carbohydrate loading.**
3. **List the roles of protein in endurance and resistance training.**
4. **Explain the rationale behind "fat loading" and why the method is out of favor.**

NUTRITION REQUIREMENTS BEFORE, DURING, AND AFTER EXERCISE

Athletes need the right types and amounts of food before, during, and after exercise to maximize the amount of energy available to fuel optimal performance and minimize the amount of gastrointestinal distress. Sports nutrition strategies should address three exercise stages: pre-exercise, exercise, and post-exercise (Fig. 7-3).

Pre-Exercise

The two main goals of a pre-exercise snack are to (1) optimize glucose availability and glycogen stores, and (2) provide the fuel needed for exercise performance. Keeping this in mind, in the days up to a week before a strenuous endurance effort, an athlete should consider what nutritional strategies might best facilitate optimal performance (see Myths and Misconceptions). For example, an athlete preparing for a long endurance event might consider the pros and cons of carbohydrate loading. On the day of the event or an important training session, the athlete should aim to eat a meal about 4 to 6 hours prior to the workout to minimize gastrointestinal distress and optimize performance. Four hours after eating, the food will already have been digested and absorbed; now liver and muscle glycogen levels are at their highest. To translate this into an everyday, practical recommendation: athletes who work out in the early afternoon should be certain to eat a wholesome carbohydrate-rich breakfast. Those who exercise in the early morning may benefit from a carbohydrate-rich snack before going to bed.

Some research also suggests that eating a relatively small carbohydrate- and protein-containing snack (e.g., 50 g of carbohydrate and 5 to 10 g of protein) 30 to 60 minutes before exercise helps increase glucose availability near the end of the workout and decrease exercise-induced protein catabolism.[19] The exact timing and size of the snack for peak performance will vary by athlete. As a general rule, athletes should try out any snacks or drinks with practice sessions prior to relying on them to help optimize athletic performance on race day.

Fueling During Exercise

The goal of fueling during exercise is to provide the body with the essential nutrients needed by muscle cells and maintain optimal blood glucose levels. During a prolonged endurance effort, such as a marathon, an athlete is at risk of "hitting the wall"—a phenomena often occurring around mile 20 in a 26-mile race. This is when extreme fatigue sets in due to drained carbohydrate

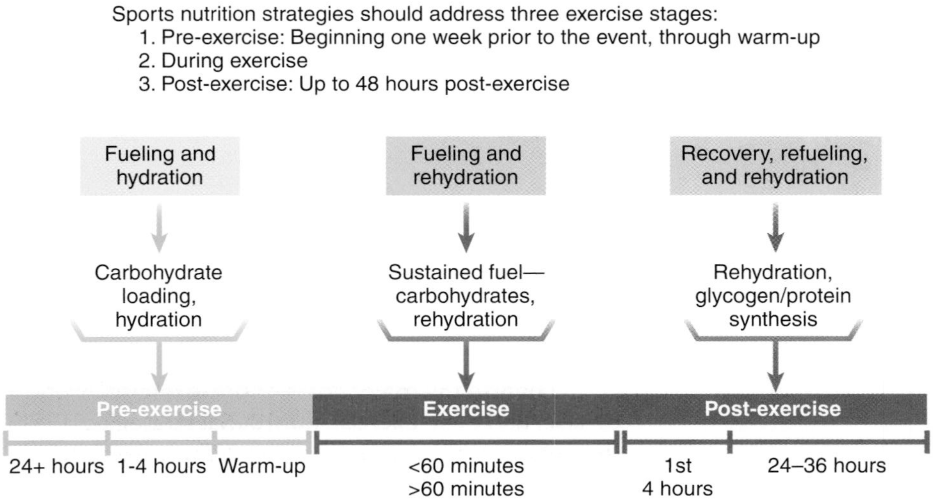

Figure 7-3. Sports nutrition strategies. *Courtesy of Fabio Comana.*

Myths and Misconceptions

Eating Sweets Before Competition Boosts Energy

The Myth

Eating sugar, honey, soft drinks, or other sweets just before competition will provide a burst of quick energy.

The Logic

Glucose is not only the body's preferred energy source, but it is also rapidly digested. Consuming a simple sugar right before exercise should make its way into the bloodstream in no time and immediately be used to fuel exercise.

The Science

It takes the body about 1 to 4 hours to digest food. Foods eaten immediately before exercise are still in the stomach at the onset of the exercise session. With good nutritional habits in the days to week preceding a prolonged endurance session, plenty of glucose will be readily available from blood and muscle glycogen to fuel the first hour of activity. By then, some of the glucose from the snack right before exercise will become available and help to optimize performance for the remainder of the workout. Box 7-1 provides tips on how to pick a pre-exercise snack to minimize gastrointestinal distress and optimize the performance benefit.

stores. But there are gradations on the physical demands of exercise based on the duration of the exercise session. Exercise lasting less than 1 hour can be adequately fueled with existing glucose and glycogen stores. No additional carbohydrate-containing drinks or foods are necessary.

To maintain a ready energy supply, athletes should consume glucose-containing beverages and snacks during prolonged exercise sessions (>60 minutes). The Academy of Nutrition and Dietetics, the Dietitians of Canada, and the American College of Sports Medicine recommend that athletes consume 30 to 60 grams of carbohydrates per hour of training.[4] For instance, an athlete who trains for 3 hours would need 90 (360 kcals) to 180 grams (720 kcals) of carbohydrates. The upper limit is especially important for prolonged exercise and exercise in extreme heat, cold, or high altitude; for athletes who did not consume adequate amounts of food or drink prior to the training session; and for athletes who did not carbohydrate load or who restricted energy intake for weight loss.

Carbohydrate consumption during prolonged exercise should begin shortly after the initiation of the workout. The carbohydrate will be more effective if the 30 to 60 grams per hour are consumed in small amounts in 15 to 20 minute intervals rather than as a large bolus after 2 hours of exercise.[4]

Box 7-1. General Guidelines for Pre-Exercise Meal or Snack

In general, a pre-exercise meal or snack should be:

- Relatively high in carbohydrate to maximize blood glucose availability
- Relatively low in fat and fiber to minimize gastrointestinal distress and facilitate gastric emptying
- Moderate in protein
- Well-tolerated by the individual

Post-Exercise Replenishment

The main goal of post-exercise fueling is to replenish glycogen stores and facilitate muscle repair. The average client training at moderate intensities every few days does not need any aggressive post-exercise replenishment. Normal dietary practices following exercise will facilitate recovery within 20 to 48 hours. But athletes following vigorous training regimens, especially those who will participate in multiple training sessions in a single day (like a triathlete), benefit from strategic refueling (see Communication Strategies).

Studies show the best post-workout meals are high in carbohydrates accompanied with some protein (e.g., 1 g/kg of carbohydrate and 0.5 g/kg of protein).[19,20] Refueling should begin within 30 minutes after exercise and be followed by a high-carbohydrate meal within 2 hours[19] (Box 7-2). The carbohydrates replenish the used-up energy that is normally stored as glycogen in muscle and the liver. The protein helps to rebuild the muscles that were broken down with exercise. The Academy of Nutrition and Dietetics recommends a carbohydrate intake of 1.5 grams/kilogram of body weight in the first 30 minutes after exercise and then every 2 hours for 4 to 6 hours.[4] After that, the athlete can resume his or her typical, balanced diet. Of course, the amount of refueling necessary depends on the intensity and duration of the training session. A long-duration, low-intensity workout may not require such vigorous replenishment.

SPEED BUMP

5. **Recognize the major goals of pre-exercise, exercise, and post-exercise nutritional strategies.**
6. **List several strategies to optimize pre-exercise, during exercise, and post-exercise nutrition.**

COMMUNICATION STRATEGIES

A Needs Assessment[21]

An acquaintance who knows that you are studying sports nutrition has asked you a laundry list of questions. Specifically, she wants to know:

- How long should she wait to exercise after eating?
- Will drinking a sports drink help her go faster on her upcoming 5-mile bike ride?
- She read that it is important to eat carbohydrates immediately after working out so she's been following every workout with a 180-calorie nutrition bar. She wants to know if this might be getting in the way of her losing weight.

Before answering each of your acquaintance's questions, conducting a brief "needs assessment" will help you to make sure you answer her questions in the most meaningful way. A needs assessment helps to identify the current knowledge and experience of a "learner" so that teaching can begin at the client's level and not at a level that is too rudimentary or too advanced. This can be represented mathematically through the following equation:

Desired knowledge, skill, attitude, or performance – Current knowledge, skill, attitude, or performance = Need for learning

For example, you might ask your friend:

"What kind of exercise do you like to do?"
"How often do you exercise?"
"How long is your typical workout?"
"You mentioned that you read that it's good to eat carbs after a workout. What else have you read on sports nutrition topics?"

This information not only helps you to most accurately answer the question, but it also helps you to answer the question at your acquaintance's level so that the information will be most meaningful to her.

Class Activity

Role play. In pairs, practice being both the health professional (choose whichever field most interests you) and the client or acquaintance who is interested in learning more about sports nutrition. As the client, ask the health professional a few nutrition questions related to the content contained in this chapter. As the health professional, practice conducting a "needs assessment" before answering the question. Then, try to provide your answer at your client's knowledge level, while being sure to stay within your scope of practice.

Box 7-2. **Post-Workout Snack and Meal Ideas**

In the several hours following a prolonged and strenuous workout, consuming snacks and meals high in carbohydrate with some protein can set the stage for optimal glycogen replenishment and subsequent performance. Here are a few snack and meal ideas that fit the bill:

Snack 1: In the first several minutes after exercise, consume 16 ounces of Gatorade or other sports drink, a power gel such as a Clif Shot or Goo, and a medium banana. This quickly begins to replenish muscle carbohydrate stores. *Carbohydrates: 73 g; protein: 1 g; calories: 288.*

Snack 2: After cooling down and showering, grab another quick snack, such as 12 ounces of orange juice and 1/4 cup of raisins. *Carbohydrates: 70 g; protein 3 g; calories: 295.*

Small meal appetizer: Enjoy a spinach salad with tomatoes, chick peas, green beans, and 3/4 cup tuna and a small whole grain baguette. *Carbohydrates: 70 g; protein: 37 g; calories: 489.*

Small meal main course: Replenish with 3/4 cup whole grain pasta with diced tomatoes. *Carbohydrates: 67 g; protein: 2 g; calories: 292.*

Dessert: After allowing ample time for the day's snacks and meals to digest, finish your refueling program with 1 cup of frozen yogurt and berries. *Carbohydrates: 61 g; protein: 8 g; calories: 280.*

CHAPTER SUMMARY

Optimal nutrition intake before, during, and after exercise helps to maintain blood glucose concentrations during exercise, maximize exercise performance, and improve recovery time.

KEY POINTS SUMMARY

1. Carbohydrates are the body's preferred energy source due to their rapid breakdown and thus quick availability of ATP, the body's usable energy. However, the body also can get energy from breakdown of fatty acids, and in less desirable situations, from the conversion of amino acids to glucose through gluconeogenesis.
2. A consumed carbohydrate passes through the gastrointestinal system, into the portal circulation to the liver, and into the systemic circulation before it reaches the exercising muscle. In the exercising muscle, it undergoes glycolysis to produce ATP.
3. Absorption of glucose from the small intestine into the portal circulation is the rate-limiting step in transforming glucose from food into fuel. The maximum rate at which glucose can pass from the small intestine into the portal circulation is 1.2 to 1.7 grams per minute.
4. Very little glucose is stored in the body. At most, slightly more than a day's worth of calories for an inactive person is available from blood glucose, liver glycogen, and muscle glycogen combined. At the lower end of muscle glycogen stores, the total calories from this stored glucose is little more than the number of calories needed to fuel a half marathon.
5. Endurance athletes can increase the amount of glucose available to fuel exercise by carbohydrate loading, which acts to help increase muscle glycogen stores. Carbohydrate loading is not without risks, though, especially the classical method. However, the current modified methods can avert some of the negative effects of carbohydrate loading. A carbohydrate loading regimen for an endurance athlete who is training for an event may best be developed with the assistance of a sports dietitian. Recommending a carbohydrate loading regimen is outside the scope of practice of most health professionals.
6. Glycemic index of carbohydrates has been explored as a possible variable in improving athletic performance, but to date the research is mixed and inconclusive.
7. The two main goals of a pre-exercise snack are to (1) optimize glucose availability and glycogen stores, and (2) provide the fuel needed for exercise performance. For peak performance, the athlete should consume a high carbohydrate diet (>60% of total calories from carbohydrates) in the week preceding the event and aim to eat a meal about 4 to 6 hours prior to the workout.
8. Eating a small carbohydrate- and protein-containing (e.g., 50 g of carbohydrate and 5 to 10 g of protein = 220–250 calories) snack 30 to 60 minutes before exercise helps increase glucose availability near the end of the workout and decrease exercise-induced protein catabolism.
9. As a general rule, athletes should try out any snacks or drinks with practice sessions prior to relying on them to help optimize athletic performance on race day.
10. The goal of fueling during exercise is to provide the body with the essential nutrients needed by muscle cells (sodium, potassium) and maintain optimal blood glucose levels.
11. To maintain a ready energy supply during prolonged exercise sessions (>60 minutes), athletes should consume 30 to 60 grams of carbohydrate per hour of training.
12. Carbohydrates consumed during exercise are most effective if the 30 to 60 grams per hour are consumed in small amounts in 15- to 20-minute intervals rather than as a large bolus.
13. Refueling should begin within 30 minutes after exercise and be followed by a high-carbohydrate meal within 2 hours. Depending on the duration and intensity of exercise, for optimal glycogen replenishment athletes should consume up to 1.5 grams/kilogram of body weight in the first 30 minutes after exercise and then every 2 hours for 4 to 6 hours.

PRACTICAL APPLICATIONS

Questions 1 to 3 are based on the following scenario:

Jack is a 20-year-old runner who consistently complains of abdominal cramping during his strenuous runs. On further questioning he tells you that he eats a 30-gram carbohydrate snack midway through a 90-minute run.

1. What is the minimal amount of time it will take for the entire snack to be oxidized to create ATP?
   A. 0 to 30 minutes
   B. 30 minutes to 1 hour
   C. 1 to 2 hours
   D. 2 to 3 hours
   E. 3 to 4 hours

2. What would be the MOST reasonable suggestion to help Jack minimize gastrointestinal distress during the workout and also improve his performance?
   A. Consume the snack early in his workout and try to have small amounts every 15 to 20 minutes instead of consuming the snack all at once in the middle of his workout.
   B. Instead of a food snack, consider drinking water only, as it will be more effectively absorbed and is associated with decreased GI distress.

C. Ask him to consider postponing his snack until the end of his workout, as he won't deplete glycogen stores in 90 minutes and so the snack will not help with his performance.
D. Ask him to consider consuming his snack 4 hours prior to exercise so that there is sufficient time for the snack to be absorbed and stored as glycogen.

3. After questioning Jack about his exercise snack, he shares with you that he usually likes to eat a couple of dates during his workout due to their high glycemic index and thus rapid energy availability. Following is a nutritional summary for dates:
Serving size 2 dates (40 g)
Calories 110
Total fat 0 g
Potassium 190 mg (5%)
Total carbohydrate 31 g (10%)
Fiber 3 g (12%)
Sugars 27 g
Protein less than 1 g
Vitamin A 0% Vitamin C 0%
Calcium 2% Iron 2%
Glycemic Index 103 (High)

Do you think the dates might be contributing to Jack's GI upset?
A. No, because the high glycemic index of dates makes them a good source of quick energy.
B. No, because the carbohydrate load averages less than 3 grams per minute of activity.
C. Yes, because the high fiber content can cause GI distress.
D. Yes, because the high sugar content irritates the stomach lining.

4. A client just signed up to participate in a century (100-mile) bike ride. She tells you that she is interested in carbohydrate loading and asks what you recommend. Which is the BEST response?
A. Share with her the basic principles behind carbohydrate loading as well as some of the risks and refer her to a sports dietitian for an individualized regimen.
B. Share with her your preferred carbohydrate loading regimen but tell her that she'll have to see a sports dietitian for a specific recommendation.
C. Tell her that it is outside your scope of practice to discuss carbohydrate loading regimens and refer her to a sports dietitian.
D. Tell her that you don't recommend carbohydrate loading and advise that she follow the MyPyramid guidelines for an optimal eating plan.

5. A client says that she has decided to consume high-protein bars during exercise because she read that consuming protein during exercise is essential to boost performance. Before responding, what further information do you MOST want to know?
A. Where she read this misleading information.
B. If she consumes adequate amounts of carbohydrate.
C. What type of protein she plans on consuming.
D. The type of physical activity she most often performs.

6. Which of the following BEST explains why fat loading is not commonly practiced?
A. Consumption of large amounts of fat increases the risk of cardiovascular disease.
B. Fat loading does not improve performance any more than carbohydrate loading.
C. Fat loading leads to dramatic decreases in energy and overall athletic performance.
D. Consumption of large amounts of fat interferes with carbohydrate oxidation.

7. What are the main goals of strategic fueling before, during, and after exercise?
A. Optimize blood glucose availability
B. Optimize liver glycogen stores
C. Optimize muscle glycogen stores
D. Optimize cerebral glucose availability

8. Which of the following foods would be the MOST appropriate as a pre-event snack for Mike, a 132-lb (60 kg) endurance-trained individual performing a 10-mile run?
A. A small apple and granola bar 4 hours prior to the event.
B. A blueberry muffin 1 hour prior to the event.
C. A banana and energy bar 1 to 2 hours prior to the event.
D. A hamburger and french fries 3 to 4 hours prior to the event.

9. You are asked to review a new product that is specially designed to provide fuel for endurance athletes (see nutrition information below). What are you looking for when rating the product?

60-g package includes 6 pieces. Serving size (3 chews) contains 100 calories, 70 mg sodium, 20 mg potassium, 24 g carbohydrate, 0 g protein, 0 g fat. Contains 95% organic ingredients. Also available with added caffeine or increased sodium. Flavors include: cola (50 mg caffeine), black cherry (50 mg caffeine), orange (25 mg caffeine), cran razz, lemon lime, mountain berry, margarita (three times more sodium than the other products).
A. The feasibility of consuming 30 to 60 grams of carbohydrate per hour
B. A high-fat content to facilitate gastric emptying
C. A high-fiber content to facilitate gastric emptying
D. Sufficient protein to optimize performance

10. Jake, a varsity swimmer, is training for his upcoming season and needs to accelerate his post-exercise recovery rates. He trains intensely for 2 hours, 5 days a week. If he weighs 155 lb (70.45 kg), which of the following nutritional strategies would BEST replenish his glycogen stores?
    A. 50 grams of carbohydrates/hour for the first 6 hours starting within 30 minutes of finishing exercise.
    B. 75 grams of carbohydrates within the first 30 minutes of finishing exercise and then every hour for the first 3 hours.
    C. 105 grams of carbohydrate per hour for 6 hours starting within the 30 minutes of finishing exercise.
    D. 105 grams of carbohydrates within 30 minutes of finishing exercise and then every 2 hours for 6 hours.

Case 1 Scott, the Professional Triathlete

Scott is a 29-year-old professional triathlete. He is 6′2″ and 170 pounds (BMI 21.8 kg/m2). Triathlon season is underway and Scott is intensifying his training to compete in the October Kona Ironman Triathlon, which is about 4 months away. Scott has already qualified for this event by completing an Ironman (2.4-mile swim, 112-mile bike ride, and 26.2-mile run) in 8 hours and 30 minutes.

Scott is at the end of the "Base" training period of his program. He will begin "building" in the next 2 weeks. His training schedule is as follows:

	MONDAY	TUESDAY	WEDNESDAY	THURSDAY	FRIDAY	SATURDAY	SUNDAY
Swim	75*		75		90	**300**	
Bike	15	180	**150**	105		**30**	
Run	3		**30**	90			
Strength	6					5.5	0
Hours	3.0	3.0	4.3	3.3	1.5		

* Each box indicates the number of minutes per workout. Those workouts in bold are bricks.

Scott has asked you for some general tips to help him with his fueling strategy for optimal performance. His total calorie needs are about 6,500 calories per day.

Nutrition Recommendation Before Exercise

1. What are the main goals of pre-exercise fueling?
2. Would carbohydrate loading be something that might be appropriate for Scott? Why or why not?
3. What are the general principles to keep in mind when considering pre-exercise fueling?
4. What are some potential snacks for pre-exercise fueling?

Nutrition Recommendation During Exercise

1. What are the main goals of during-exercise fueling?
2. Scott is trying to plan out his fueling strategy for his Wednesday workout when he will be exercising for a total of 4.3 hours. About how many grams of carbohydrates should he consume during his 150-minute bike ride, which will be immediately followed by the 30-minute run?
3. What are some potential snacks for during-exercise fueling?

Nutrition Recommendation After Exercise

1. What are the main goals of post-exercise replenishment?
2. Devise a potential post-exercise fueling regimen for Scott.

Case 2 Susan, the Middle-Age Overweight Hiker

Susan is a 55-year-old overweight teacher who is training to hike the Grand Canyon with her 17-year-old daughter and a guide. She is 5′2″ and 180 pounds (BMI 32.9 kg/m2). She has hired you to help her get in shape for this adventure. The trip is planned for late September, which is about 3 months from now. Susan anticipates that the 9.3-mile trail down will take about 6 hours and the return up about 9 hours. She plans to complete the trek over a 3-day period.

Susan's calorie needs are about 1,800 calories per day.

This is Susan's planned workout program for the next week:

	MONDAY	TUESDAY	WEDNESDAY	THURSDAY	FRIDAY	SATURDAY	SUNDAY
Morning Walk	20[a]		20		20		20
Stair Climbing		50		50			
Outdoor Hike						90	
Strength		40		40			
Hours	0.3	1.5.	0.3	1.5	0.3	1.5	0.3

a. Each box indicates the number of minutes per workout.

Nutrition Recommendation Before Exercise

1. For which workouts should Susan consider developing a pre-exercise nutrition strategy? Why?

Nutrition Recommendation During Exercise

1. For which workouts should Susan consider a during-exercise nutrition strategy? Why?
2. You notice that Susan drinks a bottle of Gatorade during each of her stair-climbing workouts. Do you think that this will improve her performance? What are some potential negative consequences? How would you best communicate this information to her?

Nutrition Recommendation After Exercise

1. What would be the best post-exercise replenishment plan for Susan? Why?

TRAIN YOURSELF: NUTRITION NEEDS BEFORE, DURING, AND AFTER EXERCISE

Calculate your caloric needs based on the Institute of Medicine energy expenditure equation provided below. If your BMI is greater than 25, base your calculated needs on a person of your height who has a BMI of 24 (use the BMI calculator at www.nhlbisupport.com/bmi/ to help determine this weight).

For men: Estimated energy expenditure = 662 – (9.53 × age in years) + PA*((15.91 × weight (kilograms)) + (539.6 × height (meters))

For women: Estimated energy expenditure = (354 – (6.91 × age in years)) + (PA*(9.36 × weight (kilograms) + 726 × height (meters))

Physical Activity (PA) Level

1.0– 1.39	Sedentary, typical daily living activities (e.g., household tasks, walking to bus)
1.4– 1.59	Low active, typical daily living activities plus 30 to 60 minutes of daily moderate activity (e.g., walking at 5 to 7 kilometers/hour)
1.6– 1.89	Active, typical daily living activities plus 60 minutes of daily moderate activity
1.9– 2.5	Very active, typical daily activities plus at least 60 minutes of daily moderate activity plus an additional 60 minutes of vigorous activity or 120 minutes of moderate activity

Workout Program

Plan your workouts for the next week. Consider the type of activity, the anticipated duration, and the anticipated intensity.

	MONDAY	TUESDAY	WEDNESDAY	THURSDAY	FRIDAY	SATURDAY	SUNDAY
Activity							
Hours							

Nutrition Recommendations Before Exercise

1. For which of your workouts should you develop a pre-exercise nutrition strategy? Why?
2. Describe your strategy, including your goal timing and amount of carbohydrate intake. If you don't think any of your workouts need a pre-exercise strategy, explain why not.
3. Make a list of potential snacks that you could use for a pre-exercise plan. Describe why you selected them.
4. Try out each of these snacks before a strenuous workout. Which is your favorite? Why is it your favorite?

Nutrition Recommendations During Exercise

1. For which of your workouts should you develop a during-exercise nutrition strategy? Why?
2. Describe your strategy, including your goal timing and amount of carbohydrate intake. If you don't think any of your workouts need a pre-exercise strategy, explain why not.
3. Make a list of potential snacks that you could use for your during-exercise plan. Describe why you selected them.
4. Try out each of these snacks during a strenuous workout. Which is your favorite? Why is it your favorite?

Nutrition Recommendations After Exercise

1. For which of your workouts should you develop a post-exercise nutrition strategy? Why?
2. Describe your strategy, including your goal timing and amount of carbohydrate intake. If you don't think any of your workouts need a post-exercise nutrition strategy, explain why not.
3. Make a list of foods that you could use for your post-exercise plan. Describe why you selected them.
4. Try out each of these snacks or meals after a strenuous workout. Which is your favorite? Why is it your favorite?

RESOURCES

Rodriguez NR, Di Marco NM, Langley S. American College of Sports Medicine position stand. Nutrition and athletic performance. *Med Sci Sports Exerc.* 2009;41:709-731.

Kreider RB, Wilborn CD, Taylor L, et al. ISSN exercise & sport nutrition review: research & recommendations. *J Int Soc Sports Nutr.* 2010;7:7.

REFERENCES

1. Jeukendrup AE, Jentjens R. Oxidation of carbohydrate feedings during prolonged exercise: current thoughts, guidelines and directions for future research. *Sports Med.* 2000;29:407-424.
2. Flatt JP. Use and storage of carbohydrate and fat. *Am J Clin Nutr.* 1995;61:952S-959S.
3. Jeukendrup AE. Carbohydrate intake during exercise and performance. *Nutrition.* 2004;20:669-677.
4. Rodriguez NR, Di Marco NM, Langley S. American College of Sports Medicine position stand. Nutrition and athletic performance. *Med Sci Sports Exerc.* 2009;41:709-731.
5. Gropper SS, Smith JL, Groff JL. *Advanced Nutrition and Human Metabolism.* Belmont, CA: Thomson Wadsworth; 2009:270.
6. Sedlock DA. The latest on carbohydrate loading: a practical approach. *Curr Sports Med Rep.* 2008;7:209-213.
7. O'Reilly J, Wong SH, Chen Y. Glycaemic index, glycaemic load and exercise performance. *Sports Med.* 2010;40:27-39.
8. Trenell MI, Stevenson E, Stockmann K, Brand-Miller J. Effect of high and low glycaemic index recovery diets on intramuscular lipid oxidation during aerobic exercise. *Br J Nutr.* 2008;99:326-332.
9. Stevenson EJ, Thelwall PE, Thomas K, Smith F, Brand-Miller J, Trenell MI. Dietary glycemic index influences lipid oxidation but not muscle or liver glycogen oxidation during exercise. *Am J Physiol Endocrinol Metab.* 2009;296:E1140-1147.
10. Donaldson CM, Perry TL, Rose MC. Glycemic index and endurance performance. *Int J Sport Nutr Exerc Metab.* 2010;20:154-165.
11. Sherman WM, Leenders N. Fat loading: the next magic bullet? *Int J Sport Nutr.* 1995;5 Suppl:S1-S12.
12. Burke LM, Hawley JA. Effects of short-term fat adaptation on metabolism and performance of prolonged exercise. *Med Sci Sports Exerc.* 2002;34:1492-1498.
13. Helge JW. Long-term fat diet adaptation effects on performance, training capacity, and fat utilization. *Med Sci Sports Exerc.* 2002;34:1499-1504.
14. Phillips SM. Dietary protein for athletes: from requirements to metabolic advantage. *Appl Physiol Nutr Metab.* 2006;31:647-654.
15. Hayes A, Cribb PJ. Effect of whey protein isolate on strength, body composition and muscle hypertrophy during resistance training. *Curr Opin Clin Nutr Metab Care.* 2008;11:40-44.
16. Gibala MJ. Protein metabolism and endurance exercise. *Sports Med.* 2007;37:337-340.
17. Joint Position Statement: nutrition and athletic performance. American College of Sports Medicine, American

Dietetic Association, and Dietitians of Canada. *Med Sci Sports Exerc.* 2000;32:2130-2145.
18. Institute of Medicine (IOM). Dietary reference intakes for energy, carbohydrate, fiber, fat, fatty acids, cholesterol, protein, and amino acids. http://fnic.nal.usda.gov/dietary-guidance/dietary-reference-intakes. Accessed April 29 2013.
19. Kreider RB, Wilborn CD, Taylor L, et al. ISSN exercise & sport nutrition review: research & recommendations. *J Int Soc Sports Nutr.* 2010;7:7.
20. Ivy JL, Goforth, Jr., HW, Damon, BM. Early postexercise muscle glycogen recovery is enhanced with a carbohydrate-protein supplement. *J Appl Physiol.* 2002;93:1337-1344. Doi:10.1152/japplphysiol.00394.2002.
21. Holli B, O'Sullivan Maillet J, Beto J, Calabrese R. *Communication and education skills for dietetics professionals.* Baltimore: Lippincott Williams & Wilkens; 2009.

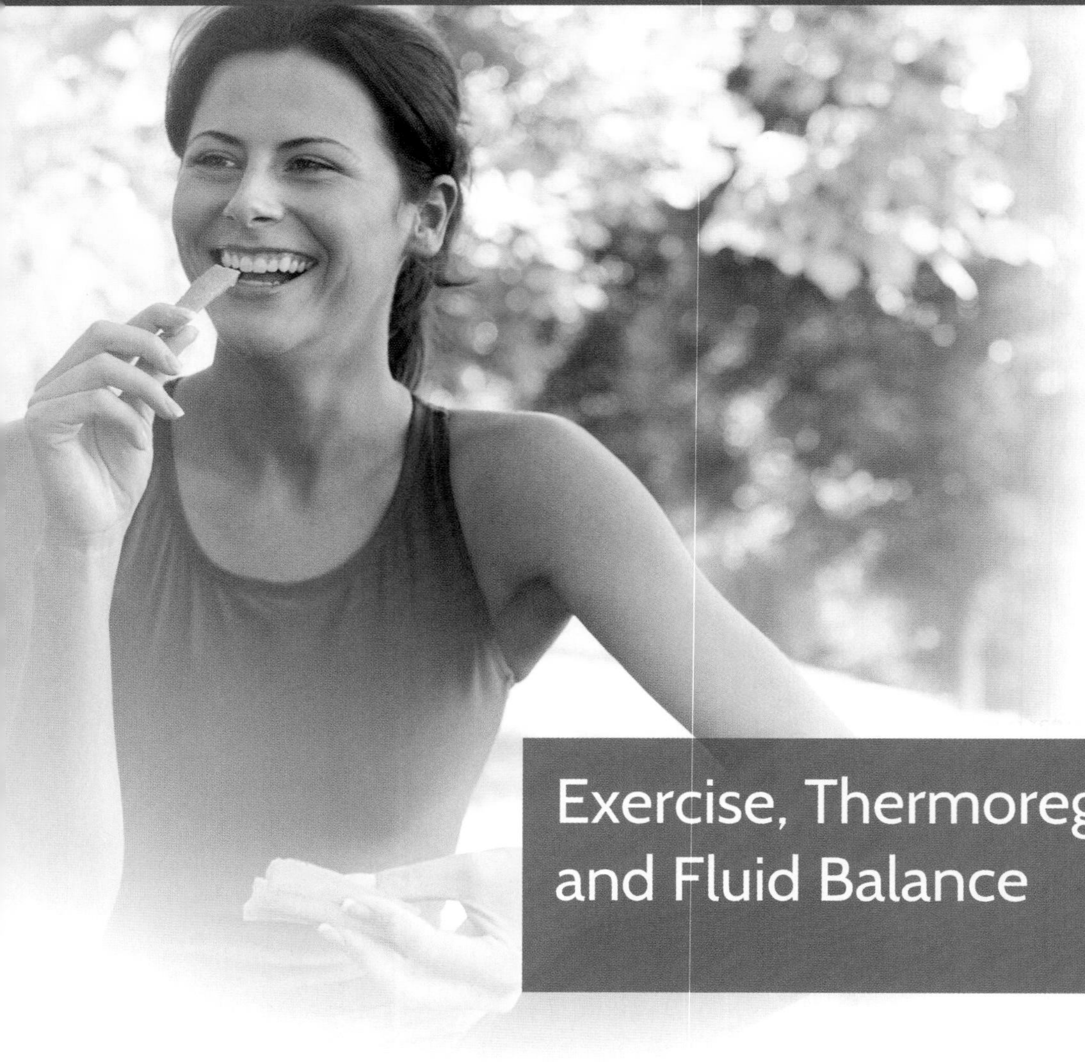

CHAPTER 8

Exercise, Thermoregulation, and Fluid Balance

CHAPTER OUTLINE

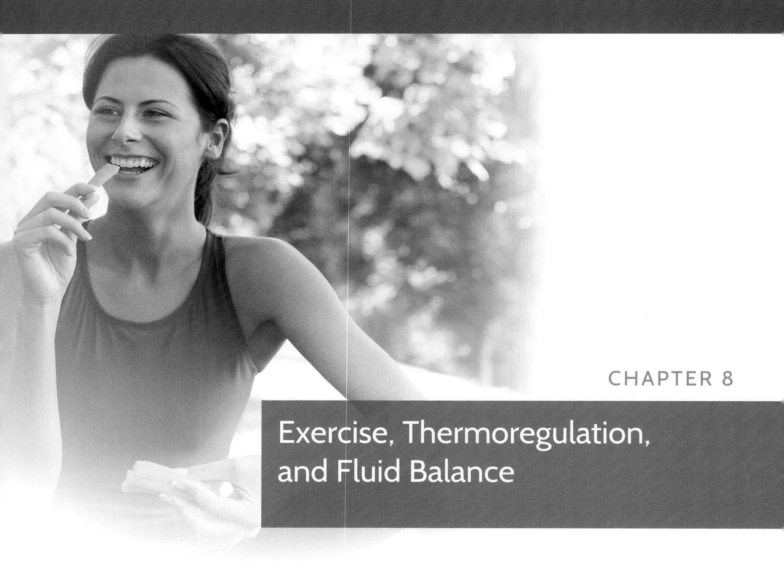

CHAPTER OUTLINE–cont'd

LEARNING OBJECTIVES

After studying this chapter, the reader should be able to:

8.1 Describe how gender, age, diet, and environment affect hydration status.

8.2 Define euhydration, hyponatremia, and dehydration.

8.3 Identify populations at greatest risk for hyponatremia and dehydration.

8.4 Identify ways to recognize and treat hyponatremia and dehydration.

8.5 List ways that hydration status affects athletic performance.

8.6 Apply the most up-to-date and scientifically sound hydration recommendations before, during, and after exercise.

8.7 Calculate sweat rate using the protocol provided by USA Track and Field.

KEY TERMS

acclimatization Physiological changes that occur in response to repeated exposure to an environmental condition such as heat or high altitude.

aldosterone A hormone released by the adrenal gland that helps to maintain normal blood sodium levels by increasing the kidney's reabsorption of sodium and decreasing the amount of sodium lost in sweat.

antidiuretic hormone A hormone released by the anterior pituitary that helps to maintain blood volume in the face of dehydration by increasing water reabsorption in the kidneys and decreasing the amount of urine produced.

cold diuresis Increased urine production and excretion that occurs in extreme cold as a result of peripheral vasoconstriction, high blood sugar, and decreased renal reabsorption of water.

diuresis Increased urine production and excretion.

encephalopathy Loss of normal function of brain tissue, which may result from a wide variety of conditions including hyponatremia.

euhydration A state of "normal" body water content ; the perfect balance between "too much" and "not enough" fluid intake.

exertional hyponatremia Abnormally low blood sodium level that results from excessive intake of low-sodium fluids during prolonged endurance activities.

heat cramps (exercise-associated muscle cramps) Muscle spasms resulting from loss of large amounts of water and electrolytes during physical exertion; typically affect the abdomen, arms, and calves.

heat exhaustion A heat-related illness that occurs after prolonged exposure to heat without adequate replacement of fluids and electrolytes; symptoms include heavy sweating, fatigue, and vomiting. Heat exhaustion is less serious than heat stroke.

heat stroke A severe heat-related illness with extreme overheating resulting from prolonged exposure to heat without adequate replacement of fluids and electrolytes; symptoms include lack of sweating, strong and rapid pulse, disorientation, and loss of consciousness. Often fatal without rapid treatment.

hypothalamus A portion of the brain responsible for regulating body temperature, among many other functions.

hypothermia Condition in which the core body temperature falls below 35°C (95°F), the minimal temperature necessary for normal metabolism and body function.

postural hypotension The pooling of blood in the legs and inadequate blood supply to the upper body that causes dizziness, weakness, and collapse; often occurs with dehydration and heat stress and may be confused with heat stroke.

rhabdomyolysis Breakdown of skeletal muscle tissue and release of contents into the bloodstream that sometimes leads to kidney failure; caused by dehydration and heat stress.

CALCULATIONS

Milliliters to ounces: 240 ml = 8 oz = 1 cup (1 oz equals 30 ml); 16 oz = 1 lb

Kilograms to pounds: 1 kg = 2.2 l bs; 1 lb = 0.45 kg

Carbohydrate concentration = grams of carbohydrate per package/total grams per package × 100

Milliequivalents to milligrams (sodium and potassium) = number of mEq × molecular weight = milligrams (23 mg/1 mEq for sodium; 39 mg/1 mEq for potassium)

Sweat rate (ml/hr) = (Weight before exercise - weight after exercise + amount of fluid consumed (ml) - amount of fluid urinated)/minutes of activity × 60

Percent body weight change = (pre-exercise weight - post-exercise weight)/pre-exercise weight × 100

1 milliliter of water = 1 gram of water

INTRODUCTION

Newspaper reports warn of the potential deadliness of underhydration or overhydration. Past headlines shared the unlikely but real tragedy of the 28-year-old novice Boston Marathon runner who suffered severe hyponatremia and later died en route to the hospital, as well as the story of the 24-year-old elite runner who collapsed from dehydration while exploring desolate trails in the Grand Canyon's summer heat without sufficient water. Mismatched fluid intake with fluid loss during exercise not only hinders athletic performance, but at its worst can lead to severe health consequences. While hearing of these stories may spook your clients, you can help to ease their fears and provide solid guidance on optimizing fluid intake with exercise.

THE PHYSIOLOGY OF EXERCISE AND HYDRATION STATUS

Water

The human body consists of between 50% to 70% water. People with more lean mass have higher water content (because muscle is 70% to 80% water), whereas those with more fat mass have lower water content (because fat is about 10% water). To put this in perspective, approximately 85 to 119 pounds (lb) of a 170-pound man is water weight. Physiologically, water has many important functions, including regulating body temperature, protecting vital organs, promoting nutrient absorption, and maintaining a high blood volume for optimal athletic performance. Water volume can be influenced by a variety of factors such as food and drink intake, sweating, urine and feces excretion, metabolic production of small amounts of water, and losses of water that occur with breathing.

These factors play an especially important role when metabolism is increased during exercise. The generated body heat is released mostly through sweat, which is a solution of water, sodium, and other electrolytes. If fluid intake is not increased to replenish the fluid lost, the body attempts to compensate by retaining more water and excreting more concentrated urine; when this happens, the person is said to be dehydrated. Severe dehydration can lead to **heat stroke** or extreme overheating, which can be fatal if not immediately treated. On the other hand, when the volume of water increases in the body compared to sodium (i.e., there is a low concentration of electrolytes resulting from overhydration), a person can become hyponatremic. The excess water circulating in the blood moves into cells to create balance. Most cells compensate by swelling with the excess water. The exception is the brain cells, which cannot expand because the skull bones confine them. This can lead to **encephalopathy**, or abnormal brain function. If left untreated, severe hyponatremia is deadly.

Thermoregulation

The body prefers to maintain a stable core temperature of about 37°C (normal range is 36.1°C to 37.8°C; this converts to 98.6°F with a range of 97°F to 100°F). To do this, the **hypothalamus**, the brain's major control center, carefully senses body temperature.

Response to Elevated Core Temperature

When a person participates in physical activity, the many biochemical reactions and muscular contractions that are essential for exercise generate large amounts of heat. This heat raises the body's core temperature. The hypothalamus senses the increase in body temperature and sends a signal to the heart and blood vessels to direct warm blood to the skin. The heart rate and stroke volume (amount of blood pumped with each heartbeat) increase and the peripheral blood vessels that supply the skin dilate. The hypothalamus also signals the sweat glands to start producing sweat. When sweat evaporates, it creates a cooling effect on the body. Sweating is especially necessary when it is hot and humid and evaporation is the main mode of heat loss. With cooler temperatures (less than body temperature), heat can be transferred from the body to the environment through other methods in addition to sweat. The most common include radiation (heat "radiates" from the warm human body to the cooler outside temperature) and convection (as cold air moves past a warm body, heat is lost to the environment). Heat loss commonly is transferred via conduction, which requires direct contact (such as transferring heat to a cold bench when sitting down to take a break). As a result of the effectiveness of losing heat through these methods, sweating rates are lower.

In addition to triggering sweat production, the hypothalamus also facilitates getting rid of excess heat by sending a signal to the pituitary gland to release **antidiuretic hormone** (ADH). ADH does what its name describes— it prevents **diuresis** by increasing water reabsorption in the kidneys. The increased water in the bloodstream helps ensure the body's ability to maintain sweat rate and stroke volume. The decreased water leaving the kidney leads to more concentrated, darker-colored urine. The hypothalamus also signals the adrenal cortex to release the hormone **aldosterone**, which increases the kidney's reabsorption of sodium and decreases the amount of sodium lost in sweat. Both of these activities help the body to retain valuable electrolytes in the face of a high sweat rate.

Response to Decreased Core Temperature

When the hypothalamus senses that core body temperature is dropping below its ideal range, it sends a signal to the body to constrict the blood vessels that supply blood to the periphery (such as the skin) and increase blood flow to the core by dilating the blood vessels that supply vital organs. The body also produces heat through shivering and as a byproduct of metabolic reactions.

Environment

The environment in which a person exercises plays a substantial role in the rate and extent of fluid losses and how well the body is able to maintain an ideal core body temperature. While a novice exerciser in any environment may struggle more than an experienced athlete, the level of **acclimatization** a person has undergone in a particular environment plays a large role in the body's response to heat, cold, and altitude stressors. Effective acclimatization usually requires exposure to and exercise in the environment over a period of days to weeks (Table 8-1).[1]

Heat

Despite the body's best efforts, athletes exercising in hot and humid environments still are susceptible to hyperthermia and heat-related illness. This is especially the case when an athlete does not drink adequate fluids to replace the fluid lost in sweat. The

Table 8-1. An Acclimatization Regimen

Regular exposure to a hot environment leads to physiological changes that enhance an athlete's performance and reduce risk of heat-related ailments when exercising in hot temperatures. These changes include: decreased core body temperature, decreased resting heart rate, increased sweat rate, decreased sodium losses in sweat and urine, and expanded blood volume. The full process of heat acclimatization takes from 1 to 2 weeks.

A Plan for Heat Acclimatization[1]

FREQUENCY	INTENSITY	TIME	TYPE
Every 3 days for 30 days OR Every day for 10 days OR Other regimen of approximately 10 workouts over no less than 1 to 2 weeks	>50% VO_2 max to induce elevation in core temperature and sweat	100 minutes	Strenuous interval training or continuous exercise

blood plasma volume shrinks, blood flow is diverted away from the skin to vital organs, and core temperature rises. In very hot and humid environments, the body is less capable of getting rid of heat. If the outside temperature exceeds body temperature, radiation no longer is an effective mode of heat loss. If outside humidity is very high, sweat cannot evaporate into the environment because the air is already too saturated with moisture (Fig. 8-1). When the body is unable to adequately cool off, an athlete can suffer **heat cramps** (also known as *exercise-associated muscle cramps*),[1] **heat exhaustion**, or heat stroke (Table 8-2).

Heat cramps have been most often attributed to electrolyte imbalances in the face of high sweat rates. However, other research suggests that muscle cramps are more likely the result of muscle fatigue.[2] The hypothesis is fatigue disrupts the balance between neural input and feedback, causing too much excitation on the muscle and not enough inhibition. Thus, a simple contraction can overstimulate the muscle, causing a cramp. Support for this hypothesis lies in the fact that the best way to get rid of a cramp is to stretch. Further research is needed. Athletes suffering from muscle cramps may experience relief with fluids and stretching.

Heat exhaustion is more serious and requires ceasing activity and quickly trying to decrease body temperature with fluids and shade. Anyone who develops signs of heat stroke needs immediate medical attention and aggressive efforts to lower body temperature such as with the use of ice packs or an ice bath. See Evaluating the Evidence, which discusses using pickle juice to prevent cramps, and Communication Strategies, which focuses on speaking to a group about hydrating for exercise in the heat.

EVALUATING THE EVIDENCE

Does Pickle Juice Prevent Exercise-Associated Muscle Cramps?[a]

About one in four athletic trainers recommends pickle juice to prevent and treat exercise-associated muscle cramps (EAMC).[b] Many believe EAMC results from electrolyte imbalances, most notably sodium losses from excessive sweating. Pickles are a high-salt food. One might reason then that pickle juice should prevent and treat EAMC. In fact, some clinicians claim that pickle juice relieves EAMC within 30 to 35 seconds.[a] However, other health professionals worry that the high-salt and low-fluid content of pickle juice can lead to dehydration-tonicity and subsequently prolong dehydration and increase risk of hyperthermia and diminished performance. Who's right?

WHAT DOES THE EVIDENCE SAY?

Researchers from North Dakota who were tired about debating the utility (or not) of pickle juice in the prevention and treatment of EAMC decided to conduct an experiment to see if the juice actually made a difference and if it caused any unwanted effects, such as worsened dehydration.[c] Nine healthy 20-something men agreed to participate in the study. Each participant drank a small volume of pickle juice, a carbohydrate-electrolyte drink, or water. Following consumption of each drink, plasma electrolytes were measured. Each of the men underwent the experiment three times (once for each of the drinks) with at least 3 days separating the trials. The researchers found that blood sodium, magnesium, calcium, osmolality, and volume did not change in the 60 minutes after ingestion. Furthermore, there were no differences in blood electrolytes between the types of drinks, except that water ingestion slightly decreased plasma potassium. The researchers concluded that at the volumes tested, drinking pickle juice or a carbohydrate-electrolyte drink would be unlikely to cause dehydration-induced hypertonicity and would also be unlikely to reverse massive electrolyte losses thought to be associated with EAMC.

1. What are the limitations to this study? What might be a better study design to answer the question, Does pickle juice prevent EAMC?
2. How might you use the results from this study when communicating with your clients?
3. Do the results of this study have clinical relevance to you and your job? That is, will this study change the way you practice your profession?

a. Based on Miller KC, Mack G, Knight KL. Electrolyte and plasma changes after ingestion of pickle juice, water, and a common carbohydrate-electrolyte solution. *J Athl Train.* 2009;44:454-461.
b. Miller KC, Knight KL, Williams RB. Athletic trainers' perceptions of pickle juice's effects on exercise associated muscle cramps. *Athl Train Today.* 2008;13:31-34.
c. Williams RB, Conway DP. Treatment of acute muscle cramps with pickle juice: a case report. *J Athl Train.* 2000;35:S24.

COMMUNICATION STRATEGIES

You've been asked by your local YMCA to give the amateur cycling club a 20-minute talk on optimal hydration for prolonged exercise in the heat. You feel like you've got the content down cold, but you're a little nervous about the public speaking component.

As a health leader in your community you may periodically be asked to give oral presentations and workshops. This offers you an exceptional opportunity to share evidence-based and credible information and also promote yourself and your services to potential clients. Delivering an effective presentation is critical. Here are a few tips to keep in mind as you prepare for these events:

- Limit your talk to a few salient points. Think about your goals for the talk in advance and then highlight three major take-home points you'd like to share.
- Know your audience. Make sure that you present in a style and level of complexity appropriate for your target audience.
- Include an introduction, body, and summary to your talk.
  - In the introduction, establish your credibility, link yourself to your audience, and let them know why they're going to leave the talk better off than when they came.
  - In the body, keep these three goals in mind:
    - The audience understands the message. To facilitate this, you should present clearly and use visual aids, handouts, or participant experiences.
    - The audience believes the message. Reinforce your credibility and back up your statements throughout the presentation.
    - The audience is comfortable enough with the speaker to ask questions and share objections. Develop rapport throughout the talk and provide ample opportunities for questions.
  - The summary should include the following ingredients:
    - Wind down. As your talk nears the end, plan for winding down or some kind of closing, such as a summary of what you discussed or a final quote or anecdote.
    - Encourage questions. If there are none, pose some yourself and ask participants to respond.
- Practice. Give your talk to family, friends, or colleagues ahead of time. This will help you feel more comfortable on the big day and also help to work out any kinks or areas that are unclear.

Class Activity

Why not give it a try? Prepare the above talk for the cycling class keeping the presentation principles in mind.

Source: Holli BB, O'Sullivan Maillet J, Beto JA, Calabrese RJ. *Communication and education skills for dietetics professionals.* 5th ed. Philadelphia: Lippincott Williams & Wilkins; 2009.

NOAA's National Weather Service
Heat Index

Temperature (°F)

Relative Humidity (%)	80	82	84	86	88	90	92	94	96	98	100	102	104	106	108	110
40	80	81	83	85	88	91	94	97	101	105	109	114	119	124	130	136
45	80	82	84	87	89	93	96	100	104	109	114	119	124	130	137	
50	81	83	85	88	91	95	99	103	108	113	118	124	131	137		
55	81	84	86	89	93	97	101	106	112	117	124	130	137			
60	82	84	88	91	95	100	105	110	116	123	129	137				
65	82	85	89	93	98	103	108	114	121	126	136					
70	83	86	90	95	100	105	112	119	126	134						
75	84	88	92	97	103	109	116	124	132							
80	84	89	94	100	106	113	121	129								
85	85	90	96	102	110	117	126	135								
90	86	91	98	105	113	122	131									
95	86	93	100	108	117	127										
100	87	95	103	112	121	132										

Likelihood of Heat Disorders with Prolonged Exposure or Strenuous Activity

Caution | Extreme caution | Danger | Extreme danger

Figure 8-1. Heat index chart. *Courtesy of the National Oceanic and Atmospheric Administration, National Weather Service.*

Table 8-2. **Signs of Heat-Related Illness**[6]

HEAT CRAMPS (EXERCISE-ASSOCIATED MUSCLE CRAMPS)		HEAT EXHAUSTION		HEAT STROKE	
Symptoms	**What to Do**	**Symptoms**	**What to Do**	**Symptoms**	**What to Do**
Muscle pain or spasm, usually in abdomen, arms, or legs	Stop all activity and sit quietly in a cool place; stretch affected muscles Drink or eat sodium-containing fluids and foods Seek medical attention if cramps persist for longer than 1 hour	Heavy sweating Paleness Muscle cramps Tiredness Weakness Dizziness, headache,nausea or vomiting; fast, weak pulse Fast, shallow breathing Fainting	Seek air-conditioned environment Drink cool, nonalcoholic beverages Rest Take a cool shower, bath, or sponge bath Wear lightweight clothing	Extremely high body temperature (above 103°F or 40°C) Red, hot, and dry skin Lack of sweat Rapid, strong pulse Throbbing headache Dizziness, nausea, confusion Unusual or irrational behavior Unconsciousness	Get person to shady area Cool rapidly using whatever methods are available (tub of cool water, cool shower, spray with hose, etc.) Monitor body temperature and continue cooling until temperature drops to 101–102°F Get medical assistance ASAP If emergency medical personnel are delayed, call hospital emergency room for further instructions

Cold

Athletes who exercise in very cold temperatures are at risk for **hypothermia**. Hypothermia occurs when the body loses heat faster than it is able to generate it. When the body experiences cold stress, blood is preferably shunted to the vital organs and away from the skin. The body perceives this as increased blood volume and instructs the kidney to produce more urine to help reduce the blood volume. This is known as **cold diuresis**. Although sweat rate is typically low in cold temperatures, an athlete still can experience dehydration from cold diuresis, increased respiratory fluid losses, and decreased incentive to drink. Further, a person exercising in cold weather with impermeable clothing—and with little outlet for heat loss through radiation and convection—could generate higher-than-expected sweat rates. When exposed to cold, the body attempts to produce and retain adequate heat to maintain core temperature in the ideal range, but if it is unsuccessful, athletes could suffer physical damage from cold exposure, including varying degrees of frostbite. Athletes can minimize this risk by dressing appropriately (Table 8-3).

Altitude

Individuals exercising at higher altitudes (>2,500 m or 8,200 ft) have increased fluid needs. This is especially the case for those people who spend most of their time at or near sea level, but then travel to and exercise in a high-altitude environment. The increased fluid losses result from increased diuresis and high respiratory fluid losses. The renal system excretes the excess circulating bicarbonate that results from excessive ventilation at high altitudes. This is important to lower the blood pH, but the increased urine output can lead to dehydration. Further, respiratory fluid losses at high altitudes may be as high as 1,900 milliliters per day in men and 850 milliliters per

Table 8-3. Dressing for Extreme Temperatures[14]

HEAT	COLD
Relatively minimal clothing to facilitate sweat evaporation	Layers to minimize sweat accumulation
Light-colored to reduce radiative heat gain	Fishnet fabrics may help facilitate sweat dissipation
Synthetic "wicking" fabrics (as opposed to cotton) to facilitate sweat evaporation	Type of fabric does not affect thermoregulation

day in women. To maintain adequate hydration for optimal kidney function and prevention of dehydration, an individual may need to consume 3 to 4 liters of fluid per day.[3]

Individual Factors

A person's susceptibility to heat-related stress and fluid imbalances is affected not only by environmental- and exercise-related factors, but importantly, also by individual factors including gender, age, and diet.

Gender

Women have a lower metabolic rate during exercise and a smaller body size when compared to men. These factors contribute to decreased sweat rates and decreased electrolyte losses, while the amount of water and electrolytes retained by the kidney during exercise is about the same. Even after adjusting for these gender differences, women still are at higher risk of developing exercise-associated hyponatremia.

Age

When working with children, keep in mind that physiologically, emotionally, and cognitively they are not just little adults. However, contrary to previous thinking, children do *not* have a less-effective ability to regulate body temperature and tolerate high levels of physical exertion when exercising in the heat compared to their adult counterparts *as long as they maintain appropriate hydration.*[15] Recommendations and strategies to help children and adolescents maintain optimal hydration during exercise are highlighted in Chapter 13.

As people age, their ability to use thirst to guide fluid intake diminishes. Thus, older adults (>65 years) not only are more likely to become dehydrated but are also not as good at knowing when and how much to drink during exercise. Encourage them to drink during and after exercise, but also be aware that excess fluid intake is more likely to lead to hyponatremia in this population because they are slower to excrete fluids.

Diet

Many foods contain large amounts of water and sodium that can help restore fluid and electrolyte losses that occur with exercise. The proportion of fat, carbohydrates, and protein in a food only minimally affects urine production at rest and with exercise. Despite the widely held belief that caffeine intake can lead to dehydration due to its diuretic effects, moderate caffeine intake (<240 mg/day, equivalent to a little more than 2 cups of coffee) has very little impact on urine losses, is unlikely to cause dehydration, and may provide a performance benefit.[4] Alcohol, on the other hand, can increase urine output and delay rehydration when consumed in large amounts. This is especially relevant during the post-exercise rehydration period when many athletes competing in endurance events celebrate with alcoholic beverages, such as at event-sponsored beer gardens.

SPEED BUMP

1. **Describe how gender, age, diet, and environment affect hydration status.**

THE NOT-SO-DELICATE BALANCE

When it comes to fluid balance during exercise it seems a lot like the proverbial double-edged sword: Drinking too little can lead to dehydration—a scary condition exercisers have been cautioned against in every text, handout, and presentation on fluid replacement. But drinking too much—out of fear of not drinking enough—could lead to hyponatremia, a condition less well known and understood but equally frightening. Here's the good news: The body is very good at handling and normalizing large variations in fluid intake. For this reason, severe hyponatremia and dehydration are rare and generally affect very specific high-risk populations during specific types of activities. Both conditions are also highly preventable. To prevent dehydration and hyponatremia, the goal is to drink just the right amount of fluid before, during, and after exercise to maintain a state of euhydration.

Euhydration

Euhydration refers to a state of "normal" body water content—the perfect balance between "too much" and "not enough" fluid intake. Clients can maintain a state of euhydration by balancing fluid losses with fluid intake. Sweat is the primary source of water loss during exercise. Other fluid losses are minor. For example, the water lost from breathing approximately equals water produced with metabolism. Gastrointestinal losses are small unless a person has diarrhea. The kidney decreases urine production during exercise and heat stress.

Sweat Rate

How much a person sweats depends on several factors including outside temperature, clothing, body size, intensity and duration of activity, metabolic efficiency (how economically the body uses energy to perform a specific exercise), genetic predisposition, and other factors. Though larger people generally tend to sweat more than smaller people, all individuals vary greatly in their sweat rates and fluid replacement should be tailored to individual needs. An evaluation of sweating rates of elite athletes in a variety of sports suggests that sweat rates are often on the order of 0.5 to 2.0 liters per hour,[6] though it's difficult to apply these findings to any one individual in an attempt to approximate sweat losses (Box 8-1).

Sweat consists of water and electrolytes including sodium, chloride, potassium, calcium, and magnesium. The absolute concentration of the different electrolytes varies from person to person. The extent of electrolyte depletion with sweating is variable and depends on total sweat losses and sweat electrolyte concentration. In general, sodium and chloride are found in the highest concentrations in sweat, although with heat acclimatization these losses can be decreased.

Fluid Needs

An athlete needs to drink just enough fluids to balance the amount of fluids lost with exercise. A small amount of water is produced from metabolic activity (only just enough to offset the water lost from respiration). The rest of the fluids need to be consumed through food and drink. If over an 8- to 24-hour period an adequate amount of fluids and electrolytes are consumed to balance the exercise losses, then a person can reestablish a state of euhydration.

Clients can test whether they've attained a baseline state of euhydration in two simple steps:

1. Measure urine-specific gravity of first morning void. Clients can purchase a container of urinalysis test strips to measure specific gravity, which is an indicator of urine concentration. A specific gravity of less than 1.020 grams per milliliter indicates euhydration. (Note: Measurement of specific gravity is the only variable of interest, although the test strips will also report urine protein, glucose, ketones, and other values. Clients should discuss any abnormalities in values with their physician.) For best results, it's important to use a first morning void, which is more indicative of a steady state hydration status compared to a random urine sample during the day.
2. Measure body weight nude after the first morning void. For men, average this value over 3 days for a baseline weight. Women may need an average over several more days because the menstrual cycle influences weight status. The averaged weight approximates euhydration. If euhydration is maintained, this weight should fluctuate less than 1%. If weight loss is greater than 1% it may be indicative of dehydration, whereas if weight gain is greater than 1% it may indicate overhydration. Of course, weight is also affected by changes in eating and stooling patterns and

Box 8-1. A Protocol to Determine Individual Fluid Needs

The Goal: Determine sweat rate.

The Calculation: Weight before exercise (g) – weight after exercise (g) + amount of fluid consumed (ml) – amount of fluid urinated, if applicable)/1 hour. Divide by 30 to determine the number of ounces of fluid needed per hour of exercise. (This assumes that 1 milliliter of sweat loss represents a 1 gram loss in body weight since the specific gravity of sweat is 1.0 g/ml.)

The Protocol:

- Warm up until you break a light sweat.
- Urinate if necessary.
- Weigh yourself naked on an accurate scale.
- Exercise for 1 hour at an intensity and in environmental conditions similar to those for your normal activity, a target race, or other event, depending on your reason for determining your sweat rate.
- Drink a measured amount of fluid, ideally the same type of beverage that you consume normally or will consume during the target race or other event. Convert ounces into pounds (16 ounces = 1 pound).
- Do not urinate during the exercise session unless you plan to measure the volume of the urine. (If you do so, convert ounces into pounds.)
- Weigh yourself naked on an accurate scale.
- Calculate sweat rate.

Protocol adapted from Casa DJ. Proper hydration for distance running—Identifying individual fluid needs: A USA Track and Field advisory. 2003. www.hartfordmarathon.com/Assets/Training%2BProgram/ProperHydrationForDistanceRunning.pdf.

so is best used in combination with urine-specific gravity.

This method is more objective and reliable than using a subjective assessment of urine color as a marker of hydration status. However, urine color can give a quick estimate of a person's hydration, with a darker, more concentrated color signaling dehydration and a clear to very light yellow indicating adequate hydration.

Hyponatremia

Hyponatremia is defined as an abnormally low concentration of blood sodium—less than 135 millimoles per liter (mmol/L). **Exertional hyponatremia** results from excessive intake of low-sodium fluids during prolonged endurance activities; that is, drinking a greater volume of fluid than the volume lost in sweat and possibly, to a lesser extent, from inappropriate fluid retention. A study of 488 Boston Marathon runners published in the *New England Journal of Medicine* found that 13% (22% of women and 8% of men) had hyponatremia and 0.6% had critical hyponatremia at the end of the race.[7] Runners with hyponatremia were more likely to be of low body mass index, consume fluids at every mile (and more than 3 liters total throughout the race), finish the race in more than 4 hours, and gain weight during the run. The greatest predictor of hyponatremia was weight gain, which researchers attributed to excessive fluid intake.[7]

Hyponatremia is not limited to runners. Anyone exercising at a low to moderate intensity for an extended period of time (generally 4 hours or more) while consuming too much water can be at risk. High-intensity exercisers are more susceptible to the other problem—dehydration.

Dehydration

Dehydration is a state of decreased total body fluid. Mild dehydration, or a 1% to 2% loss of body weight during exercise, is normal and of no great concern. In fact, most competitive marathoners are mildly dehydrated at the end of the race. However, greater losses should be avoided, as more severe dehydration is associated with alterations in cardiovascular function, thermoregulatory capacity and muscle function, and heat illness.

Dehydration during exercise results from a sweat rate that is beyond fluid replenishment. Several factors increase the likelihood of dehydration by either increasing sweat rate or decreasing fluid intake.

Increased Sweat Rate

The following factors could increase the sweat rate to the point of dehydration:

- Exercising at very high intensities or for very long periods of time. Sweat rate is increased, the time available to focus on rehydration is diminished, and the stomach and intestines are less able to process and empty fluids into the bloodstream.
- Exercising in very hot and/or humid conditions. Sweat rate is dramatically increased in an effort to rid the body of excessive heat, but when the air is heavy with water, sweat does not evaporate as readily. Therefore, the body has difficulty cooling its temperature, which may result in severe dehydration and heat stroke.
- Exercising in heavy clothing or equipment. Ideally, athletes will wear appropriate clothing to minimize sweat losses during exercise; however, in some cases excess sweat losses are inevitable, such as the case of football players practicing in the hot sun wearing a uniform and protective equipment.

Decreased Fluid Intake

Lack of fluid consumption during exercise can lead to dehydration. Poor fluid consumption may be due to:

- Inaccessibility
- A low level of fluid tolerance
- Dislike of the available beverage
- Failure to understand the importance of staying hydrated

A person who is mildly dehydrated at the onset of a workout will be at increased risk of suffering from serious dehydration during the exercise session. This is especially common in athletes who work out several times a day.

Dehydration, along with high exercise intensity, hot and humid environmental conditions, poor fitness level, incomplete heat acclimatization, and a variety of other factors can all raise body temperature and together lead to **rhabdomyolysis** (breakdown of skeletal muscle tissue and release of contents into the bloodstream that sometimes leads to kidney failure) and heat stroke. Heat stroke is rare and is often confused with a more common condition, **postural hypotension**, the pooling of blood in the legs and inadequate blood supply to the upper body, causing dizziness, weakness, and collapse.[8] Postural hypotension can be easily remedied by elevating the legs above the head for 3 to 4 minutes; nonetheless, a physician or trained health professional should be consulted to properly diagnose and treat the ailing athlete.

SYMPTOMS AND TREATMENT OF HYPONATREMIA AND DEHYDRATION

The symptoms of hyponatremia and dehydration are very similar. Symptoms of hyponatremia include nausea, vomiting, extreme fatigue, respiratory distress, dizziness, confusion, disorientation, coma, and seizures. Symptoms of dehydration include nausea, vomiting, dizziness, disorientation, weakness, irritability, headache, muscle cramps, chills, and decreased performance. The muscle cramps associated with dehydration can be especially debilitating to some athletes who practice and compete in hot and humid temperatures such as football players during preseason practice in late summer, tennis players, endurance cyclists, late-season triathletes, and soccer and beach volleyball players.[3] Because the signs of hyponatremia and dehydration are so similar, and dehydration is better understood than hyponatremia, people suffering from hyponatremia may think that they are dehydrated and consume more fluids, thus exacerbating an already severe condition.

How can you tell the difference? A simple guideline when assessing whether someone is dehydrated or hyponatremic is to look at the individual's risk profile. Is the person a recreational athlete who has been exercising for an extended period of time at a low to moderate intensity with a low sweat rate and a high consumption of fluids? If so, that individual is more likely to be suffering from hyponatremia. Or, is the person soaking in sweat from exercising at a high intensity for an extended period of time in excruciating heat and humidity with very little access to fluids? If so, dehydration is the more likely problem. While not every case will be this clear, gathering as many clues as possible will help in selecting the most appropriate next steps.

Hyponatremia should be treated by a physician who can monitor the athlete and provide sodium replacement and a diuretic to rid the body of excess fluid if necessary. Dehydration should also be treated by a physician, especially when symptoms (such as vomiting, dizziness, and disorientation) are present. The physician will treat the athlete with either oral or intravenous fluids, depending on the severity of dehydration. (Athletes who are conscious, cognizant, without gastrointestinal upset, and not at risk of hyponatremia can be encouraged to orally rehydrate themselves.)

Prevention of Fluid Disturbances

Both hyponatremia and dehydration are highly preventable. To help clients avoid either extreme it is important to (1) stay up-to-date with the latest research and guidelines, and (2) provide clients with that information. Refer to the section "Fluid Requirements for Active Adults" later in this chapter for a more detailed description of how to determine fluid needs.

> SPEED BUMP
> 2. **Define euhydration, hyponatremia, and dehydration.**
> 3. **Identify populations at greatest risk for hyponatremia and dehydration.**
> 4. **Identify ways to recognize and treat hyponatremia and dehydration.**

HYDRATION AND ATHLETIC PERFORMANCE

A smart hydration strategy contributes to improved athletic performance. Most athletes begin exercise appropriately hydrated but then over the course of the exercise session become dehydrated. This is especially common during long and intense exercise in hot and humid conditions. A minority of athletes will begin exercise dehydrated. Wrestlers, boxers, and body builders who need to meet certain weight criteria to participate are particularly susceptible because they may purposely dehydrate themselves to measure in at a lower weight. Athletes engaging in high-volume exercise with two or more exercise sessions per day or a short period between intense workouts also are more likely to begin a session dehydrated. To optimize performance, these athletes should make an attempt at rehydration during the early phase of their training session, although it is not clear how much this will actually benefit performance, and overhydration can contribute to dilutional hyponatremia.

Dehydration of greater than 2% body weight compromises aerobic exercise performance, especially in warm and humid temperatures, most likely as a result of increased core body temperature, increased strain to the heart and lungs, increased glycogen utilization, and changes to metabolic and possibly central nervous system functioning.[6] Dehydration only minimally affects aerobic performance in cold temperatures and has little to no performance effect on muscular strength or anaerobic performance.

FLUID REQUIREMENTS FOR ACTIVE ADULTS

When providing fluid recommendations to clients it is most useful to describe your suggestions in relation to the timing of exercise.

Pre-Exercise Hydration

Most people will begin exercise euhydrated, with little need for a rigorous prehydration regimen. You can assess whether an athlete is euhydrated with the specific gravity of the first morning void and body weight in comparison to baseline weight (see "Euhydration: Fluid Needs," earlier in this chapter). However, if fewer than 8 to 12 hours have elapsed since the last intense training session or fluid intake has been inadequate, then the athlete may benefit from a prehydration program.

The American College of Sports Medicine (ACSM) recommends the following regimen: An athlete should begin prehydrating about 4 hours prior to the exercise session. The athlete should aim to slowly consume about

5 to 7 milliliters of fluid per 1 kg/2.2 lbs of body weight. If after 2 hours of prehydration no urine is produced or if the urine is dark or highly concentrated, then the athlete should aim to drink an additional 3 to 5 milliliters of fluid per 1 kg/2.2 lbs of body weight 2 hours before the event. Drinking fluid that contains 20 to 50 mEq/L (460 to 1150 mg/L) of sodium or consuming salt-containing snacks at this time helps stimulate thirst and retain the consumed fluids.[6] Some athletes may try to hyperhydrate with glycerol-containing solutions, which act to expand the extra- and intracellular spaces. While glycerol may be advantageous for certain athletes who meet specific criteria, it is unlikely to be advantageous for athletes who will experience none to mild dehydration during exercise (loss of <2% body weight) and glycerol use may in fact contribute to increased risk of dilutional hyponatremia.[9]

Hydration During Exercise

The goal of fluid intake during exercise is to prevent performance-diminishing or health-altering effects from dehydration or hyponatremia. To accomplish this:

- Aim for a 1:1 fluid replacement to fluid loss ratio. Ideally, people should consume the same amount of fluid as they lose in sweat. This amount can be determined by using the United States of America Track and Field (USATF) Self-Testing Program for Optimal Hydration[10] (see Box 8-1). Or, exercisers can compare pre-exercise and post-exercise body weight. Perfect hydration is when no weight is lost or gained during exercise. The goal is to avoid weight loss greater than 2%. There is no "one size fits all" recommendation, though the ACSM position suggests that if determining individual needs is not feasible, then athletes could consider aiming for a 0.4 to 0.8 liter per hour (8 to 16 oz/h) replenishment, with the higher rate for faster, heavier athletes in a hot and humid environment and the lower rate for slower, lighter athletes in a cool environment.[6] Because people sweat at varying rates and exercise at different intensities, this range may not be appropriate for everyone. However, when individual assessment is not possible, this recommendation works for most people.
- Drink fluids with sodium during prolonged exercise sessions. If an exercise session lasts longer than 2 hours or an athlete is participating in an event that stimulates heavy sodium loss (defined as more than 3 to 4 grams [g] of sodium), then the athlete should consider consuming a sports drink that contains elevated levels of sodium. In one study, researchers did not find a benefit from sports drinks that contain only the 18 millimoles per liter (or 100 mg/8 oz) of sodium typical of most sports drinks and thus concluded that higher levels would be needed to prevent hyponatremia during prolonged exercise.[7] See Table 8-4 for the sodium content of some popular drinks.

Table 8-4. Evaluating Sports Drinks

Sports drinks play an important role in replenishing fluids, glucose, and sodium lost during exercise lasting more than 1 hour. Although sports drinks may not completely protect against hyponatremia, they serve an important purpose in endurance exercise. This table provides nutritional information for some of the most popular sports drinks.

DRINK	SERVING SIZE (OZ)	CALORIES (KCAL)	SODIUM (MG)	CARBOHYDRATE (G)	CARBOHYDRATE CONCENTRATION (%)
Gatorade	8	50	110	14	6
Gatorade Endurance Formula	8	50	200	14	6
Powerade	8	70	55	19	8
Ultima	8	12.5	37	3	1
Power Bar Endurance	8	70	160	17	7
Propel Zero	8	0	75	2	<1
Zico coconut water	8	34	91	7.4	3

Source: Compiled from sports drink websites including gatorade.com, powerade.com, ultimareplenisher.com, powerbar.com, propelzero.com, and zico.com.

The Institute of Medicine recommends that people exercising for prolonged periods in hot environments consume sports drinks that contain 20 to 30 mEq/L (450 to 700 mg/L) of sodium to stimulate thirst and replace sweat losses and 2 to 5 mEq/L (80 to 200 mg/L) of potassium to replace sweat losses.[11] Alternatively, exercisers can consume extra sodium with meals and snacks prior to a lengthy exercise session or a day of extensive physical activity. Additional sodium or supplementation with salt tablets seems to be unnecessary based on the limited research to date on this topic.[12,13]

- Drink carbohydrate-containing sports drinks to reduce fatigue. If an athlete exercises for longer than 1 hour, he or she should also obtain some additional carbohydrates with fluids. With prolonged exercise, muscle glycogen stores become depleted and blood glucose becomes a primary fuel source. To maintain performance levels and prevent fatigue, athletes should consume drinks and snacks that provide about 30 to 60 grams of rapidly absorbed carbohydrate for every hour of training. As long as the carbohydrate concentration is less than about 6% to 8%, it will have little effect on **gastric emptying**, the speed with which the stomach empties its contents into the small intestine.[3] Refer to Table 8-4 for the carbohydrate content of popular sports drinks. See Myths and Misconceptions for a discussion about beliefs related to drinking fluids before and during exercise.

Post-Exercise Hydration

Following exercise, the athlete should aim to correct any fluid imbalances that occurred during the exercise session. This includes consuming water to restore hydration, carbohydrates to replenish glycogen stores, and electrolytes to speed rehydration. If the athlete will have at least 12 hours to recover before the next strenuous workout, then rehydration with the usual meals and snacks and water should be adequate. The sodium in the foods will help retain the fluid and stimulate thirst.

Myths and Misconceptions

Drinking Fluids Before and During Exercise Causes Stomach Cramps

The Myth

Drinking fluids before and during exercise causes gastrointestinal distress.

The Logic

Because blood flow is diverted away from the gastrointestinal (GI) system during exercise, fluids consumed before or during exercise will remain in the stomach during the workout.

The Science

It is true that gastric emptying slows down during exercise. This is largely because exercise-induced sympathetic stimulation diverts blood flow from the GI system to the heart, lungs, and working muscles. As a result, athletes sometimes experience stomach cramps along with a variety of other uncomfortable GI issues such as reflux, heartburn, bloating, gas, nausea, vomiting, the urge to defecate, and diarrhea. It turns out, though, that good hydration with the right fluids can help to increase gastric emptying and lead to reduced GI problems with exercise. Gastric emptying is maximized when the amount of fluid in the stomach is high. On the other hand, high-intensity exercise, dehydration, hyperthermia, and consumption of high-energy (>7% carbohydrate) hypertonic drinks (like juices and some soft drinks) slow gastric emptying.

Here are a few practical tips to prepare the gut for competition:[a]

1. Get fit and acclimatized to heat.
2. Stay hydrated.
3. Practice drinking during training to improve race-day comfort.
4. Avoid overnutrition before and during exercise.
5. Avoid high-energy, hypertonic food and drinks before (within 30 to 60 minutes) and after exercise. Limit protein and fat intake before exercise.
6. Ingest a high-energy, high-carbohydrate diet.
7. Avoid high-fiber foods before exercise.
8. Limit nonsteroidal anti-inflammatory drugs, alcohol, caffeine, antibiotics, and nutritional supplements before and during exercise. Experiment during training to identify your triggers.
9. Urinate and defecate prior to exercise.
10. Consult a physician if GI problems persist, especially abdominal pain, diarrhea, or bloody stool.

a. Practical tips originally from Brouns F, Beckers E (1993). Is the gut an athletic organ? *Sports Medicine*, 15, 242-257. Cited in Murray R (2006). Training the gut for competition. *Curr Sports Med Rep*. 5:161-164.

If rehydration needs to occur quickly, the athlete should drink about 1.5 liters of fluid for each kilogram (or 0.75 liter of fluid for each pound) of body weight lost.[6] This will be enough to restore lost fluid and also compensate for increased urine output that occurs with rapid consumption of large amounts of fluid. A severely dehydrated athlete (>7% body weight loss) with symptoms (nausea, vomiting, or diarrhea) may need intravenous fluid replacement. Those at greatest risk of hyponatremia should be careful not to consume too much water following exercise and instead should focus on replenishing sodium.

SPEED BUMP

5. List ways that hydration status affects athletic performance.

CHAPTER SUMMARY

The human body is well equipped to withstand dramatic variations in fluid intake during exercise and at rest with little or no detrimental health effects. For this reason, most recreational exercisers will never suffer from serious hyponatremia or dehydration and should not be alarmed. It is under extreme situations of prolonged or very high intensity exercise in excessive heat and humidity that risk elevates. And even then, if athletes replenish sweat loss with equal amounts of fluid, hydration problems can be avoided and performance optimized. The key to a safe and successful finish is a few ounces of education and prevention.

KEY POINTS SUMMARY

1. Women have lower sweat rates and decreased electrolyte losses compared to men. They are at lower risk of dehydration compared with men and at higher risk of hyponatremia.
2. Children are as adept as adults at regulating body temperature as long as they are well hydrated. Attention to maintaining adequate hydration, especially in hot and humid conditions, is paramount.
3. Use particular caution when monitoring the fluid status of older adults (more than 65 years), as they are at increased risk of both dehydration and hyponatremia.
4. Caffeine intake has little effect on hydration status with exercise, while high amounts of alcohol can delay rehydration.
5. Sweat rate is highly variable and depends on many factors. Fluid replacement should be tailored to individual needs as much as possible.
6. Check for euhydration with the first morning void specific gravity and body weight. Aim for a specific gravity less than 1.020 and minimal change in body weight. Urine color can provide a rough estimate of hydration status.
7. Athletes at highest risk of hyponatremia have a low body mass index, high fluid consumption during exercise with lower sweat rate (leading to weight gain), slower pace, and prolonged duration of activity. They are most likely to be female.
8. Athletes at highest risk of dehydration exercise at high intensity in hot and humid conditions with heavy clothing and inadequate fluid intake.
9. Dehydration with less than 2% body weight loss during exercise is normal and not of great concern. Larger losses in body weight can lead to heat illness or heat stroke and can negatively affect aerobic athletic performance.
10. Symptoms of hyponatremia and dehydration are very similar. Symptoms of hyponatremia include nausea, vomiting, extreme fatigue, respiratory distress, dizziness, confusion, disorientation, coma, and seizures. Symptoms of dehydration include nausea, vomiting, dizziness, disorientation, weakness, irritability, headache, muscle cramps, chills, and decreased performance. Use a client's risk profile to help tell the difference. In either case, seek medical attention.
11. Prevent fluid disturbances by using thirst to approximate fluid needs, measuring fluid intake, and paying particular attention to environmental conditions. For optimal fluid balance, calculate a client's individual needs using the USATF Self-Testing Program for Optimal Hydration.
12. Most people begin exercise euhydrated. Those at risk for dehydration prior to an exercise session include weight-class sport athletes who purposely dehydrate themselves and those with less than an 8- to 12-hour recovery period between strenuous training sessions. These athletes should prehydrate with 5 to 7 milliliters of fluid per 1 kilogram/2.2 pounds of body weight 4 hours prior to exercise. If they do not produce urine or if the urine is dark and concentrated, then they should consume another 3 to 5 milliliters of fluid per 1 kilogram/2.2 pounds of body weight 2 hours before the exercise session. A salt-containing snack will help to retain fluid and stimulate thirst.
13. During exercise, athletes should aim to consume an amount of fluid equal to that lost in sweat. The USATF Self-Testing Program for Optimal Hydration can help to determine sweat rate. If this is not feasible, athletes should aim for 0.4 to 0.8 liter per hour (8 to 16 oz/h) fluid replenishment, the lower rate

for slower, lighter athletes in cool temperatures and the higher rate for faster, heavier athletes in a hot and humid environment.

14. Athletes exercising for prolonged periods in hot environments should consume sports drinks that contain 20 to 30 mEq/L (450 to 700 mg/L) of sodium and 2 to 5 mEq/L (80 to 200 mg/L) of potassium. Alternatively, the electrolytes can be obtained from food sources.
15. For exercise lasting longer than 1 hour, athletes should consume drinks and snacks that provide about 30 to 60 grams of rapidly absorbed carbohydrate for every hour of training. Choose drinks and snacks with less than about 6% to 8% carbohydrate concentration to reduce gastric distress.
16. After exercise, rehydrate with water, carbohydrates, and electrolytes. Most athletes can rehydrate sufficiently with usual meal, snacks, and fluids. If rehydration needs to occur within 12 hours or less, athletes should aim to drink about 1.5 liters of fluid for each 1 kilogram/ 2.2 pounds lost.

PRACTICAL APPLICATIONS

1. How can you most accurately assess if a client is euhydrated prior to an exercise session?
   A. Measure urine specific gravity and body weight.
   B. Ask the client if he or she feels thirsty.
   C. Compare body weight to body weight 1 week prior.
   D. Assess the color of the client's urine.
2. What is the main cause of hyponatremia during prolonged exercise?
   A. Insufficient glucose replenishment
   B. Excessive fluid intake
   C. Dehydration
   D. Muscle cramping
3. Which of the following exercisers is more likely to suffer from hyponatremia?
   A. A competitive marathon runner competing on a hot and humid day
   B. A moderately fit woman running a 5K who drinks 3 cups of fluid at the water stop
   C. A thin male on a 6-hour hike drinking as much as possible to prevent dehydration
   D. An overweight man on a 2-hour bike ride
4. Which of the following exercisers is most likely to suffer from dehydration?
   A. A competitive marathon runner competing on a hot and humid day
   B. A moderately fit woman running a 5K who drinks 3 cups of fluid at the water stop
   C. A thin male on a 6-hour hike drinking as much as possible to prevent dehydration
   D. An overweight man on a 2-hour bike ride
5. Which of the following is an up-to-date and sound hydration recommendation?
   A. Drink as much as possible during prolonged exercise to prevent dehydration.
   B. Do not drink fluids during exercise.
   C. Stay ahead of thirst; drink even when you're not thirsty to prevent heat stroke.
   D. Determine your approximate fluid needs based on the amount of sweat you lose during exercise. Aim for a 1:1 ratio.
6. Which of the following is NOT a true statement?
   A. Following exercise, an athlete should aim to correct any fluid imbalances that occurred during the exercise session.
   B. Because sports drinks have not been found to prevent hyponatremia, they are unnecessary, regardless of the duration of exercise.
   C. Being well hydrated before exercise will help prevent severe dehydration during exercise.
   D. Sports drinks provide rapidly absorbable energy that helps improve performance during endurance training lasting longer than 1 hour.
7. Fatigue, vomiting, dizziness, nausea, and confusion are signs of which condition(s)?
   A. Glycogen depletion
   B. Asymptomatic dehydration
   C. Asymptomatic hyponatremia
   D. Severe hyponatremia and severe dehydration
8. If a thin female client who just finished a 3-hour, 30-minute training run (20 miles) for an upcoming marathon complains of dizziness, acts confused, and believes she is dehydrated, what should you do after calling for medical attention?
   A. Provide water immediately.
   B. Give her large volumes of sports drinks to replenish glycogen stores.
   C. Attempt to assess how much fluid she drank during the run.
   D. Tell her that she is definitely hyponatremic.
9. Which of the following is NOT used to determine sweat rate?
   A. Weight before 1 hour of exercise
   B. Calories of fluid consumed during 1 hour of exercise
   C. Weight after 1 hour of exercise
   D. Amount of urine excreted during 1 hour of exercise
10. What is the sweat rate of a 130-pound female who weighs 129.5 pounds after a 1-hour bike ride and who consumed 8 ounces (120 ml) of water during the ride?
    A. 8 ounces/hour (120 ml/hour)
    B. 12 ounces/hour (180 ml/hour)
    C. 16 ounces/hour (240 ml/hr)
    D. 18 ounces/hour (270 ml/hr)

Case 1 Scott, the Professional Triathlete

Risk Profile

Scott is a 29-year-old professional triathlete. He is 6′2″ and 170 pounds (BMI 21.8 kg/m2). Triathlon season is underway and Scott is intensifying his training to compete in the October Kona Ironman Triathlon, which is about 4 months away. Scott has already qualified for this event by completing an Ironman (2.4-mile swim, 112-mile bike ride, and 26.2-mile run) in 8 hours and 30 minutes. Scott has asked you to help calculate his sweat rate during a training run.

1. Is this client more at risk for dehydration or hyponatremia? Explain.

Fluid Needs

On the morning of the training workout, Scott measured his urine-specific gravity, which was 1.015. His pre-workout weight is 170.0 pounds. During the workout, Scott ran 8 miles over the course of 60 minutes. At the completion of the workout he drank 16 ounces of water. His post-workout weight is 167.5.

1. What is Scott's percent body weight change?
2. What is Scott's calculated sweat rate?
3. How much fluid does Scott need to drink per hour to maintain euhydration?

Hydration Recommendation Before Exercise

1. What type and how much fluid would you recommend for Scott prior to a 1-hour workout similar to the one he just completed?
2. What fluid regimen would you recommend if Scott were going to do this workout 6 hours after a strenuous 20-mile bike ride?

Hydration Recommendation During Exercise

1. Based on your sweat rate calculation, how much fluid would Scott need for a 2-hour run?
2. What type of fluid would be best for this run? What is the ideal electrolyte composition?

Hydration Recommendation After Exercise

1. What would you recommend to Scott for rehydration after his 2-hour run if he wasn't planning to do his next workout for 48 hours?
2. What would you recommend if he were planning to do a 1-mile swim at 6:00 a.m. the next morning, which is 10 hours from now?

Case 2 Susan, the Middle-Age Overweight Hiker

Risk Profile

Susan is a 55-year-old overweight teacher who is training to hike the Grand Canyon with her 17-year-old daughter and a guide. She is 5′2″ and 180 pounds (BMI 32.9 kg/m2). She has hired you to help her get in shape for this adventure. The trip is planned for late September, which is about 3 months from now. Susan anticipates that the 9.3-mile trail down will take about 6 hours and the return up about 9 hours. She plans to complete the trek over a 3-day period.

1. Is this client more at risk for dehydration or hyponatremia? Explain.

Fluid Needs

On the morning of the training workout, Susan measured her urine specific gravity, which was 1.020. Her pre-workout weight is 180.0 pounds.

You choose to calculate sweat rate based on a 1-hour hike. Susan does not drink anything during the hike and she does not urinate. At the completion of the workout she drank 16 ounces of water. Her post-workout weight is 179.4 pounds.

1. What is Susan's percent body weight change?
2. What is Susan's calculated sweat rate?
3. How much fluid does Susan need to drink per hour to maintain euhydration?

Hydration Recommendation Before Exercise

1. What hydration recommendations would you offer Susan in the days prior to the Grand Canyon hike?

Hydration Recommendation During Exercise

1. About how much and what types of fluids would you recommend that Susan bring with her for her Grand Canyon hike, which is scheduled to occur over a 3-day period?

Hydration Recommendation After Exercise

1. What and how much would you advise Susan to drink in the 24 to 48 hours after she finishes her Grand Canyon hike?

TRAIN YOURSELF: CALCULATING YOUR FLUID NEEDS

1. Based on your gender, age, height, weight, typical exercise intensity and duration, and the environmental conditions, would you say that you are overall at higher risk of dehydration or hyponatremia?

Fluid Needs

1. Determine your pre-exercise hydration status. Base this on your urine specific gravity and body weight compared with a 3-day average weight.
   Urine-specific gravity: _______
   Weight (% change from 3-day average): _______
2. Calculate your individual needs using the USATF protocol to determine sweat rate during a 1-hour workout.
   a. Pre-exercise weight: ____________________
   b. Fluid intake: ____________________
   c. Post-exercise weight: ____________________
   d. Calculated sweat rate: ____________________
3. Calculate your % body weight change: ___________

Hydration Recommendation Before Exercise

1. Determine your prehydration needs based on whether or not you were euhydrated prior to exercise and the amount of time between training sessions.

Hydration Recommendation During Exercise

1. Determine how much fluid you should drink during exercise based on intensity, duration, and calculated sweat rate. Calculate how much sodium and potassium you should consume to restore electrolyte balance after a prolonged workout.

Hydration Recommendation After Exercise

1. Develop a plan for rehydration based on the amount of time between training sessions and your usual post-workout food intake.

RESOURCES

The ACSM Position Stand Exercise and Fluid Replacement (2007) offers hydration recommendations based on an evidence-based review of the existing literature. This position statement is updated periodically and offers an excellent guideline for health professionals to use when making fluid recommendations.

The ACSM Position Stand Exertional Heat Illness During Training and Competition (2007) provides detailed information about the causes, consequences, symptoms, treatment, and recommendations for returning to activity for athletes who have suffered heat-related illnesses.

USA Track and Field (www.usatf.org). Access an electronic library of information on hydration and a handout outlining the protocol for determining individual fluid needs.

REFERENCES

1. Wendt D, van Loon LJ, Lichtenbelt WD. Thermoregulation during exercise in the heat: strategies for maintaining health and performance. *Sports Med.* 2007;37(8):669-682.
2. Schwellnus, MP. Cause of exercise associated muscle cramps (EAMC—altered neuromuscular control, dehydration or electrolyte depletion? *Br J Sports Med.* 2009;43:401-408. doi:10.1136/bjsm.2008.050401.
3. Rodriguez NR, DiMarco NM, Langley S. Position of the American Dietetic Association, Dietitians of Canada, and the American College of Sports Medicine: nutrition and athletic performance. *J Am Diet Assoc.* March 2009;109(3):509-527.
4. Armstrong LE, Casa DJ, Maresh CM, Ganio MS. Caffeine, fluid-electrolyte balance, temperature regulation, and exercise-heat tolerance. *Exerc Sport Sci Rev.* July 2007;35(3):135-140.
5. Bergeron MF, Bahr R, Bärtsch P, et al. International Olympic Committee consensus statement on thermoregulatory and altitude challenges for high-level athletes. *Br J Sports Med.* 2012;46:770-779. Doi:10.1136/bjsports-2012-091296.
6. Sawka MN, Burke LM, Eichner ER, Maughan RJ, Montain SJ, Stachenfeld NS. American College of Sports Medicine position stand. Exercise and fluid replacement. *Med Sci Sports Exerc.* February 2007;39(2):377-390.
7. Almond CS, Shin AY, Fortescue EB, et al. Hyponatremia among runners in the Boston Marathon. *N Engl J Med.* April 14 2005;352(15):1550-1556.
8. Noakes T. Fluid replacement during marathon running. *Clin J Sport Med.* September 2003;13(5):309-318.
9. van Rosendal SP, Osborne MA, Fassett RG, Coombes JS. Guidelines for glycerol use in hyperhydration and rehydration associated with exercise. *Sports Med.* February 1 2010; 40(2):113-129.
10. Casa DJ. Proper hydration for distance running—Identifying individual fluid needs: A USA Track and Field advisory. 2003. www.hartfordmarathon.com/Assets/Training%2B Program/ProperHydrationForDistanceRunning.pdf.
11. Institute of Medicine. *Fluid replacement and heat stress.* Washington, DC: Institute of Medicine;1994.
12. Hew-Butler TD, Sharwood K, Collins M, Speedy D, Noakes T. Sodium supplementation is not required to maintain serum sodium concentrations during an Ironman triathlon. *Br J Sports Med.* March 2006;40(3):255-259.
13. Speedy DB, Thompson JM, Rodgers I, Collins M, Sharwood K, Noakes TD. Oral salt supplementation during ultradistance exercise. *Clin J Sport Med.* September 2002;12(5):279-284.
14. Gavin TP. Clothing and thermoregulation during exercise. *Sports Med.* 2003;33(13):941-947.
15. Bergeron MF, Devore C, Rice SG. Policy statement-Climatic heat stress and exercising children and adolescents. *Pediatrics.* Sep 2011;128(3):e741-747.

CHAPTER 9

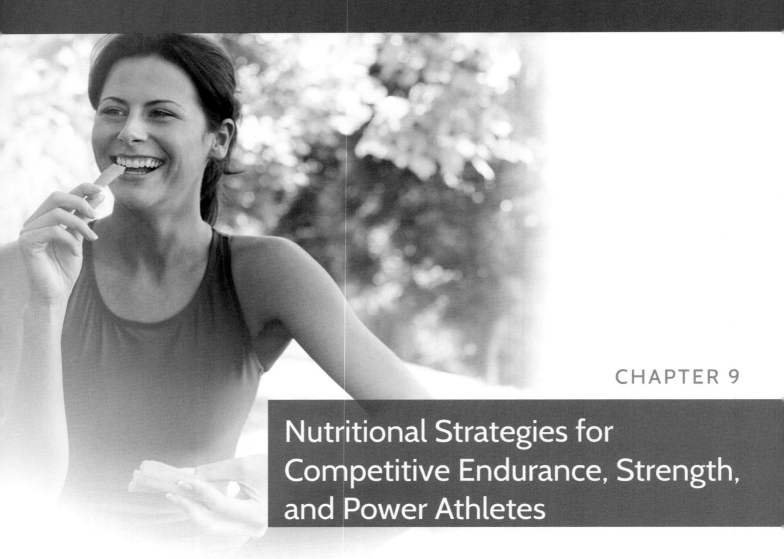

Nutritional Strategies for Competitive Endurance, Strength, and Power Athletes

CHAPTER OUTLINE

LEARNING OBJECTIVES

After studying this chapter, the reader should be able to:

9.1 List several nutrition principles that are important for athletes across disciplines.

9.2 Describe several nutritional mistakes elite athletes commonly make and potential strategies to overcome them.

9.3 Describe the important nutrition variables in influencing sports performance for endurance, strength, and power athletes and how they act to enhance athletic success.

9.4 Outline an ideal nutrition program for optimal performance in aerobic, strength, and power sports.

9.5 Given a particular sport, be able to apply the appropriate nutrition principles to provide an athlete with generalized recommendations.

KEY TERMS

aerobic power The speed at which adenosine triphosphate (ATP) is generated; increased in endurance athletes due to metabolic adaptations.

bonking Athlete fatigue in which exercise intensity dramatically decreases while the athlete's perceived effort increases. Also known as "hitting the wall."

carbonic acid An acid formed in the body that acts as an intermediate between sodium bicarbonate/hydrogen ions and carbon dioxide/water.

carnosine A dipeptide comprised of the basic amino acids alanine and histidine.

endurance sports Sports and activities lasting 30 minutes or more.

energy availability The energy available in the body to fuel physical activity and energy-requiring bodily functions. Determined by the relationship between the calories consumed in the diet and the calories expended in physical activity.

glycerol A molecule containing three carbon atoms and three OH molecules; creates an osmotic gradient in the circulation favoring fluid retention, which subsequently reduces fluid excretion from the kidneys and decreases urination; supplement is banned by the World Anti-Doping Agency.

"hitting the wall" Athlete fatigue in which exercise intensity dramatically decreases while the athlete's perceived effort increases. Also known as bonking.

hyperhydration Hydrating above currently optimal levels. By consuming large amounts of fluids prior to exercise, the athlete increases fluid reserves and delays the onset of dehydration.

hypertonic fluids Fluids that contain sodium and other electrolytes in higher concentrations than in blood.

iron depletion A state of decreased body stores of iron but normal levels of iron in the red blood cells; if not corrected, progresses to iron deficiency anemia.

isotonic fluids Fluids in which electrolyte content equals that of blood.

metabolic fatigue The fatigue that occurs when the substrates for energy production are used up. Early on in a strength workout this could be from the depletion of creatine phosphate stores, while later fatigue results from impaired energy production from glycogenolysis and anaerobic glycolysis.

muscle protein breakdown The rate of breakdown of muscle tissue into component amino acids.

muscle protein synthesis The rate of production of muscle tissue from the amino acid pool.

net protein balance The balance that exists between muscle protein synthesis and muscle protein breakdown.

neuromuscular fatigue Incompletely understood phenomena of a decrease in athletic performance with intensive activity to fatigue at some point in the pathway from initiation of exercise in the cerebral cortex to activation in the muscle cell.

nitrogen balance studies Tests that measure the amount of nitrogen in the urine, which provide an indication of whether too much, too little, or enough protein is being consumed.

periodized nutrition program A nutrition program in which calorie and macronutrient intakes vary based on the training regimen. Energy and nutrient needs are highest during peak training, somewhat decreased during taper and competition, and much lower during the transition and rest phase.

periodized training program An exercise training program that is separated into phases (periods) that vary in intensity and volume to maximize performance.

power A measure of force (strength) and speed.

power output The amount of force generated in a specified period of time.

reactive hypoglycemia Also known as rebound hypoglycemia; the drop in blood sugar that results from a surge in insulin. Theoretical concern when eating shortly before exercise because carbohydrate load and onset of exercise both cause an increase in insulin.

sodium bicarbonate A compound found naturally in blood and taken endogenously by some athletes as a supplement; helps to reduce muscle acidity by increasing the release of hydrogen ions from muscle cells.

strength The production of maximal force.

strength sports Sports that require production of maximal force for optimal performance.

ultra-endurance sports A subset of endurance sports that lasts 4 hours or more.

work-to-rest ratio The relationship of the amount of time spent in strenuous activity and the amount of time spent in rest between sets or vigorous bouts of activity.

INTRODUCTION

As two-time defending Olympic gold medalists, the women's U.S. soccer team was favored in the 2011 World Cup finals versus Japan, a team that the United States had defeated all of the last 25 matches. Up 1-0 with only 9 minutes to play, the U.S. victory was almost certain. The intensive training, diligent attention to fueling and hydration, mental focus, and teamwork were about to pay off with the first U.S. women's World Cup win in well over a decade. But then, Japan scored. Overtime. With little over 15 minutes remaining, U.S. player Abby Wambach scored to put the United States ahead 2-1. After 117 minutes of competition, with only 3 minutes left in the game, Japan scored to tie, pushing the game into a shoot-out. Ultimately, Japan dominated the United States 3-1 after two rounds of penalty kicks, winning their first World Cup. Heartbroken and exhausted, the women's U.S. soccer team was left to recover from the stinging loss, and question: What went wrong? While many factors certainly contributed, the nutritional demands and considerations of elite endurance athletes playing at the limits of their physical capacity should not be underestimated.

Determined to prove themselves after the disheartening defeat, less than 1 year later, after 123 minutes of play including overtime, the U.S. women's soccer team narrowly defeated Canada in the London Olympics semifinals. The final game posed a rematch between the United States and Japan. This time, the U.S. team beat Japan and won the Gold.

Most athletes will not go on to win a World Cup or compete in the Olympics. However, athletes of all levels strive to gain a competitive edge to perform at their highest capacity. Oftentimes an athlete's diet is as important as his or her training program in predicting success. When athletes can apply their understanding of exercise physiology and energy metabolism to making appropriate dietary choices, they set the stage to optimize athletic performance. While general nutritional and hydration considerations for active individuals are discussed in detail in Chapters 7 and 8, the application of these principles to specific sports and types of sports is the focus of this chapter.

NUTRITION FOR SPORTS PERFORMANCE

Compared to the general population, athletes have special nutritional needs including increased caloric requirements, greater amounts of protein and carbohydrates, and increased needs of some vitamins and minerals.[1] When athletes meet these nutritional needs, performance improves, recovery quickens, positive training adaptations develop, risk of injury lessens, and health improves. However, despite these potential benefits, studies of the nutrient patterns of athletes across sports have found that many athletes have long suffered from inadequate intake of many nutrients including calories, carbohydrates, and several micronutrients.[2-6] While elite athletes meticulously plan their fitness regimens, many struggle to consume the appropriate nutrients to fuel that performance, possibly owing to the difficulty of translating nutrition recommendations into a daily regimen of nutrient-dense meals and snacks. Highlighting this struggle, several common nutritional mistakes that elite athletes across all sports make (and how to overcome them) are highlighted in Box 9-1.

Ultimately, all athletes benefit from adequate caloric intake, high carbohydrate availability, tailored hydration, and an adequate intake of nutrient-dense foods. The optimal amounts, combinations, and timing of nutrient intake vary by sport and position.

SPEED BUMP

1. **List several nutrition principles that are important for athletes across disciplines.**
2. **Describe several nutritional mistakes elite athletes commonly make and potential strategies to overcome them.**

ENDURANCE SPORTS

Endurance sports are sports and activities lasting 30 minutes or more. **Ultra-endurance sports** are a subset of endurance sports which last 4 hours or more. Endurance and ultra-endurance sports include long-distance running, road cycling, long-distance swimming, and other sports and activities that rely heavily on the capacity of the aerobic system to provide adequate

Box 9-1. Common Nutritional Mistakes Athletes Make (and How to Overcome Them)

While elite athletes possess optimal fitness to excel in their respective sports, they many times encounter nutrition roadblocks to achieve peak performance. Common nutritional mistakes elite athletes make and how to overcome them include:

1. **Focusing on weight alone instead of lean mass and fat mass.**
   Many athletes are concerned with total body weight, when the strength-to-weight ratio is what is really important for athletic performance. Low lean mass may be an indicator that athletes are not meeting their energy needs, which may ultimately lower metabolic rate.[61] Energy intake sufficient to spare protein and support muscle mass can improve athletic performance, appearance, and even bone health.[62]
2. **Eating infrequently.**
   Humans are able to use only a limited amount of energy substrates at one time, and any excess macronutrients from food are stored primarily as fat.[63] Likewise, when adequate energy is not readily supplied by food, we respond by breaking down the tissue that requires energy, lean muscle.[62] Many athletes do not meet basic nutritional needs such as consuming adequate amounts of total calories and carbohydrates. In fact, one study of 52 female division I college athletes found that only 9% met calorie needs and just 25% met carbohydrate needs.[64] Increasing meal frequency and decreasing meal size improves within-day energy balance and body composition in elite athletes.[65]
3. **Unnecessary micronutrient supplementation.**
   Athletes use vitamin and mineral supplements for a variety of reasons, including to aid in bone mineral preservation, enhance performance, and fill gaps in an inadequate diet.[66] While athletes do have some higher vitamin and mineral requirements, only a limited amount can be absorbed at one time, so high-dose supplements are typically not efficiently used. In most cases, athletes should consume a diet that provides sufficient vitamins and minerals from food.[1] Exceeding vitamin and mineral requirements does not improve performance; in fact, excess micronutrient intake can negatively affect fluid balance and health.
4. **Failure to maintain adequate hydration status.**
   Fluid balance directly affects the athlete's ability to maintain adequate blood volume, which is imperative during prolonged physical activity.[1] Failure to replete both fluid and electrolytes during exercise can cause a drop in blood volume, early fatigue, and can even lead to dangerous dehydration. To maintain adequate hydration status and blood glucose levels, athletes should consume a few sips of a sports beverage containing electrolytes and carbohydrate every 15 minutes while engaging in high-intensity physical activity.
5. **Excessive energy restriction.**
   Cutting too many calories in an attempt to lose weight can actually cause a loss of lean mass and a relative increase in fat mass.[62] Insufficient energy intake results in a reduction in the amount of tissue that requires energy, lean muscle. This can ultimately lead to decreased resting metabolic rate and increased relative fat mass. To stay lean and keep metabolism up, athletes should consume sufficient energy to support physical activity, spare protein, and preserve lean tissue.

Source: Monica Grages, MS, RD, LD, past graduate research assistant in the Laboratory for Elite Athlete Performance at Georgia State University.

nutrition and oxygen to working cells over a prolonged period of time.

The Biochemistry Reviewed

While the phosphagen, anaerobic, and aerobic (or "oxidative") systems all are active in providing energy during endurance exercise, the aerobic systems predominate. Aerobic glycolysis and fatty acid oxidation metabolize glucose and fatty acids, respectively, to generate energy in the form of adenosine triphosphate (ATP). The aerobic systems have a nearly unlimited capacity to generate ATP; however, because aerobic glycolysis and fatty acid oxidation require multiple chemical reactions to generate ATP, the speed in which ATP is generated, referred to as **aerobic power**, is slower for the aerobic systems than for the anaerobic systems. Highly trained endurance athletes have increased aerobic power due to metabolic adaptations which occur in response to exercise, including increased mitochondrial concentration in muscle cells, enhanced delivery of oxygen to working cells, and more efficient utilization of fuel.

Fatigue during endurance exercise typically results from depletion of muscle glycogen and reduced blood glucose concentrations. Not only is glucose essential for aerobic glycolysis, but glucose is also necessary to metabolize fat for energy through fatty acid oxidation. When muscle and liver glycogen stores are depleted, an endurance athlete experiences extreme fatigue. Exercise intensity dramatically decreases while the athlete's perceived effort increases. This scenario is commonly referred to as **"hitting the wall"** or **bonking**; it typically occurs after several hours of continuous exercise.

Nutritional Highlights

To avoid extreme fatigue and optimize performance, the major nutritional principles for endurance athletes aim to optimize muscle and liver glycogen stores and enhance the efficiency in which glucose and fatty acids are converted to fuel.

Energy Needs

Endurance athletes engage in rhythmic, continuous movements at relatively high intensities for prolonged periods of time. Many endurance athletes require high caloric intakes to provide sufficient energy to fuel these exercise bouts. One study of elite female runners found that their average daily energy expenditure ranged from 3,000 to 3,750 kcals.[7] An ultra-endurance cyclist may need upward of 6,000 calories to fuel a prolonged training ride.[8]

Consuming sufficient calories to fuel exercise while not interfering with a training regimen or causing gastrointestinal distress may pose serious challenges for these athletes, but the consequences of inadequate caloric intake can affect athletic performance as well as overall health. When too few calories are consumed than are required to provide for basic metabolic needs and fuel exercise, the athlete is in a state of low **energy availability** and at increased risk of decreased athletic performance, muscle wasting, depressed immune function, fatigue, and injury. Female athletes with chronically low energy availability also are at risk for the **female athlete triad**, the trio of decreased energy availability, decreased bone density, and irregular menstruation.

Box 9-2 offers a few tips to help athletes meet calorie needs, while maintaining their intensive training regimen.

Optimization of Glycogen Stores and Glucose Availability

High carbohydrate availability during training increases rates of carbohydrate oxidation and the production of ATP.[9] Consequently, a major goal of fueling for endurance sports is to optimize glycogen stores and ensure a ready supply of glucose during exercise.

Carbohydrate Loading. To boost glycogen stores, athletes preparing for an event that will last longer than 90 minutes may benefit from carbohydrate loading in the days before the competition. The amount of carbohydrates required for maximal benefit depends on frequency, intensity, duration, and type of exercise that make up the athlete's training program. A typical athlete may need from 5 to 10 grams of carbohydrates per kilogram body weight per day. The increase in glycogen stores contributes to a 2% to 3% improved performance in events lasting longer than 90 minutes; it does not seem to provide benefit for shorter duration activities.[10] Carbohydrate loading also leads to water weight gain of about 3 grams per gram of glycogen stored since glucose requires water to be stored as glycogen.

Carbohydrates Prior to Exercise. A carbohydrate-rich meal 3 to 4 hours prior to competition also benefits endurance performance by increasing muscle and liver glycogen stores.[11] Carbohydrate intake on the order of 200 to 300 grams following an overnight fast helps to replenish carbohydrate reserves and increase subsequent performance. Many endurance athletes begin their training early in the morning, so carbohydrate consumption 3 to 4 hours prior to exercise is not feasible. Historically, endurance athletes had been advised to avoid carbohydrates in the

Box 9-2. Tips to Help Athletes Meet Calorie Needs While Maintaining an Intensive Training Regimen

Many athletes engaging in intensive training programs struggle to consume sufficient calories to meet nutritional needs. The following tips can help athletes overcome the challenges of fitting optimal nutrition into their daily schedules:

1. Always have a healthy snack on hand. Athletes can load up their duffel bags, backpacks, and purses with healthy snacks such as whole and dried fruit, nutrition or granola bars, and mixed nuts. This allows an athlete to always have access to a ready source of fuel when convenient. This is especially important when traveling or having uncertain access to wholesome foods.
2. Plan meals around the daily training routine. Athletes who plan in advance are more likely to eat wholesome foods and meet their nutritional needs.
3. Drink sports drinks and other easily digestible carbohydrates during training sessions lasting longer than 1 hour. The importance of nutrition support is not limited to the day of competition. Athletes should be sure to consume needed fluids and fuel during training sessions as well.
4. Choose wisely. Athletes should take special care to choose foods that are most likely to meet their nutritional needs. This means taking a conscientious approach to nutrition and nutrition labels when going grocery shopping and examining restaurant nutrition boards and menu descriptions when eating out.

hour prior to exercise—the most convenient time for many athletes to consume a pre-exercise snack—due to concern for **rebound** or **reactive hypoglycemia** and diminished performance. However, the evidence suggests that carbohydrate consumption in the hour before exercise provides more benefit than potential harm, though it probably does not provide the same performance boost as carbohydrates consumed at least 2 hours before the onset of exercise[12] (see Myths and Misconceptions).

Carbohydrates During Exercise. Carbohydrate ingestion during exercise provides both metabolic and neurological advantages. The metabolic advantages occur particularly for exercise lasting longer than 1 hour when glycogen stores and available blood glucose wane. The neuromuscular advantages of carbohydrates can occur even for short-duration and very high intensity activities. In fact, in these cases some research suggests that carbohydrate mouth rinses provide similar performance improvements to carbohydrate drinks simply from stimulation of receptors in the oral cavity.[13,14] When exercise lasts longer than 2 hours, carbohydrate ingestion is essential to provide adequate fuel.

Evolving research suggests that athletic performance improves directly with the amount of carbohydrates consumed up to the body's maximal capacity to digest and absorb the carbohydrate load. For example, a multicenter study of 51 cyclists and triathletes had the athletes complete a 2-hour ride at moderate to high intensity immediately followed by a 20-kilometer time trial. The researchers provided a range of 10 to 120 grams of carbohydrates to the athletes for each hour of exercise. Athletic performance increased in a dose-dependent manner with the amount of carbohydrates consumed, up to a rate of 60 to 80 grams per hour.[15] That is, the more carbohydrates the athletes consumed, the greater their improvement in performance.

The maximal amount of carbohydrates that can be digested, absorbed, and oxidized to create ATP is a subject of intense investigation. Carbohydrate oxidation is limited by the rate of intestinal absorption. Glucose absorption occurs in the small intestines via a SGLT1, a sodium-dependent transporter that becomes saturated with glucose at a consumption of around 1 gram per minute, or 60 grams per hour.[16] A growing body of research suggests that endurance athletes may be able to increase carbohydrate absorption and subsequent oxidation by consuming carbohydrates that rely on different transporters for absorption. Glucose, sucrose, maltose, maltodextrins (oligosaccharide), and amylopectin are rapidly absorbed, while fructose, galactose, and amylose are absorbed more slowly. Most sports drinks contain some combination of these sugars (see the beverage comparison chart at www.usaswingnet.com/gatorade_bev_chart%5B1%5D.pdf). A summary of this research and application questions are presented in Evaluating the Evidence.

While competitive athletes exercising at high levels for long periods of time may require 80 grams or more

Myths and Misconceptions

Endurance Athletes Should Avoid Carbohydrates in the Hour Prior to Exercise Due to Risk of Hypoglycemia

The rationale proceeds as follows: A carbohydrate load causes an increase in blood sugar concentration, which subsequently triggers the release of insulin. Insulin facilitates deposition of blood glucose into the cells and leads to decreased blood glucose concentration. The initiation of exercise also triggers a decrease in blood sugar levels through an insulin-independent pathway in which GLUT 4 receptors facilitate the movement of glucose from blood to the cells. Together, the rapid increase of insulin due to the carbohydrate load and the increased activity of GLUT 4 receptors in response to the onset of exercise could trigger a rebound hypoglycemia with onset occurring in the 15 to 30 minutes after beginning exercise. The athlete may then experience the uncomfortable symptoms associated with hypoglycemia such as anxiety, palpitations, nausea, and fatigue. Additionally, a high blood insulin level inhibits lipolysis and fat oxidation, potentially contributing to further reliance on carbohydrates for energy and more rapid depletion of glycogen stores.[17] Ultimately, it was believed that athletic performance would suffer.

A meta-analysis of the literature addressing this topic found that this concern has no functional significance for most athletes and no impact on performance.[12] Many athletes do not physiologically experience the rebound hypoglycemia and, of those that do, athletic performance is not compromised.[12] In practice, the increased carbohydrate availability in the 30 minutes to 1 hour prior to exercise provides more benefit to athletic performance than the potential harm of hyperinsulinemia and rebound hypoglycemia. However, some athletes may report symptoms of hypoglycemia when eating carbohydrate in the hour before exercise. These athletes may find relief from eating a low glycemic index snack such as an apple or low-fat yogurt (causing a lesser increase in blood glucose and insulin) within 15 minutes of exercise onset (when the carbohydrate functions in the same way as carbohydrates consumed during exercise).[12]

EVALUATING THE EVIDENCE

Manipulating Transporters to Increase Carbohydrate Absorption and Oxidation

Until the publication of a landmark paper by Jentjens, Moseley, Waring, Harding, and Jeukendrup, it was thought that carbohydrates consumed during exercise could be oxidized at a rate no faster than 1 gram per minute, or 60 grams per hour, regardless of the type of carbohydrate consumed.

Review the excerpted study abstract and answer the questions that follow. The complete study is available at www.pubmed.gov.

Oxidation of combined ingestion of glucose and fructose during exercise.
Jentjens RL, Moseley L, Waring RH, Harding LK, Jeukendrup AE. *J Appl Physiol.* 2004 Apr;96(4):1277-84.

Eight trained cyclists (maximal O(2) consumption: 62 +/- 3 ml × kg(-1) × min(-1)) performed four exercise trials in random order. Each trial consisted of 120 min of cycling at 50% maximum power output (63 +/- 2% maximal O(2) consumption), while subjects received a solution providing either 1.2 g/min of glucose (Med-Glu), 1.8 g/min of glucose (High-Glu), 0.6 g/min of fructose + 1.2 g/min of glucose (Fruc+Glu), or water. The ingested fructose was labeled with [U-(13)C]fructose, and the ingested glucose was labeled with [U-(14)C]glucose. Peak exogenous carbohydrate oxidation rates were approximately 55% higher (P < 0.001) in Fruc+Glu (1.26 +/- 0.07 g/min) compared with Med-Glu and High-Glu (0.80 +/- 0.04 and 0.83 +/- 0.05 g/min, respectively). Furthermore, the average exogenous carbohydrate oxidation rates over the 60- to 120-min exercise period were higher (P < 0.001) in Fruc+Glu compared with Med-Glu and High-Glu (1.16 +/- 0.06, 0.75 +/- 0.04, and 0.75 +/- 0.04 g/min, respectively). There was a trend toward a lower endogenous carbohydrate oxidation in Fruc+Glu compared with the other two carbohydrate trials, but this failed to reach statistical significance (P = 0.075). The present results demonstrate that, when fructose and glucose are ingested simultaneously at high rates during cycling exercise, exogenous carbohydrate oxidation rates can reach peak values of approximately 1.3 g/min.

1. Describe in lay terms the major findings from this study.
2. To whom are the results of this study most applicable? Why?
3. Since this study was published, many other researchers have investigated if consuming various forms of carbohydrates such as glucose and fructose lead to higher oxidation rates than use of glucose alone. Many of the studies that used total concentrations of glucose + fructose at ≤ 1g/min have found no difference in oxidation rates,[67,68] but those with glucose + fructose at ≥ 1g/min have found benefit from consuming multiple transporter carbohydrates.[69-71] Explain the potential reason for the discrepancy.
4. How might you apply these findings when providing nutrition information to endurance athletes?

of carbohydrates per hour for peak performance, an athlete engaging in moderate-intensity endurance exercise for a shorter duration or a recreational athlete may need much less. For example, very small amounts of carbohydrates in the form of a mouth rinse or drink are recommended for events of 30 to 75 minutes. At 1 to 2 hours the recommended carbohydrate intake is up to 30 grams per hour; at 2 to 3 hours up to 60 grams of carbohydrates per hour are recommended; and over 2.5 hours up to 90 grams of carbohydrates per hour are recommended. For events up to 2 hours, most forms of carbohydrates can be consumed; at 2 to 3 hours carbohydrates that are rapidly oxidized are recommended; and for events greater than 2.5 hours only multiple transportable carbohydrates are recommended.[17]

Despite the performance benefits from large amounts of carbohydrates, some athletes may hesitate to consume recommended amounts due to concerns of gastrointestinal (GI) distress. If carbohydrates are not rapidly digested and absorbed, they can contribute to performance-limiting cramps, dizziness, nausea, vomiting, and diarrhea. The likelihood of GI problems increases with consumption of fiber, fat, protein, and concentrated carbohydrate-containing foods and drinks. Up to 95% of endurance athletes have experienced GI symptoms during intense endurance sessions.[18] About 4% of marathoners and 32% of Ironman competitors experience GI distress during any given event.[19] Some preliminary research suggests that consumption of a high carbohydrate diet may upregulate carbohydrate transporters and increase carbohydrate oxidation rates[9] and decrease GI distress.

Ultimately, high carbohydrate gels, bars, and snacks extend endurance performance, even in activities lasting less than 1 hour.[20,21] Carbohydrate consumption should begin shortly after the onset of activity and every 15 to 20 minutes throughout the workout.

Box 9-3 highlights a sample nutritional plan to meet the caloric and carbohydrate needs of a triathlete who expends about 4,500 kcals per day. An approach to

Box 9-3. A Sample Meal Plan for a Triathlete Requiring 4,500 Calories per Day

Endurance athletes may have an intensive training schedule, high caloric needs, and limited time to consume the necessary calories without interfering with training. A triathlete faces special challenges as fluid and carbohydrate consumption during long training swims may be difficult. Here is a sample meal plan a triathlete with a 4,500-calorie per day requirement may follow. This plan assumes that the triathlete engages in a brick training program consisting of a 1-hour open water swim, 4-hour bike ride, and 2-hour run.

Time	Activitiy	Meal/Snack	Calories	Carbohydrate (g)
0500	Wake up	Nutrition bar 20 oz sports drink	250 135	30 35
0600	Hydrate	8 oz sports drink	53	14
0630	Start swim			
0730	End swim	12 oz sports drink 8 oz water Sports gel	80 100	21 25
0735	Start bike ride			
0750 0905 1020 1125	Hydrate	4 oz sports drink	426	112
0805 0920 1035 0820 0935 1040 0835 0950 1055 0850 1005 1110	Hydrate	2 oz water		
0935	Snack	Banana	100	27
1035		Orange	60	14
1110		Sports gel	100	25
1135	End bike ride	8 oz sports drink	53	14
1140	Start run			
1200 1300	Hydrate	4 oz sports drink, alternate	80	21
1220 1320		with 4 oz water		
1240				
1240	Snack	Nutrition bar	250	30
1340	End run			
1400	Post-workout snack	12 oz chocolate milk Peanut butter sandwich	290 400	43 30
1500	Lunch	2 cup vegetarian pasta with 100 g tofu 8 oz orange juice	550 80 135	85 3 33

Continued

Box 9-3. A Sample Meal Plan for a Triathlete Requiring 4,500 Calories per Day–cont'd

Time	Activitiy	Meal/Snack	Calories	Carbohydrate (g)
1800	Dinner	6 oz salmon	240	0
		1 cup brown rice	440	90
		1 cup broccoli	60	10
		1 cup carrots	50	12
		8 oz skim milk	90	12
2000	Snack	6 oz nonfat Greek yogurt	140	20
		½ cup granola	300	33
		½ cup raspberries	30	7
2200	Bed	8 oz water	4,492	746 *66% of total calories* *10.5 g/kg/day assuming 70 kg man*

determining calorie needs for endurance athletes is described in detail in Chapter 11.

Glycemic Index. Endurance athletes are commonly advised to consume low-glycemic index carbohydrates before exercise to optimize athletic performance. (See Chapter 1 for a complete discussion of glycemic index, how it works, and why it might impact exercise.) Despite nearly two decades of research on this topic, there is not a consensus as to whether or not glycemic index affects athletic performance.[22]

Fat Intake. Some endurance athletes adhere to a high fat diet in the days leading to a prolonged endurance event in an attempt to increase muscle triglyceride stores and spare muscle glycogen. While this practice increases intramuscular triglyceride stores, it has not been shown to improve performance and athletes report increased perceived exertion on a high-fat diet compared to a high-carbohydrate diet.[11] Overall, recommendations for fat consumption for endurance athletes parallel the recommendations for the general population.[1]

Hydration Status

During prolonged endurance exercise, sweat acts to dissipate the heat generated from the body's energy-producing metabolic reactions. Athletes with high rates of sweat loss are at increased risk of dehydration, which can impair athletic performance and contribute to fatigue.[23] The aim of hydration during exercise is to avoid significant dehydration (a loss of more than 2% to 3% of body weight). One way to do this is to begin exercise euhydrated. The American College of Sports Medicine (ACSM) recommends that athletes follow an individualized hydration regimen to ensure adequate hydration prior to exercise, which may be demonstrated by dilute urine (pale to clear-colored urine).[23] While recommendations vary by individual, the typical athlete may need about 5 to 7 ml/kg of body weight at least 4 hours prior to exercise, with another 3 to 5 ml/kg 2 hours before exercise if no urine is produced or if it is highly concentrated (dark-colored urine).[23]

Hydration needs during exercise vary considerably based on exercise time and intensity, individual factors, and environmental conditions. The most reliable method to determine fluid needs is for the endurance athlete to weigh himself or herself prior to exercise and afterward and replace losses that are greater than 2% to 3% dehydration. Addition of sodium and carbohydrate helps to increase water absorption.

Maintenance of fluid balance during exercise may not be possible for athletes with high sweat rates, as the rate of fluid loss may exceed gastric emptying rates and fluid absorption. Athletes can maximize gastric emptying by regularly drinking small sips of fluid, at least every 15 to 20 minutes, and avoiding hypertonic fluids that are greater than 8% carbohydrate. **Hypertonic fluids** contain sodium and other electrolytes in higher concentrations than blood. Athletes who are prone to dehydration during intensive training may benefit from **hyperhydration**. By consuming large amounts of fluids prior to exercise, the athlete increases fluid reserves and delays the onset of dehydration. The excess fluid also helps to offset increases in body heat (an especially serious concern when exercising in the heat) and maintain a high volume status for optimal cardiac output. Excess fluid intake also leads to increased urination, which can offset the benefits of hyperhydration. To limit urination, some athletes incorporate beverages containing **glycerol** into their hyperhydration regimen. Glycerol creates an osmotic gradient in the circulation favoring fluid retention, which subsequently reduces fluid excretion from the kidneys and decreases urination.[24] Glycerol supplementation is banned by the World Anti-Doping Agency.

Any athlete who drinks more fluid than what is lost from sweat is at increased risk of hyponatremia, or low blood sodium levels (less than 135 mEq/L); however, slower athletes are at highest risk as they are more likely to consume large amounts of **isotonic fluids** that far exceed the rate of fluid lost from sweat.[25] Exercise-related hyponatremia can be prevented by avoiding overdrinking during exercise. Hyponatremia is discussed in detail in Chapter 4.

Micronutrient Availability

Many vitamins and minerals play important roles in the body's ability to convert fuel from food into usable energy. The B vitamins are cofactors in the chemical reactions that convert food into a usable energy source. If the body has an inadequate supply of these vitamins, energy production and subsequently endurance performance are compromised. Two B vitamins of particular importance are vitamin B_{12} and folate. Deficiency of either of these nutrients can cause anemia, which impairs the ability of the blood cells to deliver oxygen to the working cells and negatively impacts endurance performance (see Figure 9-1).

Iron plays a critical role in the process of transporting oxygen to working cells. If iron is in very short supply (iron deficiency anemia), production of hemoglobin is limited. Because hemoglobin carries oxygen in the bloodstream, iron deficiency limits aerobic capacity. Iron depletion occurs when the amount of iron in the body is reduced, but the amount in red blood cells is normal. If **iron depletion** is not corrected, it progresses to iron deficiency anemia. Iron depletion is one of the most common nutrient insufficiencies, especially for female endurance athletes.1 Studies show that athletes who suffer from iron depletion, with or without anemia, may benefit from 4 to 6 weeks of iron supplementation to lessen skeletal muscle fatigue and improve endurance, increase oxygen uptake, and reduce post-endurance lactateconcentration.[26] If a health professional is concerned that a client may be at risk for iron depletion or deficiency, referral to a physician is warranted. An allied health professional should never diagnose iron depletion nor recommend supplementation. See Chapter 4 for more detailed information on iron.

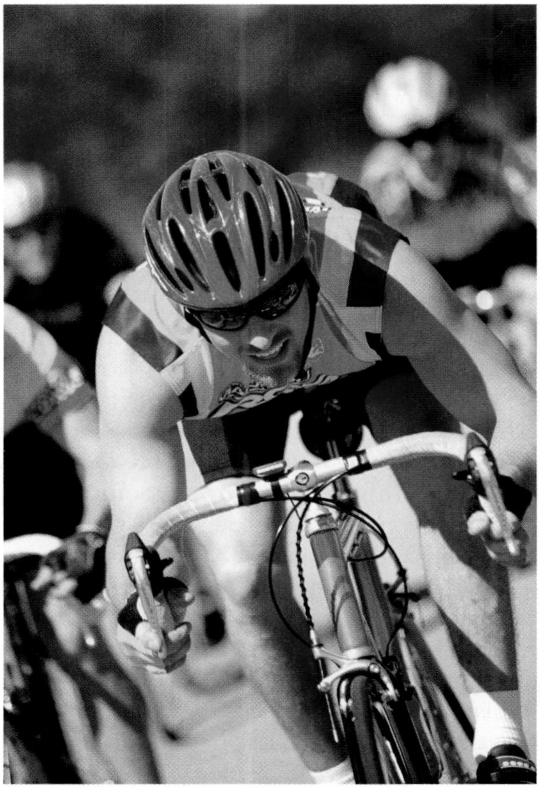

Figure 9-1. Micronutrients and endurance exercise.

Poor zinc intake is associated with decreased cardiovascular function and decreased muscle strength and endurance.[20] Zinc is a component of several enzymes important in energy metabolism, cell growth, and tissue repair. It may be depleted with prolonged exercise through excretion in sweat and urinary losses. Athletes should be cautioned against trying to meet zinc needs with supplementation as excessive zinc intake (which frequently occurs with zinc supplementation) can lower HDL cholesterol (the "good" cholesterol) and interfere with iron and copper absorption.[20]

Low magnesium intake, especially common in weight-class and body conscious sports such as wrestling, gymnastics, ballet, and tennis, compromises aerobic endurance.[1] Magnesium is a critical component to hundreds of essential biochemical reactions including the conversion of glucose to glycogen and the metabolism of glucose, amino acids, and fatty acids to produce energy.

Endurance athletes may have increased need for vitamin E. Some preliminary research suggests that antioxidants such as vitamin E reduce lipid peroxidation during aerobic exercise and may lessen DNA damage.[27] However, subsequent studies found that antioxidants like vitamin E do not prevent post-exercise peroxidation.[28] When vitamin E is taken in very large amounts (greater than the Tolerable Upper Intake Levels, which are quite high), such as may be the case with certain vitamin E supplements, it can be pro-oxidative rather than anti-oxidative, leading to potentially harmful effects.[29]

Electrolyte replenishment takes high priority for endurance athletes, especially those athletes with high rates of sweat loss. In fact, some endurance athletes may have sodium and chloride needs that are much higher than the Tolerable Upper Intake Level of 2.3 grams per day of sodium and 3.6 grams per day of chloride. The ACSM and Academy of Nutrition and Dietetics (AND) recommend that athletes who engage in endurance activity lasting longer than 1 to 2 hours consume a sports drink with carbohydrates and at least 0.5 to 0.7g/L of sodium and 0.8 to 2g/L of potassium.[1] The sports drink helps to replace sweat electrolyte losses, retain fluid and stimulate thirst, and provide energy.

Other Considerations

Caffeine. Caffeine—described in detail in Chapter 10—is the most common supplement used by endurance athletes due to its well-established ergogenic benefits. Most studies report the greatest benefit in doses of 3 to

6 mg/kg approximately 1 hour before exercise, though benefits have been reported in doses as low as 1 to 2 mg/kg.[30] Importantly, chronic caffeine users are much less likely to attain performance benefits from caffeine use compared to caffeine-naïve athletes. This is because the body has developed a tolerance to the effects of caffeine on the body. Excessive caffeine intake can be toxic.

Protein. While a high level of carbohydrate intake is essential for endurance success, sufficient protein intake also is important to provide the amino acids to repair damaged muscle tissue following an intense workout. Further, if carbohydrate intake is insufficient (less than 1.2 grams per kilogram per hour for the first 3 hours after exercise), protein co-ingestion may help to enhance glycogen replenishment.[31] (In this case, the best combination is 0.2 to 0.4 gram of protein per kilogram body weight plus 0.8 gram of protein per kilogram body weight[32]). **Nitrogen balance studies** suggest that endurance athletes need about 1.2 to 1.4 grams of protein per kilogram of body weight per day to maintain neutral nitrogen balance even though protein turnover may become more efficient with improved endurance conditioning.[1]

Body Composition. Many endurance athletes maintain an extremely lean body composition both as a result of the high level of physical activity and as a strategy to optimize performance. A detailed discussion of body composition considerations in athletes is included in Chapter 11.

SPEED BUMP

3. **Describe the important nutrition variables in influencing sports performance for endurance athletes.**
4. **Outline an ideal nutrition program for optimal performance in endurance sports.**

STRENGTH SPORTS

While all sports rely on **strength** to some degree, **strength sports** require production of maximal force for optimal performance. These sports include weightlifting, throwing events, and bodybuilding.

Because the extent of lean body tissue and muscle mass directly affects performance for these sports, most strength athletes engage in resistance training, whether that is part of the training program for a sport (such as for sprinting and throwing events) or as an integral component of the sport itself (such as for bodybuilding and weightlifting).

The Biochemistry Reviewed

Resistance training relies heavily on the phosphagen system and anaerobic glycolysis.[33] The contribution of each system is dependent on the **power output**, **work-to-rest ratio**, and muscle blood flow.[33] Fatigue during resistance exercise generally is attributable to **neuromuscular fatigue**[34] and **metabolic fatigue** leading to increased acidity in the muscle fibers.[35] Metabolic fatigue early in a strength workout typically results from depletion of phosphagen stores, while later fatigue results from impaired energy production from glycogenolysis and anaerobic glycolysis. See Chapter 6 for more information.

Nutritional Highlights

Nutrition plays an important role in primarily three domains for strength athletes: (1) fueling sport and resistance training; (2) optimizing recovery from training; and (3) promoting muscular hypertrophy.

Fueling Sport and Resistance Training

Strength athletes rely on a ready source of nutrients to optimize performance.

Calorie Needs. Competitive strength athletes typically have a large muscle mass. Because muscle mass is directly proportional to metabolic rate, strength athletes have high caloric needs to maintain body weight, although the energy expended in exercise may be less than other athletes. A compilation of studies of elite strength athletes found that the typical competitive strength athlete requires about 3,500 kcals per day, or about 43 kcals/kg of body weight to maintain weight.[36] Estimated needs by sport are included in Table 9-1. Actual needs for an individual athlete may vary significantly from this average based on age, gender, body composition, and fitness level and intensity of training.

Strength athletes need to consume sufficient calories to optimize energy availability for the body's everyday functions as well as to build muscle mass. An athlete who unintentionally loses weight during training is not eating sufficient calories to fuel optimal performance. Some athletes may need to eat four to six meals per day and snacks in between meals to meet caloric needs. An athlete attempting to gain muscle mass will need an additional 300 to 500 calories per day for a 1-pound lean weight gain per week. This can be logistically challenging for an athlete who must strategically time eating and exercise to optimize performance and also minimize the risk of gastrointestinal discomfort, which can result from eating too soon, too much, or poorly digested foods before exercise.

Protein Needs. A joint position statement of the ACSM and AND advises that strength athletes consume approximately 1.2 to 1.7 grams of protein per kilogram per day.[1] The protein needs for strength athletes are higher than for endurance athletes, as the body relies on amino acids (especially branched chain amino acids) to support muscle growth (see Chapter 2 for detailed information on the role of amino acids in muscle growth). The increased needs are especially important when a person begins a strength training program, the time when muscle growth occurs more rapidly. Protein needs may be somewhat lessened with consistent resistance training due to increased efficiency of protein utilization.[37,38] Most strength athletes consume at least

Table 9-1. Nutritional Needs for Strength Athletes[3,36]

SPORT		AVG WEIGHT KG (LB)	CALORIES (KCAL/KG)	CARBOHYDRATE G (G/KG)	PROTEIN G (G/KG)	FAT G (%E)
Throwing	Male	96 (210)	3,500 (36)	375 (3.9)	160 (1.7)	158 (41)
	Female	83 (180)	2,200 (27)	269 (3.2)	94 (1.1)	95 (38)
Sprinting	Male	67 (150)	2,650 (40)	340 (5.1)	102 (1.5)	90 (30)
	Female	54 (120)	2,400 (44)	305 (5.8)	89 (1.7)	86 (33)
Weight lifting	Male	95 (210)	3,600 (38)	392 (4.1)	161 (1.7)	160 (39)
Bodybuilding	Male	84 (185)	3,700 (44)	532 (6.9)	165 (2.1)	120 (29)
	Female	58 (130)	1,600 (28)	208 (3.6)	102 (1.8)	42 (21)
General			Male 55/kg, Female 40/kg	Male 8–9g/kg Female 5.5g/kg		

Estimates are for "national level" athletes, which describes highly skilled but not professional or elite level athletes.

the recommended amount of protein.[1] Consumption of protein beyond recommendations provides no additional strength benefit, promotes increased amino acid catabolism and protein oxidation, and may provide excess caloric intake, which is stored as fat.[39]

Carbohydrate Needs. Some research suggests that consuming carbohydrates prior to and during high volume resistance and strength training may help to maintain glycogen stores, leading to increased energy and work capacity.[40] While the precise amount and timing of carbohydrates for optimal performance varies among athletes and the type of activity, one study found that a carbohydrate snack containing about 1 g/kg of body weight prior to resistance training followed by 0.5 g/kg during resistance training improved performance.[41]

Fat. Strength athletes do not have increased needs for fat intake compared to the general population. In reality, most strength athletes consume greater than the recommendations of fat, possibly due to increased intake of animal products in an effort to increase protein intake.[37] Because many strength athletes have high caloric needs, energy-dense fat in the diet may be an important component to a strength athlete's weight management plan. However, strength athletes who are overweight or need to lose weight should monitor fat intake as it is the most energy-dense nutrient, containing 9 calories per gram (compared with 4 calories per gram for carbohydrates and protein).

Hydration. Hydration considerations for strength athletes parallel those of endurance athletes. Athletes should begin exercise euhydrated and strive to replace lost fluids during training (when possible) and after exercise.

Optimization of Recovery From Training

Ideal macronutrient distribution for strength athletes relies on a balance of carbohydrate intake to replenish depleted glycogen stores and protein intake to provide a ready source of amino acids for muscle hypertrophy. A single resistance training session can deplete glycogen stores from 24% to 40% depending on duration and intensity of the training session.[42] If these glycogen stores are not replenished prior to the next training session or competition, performance may suffer.[44]

Promotion of Muscle Hypertrophy

Muscle protein is in a state of constant flux between **muscle protein synthesis** and **muscle protein breakdown**. Muscle protein synthesis increases 40% to 150% after a single bout of resistance exercise.[45] However, in a fasted state, **net protein balance** (muscle protein synthesis – muscle protein breakdown) remains negative due to the extensive muscle protein breakdown that occurs after strength exercise. In order to shift the equation to favor hypertrophy, several nutritional factors come into play: protein source, protein quantity, timing of intake, carbohydrate intake, and supplements.[45]

Protein Source. Some evidence suggests that whey and soy protein—two high quality and rapidly digested proteins—trigger an increase in muscle protein synthesis, while consumption of the slowly digested proteins casein and milk help to decrease muscle protein breakdown.[45] Research is underway to understand which protein source ultimately is best to promote muscle hypertrophy. One study showed that milk promoted muscle synthesis more than soy among young male weight lifters.[46] Another showed that whey promoted synthesis more than casein and soy.[42] Yet another found that casein and whey were equally effective.[47] All four of these proteins are high-quality proteins that contain all of the essential amino acids.

Protein Quantity. Based on results from several laboratory and clinical studies, approximately 20 grams of intact protein or 8 to 10 grams of essential amino acids consumed after strength training seems to maximally stimulate muscle protein synthesis.[39,45] Consumption of protein in excess of the amount that can be incorporated into muscle tissue protein seems to provide no additional benefit and may lead to irreversible oxidation.[39]

Timing of Intake. The increase in muscle protein synthesis resulting from a resistance-training workout lasts approximately 24 to 48 hours. This suggests that consuming a high-quality protein at any time in this window should enhance muscle deposition. However, earlier feeding may provide the most benefit, as this is when muscle protein synthesis is most active. Studies have evaluated whey protein consumption at various times around an acute exercise bout. One study noted no difference in muscle protein synthesis when whey protein was consumed before and immediately after exercise.[48] Another study evaluating muscle protein synthesis when whey protein was consumed 1 hour and 3 hours after exercise also showed no difference.[49] These studies suggest that a wide window exists during which protein consumption provides optimal benefit following exercise. However, other research suggests that with chronic training, consuming protein immediately after exercise provides the most benefit in muscle fiber hypertrophy and lean mass.[46,50]

Carbohydrate Intake. Carbohydrate intake stimulates the release of insulin from the pancreas. Insulin is a hormone that triggers transfer of glucose from the bloodstream into the cells. It also is a known regulator of protein metabolism that enhances the uptake of amino acids into muscle tissue and stimulates muscle protein synthesis. Carbohydrate intake after exercise should be accompanied with protein. Otherwise, insufficient amino acids may be available to build muscle mass and adequately counterbalance the exercise-induced muscle protein breakdown.[45]

Supplements. Many strength athletes may rely on or experiment with a variety of supplements that claim to build muscle strength and bulk. While some may function as claimed, supplements are poorly regulated and are not without risk. Supplements are discussed in detail in Chapter 10.

SPEED BUMP

5. **Describe the important nutrition variables in influencing sports performance for strength athletes.**
6. **Outline an ideal nutrition program for optimal performance for competitive strength athletes.**

POWER SPORTS

Power is a measure of force (strength) and speed. Athletes engaged in power sports must provide a maximal amount of effort in a short period of time. Power events typically last from 1 minute to 10 minutes and require a high level of both strength and endurance. Individual sports that rely heavily on power include sprinting, middle-distance running, track cycling, rowing, canoeing/kayaking, and swimming. Power is also a major component of most team sports, which are highlighted in Box 9-4.

The Biochemistry Reviewed

Athletes who engage in power sports rely heavily on the continuum of energy systems from the creatine phosphagen system and anaerobic glycolysis to aerobic glycolysis and fatty acid oxidation. While all systems are working together at all times, the energy system that predominates depends upon the duration of exercise. At the onset of intense exercise, the muscles rely on immediate energy from the phosphagen and anaerobic systems. After the first 1 to 2 minutes of intense exercise, the aerobic system predominates,[51] though the anaerobic systems continue to be active. A summary of 30 studies with data derived from both trained and untrained individuals participating in swimming, running, benching, or cycling ergometry found that for exhaustive exercise of 0 to 15 seconds the anaerobic systems contributed 88% of energy and the aerobic systems contributed 12%; at 0 to 60 seconds the percentages were anaerobic 55% and aerobic 45%; and at 0 to 240 seconds the percentages were anaerobic 21% and aerobic 79%.[51]

During the intense anaerobic phase of exercise (the first 1 to 2 minutes of exercise), the anaerobic type II muscle fibers are highly active. This high level of anaerobic activity leads to production of the acids lactate and hydrogen ion (H+). **Carnosine**, a dipeptide found in high concentrations in skeletal muscle, especially type II muscle fibers, helps to buffer the acids and slow the decline in muscle pH. **Sodium bicarbonate**, a compound found naturally in blood and taken endogenously by some athletes as a supplement, helps to reduce muscle acidity by increasing the release of hydrogen ions from muscle cells. Sodium bicarbonate binds hydrogen ions to form **carbonic acid**, which subsequently dissociates to form carbon dioxide and water. Once the production of acid overcomes the muscle cell's capability to maintain pH (lactate threshold), the increased muscle acidity limits the repletion of phosphagen, inhibits glycolysis, decreases muscle contractility, and ultimately contributes to fatigue and cessation or greatly diminished intensity of exercise.[52] Sodium bicarbonate as a dietary supplement is described in more detail in Chapter 10.

Nutritional Highlights

Power athletes rely heavily on each of the energy systems to work at full capacity to fuel optimal performance. The nutritional regimen for these athletes must ensure high capacity of each of the energy systems, high energy availability, and quick recovery.

Periodized Nutrition to Maximize Capacity of the Energy Systems

Because they require optimum output from each of the energy systems, power athletes typically follow a

Box 9-4. Nutrition Considerations for Team Sports

Team sports are typically divided into field or court sports. Field sports are further divided into strength and power sports (football, rugby); endurance sports (soccer, field hockey, lacrosse); and batting sports (baseball, softball, cricket). Court sports include sports such as basketball, volleyball, tennis, racketball, and squash.

Team sport athletes have special nutritional needs due to the bursts of high-intensity play followed by periods of decreased activity or rest. This type of play relies heavily on both the aerobic energy systems (in which carbohydrate and fat are primary fuels) and anaerobic systems, including phosphagen system and anaerobic glycolysis (in which creatine and glucose are primary fuels). Each sport is different with varying emphasis on endurance, power, and strength, even among different positions in the same sport. Athletes should focus their nutritional approach on the type of fitness that is most essential for their particular sport and position.

Even then, nutritional needs vary based on the period of training and competition. Most team sport coaches typically plan three macrocycles per year for their teams: preseason training, competition, and off-season or transition phase. The length of each macrocycle can vary considerably by sport. For example, soccer players often have a 3-week preseason, whereas rugby players have a 4- to 5-month preseason. Energy and nutritional needs change with the different macrocycles—an athlete in preseason training engaging in two-a-day practices and intensive conditioning has greatly increased needs compared to the off-season and even the competition season. An athlete has increased energy and carbohydrate needs during match days compared to training days; however, many athletes eat less on match days due to stress, travel, or the competition schedule. Athletes who compete once per week, such as college football players, may have adequate time to recover, whereas athletes who may have multiple matches in one day, such as a high school basketball tournament, may have very little time to recover between each game.

While many of the nutritional guiding principles for individual athletes engaging in endurance, power, and strength sports apply to team sports, several nutritional considerations apply for health professionals working with sports teams. Health professionals may advise that:

- Athletes take advantage of half-time and pauses in the game to eat and drink high carbohydrate snacks and beverages to aid optimal performance.
- Nutritional recovery starts in the locker room after a competition with carbohydrate-rich snacks, bars, and gels. Including protein will help aid muscle tissue repair.
- Athletes apply general nutritional recommendations provided for the team in a way that best fits the nutritional needs for that individual athlete. Nutritional planning and recommendations are generally applied to many players who must work together for success and in the context of a multidisciplinary coaching and medical staff. Health professionals should be sensitive to their role on the team and how their nutritional recommendations may affect a diversity of people. For example, health professionals who provide nutritional coaching or information to teams should be aware if any team members have food intolerances or allergies or disordered eating or body image concerns.
- Individual athletes may consider seeking out a sports dietitian to help develop an individualized plan to achieve optimal performance in the athlete's particular position.

Source: Holway FE, Spriet LL. Sport-specific nutrition: practical strategies for team sports. *J Sports Sci.* 2011;29 Suppl 1:S115-125.

periodized training program in which athletes follow a pre-planned intensity and volume of exercise (typically including endurance exercise, high-intensity anaerobic training, and strength training) that varies and corresponds to training goals. A **periodized nutrition program**, in which calorie and macronutrient intakes vary based on the training regimen, ensures optimal fuel availability to support the athlete's specific training and competition demands. Energy and nutrient needs are highest during peak training, somewhat decreased during taper and competition, and much lower during the transition and rest phase.

Energy Availability

As for all athletes, sufficient caloric intake to fuel exercise is essential. Many power athletes engage in exceedingly intense training programs requiring high levels of caloric intake. For example, practice for an elite swimmer can last 3 hours and cover 10,000 meters. Studies suggest that caloric needs for these swimmers can range from 3,000 to 6,800 calories per day for males and 1,500 to 3,300 calories per day for females.[53] During intensive training, the typical male power athlete requires about 55 kcal/kg body weight and 40 kcal/kg body weight for females.[3] These caloric needs are considerably less during the tapering, competition, and transition phases of training.

Carbohydrate Intake. Power athletes engaging in high intensity training regimens rely heavily on carbohydrate intake to fuel performance. The typical power athlete tends to consume from 5 to 9 g/kg of carbohydrates (the lower end for females and higher end for males).[3] Insufficient carbohydrate intake, and subsequently lower concentration of muscle glycogen stores, is associated with decreased immune function, increased rates of burnout, and decreased performance.[54] For this reason, power athletes are advised to consume about 6 to 12 g/kg of carbohydrates per day and at least 30 to 60 grams of carbohydrates per hour (more for activities lasting longer than 2 hours) during intensive training. The carbohydrates help to provide energy to fuel exercise as well as reduce cognitive fatigue for those athletes engaging in technical skills such as soccer players focused on dribbling, agility, heading, and shooting.[55] While it may be difficult to consume this high amount of carbohydrates during training for some athletes, several studies have found that carbohydrate mouth washing for about 12 seconds every 7 to 10 minutes can improve performance.[54,56,57]

Protein Recommendations. Most protein recommendations refer to endurance athletes or strength athletes, without specific mention of power athletes. Endurance athletes should consume 1.2 to 1.4 g/kg of protein per day and strength athletes from 1.2 to 1.7 g/kg of protein per day. The needs of most power athletes likely fall within the midpoint of these recommendations. Protein consumption in excess of 1.7 g/kg contributes to increased protein oxidation and adipose tissue deposition.

Fat. Fat also plays an important role in fueling exercise performance for power athletes, mostly due to the intramuscular triglyceride stores, which provide nearly as much energy as stored muscle glycogen. During prolonged endurance training in which fatty acid oxidation is a major fuel source, the body relies on the stored intramuscular triglyceride as a main source of energy.

Putting all of the fueling recommendations into play during practice and training may be logistically challenging for some athletes, especially those who will engage in several meets or competitions in a single day. Box 9-5 offers practical strategies to help power athletes optimize their fueling strategy.

Recovery

The major goals of nutritional recovery for power athletes include glycogen and creatine resynthesis (which generally occurs rapidly—within 30 seconds to 1 minute) and protein repair and synthesis. Consumption of a carbohydrate-rich snack of about 1 to 1.5 g/kg body weight within 30 minutes following exercise then every 2 hours for 4 to 6 hours helps to optimize glycogen resynthesis. Inclusion of protein of about 0.3 g/kg will help to enhance muscle protein synthesis.

Box 9-5. Power Athletes and Fueling for Competition

World-class swimmer Michael Phelps won eight gold medals in the 2008 Beijing Olympics. He competed 20 times over 9 consecutive days; 5 of those days included three races each. Athletes faced with repeated intense physical challenges can optimize performance with strategic fueling and refueling. Sports nutrition experts Stellingwerff, Maughan, and Burke recommend the following approach.[54]

Before Competition	1 to 2 hours before: Consume 400 to 600 ml (13 to 20 ounces) of sports drink and/or water with electrolytes.	1 to 6 hours before: Trial several pre-competition meal and snack options that are convenient, available, and well tolerated. They should be high in carbohydrates (1 to 4 g/kg), and low in protein and fat.
After Exercise	Eat carbohydrate-rich foods of medium to high glycemic index to provide 1 to 1.5 g of carbohydrates per kilogram of body weight in the first 4 hours after competition.	
In General	Choose foods and portion sizes that are appropriate to nutritional needs. Avoid becoming overwhelmed or influenced by peers during team meals or large buffets.	When traveling, plan ahead to have ready access to well-tolerated meals and snacks. Pack favorite snacks and beverages to bring along.

Body Composition Considerations

Ideal body composition for optimal performance varies among sports, even among those sports that focus primarily on maximal power. For example, the ideal body type for a 2,000-meter rower is tall, strong, and heavier compared with a 1,500-meter runner who benefits most from a lean and svelte body composition. Some of the difference can be accounted for by whether or not the athlete has to support his or her own weight. For example, rowers and track cyclers are weight-supported, so absolute power output is most important. On the other hand, runners and swimmers need to generate enough force to support their weight and gain optimal speed. In these cases, a leaner body composition with high relative power output is ideal.

Most male elite power athletes have a body fat content of 5% to 10% and elite female athletes have a body fat content of 8% to 15%. Swimmers tend to have 4% to 8% higher body fat than endurance-matched runners.[58] These standards apply to body composition during the competitive season, but similar to physical fitness and nutrition, body composition also should vary depending on the stage of training. Research is ongoing to best elucidate what fluctuation is ideal. It seems that changes of about 3% to 5% of body weight with the leanest weight at competition season and a slightly higher and healthier weight the majority of the year is ideal.[54] Some athletes may be concerned that they will lose muscle mass as they lose weight in preparation for the competitive season. Research supports that trained athletes could lose weight and maintain a high level of muscle mass.[59] The necessary ingredients include a negative energy balance, intensive strength training, and an increased daily protein intake in the 3 to 6 weeks prior to the competitive season.[59,60]

Together, the three prongs of fitness, nutrition, and body composition set the stage for peak performance. This chapter's Communication Strategies feature offers an exercise to help health professionals help empower athletes to put the nutritional principles into practice by emphasizing the principles of adult learning in health education.

SPEED BUMP

7. Describe the important nutrition variables in influencing sports performance for power athletes.

8. Outline an ideal nutrition program for optimal performance in endurance sports.

COMMUNICATION STRATEGIES

Health Education for Adult Learners

You have been asked to lead a 20-minute educational session on eating for optimal athletic performance with your local university's female club rowing team. You feel strongly that strategic nutrition choices set the stage for optimal performance. You would like to develop a meaningful educational session for the athletes that they will remember. Rather than preparing a didactic lecture, you decide to put together a participatory workshop, keeping in mind the following principles of adult learning theory:

- New learning is built from previous knowledge and previous learning.
- Adult learners learn best when they play an engaged and participatory role in learning.
- Adult learners need information that is highly relevant and practical.
- Adult learners must perceive value to the information being shared.[73]

Use the following list to help develop your educational session.

1. What do you think are the three to four most important nutritional principles to share with the athletes?
2. How would you like to organize your session? A few ideas include a food demonstration, grocery store tour, discussion of a 1-day sample meal plan, question and answer, a case study, or other.
3. Develop an outline. Include supplies or props you may need.
4. Develop a half-page "take-away" document highlighting the tips you would like the athletes to remember.

CHAPTER SUMMARY

While all athletes require strategic fueling and refueling for optimal health and performance, strength, endurance, and power athletes each have unique nutritional needs.

KEY POINTS SUMMARY

1. Compared to the general population, athletes have special nutritional needs including increased caloric requirements, greater amounts of protein, and more carbohydrates.
2. The aerobic energy systems predominate during endurance exercise. These systems have a nearly unlimited capacity to generate ATP; however, the speed at which ATP is generated (aerobic power) is slower than for the anaerobic systems.
3. Fatigue during endurance exercise typically results from depletion of muscle glycogen and reduced blood glucose concentrations. To avoid extreme fatigue and optimize performance, the major nutritional principles for endurance athletes aim to optimize muscle and liver glycogen stores and enhance the efficiency in which glucose and fatty acids are converted to fuel.
4. The increase in muscle glycogen stores resulting from the practice of carbohydrate loading contributes to a 2% to 3% improved performance in events lasting longer than 90 minutes; however, it does not seem to provide any benefit for shorter duration activities.
5. Strength sports require production of maximal force for optimal performance. These sports include weight lifting, throwing events, and bodybuilding.
6. Nutrition plays an important role in primarily three domains for strength athletes: (1) fueling sport and resistance training; (2) optimizing recovery from training; and (3) promoting muscular hypertrophy.
7. The protein needs for strength athletes are higher than for endurance athletes as the body relies on amino acids (especially branched chain amino acids) to support muscle growth.
8. Nutritional factors important for attaining muscle hypertrophy include: protein source, protein quantity, timing of intake, carbohydrate intake, and supplementation, if any and when appropriate.
9. At the onset of intense exercise, the muscles rely on immediate energy from the phosphagen and anaerobic systems. After the first few minutes of intense exercise, the aerobic system predominates. As exercise becomes increasingly intense and the aerobic system approaches maximal capacity for oxygen consumption, the muscles rely on the anaerobic system to drive further increases in exercise intensity.
10. A periodized nutrition program, in which calorie and macronutrient intakes vary based on the training regimen, ensures optimal fuel availability to support the athlete's specific training and competition demands. Energy and nutrient needs are highest during peak training, somewhat decreased during taper and competition, and much lower during the transition and rest phase.
11. Insufficient carbohydrate intake, and subsequently lower concentration of muscle glycogen stores, is associated with decreased immune function, increased rates of burnout, and decreased performance. For this reason, power athletes are advised to consume about 6 to 12 g/kg of carbohydrate per day and at least 30 to 60 grams of carbohydrates per hour (more for activities lasting longer than 2 hours) during intensive training.
12. The major goals of nutritional recovery for power athletes include glycogen and creatine resynthesis (which generally occur rapidly—within 30 seconds to 1 minute) and protein repair and synthesis.

PRACTICAL APPLICATIONS

1. For which of the following nutrients do athletes typically have an increased requirement, when compared to the general population?
   a. Vitamins
   b. Minerals
   c. Carbohydrates
   d. Fat

2. When glycogen in muscles is depleted, it is difficult to maintain the high initial workload unless the blood glucose concentration is elevated by carbohydrate consumption. Athletes call this condition:
   a. The training effect
   b. The second wind
   c. Hitting the wall
   d. Hypoglycemia

3. It is a good idea, especially for adult women athletes, to have blood hemoglobin regularly checked to detect for a possible deficiency of what mineral?
   a. Calcium
   b. Potassium
   c. Copper
   d. Iron

4. Which of the following statements best describes the reason that carbohydrate loading days before a competition leads to weight gain in athletes?
   a. Glucose requires water to be stored as glycogen.
   b. Sodium is often found in high-carbohydrate foods, which leads to bloating.
   c. Extra carbohydrate-calorie consumption results in increased body fat.

d. Energy from carbohydrates is stored more readily as fat compared to other nutrients.

5. Which of the following statements is true regarding carbohydrate consumption and endurance athletes?
   a. A majority of athletes that have been studied experience hyperinsulinemia and rebound hypoglycemia at some point during competition.
   b. Athletes who experience the physiological symptoms of rebound hypoglycemia most often see a decrease in athletic performance.
   c. Consuming carbohydrates 1 hour prior to exercise provides more benefit to athletic performance than the potential harm of rebound hypoglycemia.
   d. Endurance athletes should avoid carbohydrate consumption in the hour prior to exercise due to the risk of rebound hypoglycemia.

6. How many additional calories per day will a strength athlete need to eat in order to gain one pound of lean muscle mass per week?
   a. 200 to 300 calories/day
   b. 300 to 500 calories/day
   c. 400 to 600 calories/day
   d. 500 to 700 calories/day

7. Which of the following statements is true regarding protein consumption and strength athletes?
   a. Strength athletes are advised to consume approximately 1.8 to 2.2 grams of protein per kilogram body weight per day.
   b. Consumption of protein beyond recommendations provides a slight additional strength benefit to athletes who lift maximum loads.
   c. Protein needs are typically increased with consistent resistance training due to increased efficiency of protein utilization.
   d. Consumption of excess protein may result in excess caloric intake, which is stored as body fat.

8. An ergogenic aid that is sometimes used by athletes in order to control lactate buildup in muscle is ______________.
   a. caffeine
   b. sodium bicarbonate
   c. anabolic steroid
   d. growth hormone

9. During which phase of a periodized nutrition program are an athlete's energy and nutrient needs the highest?
   a. Peak training
   b. Taper
   c. Competition
   d. Transition

10. Which of the following statements represents part of the major goals of nutritional recovery for power athletes?
   a. Protein repair and synthesis
   b. Antioxidant regeneration
   c. Hemoglobin production
   d. Glycogen repair and synthesis

Case 1 Scott, the Professional Triathlete

Scott is a 29-year-old professional triathlete. Scott is nearing the peak of his training for the Ironman triathlon, which is about 2 months away. Scott weighs 170 lbs, or 77 kg.

Refer to Box 9-3, which highlights a 4,500-calorie nutrient plan for a triathlete. Assume that the triathlete in the box is Scott.

1. **Planning for Optimal Performance**
   a. What is the most important consideration for endurance athletes striving for optimal athletic performance? Explain why.
   b. Scott is training for an Ironman triathlon that is far from his home. He plans to fly to the location 3 days prior to the race. What type of food should he bring with him? What advice would you offer him on choosing meals and snacks while traveling?
2. **Analyzing Intakes** (based on Box 9-3)
   a. How many grams of carbohydrates did Scott consume per hour of training? Does this amount fit within the recommendation for optimal performance for a prolonged endurance workout?
   b. What is the total fluid intake Scott consumed during training? How could you determine if this is an appropriate intake for Scott?
3. **Making Modifications**
   Use the USDA National Nutrient Database (http://ndb.nal.usda.gov/) or the USDA's Food Tracker (supertracker.usda.gov) for reference for parts a and b.
   a. List five drink/snack combinations that would provide Scott with close to the recommended 80 grams of carbohydrates per hour of training when engaging in prolonged exercise lasting longer than 2.5 hours. Be sure that the drink/snack choices are easy to consume during activity and that they will have a low likelihood of causing gastrointestinal distress.

b. Scott ate a peanut butter sandwich and drank 8 ounces of low-fat milk immediately following his workout. Does this snack provide the recommended amount of carbohydrate and protein for optimal recovery for the first hour after training for endurance athletes (include the recommended amounts in the answer)? If not, provide an example of a food Scott could add to meet requirements. Provide at least three options of other post-exercise meals or snacks that include the recommended intakes.

Case 2 Eric, the Recreational Bodybuilder

Eric is a 31-year-old competitive bodybuilder. He participates in bodybuilding competitions in the fall and trains the rest of the year.

4. **Identifying Needs**
   a. What are the major nutritional needs and considerations of bodybuilders?
   b. List several other sports that have similar nutritional considerations as bodybuilders. Explain how they are the same. Explain how they are different.
5. **Selecting Meals and Snacks**
   a. Eric asks you for ideas of snacks that would help him to meet his post-exercise nutritional needs. What ideas might you offer?
   b. Eric shares that he gets most of his protein from eating protein bars and shakes. He asks if you have a list of wholesome "real food" protein options. Provide a list of at least 10 high-protein foods, including the protein content and calories for a standard serving size (include the serving size used in your answer). Use the USDA National Nutrient Database (http://ndb.nal.usda.gov/) or the USDA's Food Tracker (supertracker.usda.gov) for nutrient information.

TRAIN YOURSELF: ACHIEVING GOALS

1. State a fitness goal. Use a SMART approach to goal setting (Specific, Measurable, Attainable, Relevant, Time-Bound). For example, I will run 30 seconds per mile faster in my next half-marathon which is in 2 months from now. I will work to achieve this goal by incorporating sprint training into my training 2 days per week.
2. Describe at least two specific changes you could make to improve your sport- or fitness-related nutrition to achieve those goals.
3. Implement the nutritional changes. Comment here on your experiences with implementing the changes and whether you believe they have helped or will help to achieve your first goal.

REFERENCES

1. Rodriguez NR, Di Marco NM, Langley S. American College of Sports Medicine position stand. Nutrition and athletic performance. *Med Sci Sports Exerc.* March 2009;41(3):709-731.
2. Iglesias-Gutierrez E, Garcia A, Garcia-Zapico P, Perez-Landaluce J, Patterson AM, Garcia-Roves PM. Is there a relationship between the playing position of soccer players and their food and macronutrient intake? *Appl Physiol Nutr Metab.* April 2012;37(2):225-232.
3. Burke LM, Cox GR, Culmmings NK, Desbrow B. Guidelines for daily carbohydrate intake: do athletes achieve them? *Sports Med.* 2001;31(4):267-299.
4. Hawley JA, Dennis SC, Lindsay FH, Noakes TD. Nutritional practices of athletes: are they sub-optimal? *J Sports Sci.* Summer 1995;13 Spec No:S75-81.
5. Hoogenboom BJ, Morris J, Morris C, Schaefer K. Nutritional knowledge and eating behaviors of female, collegiate swimmers. *N Am J Sports Phys Ther.* August 2009;4(3):139-148.
6. Drenowatz C, Eisenmann JC, Carlson JJ, Pfeiffer KA, Pivarnik JM. Energy expenditure and dietary intake during high-volume and low-volume training periods among male endurance athletes. *Appl Physiol Nutr Metab.* April 2012; 37(2):199-205.
7. Schroder S, Fischer A, Vock C, et al. Nutrition concepts for elite distance runners based on macronutrient and energy expenditure. *J Athl Train.* September-October 2008;43(5): 489-504.
8. Black KE, Skidmore PM, Brown RC. Energy intakes of ultra-endurance cyclists during competition, an observational study. *Int J Sport Nutr Exerc Metab.* February 2012;22(1):19-23.
9. Cox GR, Clark SA, Cox AJ, et al. Daily training with high carbohydrate availability increases exogenous carbohydrate oxidation during endurance cycling. *J Appl Physiol.* July 2010;109(1):126-134.
10. Hawley JA, Schabort EJ, Noakes TD, Dennis SC. Carbohydrate-loading and exercise performance. An update. *Sports Med.* August 1997;24(2):73-81.
11. Hargreaves M, Hawley JA, Jeukendrup A. Pre-exercise carbohydrate and fat ingestion: effects on metabolism and performance. *J Sports Sci.* January 2004;22(1):31-38.
12. Jeukendrup AE, Killer SC. The myths surrounding pre-exercise carbohydrate feeding. *Ann Nutr Metab.* 2010;57 Suppl 2:18-25.
13. Jeukendrup AE, Chambers ES. Oral carbohydrate sensing and exercise performance. *Curr Opin Clin Nutr Metab Care.* July 2010;13(4):447-451.
14. Rollo I, Williams C. Effect of mouth-rinsing carbohydrate solutions on endurance performance. *Sports Med.* June 1 2011;41(6):449-461.
15. Smith JW, Zachwieja JJ, Peronnet F, et al. Fuel selection and cycling endurance performance with ingestion of [13C]glucose: evidence for a carbohydrate dose response. *J Appl Physiol.* June 2010;108(6):1520-1529.
16. Wagenmakers AJ, Brouns F, Saris WH, Halliday D. Oxidation rates of orally ingested carbohydrates during prolonged exercise in men. *J Appl Physiol.* December 1993;75(6):2774-2780.

17. Jeukendrup AE. Nutrition for endurance sports: marathon, triathlon, and road cycling. *J Sports Sci.* 2011;29 Suppl 1: S91-99.
18. Pfeiffer B, Stellingwerff T, Hodgson AB, et al. Nutritional intake and gastrointestinal problems during competitive endurance events. *Med Sci Sports Exerc.* February 2012; 44(2):344-351.
19. Rehrer NJ, Brouns F, Beckers EJ, et al. Physiological changes and gastro-intestinal symptoms as a result of ultra-endurance running. *Eur J Appl Physiol Occup Physiol.* 1992; 64(1):1-8.
20. Lukaski HC. Vitamin and mineral status: effects on physical performance. *Nutrition.* July-August 2004;20(7-8):632-644.
21. Currell K, Jeukendrup AE. Superior endurance performance with ingestion of multiple transportable carbohydrates. *Med Sci Sports Exerc.* February 2008;40(2):275-281.
22. Donaldson CM, Perry TL, Rose MC. Glycemic index and endurance performance. *Int J Sport Nutr Exerc Metab.* 2010; 20(2):154-165.
23. Sawka MN, Burke LM, Eichner ER, et al. American College of Sports Medicine position stand. Exercise and fluid replacement. *Med Sci Sports Exerc.* February 2007;39(2):377-390.
24. van Rosendal SP, Osborne MA, Fassett RG, Coombes JS. Guidelines for glycerol use in hyperhydration and rehydration associated with exercise. *Sports Med.* February 1 2010; 40(2):113-129.
25. Almond CS, Shin AY, Fortescue EB, et al. Hyponatremia among runners in the Boston Marathon. *New Engl J Med.* 2005;352(12):1550-1556.
26. Brownlie Tt, Utermohlen V, Hinton PS, Haas JD. Tissue iron deficiency without anemia impairs adaptation in endurance capacity after aerobic training in previously untrained women. *Am J Clin Nutr.* March 2004;79(3):437-443.
27. Watson TA, MacDonald-Wicks LK, Garg ML. Oxidative stress and antioxidants in athletes undertaking regular exercise training. *Int J Sport Nutr Exerc Metab.* April 2005;15(2):131-146.
28. Teixeira VH, Valente HF, Casal SI, et al. Antioxidants do not prevent postexercise peroxidation and may delay muscle recovery. *Med Sci Sports Exerc.* September 2009; 41(9):1752-1760.
29. Gleeson M, Nieman DC, Pedersen BK. Exercise, nutrition and immune function. *J Sports Sci.* January 2004;22(1):115-125.
30. Cox GR, Desbrow B, Montgomery PG, et al. Effect of different protocols of caffeine intake on metabolism and endurance performance. *J Appl Physiol.* September 2002; 93(3):990-999.
31. Howarth KR, Moreau NA, Phillips SM, Gibala MJ. Coingestion of protein with carbohydrate during recovery from endurance exercise stimulates skeletal muscle protein synthesis in humans. *J Appl Physiol.* April 2009;106(4):1394-1402.
32. Beelen M, Burke LM, Gibala MJ, van Loon LJ. Nutritional strategies to promote postexercise recovery. *Int J Sport Nutr Exerc Metab.* December 2010;20(6):515-532.
33. Tesch PA, Colliander EB, Kaiser P. Muscle metabolism during intense, heavy-resistance exercise. *Eur J Appl Physiol Occup Physiol.* 1986;55(4):362-366.
34. Hakkinen K. Neuromuscular fatigue and recovery in male and female athletes during heavy resistance exercise. *Int J Sports Med.* February 1993;14(2):53-59.
35. MacDougall JD, Ray S, Sale DG, et al. Muscle substrate utilization and lactate production. *Can J Appl Physiol.* June 1999;24(3):209-215.
36. Slater G, Phillips SM. Nutrition guidelines for strength sports: sprinting, weightlifting, throwing events, and bodybuilding. *J Sports Sci.* 2011;29 Suppl 1:S67-77.
37. Phillips SM, Moore DR, Tang JE. A critical examination of dietary protein requirements, benefits, and excesses in athletes. *Int J Sport Nutr Exerc Metab.* August 2007;17 Suppl:S58-76.
38. Tipton KD, Witard OC. Protein requirements and recommendations for athletes: relevance of ivory tower arguments for practical recommendations. *Clin Sports Med.* January 2007;26(1):17-36.
39. Moore DR, Robinson MJ, Fry JL, et al. Ingested protein dose response of muscle and albumin protein synthesis after resistance exercise in young men. *Am J Clin Nutr.* January 2009;89(1):161-168.
40. Haff GG, Lehmkuhl MJ, McCoy LB, Stone MH. Carbohydrate supplementation and resistance training. *J Strength Cond Res.* February 2003;17(1):187-196.
41. Haff GG, Schroeder CA, Koch AJ, et al. The effects of supplemental carbohydrate ingestion on intermittent isokinetic leg exercise. *J Sports Med Phys Fitness.* June 2001;41(2): 216-222.
42. Koopman R, Manders RJ, Jonkers RA,et al. Intramyocellular lipid and glycogen content are reduced following resistance exercise in untrained healthy males. *Eur J Appl Physiol.* March 2006;96(5):525-534.
43. Pascoe DD, Costill DL, Fink WJ, et al. Glycogen resynthesis in skeletal muscle following resistive exercise. *Med Sci Sports Exerc.* March 1993;25(3):349-354.
44. Jacobs I, Kaiser P, Tesch P. Muscle strength and fatigue after selective glycogen depletion in human skeletal muscle fibers. *Eur J Appl Physiol Occup Physiol.* 1981;46(1):47-53.
45. Burd NA, Tang JE, Moore DR, Phillips SM. Exercise training and protein metabolism: influences of contraction, protein intake, and sex-based differences. *J Appl Physiol.* May 2009;106(5):1692-1701.
46. Hartman JW, Tang JE, Wilkinson SB, et al. Consumption of fat-free fluid milk after resistance exercise promotes greater lean mass accretion than does consumption of soy or carbohydrate in young, novice, male weightlifters. *Am J Clin Nutr.* August 2007;86(2):373-381.
47. Tipton KD, Elliott TA, Cree MG, et al. Ingestion of casein and whey proteins result in muscle anabolism after resistance exercise. *Med Sci Sports Exerc.* Dec 2004;36(12):2073-2081.
48. Tipton KD, Elliott TA, Cree MG, et al. Stimulation of net muscle protein synthesis by whey protein ingestion before and after exercise. *Am J Physiol Endocrinol Metab.* January 2007;292(1):E71-76.
49. Rasmussen BB, Phillips SM. Contractile and nutritional regulation of human muscle growth. *Exerc Sport Sci Rev.* July 2003;31(3):127-131.
50. Esmarck B, Andersen JL, Olsen S, et al. Timing of postexercise protein intake is important for muscle hypertrophy with resistance training in elderly humans. *J Physiol.* August 15 2001;535(Pt 1):301-311.
51. Gastin PB. Energy system interaction and relative contribution during maximal exercise. *Sports Med.* 2001;31(10): 725-741.
52. Hultman E, Sahlin K. Acid-base balance during exercise. *Exerc Sport Sci Rev.* 1980;8:41-128.
53. Van Handel PJ, Cells KA, Bradley PW, Troup JP. Nutritional status of elite swimmers. *J Swimming Res.* 1984;1:27-31.
54. Stellingwerff T, Maughan RJ, Burke LM. Nutrition for power sports: middle-distance running, track cycling, rowing, canoeing/kayaking, and swimming. *J Sports Sci.* 2011;29 Suppl 1:S79-89.
55. Currell K, Conway S, Jeukendrup AE. Carbohydrate ingestion improves performance of a new reliable test of soccer performance. *Int J Sport Nutr Exerc Metab.* February 2009; 19(1):34-46.
56. Carter JM, Jeukendrup AE, Jones DA. The effect of carbohydrate mouth rinse on 1-h cycle time trial performance. *Med Sci Sports Exerc.* December 2004;36(12):2107-2111.
57. Chambers ES, Bridge MW, Jones DA. Carbohydrate sensing in the human mouth: effects on exercise performance and brain activity. *J Physiol.* April 15 2009;587(Pt 8):1779-1794.
58. Fleck SJ. Body composition of elite American athletes. *Am J Sports Med.* November-December 1983;11(6):398-403.

59. Mettler S, Mitchell N, Tipton KD. Increased protein intake reduces lean body mass loss during weight loss in athletes. *Med Sci Sports Exerc.* February 2010;42(2):326-337.
60. O'Connor H, Olds T, Maughan RJ. Physique and performance for track and field events. *J Sports Sci.* 2007;25 Suppl 1:S49-60.
61. Saltzman E, Roberts SB. The role of energy expenditure in energy regulation: findings from a decade of research. *Nutr Rev.* August 1995;53(8):209-220.
62. Loucks AB. Energy balance and body composition in sports and exercise. *J Sports Sci.* January 2004;22(1):1-14.
63. Joosen AM, Bakker AH, Westerterp KR. Metabolic efficiency and energy expenditure during short-term overfeeding. *Physiol Behav.* August 7 2005;85(5):593-597.
64. Shriver LH, Betts NM, Wollenberg G. Dietary intakes and eating habits of college athletes: are female college athletes following the current sports nutrition standard? *J Am Coll Health.* 2013;61(1):10-16.
65. Deutz RC, Benardot D, Martin DE, Cody MM. Relationship between energy deficits and body composition in elite female gymnasts and runners. *Med Sci Sports Exerc.* March 2000;32(3):659-668.
66. Maughan RJ, Depiesse F, Geyer H. The use of dietary supplements by athletes. *J Sports Sci.* 2007;25 Suppl 1: S103-113.
67. Clarke ND, Campbell IT, Drust B, et al. The ingestion of combined carbohydrates does not alter metabolic responses or performance capacity during soccer-specific exercise in the heat compared to ingestion of a single carbohydrate. *J Sports Sci.* 2012;30(7):699-708.
68. Hulston CJ, Wallis GA, Jeukendrup AE. Exogenous CHO oxidation with glucose plus fructose intake during exercise. *Med Sci Sports Exerc.* February 2009;41(2):357-363.
69. Rowlands DS, Swift M, Ros M, Green JG. Composite versus single transportable carbohydrate solution enhances race and laboratory cycling performance. *Appl Physiol Nutr Metab.* June 2012;37(3):425-436.
70. Jeukendrup AE. Carbohydrate and exercise performance: the role of multiple transportable carbohydrates. *Curr Opin Clin Nutr Metab Care.* July 2010;13(4):452-457.
71. Jentjens RL, Shaw C, Birtles T, et al. Oxidation of combined ingestion of glucose and sucrose during exercise. *Metabolism.* May 2005;54(5):610-618.
72. Holway FE, Spriet LL. Sport-specific nutrition: practical strategies for team sports. *J Sports Sci.* 2011;29 Suppl 1:S115-125.
73. Knowles MS, Swanson RA, Holton EF. *The Adult Learner, Seventh Edition: The definitive classic in adult education and human resource.* Burlington, MA: Elsevier; 2011.

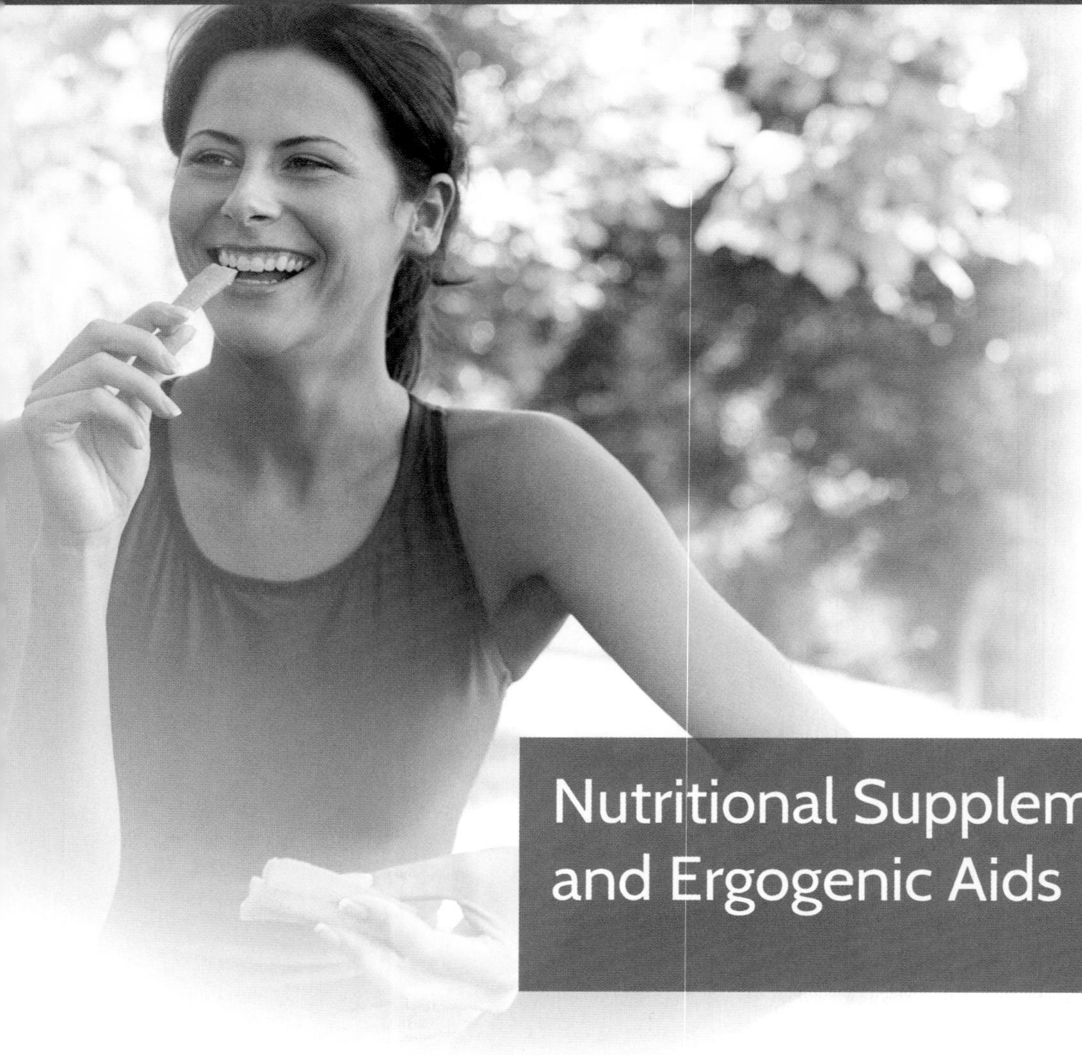

CHAPTER 10

Nutritional Supplements and Ergogenic Aids

CHAPTER OUTLINE

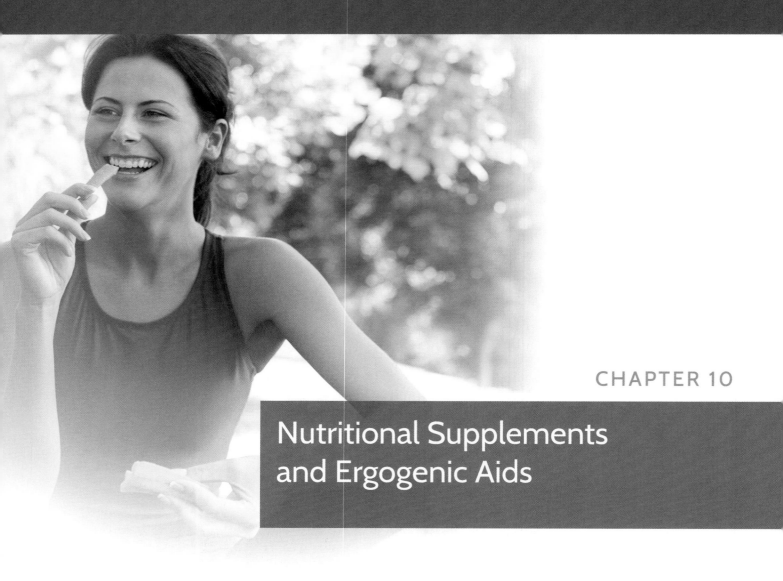

CHAPTER OUTLINE–cont'd

LEARNING OBJECTIVES

After studying this chapter, the reader should be able to:

10.1 Define what substances are considered dietary supplements.

10.2 Explain the limitations of dietary supplement regulation in the United States.

10.3 Describe the product claims, efficacy, and safety of popular, commonly used dietary supplements for weight loss, health, and performance.

10.4 Define the scope of practice for health professionals with regard to the recommendation and sale of dietary supplements.

KEY TERMS

anabolic steroids Synthetic drugs that mimic the effect of testosterone and dihydrotestosterone in the body; cause rapid strength gains but also carry significant toxic effects; expressly prohibited in sports competition.

botanical See *herbal supplements*.

contamination Inadvertent tainting of a supplement with trace amounts of another supplement without the knowledge of the manufacturer or consumer.

Current Good Manufacturing Practices (CGMPs) Regulations that ensure that dietary supplements made in the United States and abroad are consistently produced and of acceptable quality by creating manufacturing standards for all companies that test, produce, package, label, and distribute supplements in the United States.

dietary supplement A product (other than tobacco) that functions to supplement the diet and contains one or more of the following ingredients: a vitamin, mineral, herb or other botanical, amino acid, dietary substance that increases total daily intake, metabolite, constituent, extract, or some combination of the preceding ingredients.

Dietary Supplement and Health Education Act (DSHEA) Federal regulation that oversees supplement production, marketing, and safety; treats supplements more like food than medicine with limited oversight and accountability.

diuretics Medications or substances that lead to increased water loss from the kidneys.

doping The act of ingesting a substance banned by the World Anti-Doping Agency in an effort to improve athletic performance.

ergogenic A substance that increases athletic performance.

health claim A statement that suggests that a supplement may help to diagnose, prevent, mitigate, treat, or cure a specific disease.

herbal supplements Plant-derived substances used for medicinal purposes.

hormones Chemicals released by the body that affect other parts of the body; many banned synthetic hormones mimic the muscle-building effects of natural hormones, such as growth hormone, erythropoietin-stimulating hormone, and gonadotropins, which trigger increased testosterone production.

inadvertent doping When an athlete tests positive for a banned substance due to accidental ingestion, often as a result of contamination of an allowed substance.

stimulant A substance that activates the central nervous system and sympathetic nervous system. It increases heart rate and cardiac output, as well as glucose availability, and may suppress appetite.

INTRODUCTION

Eager to improve athletic performance, body composition, and overall health, many people turn to **dietary supplements** to gain an edge. Not infrequently, clients query fitness and other health professionals for information and advice about various products. All of these professionals must be well informed about dietary supplements and prepared to answer or refer these questions.

Anne Marie, a 37-year-old female, had exceeded her fitness goals, but wondered if there was anything she could take to help optimize her performance. Her personal trainer suggested that she might benefit from the supplements Thermadrene, a stimulant-containing ephedrine; Yohimbe, an extract of a tree bark that is thought to increase athletic performance; whey protein, to improve muscle strength; essential fatty acids, which can benefit heart health; and Lean Body Shake, a high-protein meal replacement.

After taking the supplements for about 3 months, Anne Marie collapsed during an early morning workout. She died later that day from a massive brain hemorrhage. The ephedra-containing Thermadrene was thought to be the most likely culprit. The Chinese botanical *ma huang*, also known as ephedra, reduces appetite but is associated with significant life-threatening side effects, including dangerously increased blood pressure, heart attacks, seizure, stroke, and serious psychiatric illness.[1] Anne Marie's pre-existing hypertension combined with physical exertion and ephedra use presumably predisposed her to the massive brain hemorrhage that took her life.[2]

Anne Marie's death resulted in the legal suit *Capati v. Crunch Fitness* in which Anne Marie's personal trainer and fitness center were sued for $320 million. Ultimately, the case was settled before going to trial, with the gym and the trainer liable for $1,750,000.

OVERVIEW OF DIETARY SUPPLEMENTS

From multivitamins and herbal supplements to weight loss pills and muscle boosters, supplements comprise a multibillion dollar industry playing to people's desire to get or stay healthy, lose weight, gain muscle, improve memory, enhance sexual function, and various other wishes. Quality studies to evaluate the effects of supplements are few and only a limited number of supplements have consistent and convincing evidence of safety and efficacy (Table 10-1). Even then, there is no guarantee that a purchased supplement actually contains the ingredients it claims. In fact, one study found that most herbal supplements are of poor quality,

Table 10-1. What Works and What Doesn't

ERGOGENIC ACIDS THAT PERFORM AS CLAIMED	ERGOGENIC ACIDS THAT MAY PERFORM AS CLAIMED, BUT FOR WHICH THERE IS INSUFFICIENT EVIDENCE	ERGOGENIC AIDS THAT DO NOT PERFORM AS CLAIMED		ERGOGENIC AIDS THAT ARE DANGEROUS, BANNED, OR ILLEGAL
Creatine	Glutamine	Some amino acids	Cytochrome C	Androstenedione
Caffeine	Beta hydroxybutyrate	Bee pollen	Dihydroxy-acetone	Dehydroepiandrosterone
Sports drinks, gels, and bars	Colostrum	Branched-chain amino acids	Gamma oryzanol	19-norandrostenedione
Sodium bicarbonate	Ribose	Carnitine	Ginseng	19-norandrostenediol
Some protein and amino acid supplements		Chromium picolinate	Medium-chain triglycerides	Other anabolic, androgenic steroids
		Cordycemps	Pyruvate	Tribulis terestris
		Coenzyme Q10	Oxygenated water	Ephedra
		Conjugated linoleic acid	Vanadium	Strychnine
				Human growth hormone

Source: Rodriguez NR, Di Marco NM, Langley S. American College of Sports Medicine position stand. Nutrition and athletic performance. *Med Sci Sports Exerc.* March 2009;41(3):709-731.

contaminated, and diluted with use of fillers.[51] In the occasional instance when a supplement is efficacious, consumers should purchase and use these products cautiously as, unlike medicines, they are not closely regulated by the Food and Drug Administration (FDA), though they can be just as dangerous when used imprudently.

SUPPLEMENT REGULATION

Supplement regulation has been an ongoing source of controversy and debate. Though 38 million people spend approximately 17 billion dollars per year on supplements, not including vitamins and minerals,[3] the federal government has relatively loose standards to ensure supplement quality and safety. The 1994 **Dietary Supplement and Health Education Act** and the 2007 **Current Good Manufacturing Practices** dictate the government's approach to supplements. Several monitoring systems are in place to help ensure compliance with FDA regulations. However, the regulations are loose and do not ensure supplement safety. While legislation such as the Dietary Supplement Act of 2011 and the Dietary Supplement Labeling Act of 2013 had been proposed to improve the safety of dietary supplements, none has been enacted as of the publication date of this text.

The Dietary Supplement and Health Education Act

The Dietary Supplement and Health Education Act (DSHEA) of 1994 dictates supplement production, marketing, and safety guidelines.

Following are the basic highlights of the DSHEA:[4]

- The Act established that a dietary supplement is defined as "a product (other than tobacco) that functions to supplement the diet and contains one or more of the following ingredients: (A) a vitamin; (B) a mineral; (C) an herb or other botanical; (D) an amino acid; (E) a dietary supplement used by man to supplement the diet by increasing the total dietary intake; or (F) a concentrate, metabolite, constituent, extract, or combination of any ingredient described in clause (A), (B), (C), (D), or (E)."
- Supplements must contain an ingredient label including the name and quantity of each dietary ingredient (Fig. 10-1). The label must also identify the product as a "dietary supplement."
- Safety standards provide that the Secretary of the Department of Health and Human Services may declare that a supplement poses imminent risk or hazard to public safety. A supplement is considered *adulterated*, or unsafe, if it or one of its ingredients presents a "significant or unreasonable risk of illness or injury" when used as directed, or under normal conditions. It may also be considered adulterated if too little information is known about the risk of an unstudied ingredient.
- Retailers are allowed to display third-party materials, such as an article or a chapter in a book, that provide information about the health-related benefits of dietary supplements. The Act stipulates the guidelines the literature must follow, including that it must not be false or misleading and cannot promote a specific supplement brand.
- Supplements cannot make **health claims**—statements that suggest that the supplement may help to diagnose, prevent, mitigate, treat, or cure a specific disease. Instead, they may describe the supplement's effects on the "structure or function" of the body or the "well-being" achieved by consuming the substance. For example, an allowable structure/function claim for a calcium supplement may state that calcium

Dietary supplement of amino acids:

Supplement Facts
Serving Size 1 Tablet

Amount Per Tablet	
Calories	15
Isoleucine (as L-isoleucine hydrochloride)	450 mg*
Leucine (as L-leucine hydrochloride)	620 mg*
Lysine (as L-lysine hydrochloride)	500 mg*
Methionine (as L-methionine hydrochloride)	350 mg*
Cystine (as L-cystine hydrochloride)	200 mg*
Phenylalanine (as L-phenylalanine hydrochloride)	220 mg*
Tyrosine (as L-tyrosine hydrochloride)	900 mg*
Threonine (as L-threonine hydrochloride)	300 mg*
Valine (as L-valine hydrochloride)	650 mg*

*Daily Value not established

Other ingredients: Cellulose, lactose, and magnesium stearate.

What must be included in a supplement label?

General information
- Name of product (including the word "supplement" or a statement that the product is a supplement)
- Amount of contents
- Name and place of business of manufacturer, packer, or distributor
- Directions for use

Supplement Facts panel (see left)
- Serving size, list of dietary ingredients, amount per serving size (by weight), percent Daily Value (%DV), if established
- If the dietary ingredient is a botanical, the scientific name of the plant or the common or usual name
- If the dietary ingredient is a proprietary blend (a blend exclusive to the manufacturer), the total weight of the blend and the components of the blend in order of predominance by weight

Other Ingredients
- Non-dietary ingredients such as fillers, artificial colors, sweeteners, flavors, or binders; listed by weight in descending order of predominance and by common name or proprietary blend

Figure 10-1. The supplement label. *From Office of Dietary Supplements, National Institutes of Health. Dietary supplements. 2011. http://ods.od.nih.gov/factsheets/DietarySupplements/. Accessed April 14, 2013.*

builds strong bones. The manufacturer need only state alongside the claim: *This statement has not been evaluated by the Food and Drug Administration. This product is not intended to diagnose, treat, cure, or prevent any disease.* A calcium supplement could not legally claim to prevent osteoporosis, an illness that may result at least in part due to low-calcium intake[5] (Table 10-2).

In contrast to the approval process for new medicines, which undergo extensive testing for safety and efficacy before the FDA approves their use, supplement manufacturers must simply notify the FDA 75 days before marketing a new product to the public. Manufacturers are asked to include with the notification a statement that the product is thought to be generally safe to the consumer. Beyond that, the FDA does not play a major role in preventing the distribution of fraudulent supplements in the marketplace. It does, however, monitor those supplements that are available to the consumer and investigate those with high suspicion for health or safety threats (see Myths and Misconceptions).

Overall, while the DSHEA was intended to help protect consumers, safety and legitimacy of any supplement cannot be assumed. Box 10-1 offers a strategy to help protect consumers from experiencing harm from supplements.

Current Good Manufacturing Practices

In June 2007, the FDA issued regulations that require Current Good Manufacturing Practices (CGMPs) for dietary supplements. The CGMPs ensure that dietary supplements made in the United States and abroad are consistently produced and of acceptable quality.

Table 10-2. Structure/Function Versus Health Claims[a]

FDA APPROVAL NOT NEEDED (STRUCTURE/FUNCTION CLAIM)	FDA APPROVAL NEEDED (HEALTH CLAIM)
Enhances muscle tone or size	
Improves memory	
Helps maintain normal cholesterol levels	Lowers cholesterol
Provides relief of occasional constipation	Provides relief of chronic constipation
Suppresses appetite to aid weight loss	Suppresses appetite to treat overweight or obesity
Supports the immune system	Supports the body's antiviral abilities
Relief of occasional heartburn or acid indigestion	Helps relieve persistent heartburn or acid indigestion
Relief of occasional sleeplessness	Helps reduce difficulty in falling asleep
Arouses sexual desire	Restores sexual energy, strength, and performance
Maintains healthy lung function	Retains healthy lung function in smokers
Improves strength	
Promotes digestion	
Boosts stamina	
For common symptoms of PMS	
For hot flashes	
Helps you relax	
Relieves stress	
Helps promote urinary tract health	
Maintains intestinal flora	
For hair loss associated with aging	
Prevents wrinkles	
For relief of muscle pain after exercise	
To treat or prevent nighttime leg muscle cramps	

a. www.fda.gov/food/dietarysupplements/guidancecomplianceregulatoryinformation/ucm107336.htm

Myths and Misconceptions

If Science Backs It, It Must Work

The Myth

If scientific research shows that the supplement is effective, then the supplement must be effective.

The Logic

Scientific research helps uncover truths. If research shows that a product works as described, then that is convincing evidence that the product may actually work.

The Science

A body of high-quality scientific research performed on individuals in the same target population as the individual taking the supplement provides convincing evidence whether or not a supplement works as described. Individual studies taken alone are less convincing, and "scientific" studies conducted by product manufacturers are the least credible. For example, a Cochrane review of 48 studies found that industry-sponsored studies were more likely to overstate product efficacy, understate risks, and show less agreement between study results and study conclusions.[34] Before believing the scientific evidence cited as support for a particular supplement, it is important to consider the source.

CGMPs apply to all companies that test, produce, package, label, and distribute supplements in the United States. The CGMPs include regulations related to:

- The design and construction of physical plants that facilitate maintenance
- Cleaning
- Proper manufacturing operations
- Quality control procedures
- Testing final product or incoming and in-process materials
- Handling consumer complaints
- Maintaining records

All companies were required to be in compliance with the CGMPs by mid-year 2010. The benefits to the consumer include assurance that supplements are of acceptable quality and accurately labeled, and of consistent identity, purity, strength, and composition. The CGMPs do not address supplement safety or their effect on health. The goals of the CGMPs are to prevent:

- Imprecise dosages of ingredients
- Wrong ingredients
- Contaminants (e.g., bacteria, pesticide, glass, lead)
- Foreign material in a dietary supplement container
- Improper packaging
- Mislabeling[6]

Monitoring Systems

Several nongovernmental organizations implement monitoring systems to help ensure compliance with FDA regulations. The United States Pharmacopeia (USP) is a nonprofit organization that offers a set of

Box 10-1. Key Points to Ponder[a]

- **Think twice about the latest headline.** Sound health advice is generally based on research over time, not a single study. Be wary of results claiming a quick fix that departs from scientific research and established dietary guidance. Science does not generally proceed by dramatic breakthroughs, but rather by taking many small steps, slowly building toward scientific agreement.
- **Some people may think, *Even if a product may not help me, it at least won't hurt me.* It's best not to assume that this will always be true.** Some product ingredients, including nutrients and plant components, can be toxic based on their activity in the body. Some products may become harmful when consumed in high enough amounts, for a long enough time, or in combination with certain other substances.
- **The term *natural* does not always mean safe.** Use of this term to describe products does not assure wholesomeness or that these products have milder effects, making them safer to use than prescribed drugs. For example, many weight-loss products claim to be *natural* or *herbal*, but this doesn't necessarily make them safe. The products' ingredients may interact with drugs or may be dangerous for people with certain medical conditions.
- **Spend money wisely.** Some supplement products may be expensive and may not work, given an individual's specific condition. Be wary of substituting a product or therapy for prescription medicines. Discuss supplements with your health-care team to determine what is best for your overall health.
- **Safety first.** Resist pressure to decide immediately about trying an untested product or treatment. Ask for more information and consult your doctor, nurse, dietitian, pharmacist, and/or caregiver about whether the product is right for you and safe for you to use.

a. www.fda.gov/Food/DietarySupplements/ConsumerInformation/ucm110493.htm.

guidelines for the quality, purity, strength, manufacturing practices, and ingredients in dietary supplement products. Dietary supplement manufacturers can choose to voluntarily subject their products to USP testing. If the supplement passes the testing, the manufacturer is authorized to display the USP symbol on their labels. ConsumerLab.com also offers supplement testing and a ready source of supplement information for subscribers.

Sports organizations such as Major League Baseball, the National Football League, the National Collegiate Athletic Association, and their players' associations have partnered with companies like the nonprofit NSF International that test and certify dietary supplements. NSF screens supplements for banned substances such as steroids, stimulants, and hormones, and monitors manufacturing facilities for compliance with the U.S. Food and Drug Administration's Good Manufacturing Practices. NSF's certification service includes product testing, good manufacturing practices inspections, and ongoing monitoring. Supplements that pass NSF testing may be eligible for NSF certification, a recognizable seal of approval (more information is available at www.nsf.org).

SPEED BUMP

1. **Define what substances are considered dietary supplements.**
2. **Explain the limitations of dietary supplement regulation in the United States.**

WEIGHT-LOSS SUPPLEMENTS

With millions of Americans on a diet at any given time, weight-loss supplements are top sellers. Manufacturers claim the supplements can aid fat loss, enhance metabolism, suppress appetite, and promote weight loss, sometimes without significant changes to physical activity or dietary intake. Some are considered to be *thermogenic*, meaning "they increase production of heat in the body." The claim is that thermogenic products alter the metabolism in a way that causes the body to use more energy. The claims are largely unsubstantiated and the supplements poorly regulated. Ultimately, the safety and efficacy of weight-loss supplements is largely unknown. Anyone considering using a weight-loss supplement should discuss this first with his or her physician, especially if the person is taking prescription or over-the-counter medications or other supplements. Most weight-loss supplements contain several ingredients, including herbs and botanicals, vitamins, minerals, and sometimes caffeine or laxatives. These chemicals can interact with other medications and supplements, causing harmful consequences.

Table 10-3 highlights the characteristics of some of the most commonly used weight-loss substances, though the list is far from exhaustive. Health professionals should feel confident in sharing this information

Table 10-3. Weight-Loss Supplements[a]

PRODUCT	CLAIM	EFFECTIVENESS	SAFETY
Alli, over-the-counter version of prescription drug orlistat (Xenical)	Decreases fat absorption	Effective though weight loss usually less for OTC versus prescription	FDA investigating reports of liver injury
Bitter Orange	Aids weight loss	Insufficient evidence to confirm health benefit	Similar to ephedra, and insufficient information to say if safer; unsafe for many, including those with hypertension
Conjugated Linoleic Acid (CLA)	Reduces body fat and builds muscle	Possibly effective for weight loss	Possibly safe
Ephedra	Decreases appetite	Possibly effective	Likely unsafe and banned by FDA
Green Tea Extract	Increases calorie and fat metabolism and decreases appetite	Insufficient reliable evidence to rate	Possibly safe
Human Chorionic Gonadotropin (hCG)	"Resets metabolism" and changes "abnormal eating patterns"	No evidence that it increases weight loss more than restricting calories (which manufacturers typically advise in conjunction with pill)	Sold illegally with unsubstantiated claims, target of FDA investigation
Hoodia	Decreases appetite	Insufficient reliable evidence to rate	Insufficient information

a. National Center for Complementary and Alternative Medicine (http://nccam.nih.gov/health/).

with clients but also should direct clients to their primary care physician for further discussion of whether or not it is safe for a client to consume any of these supplements.

HEALTH SUPPLEMENTS

From vitamins and minerals to proteins, essential fatty acids, and various herbs, many supplements claim to improve health. While some may provide health benefits, supplements do not substitute for a healthy diet. Whole foods offer important benefits over dietary supplements such as a being a source of a variety of important nutrients (rather than just one) including health-promoting fiber and phytochemicals, which are naturally occurring protective substances that may help protect against myriad diseases and conditions. It is very unlikely to over- or under-consume important vitamins and minerals with a balanced, healthy diet. Still, in some cases supplements may benefit overall health, while in others they may do harm or contribute to health in some way that is not yet understood. Often, whole foods inspire the development of food-based supplements, such as in the case of the exotic fruit juice supplement industry. Little human research has been done to support or reject industry assertions that these supplements improve health. Some of the most common exotic fruit juice supplements are described in Table 10-4.

Vitamin and Mineral Supplements

Physicians, scientists, dietitians, and other health professionals have long stressed the importance of adequate intake of vitamins and minerals to overall health. To meet or exceed these requirements, many people take daily vitamin and mineral supplements. However, the latest research, which has mostly been done to evaluate whether megadoses of vitamins offer additional benefits, has largely been disappointing.

A study of 161,000 older women enrolled in the Women's Health Initiative found that after 8 years there was no difference in rates of heart disease and cancer in women who took a multivitamin compared to those who did not.[7] A study of 15,000 physicians from the Physician's Health Study found no difference in heart disease in men taking vitamins E and C compared to those taking a placebo.[8] Another study failed to show that vitamin E and selenium supplements change the risk of developing prostate cancer in older men,[9] while other research has shown that megadoses of vitamins may actually be harmful.[10,11] An analysis of randomized-controlled trials (the gold standard in research design) studying the role of antioxidants in disease found that people who take antioxidant supplements, especially vitamin A, beta carotene, and vitamin E, had higher mortality rates, while vitamin C and selenium supplements seemed to provide no benefit or harm.[12]

Some researchers had held out hope that vitamin D supplements might help ward off a variety of health conditions, but so far the research is lacking.[13] In fact, authors of a 2014 review on the topic concluded "vitamin D supplementation with or without calcium does not reduce skeletal or non-skeletal outcomes in unselected community-dwelling individuals by more than 15%. Future trials with similar designs are unlikely to alter these conclusions."[52]

Overall, most studies have shown no significant association between vitamin supplements and improved health, with the exception of folic acid supplementation in pregnant women. A U.S. Preventive Services Task Force review concluded that there is insufficient scientific evidence to recommend vitamins for the prevention of cardiovascular disease or cancer.[53] This and two other studies[54,55] published in Annals of Internal Medicine also showed little benefit from vitamins compelled a group of well-respected researchers to comment in an accompanying editorial: ". . . we believe that the case is closed— supplementing the diet of well-nourished adults with (most) mineral or vitamin supplements has no clear benefit and might even be harmful. These vitamins should not be used for chronic disease prevention. Enough is enough."[56]

Many athletes suffer from iron deficiency due to inadequate intake or excessive iron losses, which can occur with exercise. Iron is necessary for optimal oxygen delivery to working cells. When iron levels fall, aerobic athlete performance falters. Some athletes may require iron supplementation to restore normal levels. This should be discussed with a registered dietitian or a physician.

Ultimately, clients who consume a balanced diet that provides adequate vitamins and minerals to prevent an overt nutritional deficiency probably do not need vitamin or mineral supplementation (Tables 10-5 and 10-6). Clients who suspect that they may suffer from an overt nutritional deficiency should discuss this with a qualified professional to determine whether or not supplementation beyond a multivitamin is advantageous.

Macronutrient Supplements

Some clients may take macronutrient supplements such as soy protein or essential fatty acids in an effort to improve health.

Soy Protein Supplements

Soy isolates, which are 90% protein and contain isoflavones (phytoestrogens that mimic estrogen), are highly digestible and easily added to sports drinks, health beverages, and infant formulas.[14] Early studies suggested that isolated soy protein might lower low-density lipoprotein (LDL) cholesterol and blood pressure, potentially protect against breast cancer, maintain bone density, and decrease menopausal symptoms.[15] Given what seemed to be compelling evidence of benefit, in 1999

Table 10-4. **Supplement-Inspiring Fruits**

FRUIT	ORIGIN	NUTRIENTS	CLAIMS	EVIDENCE FROM HUMAN STUDIES	COST PER 8 OZ
Pomegranate 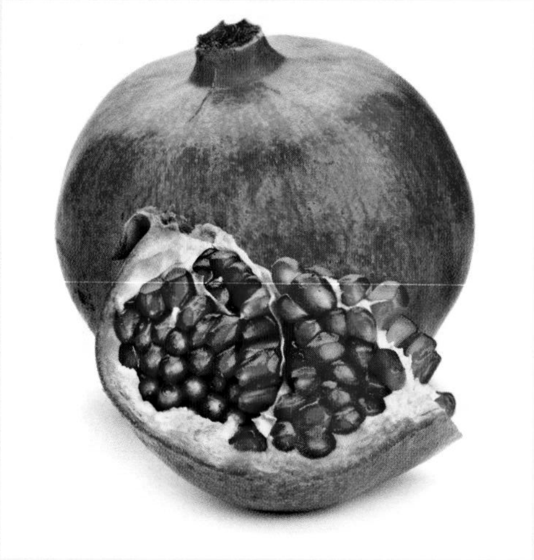	Mediterranean, India, Israel, China, Japan, Russia, Afghanistan, U.S. (CA and AZ)	Highest concentration of antioxidants, specifically ellagitannins and anthocyanins	Decreased risk of cardiovascular disease, decreased periodontal disease, decreased erectile dysfunction	All from small studies: Improved blood flow in men with cardiovascular disease,[38,39] reduced atherosclerosis and blood pressure,[40] improved cholesterol,[41] no effect on erectile dysfunction	$2.50
Acai (ah-SIGH-ee) 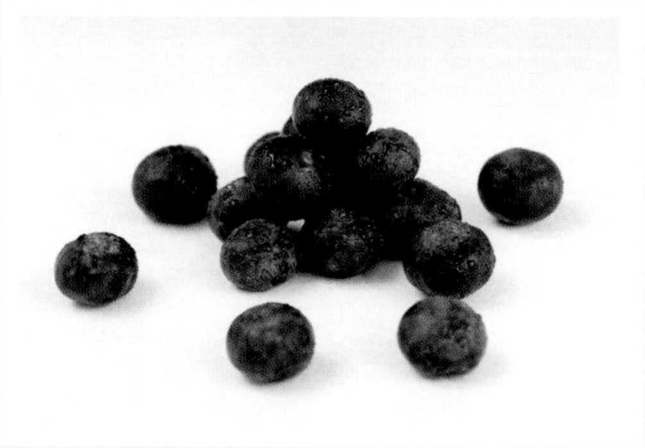	Brazil	Antioxidants, monounsaturated fat, 19 amino acids, dietary fiber, phytosterols, many vitamins and minerals	Removes wrinkles, cleanses body of toxins, quickens weight loss	Two small studies showed increased serum antioxidant capacity following consumption of acai juice[42,43]	$7.50

Goji Berries (Go-jee) 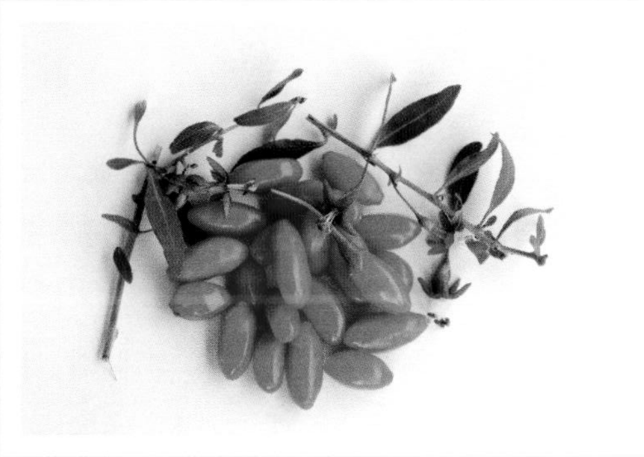	China	Antioxidants beta-carotene and lycopene, 19 amino acids, 21 trace minerals, protein, high vitamin C, vitamin E, essential fatty acids (in seeds)	Varied, including: anti-aging; prevention and treatment of cancer, diabetes, arthritis, and digestive problems; and weight loss	1 small study paid for and conducted by a company that sells goji juice reported increased feelings of well-being, reduced fatigue and stress, and improved regularity of gastrointestinal function after 15 days of 4 oz goji juice daily[44]	$13.30
Mangosteen 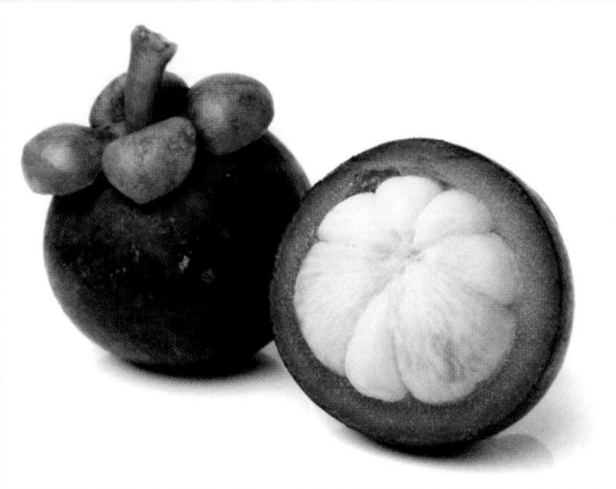	Southeast Asia/India	Xanthone antioxidant, otherwise lacking in vitamin and mineral content	Maintains intestinal health, neutralizes free radicals, supports cartilage and joint function, promotes healthy seasonal respiratory system, and myriad traditional medicinal properties	1 human study in 1932 showed benefit in treating dysentery in Singapore[45]	$35 (25 oz)
Noni (NO-knee) 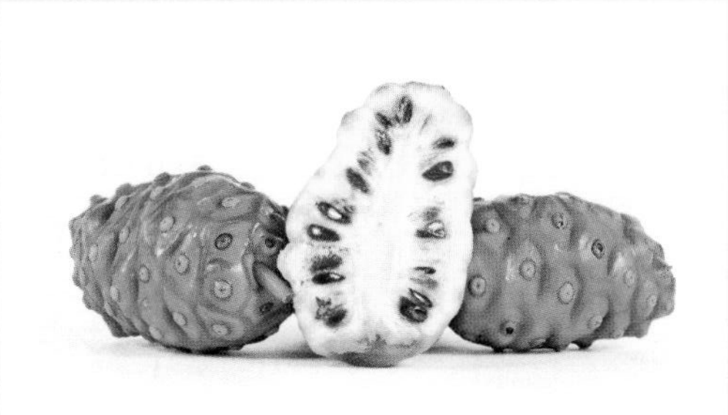	Tropical Asia, Pacific Islands	"Mystery ingredients"; a small amount of vitamins and minerals, moderate antioxidant potency	Boosts immune system, delivers superior antioxidants, increases energy and physical performance, and many users believe it helps to cure cancer	None found	$11.20

Table 10-5. Vitamin Facts

VITAMIN	RDA/AI		BEST SOURCES	FUNCTION
	Men[a]	Women[a]		
A (carotene)	900 µg	700 µg	Yellow or orange fruits and vegetables, green leafy vegetables, fortified oatmeal, liver, dairy products	Formation and maintenance of skin, hair, and mucous membranes; helps people see in dim light; bone and tooth growth
B_1 (thiamine)	1.2 mg	1.1 mg	Fortified cereals and oatmeal, meats, rice and pasta, whole grains, liver	Helps the body release energy from carbohydrates during metabolism; growth and muscle tone
B_2 (riboflavin)	1.3 mg	1.1 mg	Whole grains, green leafy vegetables, organ meats, milk, eggs	Helps the body release energy from protein, fat, and carbohydrates during metabolism
B_6 (pyridoxine)	1.3 mg	1.3 mg	Fish, poultry, lean meats, bananas, prunes, dried beans, whole grains, avocados	Helps build body tissue and aids in metabolism of protein
B_{12} (cobalamin)	2.4 µg	2.4 µg	Meats, milk products, seafood	Aids cell development, functioning of the nervous system, and the metabolism of protein and fat
Biotin	30 µg	30 µg	Cereal/grain products, yeast, legumes, liver	Involved in metabolism of protein, fats, and carbohydrates
Choline	550 mg	425 mg	Milk, liver, eggs, peanuts	A precursor of acetylcholine; essential for liver function
Folate (folacin, folic acid)	400 µg	400 µg[b]	Green leafy vegetables, organ meats, dried peas, beans, lentils	Aids in genetic material development; involved in red blood cell production
Niacin	16 mg	14 mg	Meat, poultry, fish, enriched cereals, peanuts, potatoes, dairy products, eggs	Involved in carbohydrate, protein, and fat metabolism
Pantotheric Acid	5 mg	5 mg	Lean meats, whole grains, legumes	Helps release energy from fats and vegetables
C (ascorbic acid)	90 mg	75 mg	Citrus fruits, berries, and vegetables— especially peppers	Essential for structure of bones, cartilage, muscle, and blood vessels; helps maintain capillaries and gums and aids in absorption of iron
D	5 µg	5 µg	Fortified milk, sunlight, fish, eggs, butter, fortified margarine	Aids in bone and tooth formation; helps maintain heart action and nervous system function
E	15 mg	15 mg	Fortified and multigrain cereals, nuts, wheat germ, vegetable oils, green leafy vegetables	Protects blood cells, body tissue, and essential fatty acids from harmful destruction in the body
K	120 µg	90 µg	Green leafy vegetables, fruit, dairy, grain products	Essential for blood-clotting functions

a. RDAs and AIs given are for men aged 31 to 50 and nonpregnant, nonbreastfeading women aged 31 to 52; mg = milligrams; µg = micrograms.

b. This is the amount women of childbearing age should obtain from supplements or fortified foods.

Source: Reprinted with permission from Dietary Reference Intakes (various volumes). Copyright 1997, 1998, 2000, 2001 by the National Academy of Sciences. Courtesy of the National Academics Press, Washington, DC.

Table 10-6. Mineral Facts

VITAMIN	RDA/AI		BEST SOURCES	FUNCTION
	Men[a]	**Women**[a]		
Calcium	1,000 mg	1,000 mg	Milk and milk products	Strong bones, teeth, muscle tissue; regulates heartbeat, muscle action, and nerve function; blood clotting
Chromium	35 μg	25 μg	Corn oil, clams, whole-grain cereals, brewer's yeast	Glucose metabolism (energy); increases effectiveness of insulin
Copper	900 μg	900 μg	Oysters, nuts, organ meats, legumes	Formation of red blood cells; bone growth and health; works with vitamin C to form elastin
Fluoride	4 mg	3 mg	Fluorinated water, teas, marine fish	Stimulates bone formation; inhibits or even reverses dental caries
Iodine	150 μg	150 μg	Seafood, iodized salt	Component of hormone thyroxine, which controls metabolism
Iron	8 mg	18 mg	Meats, especially organ meats, legumes	Hemoglobin formation; improves blood quality; increases resistance to stress and disease
Magnesium	420 mg	320 mg	Nuts, green vegetables, whole grains	Acid/alkaline balance; important in metabolism of carbohydrates, minerals, and sugar (glucose)
Manganese	2.3 mg	1.8 mg	Nuts, whole grains, vegetables, fruits	Enzyme activation; carbohydrate and fat production; sex hormone production; skeletal development
Molybdenum	45 μg	45 μg	Legumes, grain products, nuts	Functions as a cofactor for a limited number of enzymes in humans
Phosphorus	700 mg	700 mg	Fish, meat, poultry, eggs, grains	Bone development; important in protein, fat, and carbohydrate utilization
Potassium	4700 mg	4700 mg	Lean meat, vegetables, fruits	Fruit balance; controls activity of heart muscle, nervous system, and kidneys
Selenium	55 μg	55 μg	Seafood, organ meats, lean meats, grains	Protects body tissues against oxidative damage from radiation, pollution, and normal metabolic processing
Zinc	11 mg	8 mg	Lean meats, liver, eggs, seafood, whole grains	Involved in digestion and metabolism; important in development of reproductive system; aids in healing

a. RDAs and AIs given are for men aged 31 to 50 and nonpregnant, nonbreastfeeding women aged 31 to 50; mg = milligram; μg = micrograms.

Source: Reprinted with permission from Dietary Reference Intakes (various volumes). Copyright 1997, 1998, 2000, 2001 by the National Academy of Sciences. Courtesy of the National Academics Press, Washington, DC.

the Food and Drug Administration approved labeling for food containing soy protein as protective against heart disease. Shortly thereafter, the American Heart Association (AHA) released a statement concluding that "it is prudent to recommend including soy protein foods in a diet low in saturated fat and cholesterol."[15] Food manufacturers eagerly diversified soy product offerings (including various soy supplements and additives) and grocery stores and consumers readily boosted their soy consumption. However, after a comprehensive review of the scientific studies available at that time, the Nutrition Committee of the American Heart Association released an updated statement in 2006, concluding that "the direct cardiovascular benefit of soy protein or isoflavone supplements is minimal at best."[16] The authors recommended against use of soy protein isolates (with isoflavones) in foods or pills, but did continue to encourage consumption of *whole* soy products such as tofu, soy burgers, and soy nuts, which contain high levels of nonprotein nutrients including heart-healthy polyunsaturated fats, fiber, vitamins, and minerals and low levels of saturated fat.[16]

The scientific research on soy in general and soy protein and isoflavone in particular continues to evolve, with mostly conflicting findings. For example, the 1999 FDA health claim linking soy protein consumption to decreased cardiovascular disease has not been retracted despite the AHA's serious concerns about its validity.

Omega-3 Essential Fatty Acids

Consumer interest in the health benefits of omega-3 essential fatty acids has motivated food manufacturers to add the fatty acids to a variety of foods and to produce omega-3 supplements, which are widely available. A growing body of research and media attention suggests that omega-3 fatty acids offer numerous health benefits including decreased risk of heart disease, improved brain development in fetuses and young children, and reduced disability from mental illnesses such as depression and attention deficit and hyperactivity disorder.[17] Omega-3s reduce blood clotting, dilate blood vessels, and reduce inflammation. Natural food sources include egg yolks and cold water fish like tuna, salmon, mackerel, cod, crab, shrimp, and oysters. Some evidence suggests that people who do not meet this recommendation may benefit from supplementation or from fortified foods.

While there is no established dietary reference intake for the optimal amount of omega-3 intake, some expert panels have recommended an intake between 250 to 500 milligrams per day.[18] This dosage is likely safe and effective to achieve the benefits of omega-3s without increased risk of complications such as bleeding. Clients who are considering fish oil supplementation should talk with their physician and pay close attention to the dosage of omega-3s in the supplement. See Chapter 3 for more detailed information on essential fatty acids.

Herbal Supplements

Herbal supplements, or botanicals, are plant-derived substances used for medicinal purposes. Plants have been used as medicine for thousands of years, long before Westernized medicine evolved. Community healers throughout the world continue to prescribe plant extracts to fend off physical and mental ailments. Meanwhile, a large number of people in Western countries have turned to herbal supplements for a more "natural" way to heal. The two major problems are that (1) herbal supplements have not been as thoroughly studied and evaluated as medications to understand their effects on health, and (2) herbal supplements are not as closely regulated as medications and, as a result, consumers cannot know for certain that the supplement they take is not adulterated, contaminated, or otherwise different from the supplement that they thought they purchased.

The most commonly used herbal supplements that health professionals are likely to encounter include gingko biloba, an herb thought to improve memory; St. John's Wort for depression; echinacea to fight off cold symptoms and improve the immune system; and flaxseed and flaxseed oil, which provide the essential fatty acids (omega-3 and omega-6) to improve cardiovascular health. The characteristics of each of these and other popular herbal supplements are highlighted in Table 10-7. For information on herbal supplements not specifically described here, health professionals (and their clients) should refer to the Office of Dietary Supplements of the National Institutes of Health at http://ods.od.nih.gov/ or the National Center for Complementary Medicine of the National Institutes of Health at http://nccam.nih.gov/.

SUPPLEMENTS FOR ATHLETIC PERFORMANCE

Numerous supplements claim **ergogenic** effects from enhanced cardiovascular endurance to a boost in muscular hypertrophy and strength. These promises of increased athletic performance appeal to athletes from recreational to professional and Olympic contenders who strive to beat their personal records and achieve athletic success.

Banned Substances and Doping

The International Olympic Committee, the British Olympic Association, professional sports organizations, and other organizations have published position statements describing the risks and restrictions of supplement use for athletes. The World Anti-Doping Agency (WADA) code explicitly describes those supplements that are banned from use. Readers are advised to access

Table 10-7. Commonly Used Herbal Supplements[46,47,a]

HERB	SOURCE	CLAIM	EFFECTIVENESS	SAFETY
Arnica	Flowering head of the plant	Anti-inflammatory and antimicrobial activity; used as a remedy for sports injuries and to reduce delayed onset muscle soreness	Topical herbal cream widely used and minimally studied; Homeopathic oral preparation, with unproven effectiveness	Topical herbal cream, safety unknown; homeopathic oral supplement, highly diluted and safe for oral use
Bee Pollen	Pollen granules from stamens of flowers and flower nectar collected by bees	"Super food" that boosts athletic performance	Minimal effect	Generally safe but may cause anaphylaxis in those with bee allergy
Echinacea	Coneflower found in the U.S. and southern Canada	Treatment and prevention of colds, flu, and other infections	May be beneficial in treating upper respiratory infections, but study results are mixed	Usually no side effects if taken by mouth, though some people experience allergic reactions
Flaxseed and Flaxseed Oil	Oil of the flaxseed which is the seed of the flax plant	Laxative effects, arthritis relief, treatment of hot flashes and breast pain, treatment of high cholesterol, cancer prevention	Study results are mixed whether flaxseed claims are accurate; probably does have a laxative effect due to fiber content	Generally well tolerated with few side effects
Ginseng	Chinese herb	Improves cardiorespiratory function, increases aerobic and anaerobic performance, improves mental acuity	Claims have not been substantiated	Easily contaminated, little standardization of ingredients
Gingko Biloba	Eastern Asia Maidenhair tree	Aids memory, improves circulation, prevents altitude sickness	Research ongoing, large study showed no improvement in memory, Alzheimer's disease risk, cognitive function, blood pressure, or hypertension	Side effects include headache, nausea, GI upset, dizziness, and allergic reactions; may increase bleeding risk
Garlic Powder	Herb grown in many countries	Prevents fatigue	May improve circulation and slightly lower blood pressure; could help prevent colorectal and stomach cancer	Safe for most adults; may thin blood; side effects include breath and body odor, stomach upset, and allergic reactions
Guarana	Climbing plant in Amazon Basin	Reduced fatigue, increased alertness, ergogenic aid	Stimulant with twice the amount of caffeine as the coffee bean	Generally safe, but lethal overdose possible
St. John's Wort	Yellow flowering plant, medicinal use first recorded in ancient Greece	Treatment of depression, anxiety, and sleep disorders; balm for wounds, burns, and insect bites	Mixed results in treatment of depression	Interacts with many medications, which could lead to serious side effects

a. National Center for Complementary and Alternative Medicine (www.nccam.nih.gov).

the report at www.wada-ama.org for a complete listing of banned substances. Despite the ban, athletes frequently get caught with low levels of banned substances in their blood and urine during random testing.

Doping, the act of ingesting a banned substance in an effort to improve athletic performance, is relatively common among elite athletes and has especially plagued the Tour de France, with only four of the winners between 1995 and 2013 *not* involved in controversies surrounding performance-enhancing drugs. In the most widely publicized downfall of a world-class athlete, seven-time Tour de France winner Lance Armstrong was stripped of his medals after he was exposed for what the United States Anti-Doping Agency called "the most sophisticated, professionalized and successful doping program that sport has ever seen." Armstrong ultimately admitted to using blood doping and a cocktail of banned substances including erythropoietin (EPO), testosterone, cortisone, and human growth hormone.[19] Another disgraced Tour de France "winner," Alberto Contador, was stripped of his 2010 victory after he screened positive for the performance-enhancing and illegal drug clenbuterol; he says it was a contaminant in a cut of steak he ate. (Sometimes cattle are given the drug to improve their value, but investigators found no evidence that the meat was tainted.) For Armstrong, Contador, and other athletes found guilty of doping, a lifetime of intense physical training, competition, and success is nullified by cheating.

While some athletes may blatantly violate the rules, many other athletes have been expelled from their sport due to **inadvertent doping**. Because supplements are not closely regulated and rates of **contamination** are high, some athletes test positive for banned substances without being aware of the ingestion. The rates of inadvertent doping are highest with the banned stimulants ephedrine, sibutramine, and methylhexaneamine.[20] Products containing ephedrine often are labeled with the herbal names *Ma Huang* or *ephedra sinica* and not by the more easily identifiable names of ephedrine, pseudoephedrine, or methylephedrine. The unclear labeling poses a trap for less sophisticated athletes. Due to its potent potential side effects, such as stroke and heart attack in certain individuals, sibutramine is approved as a prescription-only medication for weight loss. When it is contained within a supplement, a consumer may only know that the product has "pure herbal ingredients" and that it is advertised to induce weight loss. The supplement name and ingredient list may not say the word "sibutramine" anywhere, leaving it up to the athlete to recognize that the banned substance sibutramine may be a hidden ingredient. Methylhexaneamine is frequently inadvertently ingested due to confusing labeling. The same substance can be found on supplement labels as dimethylamylamine, dimethylpentylamine, pentylamine, geranamine, and forthane, among others. On the WADA's 2014 prohibited list only the names methylhexaneamine and dimethylpentylamine are mentioned.[21,57]

Steroids

Anabolic steroids are strictly prohibited by the WADA code. Steroids quickly and dangerously build muscle mass and strength. Their use is accompanied with serious adverse effects including high blood pressure, rage, gynecomastia (enlarged breast size), and decreased testicle size in men; and increased testosterone, facial hair growth, and deepening of the voice in women. While most elite and recreational athletes know to avoid these substances, many supplements are on the market that contain anabolic steroid contaminants, possibly intentionally.[20] Consumers should proceed with caution when considering trying any product that boasts of its ability to quickly boost muscle mass.

Androstenedione, a precursor to testosterone, is commonly referred to as a "natural alternative" to anabolic steroids. Androstenedione supplements claim to increase testosterone levels and promote muscle size and strength. Research in men does not support these claims,[22] while the effect of androstenedione intake in women has not been studied. Repeated use of androstenedione supplements poses significant health risks including decreased high-density lipoprotein (HDL, the "healthy" cholesterol) levels and increased cardiovascular disease risk; increased risk of prostate cancer and pancreatic cancer; baldness; and gynecomastia in men.[22] While androstenedione is not banned by Major League Baseball, the National Basketball Association, or the National Hockey League, it is banned by the WADA and the International Olympic Committee (IOC), the National Collegiate Athletic Association (NCAA), and the National Football League. The FDA has also banned the sale of androstenedione in the United States.

Similar to androstenedione, dehydroepiandrosterone (DHEA) is a precursor to testosterone. Despite claims of promoting youthfulness, virility, and enhanced strength, research consistently shows that it does not affect strength, lean body mass, or athletic performance.[23] DHEA is banned by the WADA.

Hormones

Some athletes turn to **hormones** to gain an unfair athletic advantage. From erythropoesis-stimulating hormones, which lead to increased red blood cell production and consequently increased oxygen-carrying capacity, to growth hormones and sex hormones that boost testosterone levels, most hormone supplements are strictly banned and should be avoided by all athletes.

Diuretics

Diuretics are medications or substances that lead to increased water loss. Athletes trying to make weight frequently abuse diuretics. Again, use of these substances is strictly prohibited by the WADA.

Stimulants

A **stimulant** is a substance that activates the central nervous system and sympathetic nervous system. It increases heart rate, cardiac output, and glucose availability, and may even suppress appetite. In addition to their potential performance-enhancing attributes, stimulants also can have serious and significant side effects. With the exception of caffeine, the WADA prohibits stimulant use during competition.

Caffeine

Caffeine is now found in soap, lip balm, and chewing gum in addition to coffee, tea, chocolate, and 60 plus other plants and artificially injected foods and drinks. Countless caffeine-loaded products promise to enhance performance and stimulate the metabolism. Caffeine's potent ability to ward off sleep, improve athletic performance, decrease pain and fatigue, boost memory, and enhance mood[24] makes it America's drug of choice. Over 90% of Americans admit to regular caffeine use,[25] and 20% to 30% consume 600 milligrams (equivalent to about 6 cups of coffee) or more each day.[24]

Caffeine rapidly enters the bloodstream and within a short 40 to 60 minutes reaches all organs of the body, causing physiological changes that last for up to 6 hours.[26] Due to its lipophilic or "fat-loving" chemical structure, caffeine easily crosses the blood-brain barrier, the brain's security system aimed to prevent water-soluble toxins from damaging the all-important organ. To a nerve cell, caffeine resembles adenosine, a molecule that slows down the nervous system, dilates blood vessels, and allows sleep. The nerve's adenosine receptor cannot tell the difference between the two molecules, so caffeine and adenosine compete for receptor binding. When caffeine wins, an exaggerated stress response takes hold. The cell activity speeds up, the brain's blood vessels constrict, and neuron firing increases. The pituitary gland responds to the increased activity by sending a message to the adrenal glands to produce adrenaline, the "fight or flight" hormone. Pupils and breathing tubes dilate. Heart rate increases. Blood flow shunts to the muscles. Blood pressure rises. Muscles contract. The liver releases extra glucose into the bloodstream to fuel the "fight or flight" response, thus sparing muscle glycogen stores.[2]

Given the physiological response to caffeine, it comes as no surprise that the research findings on caffeine are so consistent and clear: caffeine enhances athletic performance. Caffeine sustains or improves exercise performance, maximizes effort at 85% VO_2 max in cyclists, and quickens speed in an endurance event.[26] Perceived exertion decreases and high intensity efforts seem less taxing.[24] Contrary to popular opinion, research suggests that caffeine use combined with exercise does not cause negative effects like water-electrolyte imbalances, hyperthermia, or reduced exercise-heat tolerance.[24] Athletes are taking note— nearly 70% of athletes in one study reported regular caffeine use.[26] The NCAA and the IOC allow intake of the ubiquitous and relatively harmless substance up to an approximately 800 milligram dose (cut-offs are based on caffeine amounts in urine testing). Notably, most research studying the ergogenic potential of caffeine has used dosages around 400 to 600 milligrams in capsule form, though benefits have been seen at doses as low as 250 milligrams.[26]

Here's the catch: performance-enhancing benefits of caffeine are stronger in nonusers (<50 mg/day) than regular users (>300 mg/day).[27] That's because the brain adapts to chronic caffeine use by producing more adenosine receptors for adenosine binding. Caffeine's effects are lessened and the same dose produces fewer desirable physiological changes. In a chronically sleep-deprived, high-achieving culture, a common response to increased caffeine tolerance is consumption of more caffeine. While the extra caffeine binds up the newly created adenosine receptors, the brain gets back to work increasing receptor production. As the dose continues to increase in pursuit of the invigorating caffeine jolt, risk of severe consequences multiply. In addition to its toxicity at high doses, when combined with other substances like alcohol, ephedrine, or anti-inflammatory medications, even moderate caffeine use can be dangerous.

On top of tolerance, chronic caffeine use contributes to high blood pressure, high blood sugar, decreased bone density in women, jittery nerves, sleeplessness, and for many, withdrawal symptoms after a brief respite from the stimulant including headache, irritability, increased fatigue, drowsiness, decreased alertness, difficulty concentrating, and decreased energy and activity levels.[26]

Proteins and Amino Acids

Proteins and amino acids are among the most popular and commonly used supplements.

Whey and Casein

Two forms of commonly supplemented proteins include the milk proteins whey and casein. Whey is the liquid remaining after the milk has been curdled and strained. There are three varieties of whey: whey protein powder, whey protein concentrate, and whey protein isolate, all of which provide high levels of the essential and branched-chain amino acids, vitamins, and minerals. Whey powder is 11% to 15% protein and is used as an additive in many food products. Whey concentrate is 25% to 89% protein, whereas whey isolate is more than 90% protein. Both are commonly used in dietary supplements. It should be noted that while the isolate form is nearly pure whey, some of the proteins can be lost during the manufacturing process. Unlike the other whey forms, the isolate is lactose-free. Whey contains high levels of the amino acids that play an important role in muscle hypertrophy. It is also rapidly digested and absorbed, and effectively stimulates muscle protein synthesis.

Casein, which gives milk its white color, accounts for 70% to 80% of milk's protein. Casein possesses a property that allows the protein to provide a sustained slow release of amino acids into the bloodstream, sometimes lasting for hours. Some studies suggest that combining casein and whey may produce the greatest muscular strength improvements after an intensive resistance-training program.[28]

Amino Acids

Branched-chain amino acids (leucine, isoleucine, and valine) play important roles in muscle building. Some researchers have found that following exercise the branched-chain amino acids, especially leucine, increase the rate of protein synthesis and decrease the rate of protein catabolism.[29] The supplement industry has been quick to respond; leucine supplements are widely available in health food stores, with a cost upwards of $50 per container. However, because the research findings are inconsistent and little is known about the safety of these products, the Academy of Nutrition and Dietetics advises against individual amino acid supplementation and protein supplementation overall.[30] Arginine and aspartate/aspartic acid are additional frequently supplemented amino acids, but supplementation is likely unnecessary to achieve the purported benefits. It may be that food sources of these proteins and amino acids provide the same effect for a small fraction of the cost. Table 10-8 highlights readily available amino acid supplements.

Creatine

A large body of research has proven creatine (sold as creatine monohydrate) effective in building muscle mass, especially when combined with intensive strength training.

Table 10-8. Readily Available Amino Acid Supplements[23,48,49]

AMINO ACID	CLASSIFICATION	ERGOGENIC FUNCTION	DESCRIPTION	EFFICACY OF SUPPLEMENTATION
Alanine (and Dipeptide Carnosine)	Nonessential	Combines with histidine to form carnosine; synthesis of carnitine dependent on availability of alanine; increases muscle buffering capacity	Buffer	Attenuates fall in blood pH during high-intensity exercise, leading to increased capability to perform strenuous exercise
Valine	Essential	Stimulates protein synthesis in muscle	Branched-chain amino acid	After exercise, shown to increase rate of protein synthesis and decrease protein catabolism, especially leucine
Leucine	Essential	Stimulates protein synthesis in muscle	Branched-chain amino acid	
Isoleucine	Essential	Stimulates protein synthesis in muscle	Branched-chain amino acid	
Arginine	Nonessential	Facilitates vasodilation as nitrous oxide precursor and improved muscle strength as substrate for creatine formation	Formed in urea cycle, essential for nitric oxide signaling pathway; necessary for creatine formation; may stimulate growth hormone and recovery of muscle after exercise	Could enhance muscle gain from resistance training but effect may be minimal in athletes who already eat enough protein; supplementation unnecessary for most
Aspartic Acid/ Aspartate	Nonessential	Glucose production	Easily converted to oxaloacetate intermediary of citric acid cycle	Supplementation increased time to exhaustion when combined with asparagine in rat studies but results not confirmed in human study of triathletes

Table 10-8. Readily Available Amino Acid Supplements[23,48,49]—cont'd

AMINO ACID	CLASSIFICATION	ERGOGENIC FUNCTION	DESCRIPTION	EFFICACY OF SUPPLEMENTATION
Glutamic Acid/ Glutamine	Nonessential	Increases athletic performance	Many metabolic roles; excitatory neurotransmitter; food flavoring "umami"	No evidence of efficacy when used alone but significant improvements when combined with carbohydrate or other amino acids
Cysteine	Essential (in infants and those with chronic disease)	Increases exercise performance	Essential for glutathione synthesis (important antioxidant in cellular signaling)	May be beneficial due to its ability to increase levels of glutathione

Creatine, a derivative of three amino acids and a source of rapid energy, is stored in the muscles in small amounts. With creatine loading or supplementation, athletes increase muscle stores of the energy-containing compound, which then can be used to provide an extra boost for a high-intensity weight-lifting session. Studies support that ingestion of a relatively high dose of creatine (20 to 30 grams per day for up to 2 weeks) increases muscle creatine stores by 10% to 30% and can boost muscle strength by about 10% when compared with resistance training alone.[31,32] Because creatine is a natural substance that is produced by the body, it is not included on any doping lists. It has limited known side effects, with some anecdotal reports of muscle cramping and liver metabolism, although the research has not confirmed these findings.[32] People with potential risk of renal dysfunction, such as those with diabetes, hypertension, and decreased kidney function, should not use creatine unless its use is advised or cleared by a physician. Anyone who uses creatine on a long-term basis should undergo routine monitoring by a physician.

Other Popular Ergogenic Aids

Several other categories of ergogenic aids show promise in their ability to boost athletic performance without major safety risks. For example, sodium bicarbonate and sodium citrate effectively buffer the metabolic acidosis that occurs with intense physical activity. Consequently, these substances help to reduce or delay the fatigue associated with lactate-induced acidosis. Nitrates also show promise in their ability to reduce the oxygen cost of physical activity. These and other potential performance-enhancing supplements are described in Table 10-9. This chapter's Evaluating the Evidence describes the evolving research surrounding the performance-enhancing capabilities of beetroot juice, a natural nitrate-containing compound.

SPEED BUMP

3. Describe the product claims, efficacy, and safety of the most commonly used dietary supplements for weight loss, health, and performance.

EVALUATING THE EVIDENCE

Boost Athletic Performance With a Big Gulp of *Beetroot Juice*?

A group of British researchers may have discovered the next popular all-natural, performance-enhancing–*vegetable*? Lead author Katherine Lansley and her mentor Andrew Jones' research team at the University of Exeter have been conducting a series of experiments looking at the impact of beetroot juice on exercise performance.

In one study, the researchers gave a group of competitive male cyclists either 16 ounces of beetroot juice or 16 ounces of a nitrate-free placebo beetroot juice about 2.5 hours before completing a 4-kilometer or a 16.1-kilometer timed trial. Two to 3 days later, each athlete completed the workout again, this time with a different drink-distance combination. In all, each of the athletes completed four trials with 2 to 3 days separating the workouts. Once the times were tallied, the researchers found that beetroot juice improved trial time by about 2% to 3% in both the short- (lasting about 5 minutes) and longer-distance (lasting about 30 minutes) trials when compared to the nitrate-free placebo.[35]

The authors credit the nitrate in beetroot juice for the improved performance. The thinking is that the body converts high levels of inorganic nitrate (found in high levels in beets as well as most green leafy vegetables) into

Continued

EVALUATING THE EVIDENCE—cont'd

bioactive nitrite. (Blood nitrite levels more than doubled in the beetroot juice group compared to the placebo group in the study of cyclists.) The body converts the nitrite to nitric oxide. Nitric oxide is well known to improve vasodilation and blood flow in vessels. This could provide a mechanism for decreased oxygen cost of exercise and thus increased athletic performance.

This research team also looked at the effects of beetroot juice on blood pressure; mitochondrial oxidative capacity, a marker of how efficiently and effectively the body converts food to fuel; and physiological responses, such as how much oxygen is required to fuel walking and moderate- to high-intensity running, and how long a participant could exercise before exhaustion. The researchers found that participants who consumed the beetroot juice had lower blood pressure and lower oxygen cost of exercise. In fact, walkers had a significant 12% to 14% decrease in the amount of oxygen needed. The authors point out that this could have significant implications for improving exercise capacity in people who suffer from certain cardiovascular and pulmonary diseases. The participants also had decreased overall maximal oxygen consumption (VO_2 max), but this was compensated for with an increased time to exhaustion.[36]

1. What are some limitations to the studies cited?
2. What are the benefits and risks of beetroot juice supplementation?
3. Is this research compelling enough for you to want to try to beetroot juice in an effort to improve performance? Why or why not?
4. What would you tell your clients about beetroot juice?

Sidebar: What's in a Beet?

Beetroot juice is the blended, liquefied version of the beet. While the taste might take a little getting used to (for best results, most raw food connoisseurs recommend a 4:1 dilution with the juice of other, preferably sweeter, vegetables and fruits), the juice from this vegetable is packed with a nutritional punch and a long list of health benefits including increased performance, decreased blood pressure, and overall improved cardiovascular health.[37] (Note: Eating beets or drinking beetroot juice may cause urine to turn pink).

Nutritional Content of Beets

Nutrient	100 g of raw beet (approx. 1½ to 2″ diameter beets or 4 oz of juice)
Calories	43
Carbohydrate	10 g
Sugars	7 g
Dietary fiber	3 g
Protein	2 g
Fat	0 g
Potassium	325 mg (7%)
Folate	27%
Vitamin B_6	5%
Vitamin C	6%
Iron	0.8 mg (6%)
Magnesium	23 mg (6%)
Phosphorus	40 mg (6%)

Source: USDA Nutrient Database.

Table 10-9. Performance-Enhancing Supplements [37,47,49,50]

	CLAIM	EFFECTIVENESS	SAFETY
	Used Most By Strength/Power Athletes		
Androstenedione	Promotes muscle size and strength	No more effective than resistance training alone	May increase risk of cardiovascular disease, cancer, baldness, and gynecomastia (development of breast tissue)
Beta Hydroxymethyl Butyrate	Increases muscle size and strength and decreases muscle damage and soreness associated with resistance training	May slightly enhance strength-training adaptations in untrained athletes and negligibly in trained athletes	Short-term supplementation appears safe
Bovine Colostrum	Contains growth factors that mediate protein synthesis	Limited studies, but may provide ergogenic benefits	No safety information
Branched-Chain Amino Acids	Increases the rate of protein synthesis and decreases protein breakdown following exercise	Unlikely to provide benefit	Uncertain
Chromium Picolinate	Increases muscle mass, decreases fat mass, and improves blood glucose and cholesterol	No benefit	Safety uncertain
Conjugated Linoleic Acid (CLA)	Reduces body fat and builds muscle	Not effective to build muscle mass; possibly effective to reduce body fat	Possibly safe
Creatine	Improves athletic performance for high-intensity exercise, especially when combined with resistance training	Consistently provides benefit	Appears safe
Dehydroepiandrosterone (DHEA)	Enhances muscle strength and lean body mass	Consistently provides NO benefit	Possibly safe for short-term use, and possibly unsafe for long-term use
Gamma Oryzanol	Increases testosterone levels in the body leading to muscle and strength gains, improved recovery time, and decreased body fat	Not effective	Possibly safe
Glutamine	Taking the amino acid after intense exercise decreases muscle breakdown after intense activity	No evidence of efficacy when used alone but significant improvements when combined with carbohydrate or other amino acids	Possibly safe

Continued

Table 10-9. **Performance-Enhancing Supplements Continued[37,47,49,50]—cont'd**

	CLAIM	EFFECTIVENESS	SAFETY
Human Growth Hormone (HGH)	Increases muscle mass, strength, and power; enhances fat loss	Effective	Dangerous, banned, illegal
Protein Powder (whey, casein, certain amino acids)	Increases strength, increases muscle growth	Provides benefit	Appears safe
Ribose	Increases the rate of ATP resynthesis and the speed of recovery following high-intensity exercise	Little published evidence to suggest benefit	Appears safe, even at high doses
Steroids	Increases muscle mass and strength	Effective	Dangerous, banned, and illegal
Vanadium/Vanadyl Sulfate	Increases muscle definition by making muscle look fuller and larger due to insulin-like properties which shuttle increased glucose for glycogen storage and amino acids into the muscle cell	No evidence for benefit	Toxicity at high doses
	Used Most By Endurance Athletes		
Bee Pollen	Its combination of nutrients, including saccharides, amino acids, vitamins, and minerals enhances endurance and strength performance	Not effective	Generally safe, though may induce anaphylaxis in individuals allergic to bees
Caffeine	Improves athletic capacity and performance	Effective	May develop dependency, toxic at very high doses
Coenzyme Q10	Enhances exercise capacity, improves athletic performance, and protects against oxidative muscle damage, due to its antioxidant properties	Equivocal research findings with some studies showing worsened performance; likely ineffective	Appears safe, some research suggests use could increase muscle damage in response to exercise
Cytochrome C	Increases maximum oxygen-carrying capacity, reduces lactate, and increases anaerobic threshold	Not effective	Possibly safe
Dihydroxyacetone	When combined with pyruvate (then known as DHAP), can increase time to exhaustion during endurance activities	Not effective	Probably safe
Ginseng	Increases stamina, immune function, and ability to adapt to training stressors	No evidence to support	Easily contaminated, nonstandardized ingredients

Table 10-9. Performance-Enhancing Supplements Continued[37,47,49,50]–cont'd

	CLAIM	EFFECTIVENESS	SAFETY
Glycerol	Improves performance by decreasing risk of heat stress through "hyperhydration" before exercise	Uncertain effectiveness	Banned by IOC/WADA. Many side effects including nausea, lightheadedness, and GI symptoms
L-carnitine	Increases rates of carbohydrate and fatty acid oxidation and thus increases energy available for exercise	20 years of research finds no consistent evidence for benefit to athletic performance	Safe at most doses. May cause nausea, vomiting, abdominal cramps, diarrhea, and a "fishy" body odor at higher doses (about 3 g/d)
Medium Chain Triglycerides	Providing a ready source of easily metabolized fatty acids; spares glycogen and thus improves endurance capacity	No evidence to support claims	May cause GI distress and cramping
Nitrates	Reduces oxygen cost of activity and could improve exercise performance	Studies to date support claims	Nitric oxide-induced vasodilation could lead to a drop in blood pressure
Pyruvate	No plausible ergogenic mechanism, but marketed to improve athletic performance and enhance weight loss	No scientific basis as ergogenic aid	Appears safe
Sodium Tablets	Prevents hyponatremia during prolonged endurance activities by supplying sodium	Effective	May cause diarrhea or cramping
Sodium Bicarbonate and Sodium Citrate	By buffering metabolic acidosis, reduces or delays onset of fatigue during strenuous exercise	Effective, especially at optimal amounts of 0.3 g/kg body weight	May contribute to GI upset
Sports Drinks, Gels, Bars	Improves endurance and reduces fatigue by replenishing carbohydrate stores, replacing electrolytes, and supplying fluid	Effective	Safe

SCOPE OF PRACTICE

Health professionals play an important role in helping to inform and educate athletes and the general population about supplements. While health professionals should not specifically endorse or recommend any supplement, they can help clients collect the right information to make their own informed decision, with the help of their physician or dietitian, when appropriate.

Evaluating Supplements

Developing an approach to learning about and evaluating supplements will not only be useful to share with clients so that they can do their own research on supplements, but is also useful for health professionals to inform their own opinions and views on supplements that are readily available in the marketplace.

Understand the Claim

The first step to evaluating a supplement is to understand the claim. Why do people take the supplement? What does the supplement manufacturer state or imply that the supplement will do? Many supplements promise multiple benefits. Which is the most compelling or relevant claim for the goal the client is trying to achieve? Start this process by going directly to the source. How do supplement manufacturers market the product? Go to the manufacturer's website or carefully read the supplement packaging and insert.

Assess the Credibility

A quick Web search will reveal many credible websites along with many more sites with marginal quality and a hidden (or sometimes overt) agenda. Generally, the Office of Dietary Supplements (www.ods.od.nih.gov), the National Center for Complementary and Alternative Medicine (www.nccam.nih.gov), and the Food and Drug Administration (www.FDA.gov) offer unbiased information to understand the validity of claims as well as risks and benefits from taking supplements. Because the sites are credible and in the public domain, health professionals can freely distribute and share the information contained on these sites.

Assess the Relevance

After gaining an understanding of the product claims and their validity, consider whether or not the claims are relevant to the specific situation. For example, it may not make sense for an endurance athlete who does not do any resistance training to take a creatine supplement, as creatine builds muscle strength and hypertrophy only when combined with intensive strength training. Vitamin C supplements would not be necessary for a person who already consumes a diet that is rich in vitamin C, as excess intake of water-soluble vitamins is excreted in the urine (and at very high doses, vitamin C can cause harmful effects such as bladder irritation and kidney stones).

On the other hand, certain populations may benefit substantially from supplementation. For example, individuals who severely restrict intake of certain food groups, such as vegans; some people with celiac disease or gluten intolerance on a gluten-free diet; or individuals on a very low calorie diet, may be advised by a physician to take vitamin and mineral supplements to avoid nutrient deficiencies. The Centers for Disease Control and Prevention recommends that all women of childbearing age who could become pregnant take a folic acid supplement to prevent neural tube defects in a developing fetus. Elderly people with poor dietary intake or illness may need supplementation to prevent deficiency and improve overall health. Excessive alcohol intake and alcoholism contribute to vitamin deficiency due to inadequate dietary intake and compromised vitamin absorption. Often, vitamin supplementation is necessary to prevent serious disability in people with alcoholism. A client's personal physician can be an excellent resource to help determine when and if supplementation is advised.

Evaluate the Safety

Supplements are not closely regulated by the federal government; therefore, ensuring supplement safety is primarily the responsibility of the product manufacturer. Government intervention occurs only once significant harm has been established, clearly too late for those people who already have been harmed by a supplement. Prior to taking a supplement, consumers should be aware of the safety record of the particular product. Safety information is available on the government websites mentioned previously. Individuals who spend a large portion of their time discussing supplements may consider a subscription to the *Natural Medicines Comprehensive Database* (www.naturaldatabase.com), a resource that provides credible evidence-based information on many commonly used supplements.

Athletes should also check the *Dietary Supplements Label Database* (www.dietarysupplements.nlm.nih.gov) for a complete listing of known ingredients in specific supplements and U.S. Pharmacopeia (www.usp.org), ConsumerLab.com (www.consumerlab.com), or NSF International (www.nsf.org) to determine supplement compliance with FDA and professional regulatory body rules, such as WADA, NCAA, IOC, and United States Olympic Committee (USOC), or USA Track & Field, as applicable.

Evaluate the Risks Versus Benefits

Some dietary, weight loss, and ergogenic supplements may provide benefit, while others may cause harm, including severe disability or death. Many times the risk or benefit of a supplement depends in large part on certain individual factors like age, health status, diet, and effects of other medications and supplements. Clients scheduled for surgery should also be aware that certain supplements can cause complications before, during, or after surgery. For example, a 2001 study in the *Journal of the American Medical Association* of eight commonly used supplements (echinacea, ephedra, garlic, gingko, ginseng, kava, St. John's wort, and valerian) attributed the supplement use to increased risk of bleeding, cardiovascular instability, hypoglycemia, and alterations in metabolism of anesthetic agents and other drugs used during surgery.[33] The best person to help a client evaluate the risks and benefits of supplement use is the primary care physician (or surgeon for those undergoing surgery), or in some cases a registered dietitian. If a client is seriously considering taking supplements, a referral to a qualified heath provider is in order.

Consider Possible Drug, Supplement, and Nutrient Interactions

Many supplements interact with each other and with medications. Clients and their physicians should seriously evaluate these possible interactions prior to starting a supplement. Some common medication/supplement interactions are listed in Box 10-2. Clients should also be reminded to be forthright with their physician in discussing any supplement use, as many doctors may not specifically ask about or consider existing supplement use when making medication recommendations.

Make an Informed Decision

After gathering all of the available information about a supplement, a client can decide whether or not to use it. Ideally, this situation will be based on a thoughtful analysis and discussion with a qualified health professional. While health professionals play an important role in helping a client to gather the information to make this decision, health professionals who are not a physician or registered dietitian should not specifically recommend or advise a client to take a supplement. Not only does this fall outside the scope of practice and put the health professional at legal risk, but it may also put the client at increased risk for a negative effect and compromise the professional-client relationship.

Continuously Evaluate the Need (or Lack of Need) for Supplementation

If a client begins to take a supplement, the plan for the duration of supplementation should not be indefinite. The process of evaluating the need for supplementation should help a client to have a specific purpose for taking the supplement and a predetermined (though possibly flexible) duration of supplementation. The health professional should periodically check in with the client to understand the client's plan and when it is time to stop a supplement. Of course, supplements should be stopped sooner than planned if negative side effects occur.

Clients should understand that the process to evaluate the safety and efficacy of a supplement by necessity must be much more thorough and comprehensive than the process of understanding a medication because the government regulations for medications are much more strict and comprehensive.

The Bottom Line

Ultimately, while health professionals play an important role in helping clients to understand the risks and potential benefits of supplements, *no matter how harmless a supplement seems, health professionals who are not registered dietitians or physicians should never recommend supplements to clients. Not only is it outside the scope of practice, but recommending supplements without a full medical history and physical exam is dangerous* (see Communication Strategies).

SPEED BUMP

4. Define the scope of practice for allied health professionals with regard to the recommendation and sale of dietary supplements.

Box 10-2. Examples of Drug Interactions with Dietary Supplements[a]

St. John's Wort (*Hypericum perforatum*): This herb is considered an inducer of liver enzymes, which means it can reduce the concentration of medications in the blood. St. John's wort can reduce the blood level of digoxin (Lanoxin), which is used to treat heart failure and atrial fibrillation (irregular, fast heartbeat); the cholesterol-lowering drug lovastatin (Mevacor, Altocor); and the erectile dysfunction drug sildenafil (Viagra).

Vitamin E: Taking vitamin E with a blood-thinning medication such as Coumadin (warfarin) can increase anti-clotting activity and may cause an increased risk of bleeding.

Ginseng: This herb can interfere with the bleeding effects of Coumadin (warfarin). In addition, ginseng can enhance the bleeding effects of heparin, aspirin, and nonsteroidal anti-inflammatory drugs such as ibuprofen, naproxen, and ketoprofen. Combining ginseng with MAO inhibitors such as Nardil (phenelzine) or Parnate (tranylcypromine) may cause headache, trouble sleeping, nervousness, and hyperactivity.

Ginkgo Biloba: High doses of the herb ginkgo biloba could decrease the effectiveness of anticonvulsant therapy in patients taking the following medications to control seizures: Tegretol, Equetro, or Carbatrol (carbamazepine), and Depakote (valproic acid).

a. Food and Drug Administration. www.fda.gov/forconsumers/consumerupdates/ucm096386.htm#supplements.

COMMUNICATION STRATEGIES

Discussing Supplements

Health professionals work with both athletes and the general population–many of whom will be taking, have tried, or are considering trying a vitamin, herbal, or ergogenic supplement. These encounters provide a valuable opportunity to share information with clients about supplements. However, allied health professionals must also be careful not to step outside their scope of practice.

1. Working together with a partner, make a list of five scenarios in which an allied health professional may be in the position to discuss supplements. For each scenario, develop an acceptable response and an unacceptable response to the situation. For example, an acceptable response to a client who is considering creatine supplementation could be, "Some studies have shown that creatine supplementation improves athletic performance." An unacceptable response would be, "Creatine supplementation works. You should try it."
2. What is the difference between an acceptable and an unacceptable response?
3. Choose two of the scenarios to role play. Each student should have the opportunity to role play as both a client and a health professional. What challenges did you face? What insights did you gain from the simulation?

KEY POINTS SUMMARY

1. Supplements are not closely regulated by the federal government and should be used with extreme caution.
2. The existing legislation, including the Dietary Supplement and Health Education Act (DSHEA) and the Current Good Manufacturing Practices (CGMPs), dictate the government's approach to supplements. The DSHEA outlines supplement production, marketing, and safety guidelines. CGMPs assure that dietary supplements are consistently produced and of acceptable quality. Other more stringent laws have been proposed, but as of the publication of this text, have not been passed.
3. Many people use supplements with claims of weight loss. The safety and efficacy of these supplements are poorly understood. Health professionals should be aware of the commonly used weight loss supplements, their claims, efficacy, and safety.
4. Whole foods provide the majority of vitamins and minerals needed for optimal health. Most supplements that aim to improve health do not provide benefit beyond a wholesome, balanced eating plan. However, many people do not consume adequate amounts of nutrients such as vitamin D and DHA/omega-3 fatty acids and folic acid in pregnant women, suggesting that in some cases, supplementation may be beneficial.
5. Herbal supplements are plant-derived substances used for medicinal purposes. Like other supplements, they are not closely regulated and safety and purity are not certain.
6. Many of the most profitable supplements include those that boast enhanced athletic performance for strength/power athletes, endurance athletes, or both. Despite the large revenue they generate, only a select few supplements have strong evidence to support their efficacy (and safety).
7. Many supplements that have proven effective are also toxic, dangerous, and banned (such as anabolic steroids). Other banned substances such as androstenedione and DHEA do not provide rapid muscle gains. An alarming number of athletes use the illegal substances to gain a competitive edge. This is referred to as doping. Some athletes have been expelled from their sports for inadvertent doping, consuming a banned substance added without their knowledge to a legal supplement or food.
8. In addition to steroids, some athletes also use illegal hormones, diuretics, and stimulants to improve performance.
9. Caffeine is an allowed (to a certain level) stimulant that is proven effective in improving athletic performance. It can be toxic at high levels.
10. Some protein supplements such as whey protein powder may facilitate increased athletic performance and improved muscle mass. However, others, such as individual amino acid supplements, probably do not provide much additional benefit beyond a balanced protein-sufficient eating plan.
11. Creatine supplementation when combined with intense exercise training improves muscle mass. It is generally considered to be safe, though clients should not begin creatine supplementation without first discussing this with a physician.

12. Consumers and health professionals should develop a systematic approach to evaluating supplements. Be sure to understand the claim, assess the credibility and relevance, evaluate the safety and risks versus benefits, consider possible interactions, make an informed decision, and continuously evaluate the need (or lack of need) to use a supplement.
13. Health professionals should be keenly aware of their scope of practice when discussing sports nutrition with clients, especially in the case of discussing supplements. Health professionals who are not physicians or registered dietitians should not recommend that a client begin a supplement. Rather, the client should first discuss this with the appropriate licensed, qualified professional.

PRACTICAL APPLICATIONS

1. Jack's new personal training client, Alexi, is a strong believer in the practice of vitamin supplementation. After reviewing her 3-day food diary, which includes her supplement schedule, Jack noted that Alexi is taking megadoses of vitamin A and niacin. Which of the following statements would be the most appropriate for Jack to make in addressing Alexi regarding her supplementation practice?
   A. "After looking at your food diary, I realized that you are taking megadoses of certain vitamins. I advise you to stop taking supplements immediately and improve your diet by eating more whole grains, fruits, and vegetables."
   B. "Your food diary revealed that you are taking an amount of vitamins that could potentially lead to health problems. I encourage you to adopt a well-balanced, nutrient-dense diet and discuss your supplementation habits with your physician."
   C. "I realize that you feel strongly about taking your vitamin supplements, but as we have discussed before, you really shouldn't need to take any supplements if you're eating a well-balanced diet."
   D. "Unfortunately, we are going to have to postpone our training sessions until you discuss your vitamin supplementation practices with your physician."

2. After several months of sticking to his exercise program, Mark informs his personal trainer that he is pleased with his progress and would like to enhance his rate of muscle building by incorporating creatine supplementation into his current program. From the personal trainer's perspective, which of the following responses to Mark's inquiry about creatine is the most appropriate?
   A. "While some research shows that creatine may enhance muscular performance, it would be best for you to discuss supplementation with your physician prior to taking it."
   B. "Taking creatine supplements is a good strategy as long as you follow the dosage instructions carefully and monitor yourself for any unwanted symptoms."
   C. "Try taking 3 grams of creatine per day for approximately 1 month. If you experience any gastrointestinal discomfort, decrease the dose and contact your physician."
   D. "Inform your physician that I recommend you start a creatine supplementation program and let me know if he or she advises any precautions or limitations for you."

3. Ben has just purchased a daily multivitamin supplement per the recommendation of his physician. The label on the bottle carries the United States Pharmacopeia (USP) seal. What does the USP seal mean as it relates to the product in the bottle?
   A. This vitamin supplement is regulated by the federal government.
   B. The dietary supplement manufacturer chose to subject this product to USP testing and successfully passed the test.
   C. The health claims made in the promotion of the product are guaranteed by the manufacturer to produce the desired effects.
   D. This product is safe and effective for use by all populations.

4. Which of the following dietary supplementation practices is best supported by evidence from scientific research?
   A. Multivitamin supplementation in older women to reduce their risk for heart disease
   B. Vitamin C supplementation in men and women to decrease premature mortality
   C. Vitamin D supplementation in men and women to improve health and decrease morbidity
   D. Folic acid supplementation in pregnant women to reduce risk of birth defects

5. Which of the following dietary supplements has been associated with numerous health benefits including decreased risk of heart disease, improved brain development in fetuses and young children, and reduced disability from mental illnesses such as depression?
   A. Soy protein
   B. Botanicals
   C. Omega-3 essential fatty acids
   D. Iron

6. Which of the following substances easily crosses the blood-brain barrier and produces the "fight or flight" response?
   A. Creatine
   B. Caffeine
   C. Diuretics
   D. Amino acids

7. Which of the following statements about weight-loss supplements is true?
   A. The manufacturer's claims are largely unsubstantiated and the supplements are poorly regulated.
   B. Thermogenic weight-loss supplements alter metabolism in a way that causes the body to use more energy.
   C. Herbal weight-loss substances are generally recognized as safe and are effective at promoting body-fat reduction.
   D. Weight-loss supplements approved by the United States Pharmacopeia (USP) are less likely to interfere with other medications.

8. Mitch is a competitive wrestler who was recently disqualified from participation because he had tested positive for the banned substance, ephedrine. Mitch denies all claims of using an ergogenic aid to enhance performance. Upon further evaluation, Mitch discovered that, without his knowledge, a weight-loss supplement he was taking contained Ma Huang, which is another name for ephedrine. Mitch's case is an example of:
   A. Cross contamination
   B. Illegal supplementation
   C. Blatant violation
   D. Inadvertent doping

9. Which of the following ergogenic aids has been shown to perform as claimed?
   A. Ginseng
   B. Coenzyme Q10
   C. Caffeine
   D. Chromium picolinate

10. In general, which of the following health-care professionals is the most qualified to help a consumer evaluate the risks and benefits of supplement use relative to individual needs?
   A. Primary care physician
   B. Registered nurse
   C. Nurse practitioner
   D. Nutritionist

Case 1 Scott, the Professional Triathlete

Scott is a 29-year-old professional triathlete. He is 6′2″ and 170 pounds (BMI 21.8 kg/m2). Triathlon season is underway and Scott has intensified his training to compete in the Kona Ironman Triathlon.

1. On the initial intake interview, Scott shares that he takes several supplements. He says that he takes iron supplements to prevent nutritional deficiency given his rigorous endurance training, a multivitamin to ensure adequate nutrient intake, caffeine to help improve performance, and glutamine because all of his colleagues swear by it.
   a. What is your approach to a client who takes a supplement to prevent or treat nutritional deficiency?
   b. If Scott asks you what you think about the use of multivitamins to provide a more convenient form of nutrients, what will you tell him?
   c. What are a few important considerations for clients taking supplements to improve athletic performance?
   d. What is your response to a client taking a supplement because "everyone else is doing it"?
2. Scott tells you that he is planning to try an ergogenic supplement, but before he takes it he wants to be certain that this supplement is safe and effective. What process might you recommend that he undertake to get information on the safety and efficacy of the supplement? How is this process different from the process he might take to understand the safety and efficacy of a medication prescribed by his physician?

   Now, choose a supplement that you are interested in learning more about. Research whether it is considered to be safe and effective. (Go through the process you would recommend to this client). What did you find?

Case 2 Eric, the Recreational Bodybuilder

Eric is a 31-year-old competitive bodybuilder. He participates in bodybuilding competitions in the fall and trains the rest of the year. He is 5′11″ and weighs 184 pounds. He currently is in summer training. Eric tells you that he takes several performance-enhancing supplements including creatine androstenedione and L-arginine.

1. Eric takes 30 grams of creatine per day. He says that while this is working for him, he is thinking about increasing his intake to 45 grams of creatine per day. He asks if you think the increased dosage will lead to further enhanced performance.

   Health professionals are often asked to comment on the usefulness of taking various supplements. What is the scope of practice related to nutrition advice in your state? Describe several ways you may talk about supplements with your clients while staying within your scope of practice. Describe how you might answer Eric's question.

Refer to the Commission on Dietetic Registration website (www.cdrnet.org) to get started.

2. Several of your clients take L-arginine supplements to boost muscular strength before workouts. To learn more about this supplement, you look at the supplement nutrition label and ingredient list on several L-arginine supplements. Below is an example label:

Supplement Facts
Serving Size: 10 Grams (1 Level Scoop)
Servings Per Container: 30

	Amount Per Serving	%DV*
Calories	5	
Total Carbohydrate	1 g	0%
Total Fat	0 g	0%
Vitamin C (as ascorbic acid)	60 mg	100%
Vitamin D (as cholecalciferol)	2,500 IU	625%
Vitamin K (as phytonadione)	20 mcg	25%
Vitamin B6 (as pyridoxine hcl)	2 mg	100%
Folate (Folic Acid)	400 mcg	100%
Vitamin B12 (as cyanocobalamin)	15 mcg	250%
Magnesium Citrate	20 mg	5%
Chromium Aminonicotinate	200 mcg	167%
L-Arginine	5,000 mg	**
L-Citrulline	1,000 mg	**
Resveratrol	100 mg	**
Astaxanthin (Haematococcus pluvialis)	8 mg	**

* % Daily Value based on a 2,000 calorie diet.
** Daily Value not established.

Other Ingredients: Citric Acid, Natural Flavors, Vegetable Juice Color, Tricalcium Phosphate, Stevia.

a. How is this label different from the nutrition label on foods?

b. What information on the label could be a potential source of concern?

TRAIN YOURSELF

1. Do you take or have you ever taken any supplements? If yes, why did you take the supplement? Did you experience any beneficial or harmful effect from the supplement? What is your current opinion of the supplement?
   If you have never taken any supplements, have you ever considered taking a supplement? Why did you decide not to take it? While reviewing this chapter, were there any supplements that seemed appealing to you? Why or why not? Do you think you will try any of the supplements described?
2. You were recently offered a job working at a popular gym in town. During your tour and interview of the facility, you notice that the gym sells a variety of supplements. How do you feel about this? What questions would you ask your potential employer? How would this affect your decision, if at all, whether or not to work at the gym?

RESOURCES

Dietary Supplements Labels Database (www.dietarysupplements.nlm.nih.gov/). The database has information on the ingredients for thousands of dietary supplements sold in the United States. Look up products by brand name, uses, active ingredient, or manufacturer.

Office of Dietary Supplements of the National Institute of Health (http://ods.od.nih.gov/). Aims to strengthen knowledge and understanding of dietary supplements by evaluating scientific information, stimulating and supporting research, disseminating research results, and educating the public to foster an enhanced quality of life and health for the U.S. population.

National Center for Complementary and Alternative Medicine (NCCAM) of the National Institutes of Health (http://nccam.nih.gov). The NCCAM maintains a list of supplements that are under regulatory review or that have been reported to cause adverse effects in addition to a general listing of dietary and herbal supplements.

Food and Drug Administration (FDA) Dietary Supplements Alerts and Safety Information (www.fda.gov/Food/DietarySupplements/Alerts/default.htm). The FDA website provides information and updates regarding supplement regulations and safety issues.
The following three organizations provide supplement testing and assurances of compliance with FDA regulations:

- **U.S. Pharmacopeia** (www.usp.org)
- **ConsumerLab.com** (www.consumerlab.com)
- **NSF International** (www.nsf.org)

Pubmed Dietary Supplement Subset (http://ods.od.nih.gov/Research/PubMed_Dietary_Supplement_Subset.aspx) Pubmed provides an easy-to-use search engine to identify published scientific literature of interest. The subset is designed to limit search results to citations from a broad spectrum of dietary supplement literature including vitamin, mineral, phytochemical, ergogenic, botanical, and herbal supplements in human nutrition and animal models.

REFERENCES

1. Jenkinson DM, Harbert AJ. Supplements and sports. *Am Fam Physician*. November 1 2008;78(9):1039-1046.
2. O'Neill A. Fatal choice. *People Magazine*. Vol. 52;1999.
3. Nahin RJ, Barnes PM, Stussman BJ, Bloom B. *Cost of Complementary and Alternative Medicine (CAM) and Frequency of Visits to CAM Providers*. National Health Statistics Reports; July 30 2009.
4. Commission on Dietary Supplement Labels. Chapter 1. Dietary supplement health and education act of 1994. www.health.gov/dietsupp/ch1.htm. Accessed April 14, 2013.
5. Dietary Supplement Health and Education Act of 1994. In: Congree R, Ed. *Public Law 103-417*, 1994.

6. Food and Drug Administration. Dietary Supplement Current Good Manufacturing Practices and Interim Final Rule Facts; 2007.
7. Neuhouser ML, Wassertheil-Smoller S, Thomson C, et al. Multivitamin use and risk of cancer and cardiovascular disease in the Women's Health Initiative cohorts. *Arch Intern Med.* February 9 2009;169(3):294-304.
8. Sesso HD, Buring JE, Christen WG, et al. Vitamins E and C in the prevention of cardiovascular disease in men: the Physicians' Health Study II randomized controlled trial. *JAMA.* November 12 2008;300(18):2123-2133.
9. Gaziano JM, Glynn RJ, Christen WG, et al. Vitamins E and C in the prevention of prostate and total cancer in men: the Physicians' Health Study II randomized controlled trial. *JAMA.* January 7 2009;301(1):52-62.
10. Mursu J, Robien K, Harnack LJ, Park K, Jacobs DR, Jr. Dietary supplements and mortality rate in older women: the Iowa Women's Health Study. *Arch Intern Med.* October 10 2011;171(18):1625-1633.
11. Klein EA, Thompson IM, Jr., Tangen CM, et al. Vitamin E and the risk of prostate cancer: the Selenium and Vitamin E Cancer Prevention Trial (SELECT). *JAMA.* October 12 2011;306(14):1549-1556.
12. Bjelakovic G, Nikolova D, Gluud LL, Simonetti RG, Gluud C. Mortality in randomized trials of antioxidant supplements for primary and secondary prevention: systematic review and meta-analysis. *JAMA.* February 28 2007;297(8): 842-857.
13. Slomski A. IOM endorses vitamin D, calcium only for bone health, dispels deficiency claims. *JAMA.* February 2 2011;305(5):453-454, 456.
14. Hoffman JR, Falvo MJ. Protein: which is best? *J Sport Sci Med.* 2004;3:118-130.
15. Erdman JW, Jr. AHA Science Advisory: soy protein and cardiovascular disease: a statement for healthcare professionals from the Nutrition Committee of the AHA. *Circulation.* November 14 2000;102(20):2555-2559.
16. Sacks FM, Lichtenstein A, Van Horn L, Harris W, Kris-Etherton P, Winston M. Soy protein, isoflavones, and cardiovascular health: an American Heart Association Science Advisory for professionals from the Nutrition Committee. *Circulation.* February 21 2006;113(7):1034-1044.
17. Riediger ND, Othman RA, Suh M, Moghadasian MH. A systemic review of the roles of n-3 fatty acids in health and disease. *J Am Diet Assoc.* April 2009;109(4):668-679.
18. Kris-Etherton PM, Grieger JA, Etherton TD. Dietary reference intakes for DHA and EPA. *Prostaglandins Leukot Essent Fatty Acids.* August-September 2009;81(2-3):99-104.
19. USADA. Statement from USADA CEO Travis T. Tygart regarding the U.S. Postal Service pro cycling team doping conspiracy. Statement released 10-10-12. http://cyclinginvestigation.usada.org/. Accessed April 14, 2013.
20. *The World Anti-Doping Code: The 2012 Prohibited List: International Standard.* World Anti-Doping Agency; 2012.
21. Burke LM, Castell LM, Stear SJ. BJSM reviews: A-Z of supplements: dietary supplements, sports nutrition foods and ergogenic aids for health and performance part 1. *Br J Sports Med.* October 2009;43(10):728-729.
22. Currell K, Syed A, Dziedzic CE, et al. BJSM reviews: A-Z of nutritional supplements: dietary supplements, sports nutrition foods and ergogenic aids for health and performance part 12. *Br J Sports Med.* 2010;44:905-907.
23. Armstrong LE, Casa DJ, Maresh CM, Ganio MS. Caffeine, fluid-electrolyte balance, temperature regulation, and exercise-heat tolerance. *Exerc Sport Sci Rev.* July 2007;35(3): 135-140.
24. Frary CD, Johnson RK, Wang MQ. Food sources and intakes of caffeine in the diets of persons in the United States. *J Am Diet Assoc.* January 2005;105(1):110-113.
25. Keisler BD, Armsey TD, 2nd. Caffeine as an ergogenic aid. *Curr Sports Med Rep.* June 2006;5(4):215-219.
26. Bell DG, McLellan TM, Sabiston CM. Effect of ingesting caffeine and ephedrine on 10-km run performance. *Med Sci Sports Exerc.* February 2002;34(2):344-349.
27. Kerksick CM, Rasmussen CJ, Lancaster SL, et al. The effects of protein and amino acid supplementation on performance and training adaptations during ten weeks of resistance training. *J Strength Cond Res / Nat Strength & Cond Assoc.* August 2006;20(3):643-653.
28. Blomstrand E. A role for branched-chain amino acids in reducing central fatigue. *J Nutr.* February 2006;136(2): 544S-547S.
29. Rodriguez NR, Di Marco NM, Langley S. American College of Sports Medicine position stand. Nutrition and athletic performance. *Med Sci Sports Exerc.* March 2009;41(3):709-731.
30. Rawson ES, Volek JS. Effects of creatine supplementation and resistance training on muscle strength and weightlifting performance. *J Strength Cond Res / Nat Strength & Cond Assoc.* November 2003;17(4):822-831.
31. Poortmans JR, Rawson ES, Burke LM, Stear SJ, Castell LM. A-Z of nutritional supplements: dietary supplements, sports nutrition foods and ergogenic aids for health and performance Part 11. *Br J Sports Med.* August 2010;44(10):765-766.
32. Lansley KE, Winyard PG, Bailey SJ, et al. Acute dietary nitrate supplementation improves cycling time trial performance. *Med Sci Sports Exerc.* June 2011;43(6):1125-1131.
33. Ang-Lee MK, Moss J, Yuan C. Herbal medicines and perioperative care. *JAMA.* 2001;286(2):208-216.
34. Lundh A, Sismondo S, Lexchin J, Busuioc OA, Bero L. Industry sponsorship and research outcome. *Cochrane Database of Systematic Reviews.* December 12 2012;12:MR000033.
35. Lansley KE, Winyard PG, Fulford J, et al. Dietary nitrate supplementation reduces the O_2 cost of walking and running: a placebo-controlled study. *J Appl Physiol.* March 2011;110(3):591-600.
36. Lundberg JO, Carlstrom M, Larsen FJ, Weitzberg E. Roles of dietary inorganic nitrate in cardiovascular health and disease. *Cardiovasc Res.* February 15 2011;89(3):525-532.
37. Rodriguez NR, Di Marco NM, Langley S. American College of Sports Medicine position stand. Nutrition and athletic performance. *Med Sci Sports Exerc.* March 2009;41(3):709-731.
38. Sumner MD, Elliott-Eller M, Weidner G, et al. Effects of pomegranate juice consumption on myocardial perfusion in patients with coronary heart disease. *Am J Cardiol.* September 15 2005;96(6):810-814.
39. Aviram M, Rosenblat M, Gaitini D, et al. Pomegranate juice consumption for 3 years by patients with carotid artery stenosis reduces common carotid intima-media thickness, blood pressure and LDL oxidation. *Clin Nutr.* June 2004; 23(3):423-433.
40. Rosenblat M, Hayek T, Aviram M. Anti-oxidative effects of pomegranate juice (PJ) consumption by diabetic patients on serum and on macrophages. *Atherosclerosis.* August 2006;187(2):363-371.
41. Mertens-Talcott SU, Rios J, Jilma-Stohlawetz P, et al. Pharmacokinetics of anthocyanins and antioxidant effects after the consumption of anthocyanin-rich acai juice and pulp (Euterpe oleracea Mart.) in human healthy volunteers. *J Agric Food Chem.* September 10 2008;56(17):7796-7802.
42. Jensen GS, Wu X, Patterson KM, et al. In vitro and in vivo antioxidant and anti-inflammatory capacities of an antioxidant-rich fruit and berry juice blend. Results of a pilot and randomized, double-blinded, placebo-controlled, crossover study. *J Agric Food Chem.* September 24 2008; 56(18):8326-8333.
43. Amagase H, Nance DM. A randomized, double-blind, placebo-controlled, clinical study of the general effects of a standardized Lycium barbarum (Goji) Juice, GoChi. *J Altern Complement Med.* May 2008;14(4):403-412.
44. Pedraza-Chaverri J, Cardenas-Rodriguez N, Orozco-Ibarra M, Perez-Rojas JM. Medicinal properties of mangosteen

(Garcinia mangostana). *Food Chem Toxicol.* October 2008; 46(10):3227-3239.
45. Stear S, Burke L, Castell LM. BJSM reviews: A-Z of nutritional supplements: dietary supplements, sports nutrition foods and ergogenic aids for health and performance part 3. *Br J Sports Med.* 2009;43:890-892.
46. Burke L, Castell LM, Stear S, et al. BJSM reviews: A-Z of nutritional supplements: dietary supplements, sports nutrition foods and ergogenic aids for health and performance part 4. *Br J Sports Med.* 2009;43:1088-1090.
47. Castell LM, Burke L, Stear S, McNaughton LR, Harris RC. BJSM reviews: A-Z of nutritional supplements: dietary supplements, sports nutrition foods and ergogenic aids for health and performance part 5. *Br J Sports Med.* 2010;44: 77-78.
48. Newsholme P, Krause M, Newsholme EA, Stear S, Burke L, Castell LM. BJSM reviews: A to Z of nutritional supplements: dietary supplements, sports nutrition foods and ergogenic aids for health and performance part 18. *Br J Sports Med.* 2011;45:230-232.
49. Castell LM, Burke L, Stear S. BJSM Reviews: A-Z of supplements: dietary supplements, sports nutrition foods and ergogenic aids for health and performance part 2. *Br J Sports Med.* 2009;43:807-810.
50. Stear S, Castell LM, Burke L, et al. BJSM reviews: A-Z of nutritional supplements: dietary supplements, sports nutrition foods and ergogenic aids for health and performance part 10. *Br J Sports Med.* 2010;44:688-690.
51. Newmaster, S.G., Grguric, M, Shanmughanandhan, D., et al. DNA barcoding detects contamination and substitution in North American herbal products. *BMC Medicine.* 2013; 11: 222.
52. Bolland, M.J., Grey, A., Gamble, G.D., Reid, I.R. The effect of vitamin D supplementation on skeletal, vascular, or cancer outcomes: a trial sequential meta-analysis. *The Lancet Diabetes & Endocrinology.* Early online publication 24 January 2014 doi: 10.1016/S2213-8587(13)70212-2.
53. Fortmann, S.P., Burda, B.U., Senger, C.A., et al. Vitamin and mineral supplements in the primary prevention of cardiovascular disease and cancer: an updated systematic evidence review for the U.S. Preventive Services Task Force. *Annals of Internal Medicine.* 2013; 159(12): 824-834.
54. Grodstein, F., O'Brien, J., Kang, J.H., et al. Long-term multivitamin supplementation and cognitive function in men. A randomized trial. *Annals of Internal Medicine.* 2013; 159, 806-814.
55. Lamas, G.A., Boineau, R., Goertz, C., et al. Oral high-dose multivitamins and minerals after myocardial infarction. A randomized trial. *Annals of Internal Medicine.* 2013; 159(12): 797-804.
56. Guallar, E., Stranges, S., Mulrow, C., et al. Enough is enough: stop wasting money on vitamin and mineral supplements. *Annals of Internal Medicine.* 2013; 159(12): 850-851.
57. World Anti-Doping Agency. The world anti-doping code. The 2014 prohibited list. International Standard. Available at http://www.wada-ama.org/Documents/World_Anti-Doping_Program/WADP-Prohibited-list/2014/WADA-prohibited-list-2014-EN.pdf; retrieved February 11, 2014.

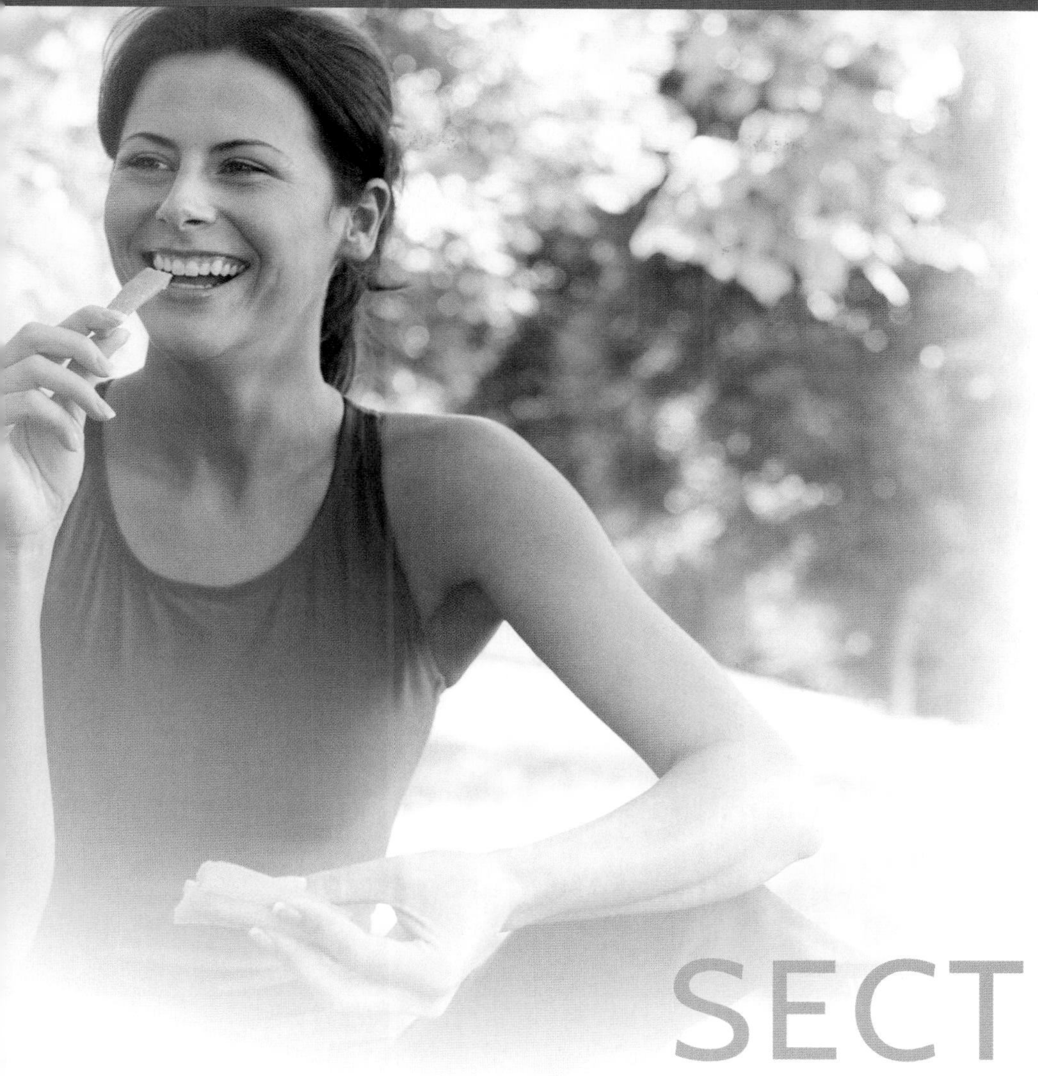

SECTION 3

Evaluation of Nutritional Status

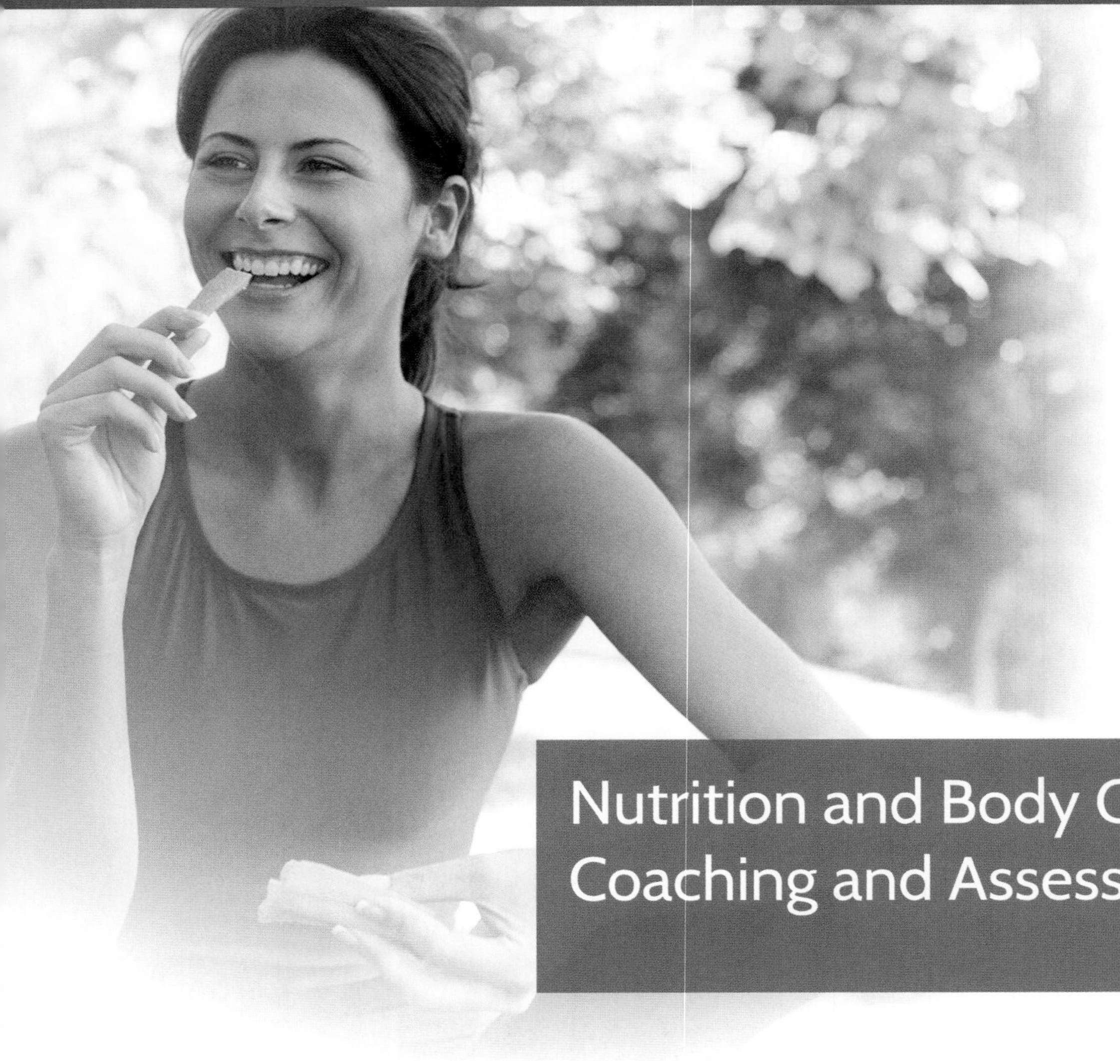

CHAPTER 11

Nutrition and Body Composition Coaching and Assessment

CHAPTER OUTLINE

CHAPTER OUTLINE—cont'd

LEARNING OBJECTIVES

After studying this chapter, the reader should be able to:

11.1 Describe the procedures, benefits, uses, and limitations of indirect, direct, and reference methods of assessing body composition.

11.2 Outline the process of a nutrition assessment and explain which components are within and outside the health professional's scope of practice.

11.3 Explain how a health professional might help to coach a client to achieve an improved body composition.

KEY TERMS

air displacement plethysmography (ADP) (brand name is BodPod) A device that uses the displacement of air to measure body volume and density; compare to hydrostatic weighing which uses the displacement of water to estimate body composition.

android obesity Excess weight distributed mostly in the abdomen ("apple shape").

bioelectrical impedance analysis An indirect measure of body composition that measures the conduction of current through muscle and fat, and inserts data into a predictive equation to estimate fat mass and lean mass.

body composition The proportion of fat and lean mass.

body density Calculated by dividing body weight by body volume; an intermediary to convert circumference measurements to body fat percentage.

body mass index Weight in kilograms divided by height in meters squared; a proxy for measurement of body composition.

certified specialist in sports dietetics Working as a registered dietitian for a minimum of 2 years applying evidence-based nutrition knowledge in exercise and sports and having received a passing score on a board-certifying exam. They assess, educate, and counsel athletes and active individuals. They design, implement, and manage safe and effective nutrition strategies that enhance lifelong health, fitness, and optimal performance (definition from the Commission on Dietetic Registration, www.cdrnet.org).

decisional balance The weighing of pros and cons when considering a behavior change.

dual-energy x-ray absorptiometry (DXA) A method of body composition assessment that maps the bone density, fat mass, and fat-free tissue mass using two low-dose x-rays from different sources that measure bone and soft tissue mass simultaneously.

ectomorph Body type characterized by thinness with lean muscles, fast metabolism, and difficulty gaining weight.

empathic statements Statements that express an attempt to understand what another person is experiencing.

endomorph Body type characterized by a slow metabolism and propensity to gain fat.

essential fat The fat required for normal body functioning including that of the brain, nerves, heart, lungs, and liver; typically 3% to 5% in men and 10% to 15% in women.

field methods Techniques health professionals commonly use to measure body composition.

food frequency questionnaire A method used to identify typical eating habits, which is composed of a checklist of foods and beverages with a section for the client to mark how often each of the listed foods are eaten.

food record A written report of all of the foods consumed in a pre-defined period of time, usually 3 days with at least 1 weekend day. Also includes the time of day, mood, and level of hunger when consuming each food.

gravitational sport A sport in which the force of gravity combined with an athlete's body mass impacts performance; examples include long-distance running, road cycling, and ski jumping.

gynoid obesity Excess weight distributed mostly in the hips and thighs ("pear shape").

health history questionnaire A form that aims to gather information about an individual's past medical history and family history to assess a client's health risk and determine need for evaluation by a medical professional.

Health Insurance Portability and Accountability Act (HIPAA) Federal legislation that requires express written permission from a patient or client authorizing sharing of health information among health professionals and institutions.

health screening A systematic assessment of a client's health history and risk factors to identify clients who may require evaluation by other health professionals before beginning a nutrition or activity program.

hydrostatic weighing Also known as underwater weighing and hydrodensitometry; measures body composition by comparing the weight of a person in water and on land.

indirect calorimetry A noninvasive study that estimates energy needs based on the use of oxygen and production of carbon dioxide.

laboratory methods Techniques to measure body composition, generally in a research or laboratory setting; methods include hydrodensitometry, air displacement plethysmography, isotope dilution, and dual-energy x-ray absorptiometry

mesomorph Body type characterized by an athletic and muscular physique.

multi-component model A reference method of assessing body composition that bases an estimate of fat and lean mass on measurements from several methods; the four-component equation is the leading reference method. The variables include body volume, total body water, bone mineral, and body mass.

near-infrared interactance Estimates body composition using the optical densities of skin, fat, and lean tissue as an infrared light probe is reflected off bone and back to the probe.

nonessential fat Triglycerides and other fatty tissue stored in muscle, around vital organs, and within subcutaneous tissue.

nutrition assessment Evaluation of nutrition status and nutritional needs.

power-to-weight ratio The amount of force generated divided by body mass, or force adjusted by weight; a high ratio especially benefits athletic performance in gravitational sports like long-distance running and road cycling.

rapport Relationship of trust and respect.

reference methods The most accurate, but least practical, methods used to measure body composition; infrequently used in practice or in research studies of body composition; includes CT scan, MRI, and multi-component models.

registered dietitian A health professional with specialized training in nutrition who has completed the minimum requirements for the credential including a bachelor degree, completion of an accredited program in nutrition and 1,200 hours of an approved supervised internship in nutrition, and passed a national examination. The registered dietitian is an expert in nutrition and is qualified to provide individualized nutrition assessment and recommendations, and to provide medical nutrition therapy.

reliability The reproducibility of a measure.

resting energy expenditure (REE) The number of calories expended at rest to maintain normal vital function. Also referred to as resting metabolic rate (RMR).

screening tool A test that is useful in identifying nearly all people who have a condition, but that typically has a high "false positive" rate in that not everyone who tests "positive" actually has the condition.

skinfold calipers A hand-held device used to measure in millimeters the thickness of subcutaneous fat at standardized locations in the body.

somatotype Body type.

stages of change Also known as transtheoretical model, a theory of behavior change which posits that people progress through a series of stages as they ready themselves to make a behavioral change, such as modification to nutrition or physical activity behaviors.

SuperTracker An online tool from the U.S. Department of Agriculture that can be used to track, analyze, and evaluate nutrition and physical activity.

three-dimensional photonic scanning Uses a low-power laser light and digital cameras to rapidly produce a 3-D digital model of the human body, which is used to approximate lean and fat mass.

24-hour recall A method of gaining information about a client's eating habits by asking for detailed information about the foods and drinks the client consumed in the 24 hours prior to the consultation.

validity The accuracy of a measure.

waist-to-hip ratio Waist circumference divided by hip circumference; a number greater than or equal to 1.0 confers increased health risk; a ratio of 0.9 or less in men and 0.8 or less in women is considered safe.

INTRODUCTION

Retired NBA Hall-of-Fame athlete Charles Barkley prevailed on the basketball court. Small for a power forward at 6′6″ and 252 pounds, Barkley still dominated his opponents, becoming only the fourth NBA player to accumulate 20,000 points, 10,000 rebounds, and 4,000 assists. At the elite level of an NBA star with unlimited access to myriad premier coaches, sports dietitians, athletic trainers, chefs, and other health professionals and supporters, Barkley maintained a high level of fitness and nutrition to match his level of intense exercise and athletic performance. But after his retirement, with a minimal fitness routine and dietary habits that no longer matched his nutritional needs, Barkley publicly battled a rapidly changing body composition and gained over 100 pounds.

Barkley provides an example of an athlete who struggled to apply his understanding of nutrition and body composition to making healthful nutritional choices to match nutritional needs. Many athletes of all levels suffer from suboptimal nutrition knowledge and significant difficulties in translating nutrition information into a healthy and appropriate eating plan. Qualified health professionals can help to fill the gap and prepare athletes to make smart nutritional choices, not only to fuel peak athletic performance, but also to maintain a healthy lifestyle at all levels of physical fitness.

NUTRITION AND BODY COMPOSITION COACHING AND HEALTH PROFESSIONALS

While elite athletes may have access to sports dietitians to help them develop a meal plan that is in perfect alignment with their fitness program, many amateur and recreational athletes either do not have access to or may not have the resources to afford the individualized and specialized attention of these professionals. In other cases, athletes work with a **registered dietitian** who is board certified in sports dietetics, but still rely on other health professionals to provide nutrition information, tips, and resources. In either case, widespread access to credible nutrition information and knowledge prepares athletes not only for peak athletic performance but also to make healthful nutrition choices, set and achieve body composition goals, and fuel a healthy and active lifestyle.

In many cases an athlete strives to optimize nutrition to directly improve performance and also to improve or modify **body composition**, an important predictor of athletic success for many sports. By being prepared to include body composition assessment, education, and coaching in a conversation or consultation related to nutrition, a health professional provides the athlete a valuable service and further links the critical components of optimal athletic performance: fitness training with strategic fueling and hydration.

In some cases an athlete will require comprehensive, individualized assessment and consultation to meet nutritional needs, achieve body composition goals, help manage an underlying medical or nutritional disorder, or receive treatment or therapy for an eating or exercise disorder. There may be many additional situations in which the athlete's needs are best met through consultation or in collaboration with another health professional, such as a registered dietitian, physician, or mental health professional. A health professional can identify those clients who require specialized attention or referrals through an initial **health screening**. Health screening is the systematic assessment of the client's health history and risk factors to identify clients who may require evaluation by other health professionals before beginning a nutrition or activity program. The Communication Strategies feature and Figure 11-1 provide an overview of the health screening as well as a sample **health history questionnaire** to help guide health professionals through the initial interview.

Regardless of the profession chosen, it is essential for a health professional to be able to recognize when a client's interests are best met with the services of a specially trained and qualified professional. Common situations in which a referral is indicated—and to whom these athletes should be referred—are highlighted in Table 11-1. While a client may initially require referral to a physician or registered dietitian, in many cases the client may only require a one-time evaluation or consultation and then be referred back to the health professional. Other times, the client may require ongoing assessment or treatment before he or she is cleared to participate in sports or follow a general nutrition plan. Prior to initiating referrals to other health professionals, it is essential to ask a client to sign a **Health Insurance Portability and Accountability Act** (HIPAA) release form, which provides authorization to share certain health information. A sample form is included in Figure 11-2. If this form is not available, or if a client declines to sign it, the health professional can verbally recommend to the client to see his or her primary care physician and arrange for follow-up once the client has documented clearance from the health provider.

SPEED BUMP

1. **List the essential components of the initial interview.**
2. **Describe the importance of health screening.**
3. **List several situations in which a client should be referred to another health professional.**

BODY COMPOSITION ASSESSMENT

The nutritional goals and objectives for many athletes and recreational exercisers are directly tied to weight management and optimization of body composition. Whether the athlete's goal is to lose weight in general,

CONFIDENTIAL

Health, Nutrition, and Fitness Questionnaire

Name ______________________ Age ______ Gender ________ Date ________

Email ______________________ Phone number ____________

Health Goals

1. Please describe your major health, nutrition, and/or fitness goals: ______________
2. What are the two to three biggest barriers to achieving these goals? ______________
3. What are the two to three greatest strengths that will help you to achieve these goals? ______________
4. Please check the box that best describes how ready you are to make changes to your lifestyle to achieve these goals:
   ☐ Do not believe I need to change ☐ Would like to change, but don't think that I can ☐ Would like to intensify changes
   ☐ Will make changes soon ☐ Recently started to make changes (past 6 months) ☐ Made changes, but relapsed
5. On a scale of 1-10, how important is this change to you? ______
6. On a scale of 1-10, how confident are you that you will achieve this change? ______

Medical Information

7. How would you describe your health? Excellent Good Fair Poor
8. Are you taking any prescription or over-the-counter medications or dietary herbs or supplements? Yes No
   If yes, please list the medications and state the reason for taking: ______________
9. When was the last time you visited your physician? ______________
10. Do I have permission to communicate with your physician? Yes No If yes, please state your physician's name and contact phone number. (See HIPPA release form.) ______________
11. Do you have or has your doctor or another licensed health-care professional told you that you have any of the following conditions?
   - ☐ Allergies (specify: ________)
   - ☐ Amenorrhea or absence of menstrual period >3 months
   - ☐ Anemia
   - ☐ Anxiety
   - ☐ Arthritis
   - ☐ Asthma
   - ☐ Cancer
   - ☐ Cardiovascular disease
   - ☐ Celiac disease
   - ☐ Chronic sinus condition
   - ☐ Cigarette smoker
   - ☐ Crohn's disease
   - ☐ Depression
   - ☐ Diabetes
   - ☐ Disordered eating
   - ☐ Intestinal problems
   - ☐ Gastroesophageal reflux (GERD)
   - ☐ High blood pressure/hypertension
   - ☐ High cholesterol
   - ☐ Hyper/hypothyroidism
   - ☐ Insomnia
   - ☐ Intestinal problems
   - ☐ Irritable bowel syndrome
   - ☐ Osteoporosis
   - ☐ Polycystic ovary disease
   - ☐ Currently pregnant or <3 months post-partum
   - ☐ Skin problems. Describe: ________
   - ☐ Surgeries. Describe: ________
   - ☐ Past injuries. Describe: ________
   - ☐ Describe any other health conditions you have, or for which you take medication: ________
12. Has anyone in your immediate family been diagnosed with any of the following? If yes, please describe

	Relationship (e.g., father)	Age of diagnosis		Relationship (e.g., father)	Age of diagnosis
Heart disease	________	________	Cancer	________	________
High cholesterol	________	________	Diabetes	________	________
High blood pressure	________	________	Osteoporosis	________	________

Nutrition History

13. Have you ever followed a modified diet to manage a health condition? Yes No If yes, please describe:
    ____
14. Do you follow a specialized diet (low carb, gluten-free, vegan, etc)? Yes No If yes, please describe the diet and reasons for following: ______________
    Was the diet prescribed by a physician? Yes No
15. Who purchases and prepares your food? ______________

Physical Activity History

16. Are you currently physically active? Yes No If yes, please describe:
    ______ minutes of cardiovascular activity, ______ times per week
    ______ minutes of strength or resistance training, ______ times per week
    ______ minutes of flexibility training, ______ times per week
17. Please list your favorite physical activites or sports in which you participate or compete, and the level of competition (if applicable):
    ____

Weight History

18. What would you like to do with your weight? ☐ lose ☐ maintain ☐ gain
19. What was your lowest weight in the past five years? ______ Your highest? ______
20. What is your current weight? ______ What is your height? ______

Other

Is there any other information you think I should know? Please use this space.

____

Thank you for your time and for sharing this information. It will be used to help develop a plan that will best meet your needs and help you to achieve your goals.

Figure 11-1. Health history questionnaire.

COMMUNICATION STRATEGIES

The Initial Interview and the Health History Questionnaire

The initial interview provides a health professional an opportunity to build **rapport** with clients. Similar to working with athletes in other roles of allied health, to be effective in helping an athlete to achieve nutrition and body composition goals it is essential to have a trusting relationship with the client. A health professional can begin to build rapport with a client from the start of the initial interview with a warm welcome and use of active listening techniques including use of open-ended questions, reflections, affirmations, summarizing, and empathic statements.

After the initial introductions and greetings, the health professional may ask the client to complete a health history questionnaire (Fig. 11-1). Alternatively, the client may have received and completed the questionnaire prior to the initial meeting. In either case, the initial interview should include discussion of the questionnaire to identify health risks, such as body composition and nutrition assessment, goal setting, and health education that may require evaluation by another health professional prior to initiating the nutrition coaching. In addition to the health history, the questionnaire in Figure 11-1 also asks nutrition, physical activity, and behavioral questions to better understand the client's motivation for seeking help. A "yes" answer to any of the medical or family history questions should warrant further evaluation by a physician.

CLASSROOM EXERCISE

In groups of two, conduct a mock initial intake with one student role-playing the nutrition coach and the other role-playing the athlete seeking nutrition consultation. Include an initial phase of rapport-building, discussion of the health history questionnaire, and an overview of the body composition and nutrition assessment process.

Table 11-1. **Making Referrals**

CONCERN	REFER TO . . .
Requests comprehensive individualized sports nutrition program for optimal athletic performance	Registered dietitian who is a board-certified specialist in sports dietetics (CSSD)
Demonstrates signs or symptoms of an eating disorder	Primary care physician, mental health specialist, registered dietitian with focus in eating disorders
Any significant underlying medical condition such as cardiovascular problems, hypertension, kidney disease, diabetes, arthritis, gastrointestinal problems	Primary care physician
Takes multiple medications or supplements or is considering starting new supplement	Primary care physician, registered dietitian
Pregnant or lactating	Primary care physician, registered dietitian
Recent injury and would like nutrition plan to enhance healing and recovery	Primary care physician, registered dietitian
Child, adolescent, or adult with obesity	Primary care physician

lose body fat, gain muscle mass, or maintain current weight, a discussion of body composition and goal setting to achieve realistic ideals is an important component of the fitness and nutrition plan for nearly all athletes. Many health professionals of varying backgrounds use body composition assessment to gain baseline information on a client's current weight status. Though body composition is only one marker of fitness—the others being cardiovascular endurance, muscle strength and endurance, and flexibility—it is generally the most convenient to assess (though not always the most accurate) and the most relevant to many clients (but not all of them). Box 11-1 highlights a few situations in which a discussion of body composition may best be deferred to a later date or skipped altogether.

Understanding Body Composition

Body composition refers to a person's proportion of fat; lean tissue, such as bone, muscle, and connective tissue; and water. Fat mass includes **essential fat**, the fat required for normal body functioning including that of the brain, nerves, heart, lungs, and liver; and

Authorization to Share Health Information

I, ____________________(client's name), authorize ____________________
(allied health professional's name) to share the following information:

☐ nutrition intake	☐ nutrition concerns	☐ eating behaviors
☐ body composition assessment results	☐ medication and supplement use	
☐ nutrition and body composition goals	☐ any information deemed necessary to improve health or athletic performance	

With the following individual or organization:
(Insert name, address, and phone number of individual or organization with whom the information will be shared)

____
____
____

This consent will be revoked on: ____________________
If no date is listed, it will be revoked in one year of the date of signature.

Athlete's signature: ____________________ Date: ____________

Figure 11-2. Sample HIPAA release form.

Box 11-1. When Body Composition Assessment Is Best Deferred

Most clients benefit from assessment of baseline body composition to help inform goals and provide a marker by which to judge success. However, in some cases the discussion and measurement of body composition may best be deferred to a later date. Health professionals should consider these potential scenarios when considering body composition assessment and coaching with clients, and make an informed decision as to whether or not to proceed.

- The severely obese client who is new to exercise. Many obese clients already know that their body composition is above the normal range. An initial detailed body composition assessment may not provide them with productive and meaningful information. Once the client has achieved considerable success, such as by improved health markers, decreased clothes size, and/or improved self-confidence, he or she may welcome a discussion of body composition and baseline measurement.
- A client struggling with an eating or exercise disorder or a client who perseverates about a number on a scale may be harmed more than helped by providing an extensive body composition evaluation. After the client has developed a healthier relationship with food and body image, body composition assessment may be a useful tool.
- Limited experience or confidence of assessor or questionable quality or reliability of the body composition assessment tool. In most cases, forgoing body composition assessment is more productive for the client than engaging in the assessment when the results may be significantly skewed.

nonessential fat, primarily triglycerides which are stored in muscle tissue (intramuscular triglycerides), around vital organs (visceral fat), and within subcutaneous tissue (adipose tissue). Essential body fat ranges from 3% to 5% for men and 12% to 14% for women.[1] Women have higher essential fat requirements than men to support menstrual function, childbearing, and lactation. Table 11-2 highlights approximate age- and gender-specific body composition norms.

Body composition is determined by both modifiable and nonmodifiable factors. Modifiable factors include a person's fitness training regimen and dietary habits. Nonmodifiable factors include gender, age, ethnicity, **somatotype** (body type), and distribution of type 1 versus type 2 muscle fibers. The three somatotypes—**mesomorph**, **endomorph**, and **ectomorph**—and the sports in which each body type is likely to dominate are described in Box 11-2. Most people express some

Table 11-2. Percent Body Fat Norms for Men and Women

CLASSIFICATION	MEN				WOMEN			
	12–18 years	**20–40 years**	**40–60 years**	**60–80 years**	**12–18 years**	**20–40 years**	**40–60 years**	**60–80 years**
Very lean (95–99%)	8–9%	4–10 %	9–14%	11–16%	12–18%	10–14%	13–17%	14–17%
Excellent (80–90%)	9–11%	8–15%	15–19%	17–20%	15–23%	15–17%	17–23%	20–24%
Good-Fair (40–75%)	14–22%	16–21%	20–25%	21–25%	19–28%	17–25%	21–30%	25–32%
Poor (<40%)	>22%	>21%	>25%	>25%	>28%	>25%	>30%	>33%

Norms presented are based on body composition values collected from the Cooper Institute. Percentiles indicate the percentage of the population with a higher proportion of body fat. Values are approximate. Classification and table adapted from American College of Sports Medicine Guidelines for Exercise Testing and Prescription (2010)[1] and Laurson, KR et al. (2011) *Amer J Prev Med;* 41(4S2):S87-S92.[2]

Box 11-2. Somatotypes and Sports Performance

Three somatotypes—ectomorph, endomorph, and mesomorph—have been well described. The mesomorph body type is most conducive to athletic performance given the high metabolism, low body fat, and propensity to gain muscle. The average person encompasses a hybrid of the three types, so that an individual's body type falls along a continuum. While body type is genetically determined to an extent, with conscientious training and nutrition an athlete can train to achieve his or her full genetic potential.

BODY TYPE	SPORTS
Mesomorph 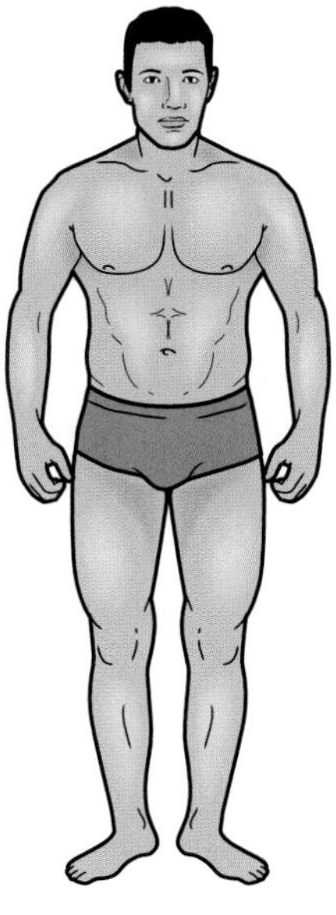 Mesomorph	• *Sports challenges:* Medium structure and height limits performance in sports that require very large or tall build such as football lineman or basketball forward or center • *Sports strengths:* Agility and speed; gain muscle easily; easy to lose and gain weight • *Ideal sports:* Power sports such as sprinting, mid-distance swimming, most team sports; gravitational sports that emphasize high strength-to-weight ratio such as distance running, cycling, triathlon, weightlifting

Continued

Box 11-2. Somatotypes and Sports Performance–cont'd

BODY TYPE	SPORTS
Ectomorph 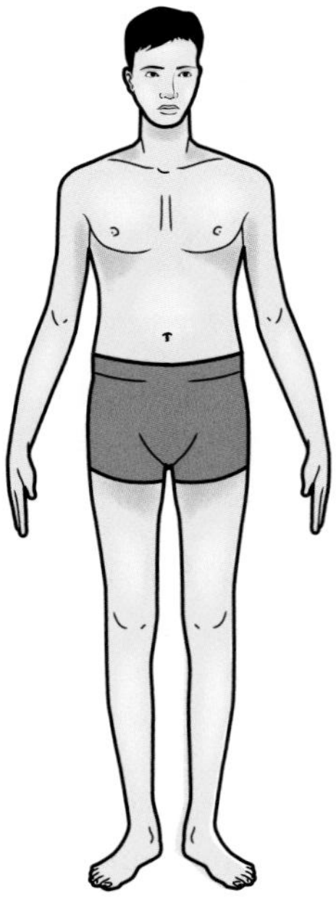 Ectomorph	• *Sports challenges:* Limited ability to gain mass restricts performance in power or strength sports • *Sports strengths:* Lean and thin enhances performance in gravitational sports • *Ideal sports:* Distance running, ultra-endurance events, aesthetic sports
Endomorph 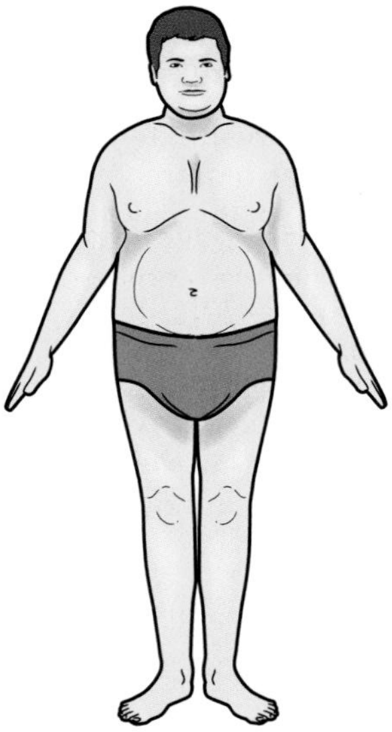 Endomorph	• *Sports challenges*: Agility and speed, sustained weight-bearing cardiovascular activities such as running; lose conditioning quickly once training/activity ceases • *Sports strengths*: Strong, large lung capacity • *Ideal sports*: Power lifting, football lineman, wrestling

combination of the somatotypes, such as endomorph-mesomorph or ectomorph-mesomorph. Somatotype is genetically determined; however, a strategic fitness training and nutrition program can help an athlete to optimize genetic potential.

Many elite athletes—especially those who engage in endurance, aesthetic, and **gravitational sports** such as long-distance running, road cycling, and ski jumping—have very low levels of body fat (Table 11-3). For these sports, a low weight, high muscle density, and low level of body fat contribute to a high **power-to-weight ratio** and improved performance. Other athletes, such as bodybuilders, strive for a high weight, high muscle density, and a low level of body fat to generate maximal muscular force. Athletes who compete in sports with specific weight requirements, such as wrestling, weight lifting, lightweight rowing, and many disciplines within martial arts, focus intensely on optimizing muscle mass and minimizing fat mass to achieve that weight. For athletes, the genetically determined components of body composition undoubtedly contribute to their success, but their attention to modifiable dietary habits and activity enable them to excel.

SPEED BUMP

4. Describe the major determinant of an individual's body composition.

Assessment Methods

Assessment of body composition by an appropriately trained and qualified professional provides useful information about health risk and a baseline to assess progress. Several **field methods** to measure body composition are currently used in practice, each with its own strengths and limitations. While these methods are the most practical, they also have the highest margin of error. Though more reliable than field methods, **laboratory methods** for assessing body composition tend to be more expensive and less accessible to the average athlete. The results attained using both field and laboratory methods are judged against **reference methods** to establish **reliability** and **validity**.[2]

Field Methods

Field methods are the body composition assessment methods most familiar to the majority of recreational and competitive athletes. The field methods include tools typically used for population screening, such as height and weight tables and body mass index, as well as the more informative tools of girth measurement, skinfolds, and bioelectrical impedance analysis.

Height and Weight Tables. Height and weight tables historically were the measures used to determine whether a person was classified as underweight, normal weight, or overweight based on weight, height, and frame size. They were initially developed in the 1940s by the MetLife Insurance Company to estimate the life expectancy for life insurance applicants. Currently, the height and weight tables are rarely used in practice and have largely been replaced by measurement of body mass index.

Body Mass Index. **Body mass index** (BMI) estimates a person's body composition by evaluating weight (in kilograms) divided by height (in meters) squared. BMI is a measure based exclusively on height and weight and does not assess fat mass, lean mass, or water weight. It is commonly evaluated in physician's offices and by other health-care providers to characterize a person as underweight (BMI <18.5), normal weight (BMI 18.5 to <25), overweight (BMI ≥25), or obese (BMI ≥30). While it is a useful **screening tool** to approximate body fat and better understand a person's health risk related to weight, it may falsely categorize certain individuals, especially those with high muscle mass (e.g., many athletes) and those with low weight but high fat mass (e.g., many older adults). Evaluating the Evidence highlights how body weight and body mass index are not necessarily correlated with fat mass.

EVALUATING THE EVIDENCE

The Relationship of BMI and Body Fatness Among Elite Female Athletes

The Study

Klungland Torstveit, M. and Sundgot-Borgen, J (2012). "Are under- and overweight female elite athletes thin and fat? A controlled study." ***Medicine & Science in Sports & Exercise,*** 44, 5, 949-957.[21]

Purpose

Compare BMI classification with body composition measured with dual-energy x-ray absorptiometry (DEXA) in elite female athletes and nonathletic controls.

Population and Methods

Norwegian females aged 13 to 39 years. A total of 186 elite athletes representing 46 sports and 145 controls participated in all three phases of the study (questionnaire, body composition measurement, and clinical interview).

The authors compared BMI and body composition of athletes and controls. They also compared body composition of athletes in technical sports, weight class sports, ball game sports, power sports, and gravitational sports. Results are summarized in the following table.

	DEXA BODY FAT 12% (EXTREMELY LEAN)	DXA BODY FAT ≥33% (OBESE)
	Athletes	
BMI 18.5–24.9 kg/m2	2%	6.7%
BMI ≥25 kg/m2	0%	58.8%
	Controls	
BMI 18.5–24.9 kg/m2	0%	50%
BMI ≥25 kg/m2	0%	97.1%

Continued

EVALUATING THE EVIDENCE–cont'd

Authors' Stated Conclusion

"Our data show BMI is not a valid measure for assessing or monitoring body composition in elite female athletes, and it should be used carefully in female nonathletes."

Critical Thinking Questions

1. In your own words, summarize the intention of this study.
2. If you were to conduct this study, what would be your hypothesis?
3. Explain–as if you were discussing with your neighbor or a lay person–the results from this study.
4. The authors conclude that BMI is not valid in athletes and limited in nonathletes. Explain why you agree or disagree with these findings.
5. List several potential limitations to this study.

Girth Measurements. Girth measurements are a useful tool for both recreational exercisers and elite athletes. For recreational exercisers, girth measurements are a minimally invasive approach to evaluate body size at various locations and monitor changes, especially in the waist and hips, where fat deposition is most likely to fluctuate. For elite athletes, circumference measurements may be most useful to identify body areas that are underdeveloped or overdeveloped, or to evaluate the effect of a training regimen on body size. To be useful, girth measurements must be collected using precise anatomical landmarks (Fig. 11-3). Apply the measuring tape lightly to the skin surface; the tape should be taut but not tight. Make duplicate measurements and calculate an average for reporting.

Circumference measures can be used to approximate body fat percentage. First, the values are used to calculate **body density**, which then is converted to body fat percentage. A regression equation to do this is shown in Box 11-3. The margin of error is about 2.5% to 4% for most people.[3,4] Measurements of very thin, very muscular, or very obese individuals substantially increase margins of error.

The waist and hip measurements can be used to calculate a **waist-to-hip ratio** (waist circumference/hip

Table 11-3. Body Mass Index

	NORMAL						OVERWEIGHT					OBESE					
BMI	**19**	**20**	**21**	**22**	**23**	**24**	**25**	**26**	**27**	**28**	**29**	**30**	**31**	**32**	**33**	**34**	**35**
HEIGHT (INCHES)	BODY WEIGHT (POUNDS)																
58	91	96	100	105	110	115	119	124	129	134	138	143	148	153	158	162	167
59	94	99	104	109	114	119	124	128	133	138	143	148	153	158	163	168	173
60	97	102	107	112	118	123	128	133	138	143	148	153	158	163	168	174	179
61	100	106	111	116	122	127	132	137	143	148	153	158	164	169	174	180	185
62	104	109	115	120	126	131	136	142	147	153	158	164	169	175	180	186	191
63	107	113	118	124	130	135	141	146	152	158	163	169	175	180	186	191	197
64	110	116	122	128	134	140	145	151	157	163	169	174	180	186	192	197	204
65	114	120	126	132	138	144	150	156	162	168	174	180	186	192	198	204	210
66	118	124	130	136	142	148	155	161	167	173	179	186	192	198	204	210	216
67	121	127	134	140	146	153	159	166	172	178	185	191	198	204	211	217	223
68	125	131	138	144	151	158	164	171	177	184	190	197	203	210	216	223	230
70	132	139	146	153	160	167	174	181	188	195	202	209	216	222	229	236	243
71	136	143	150	157	165	172	179	186	193	200	208	215	222	229	236	243	250
72	140	147	154	162	169	177	184	191	199	206	213	221	228	235	242	250	258
73	144	151	159	166	174	182	189	197	204	212	219	227	235	242	250	257	265
74	148	155	163	171	179	186	194	202	210	218	225	233	241	249	256	264	272
75	152	160	168	176	184	192	200	208	216	224	232	240	248	256	264	272	279
76	156	164	172	180	189	197	205	213	221	230	238	246	254	263	271	279	287

Adapted from Clinical Guidelines on the Identification, Evaluation, and Treatment of Overweight and Obesity in Adults: The Evidence Report.

circumference). Individuals with a ratio greater than 1.0 are at increased risk for cardiovascular disease and health problems. This is indicative of increased abdominal obesity (**android obesity** or "apple shape") as compared to **gynoid obesity** ("pear shape") in which more fat is deposited in the hips and thighs. A waist-to-hip ratio of 0.9 or less in men and 0.8 or less in women is considered "safe," though health risk is elevated for obese individuals in general.[5]

Skinfold Measurements. Skinfold measurements approximate body fat by measuring the amount of subcutaneous fat in various locations throughout the body. The thickness of the subcutaneous fat is measured to the nearest 1 millimeter with **skinfold calipers**. This method assumes that subcutaneous fat composition reflects internal fat composition.

The U.S. Olympic Committee advocates measurement of seven skinfold sites: abdomen, biceps, anterior thigh, medial calf, subscapular, supraspinale, and triceps, measured according to the standards set forth by the International Society for the Advancement of Kinanthropometry (ISAK).[6,7] A bullet-point overview of the standards is highlighted in Box 11-4. Figures 11-4 through 11-11 provide descriptions for measurement of each of the seven standard sites as well as chest measurement, which is not included in the seven-site recommendations but is frequently measured in the field. Health professionals working with elite athletes should become familiar with, and adhere to, these standards.

In practice, most health professionals use the three-site method: measuring chest, thigh, and abdomen in men and triceps, thigh, and supraspinale in women. While skinfold measurements can be entered into a prediction equation to estimate body fat, the estimates are prone to error. In fact, more than 100 such equations have been developed with only three deemed reliable for use in athletes.[8] Box 11-5 provides the commonly adapted Jackson-Pollock three-site equation. Though rates of error have the potential to be high, when assessors are trained and the retest measurements are obtained by the same individuals, the results can be meaningful and measurement error is about 3% to 3.5%.[2]

In addition to using skinfold measurement to estimate body fat, the sum of skinfold of the seven sites can be used as a marker to assess progress within a training program or to compare to age, gender, and sport norms. Ultimately, due to the low expense and convenience of this method, skinfold measurement is one of the methods of

				EXTREME OBESITY														
36	**37**	**38**	**39**	**40**	**41**	**42**	**43**	**44**	**45**	**46**	**47**	**48**	**49**	**50**	**51**	**52**	**53**	**54**
BODY WEIGHT (POUNDS)																		
172	177	181	186	191	196	201	205	210	215	220	224	229	234	239	244	248	253	258
178	183	188	193	198	203	208	212	217	222	227	232	237	242	247	252	257	262	267
184	189	194	199	204	209	215	220	225	230	235	240	245	250	255	261	266	271	276
190	195	201	206	211	217	222	227	232	238	243	248	254	259	264	269	275	280	285
196	202	207	213	218	224	229	235	240	246	251	256	262	267	273	278	284	289	295
203	208	214	220	225	231	237	242	248	254	259	265	270	278	282	287	293	299	304
209	215	221	227	232	238	244	250	256	262	267	273	279	285	291	296	302	308	314
216	222	228	234	240	246	252	258	264	270	276	282	288	294	300	306	312	318	324
223	229	235	241	247	253	260	266	272	278	284	291	297	303	309	315	322	328	334
230	236	242	249	255	261	268	274	280	287	293	299	306	312	319	325	331	338	344
236	243	249	256	262	269	276	282	289	295	302	308	315	322	328	335	341	348	354
250	257	264	271	278	285	292	299	306	313	320	327	334	341	348	355	362	369	376
257	265	272	279	286	293	301	308	315	322	329	338	343	351	358	365	372	379	386
265	272	279	287	294	302	309	316	324	331	338	346	353	361	368	375	383	390	397
272	280	288	295	302	310	318	325	333	340	348	355	363	371	378	386	393	401	408
280	287	295	303	311	319	326	334	342	350	358	365	373	381	389	396	404	412	420
287	295	303	311	319	327	335	343	351	359	367	375	383	391	399	407	415	423	431
295	304	312	320	328	336	344	353	361	369	377	385	394	402	410	418	426	435	443

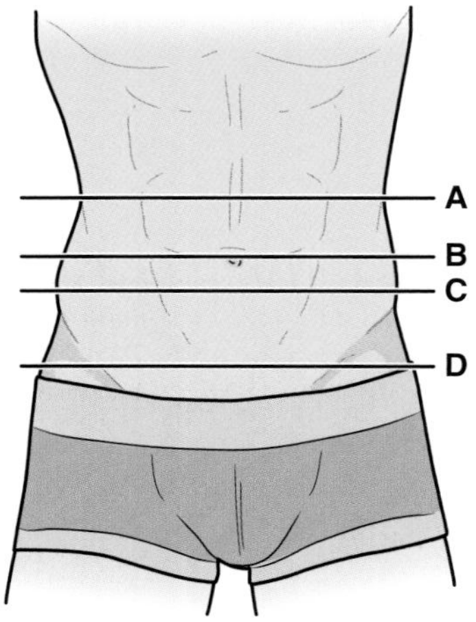

Figure 11-3. Circumference measurement landmarks. A. Waist circumference measurement is taken at the narrowest part of the torso. B. Abdominal circumference measurement is taken at the level of the navel. C. Iliac circumference measurement is taken level with the iliac crests. D. Hip circumference measurement is taken at the location with the largest circumference of the gluteals.

Box 11-3. Converting Circumference Measurements to Body Fat Percentage

1. Calculate body density (BD)
   For women:
   BD = 1.168297 – (2.824 × [MD3]10^{-3} × abdomen circumference (cm)) + (1.22098 × 10^{-5} × abdomen circumference (cm)^2) – [MD4](7.33128 × 10^{-4} × hip circumference (cm)) + (5.10477 × 10^{-4} × height (cm)) – 2.16161 × 10^{-4} × age)
   For men:
   BD = 1.21142 + (8.5x10^{-4} × weight (kg)) – (5.0 × 10^{-4} × iliac (cm)) – (6.1 × 10^{-4} × hip circumference (cm)) – (1.38 × 10^{-3} × abdomen circumference (cm))
2. Convert BD to percent fat
   Percent fat = (495/BD) – 450

estimating body fat composition most often used in practice. Health professionals planning to measure body composition with clients should consider undergoing in-person training to increase accuracy and reliability of measures and, consequently, usefulness of results.

Bioelectrical Impedance Analysis. Relying on a complex mathematical formulation translating the conduction of an electrical current through muscle (fast) compared with fat (slower), **bioelectrical impedance analysis** (BIA) provides a digital report of lean body tissue (Fig. 11-12). The most reliable BIA machine requires that a wrist and ankle electrode be placed on the participant. The participant remains still while the electrical current passes from the wrist through the body and into the foot. An accurate BIA reading relies heavily on adequate hydration status, among a variety of other factors highlighted in Box 11-6. Prerequisites for accurate BIA reporting may make the method unreasonable for highly competitive or elite athletes. When the corrective predictive equation is selected and the established protocol is followed, accuracy of BIA is similar to skinfold measurement with a standard error of about 3.5%.[2]

While most of the research evaluating the accuracy of BIA has been conducted on the standard BIA equipment, other less-expensive forms of BIA are available, including a scale-only and a hand-held device. These devices generally are not reliable due to their inability to differentiate between body types or provide consistent results.

Laboratory Methods

In addition to the body composition methods described above, which are used most frequently in practice, several other methods with lower rates of error are used as laboratory methods, mostly in research studies and in large medical centers or other facilities with financial support and access to resources.

Hydrostatic Weighing. **Hydrostatic weighing** was until recently considered the gold standard in the evaluation of body composition. This is the reference method against which many of the field methods have been judged in the scientific literature. With this method, the athlete, who is seated in a chair attached to a scale, is submerged in a tank of water. Body density is calculated by assessing the relationship of the person's weight on land with his or her weight in water. The method is most accurate when underwater weight is taken after a complete expiration. Total body water—comprising about 50% to 70% of the human body, about 70% to 80% of muscle mass, and 10% to 20% of fat mass—is used to estimate fat mass and fat-free mass. Figure 11-13 demonstrates a typical hydrostatic weighing device.

Air Displacement Plethysmography (BodPod). **Air displacement plethysmography** (ADP) uses whole body air displacement to measure body volume and density. In comparison to hydrostatic weighing, ADP is quick and suitable for a broader range of people. However, its results are affected by moisture in hair or skin, clothing (participants are instructed to wear swimwear), and ambient air temperature and humidity. ADP tends to underestimate total body fat, especially for lean athletes.[2] Figure 11-14 shows a picture of the ADP, under the brand name BodPod.

Dual-Energy X-Ray Absorptiometry. **Dual-energy x-ray absorptiometry** (DXA) scanning has emerged as the premier method for assessing body composition. Initially developed to measure bone density (and commonly prescribed by the physician for this purpose in older female athletes and women with signs of the female athlete triad), the full-body x-ray maps the bone density, fat mass, and fat-free tissue mass using two low-dose x-rays from

Box 11-4. Standard Procedure for Obtaining Skinfold Measurements

1. Take all measurements on the right side of the body.
2. Carefully identify landmarks and mark location of measurement.
3. Advise the client to relax muscles at the measurement site.
4. Grasp the skinfold firmly between the left thumb and index finger, which should be approximately 8 cm apart on a line perpendicular to long axis of the skinfold.
5. Lift the skinfold 1 cm and place caliper jaws perpendicular to the fold and approximately 1 cm below the thumb and index finger. Do not release the skinfold while taking the measurement. Slowly close jaws on skinfold. Take skinfold measurement approximately 4 seconds after the pressure is released.
6. Take a minimum of two measurements at each site. If values differ by more than 10%, take additional measures until two recorded measures are within 10%. It is preferable to rotate measurement sites and then repeat measurements, rather than taking two measurements consecutively at the same site.
7. Do not measure skinfolds immediately after exercise, as fluid shifts to the skin will compromise accuracy.
8. Provide results as a range rather than a specific number.

Rodriguez NR, Di Marco NM, Langley S. American College of Sports Medicine position stand. Nutrition and athletic performance. *Med Sci Sports Exerc.* March 2009;41(3):709-731.

American College of Sports Medicine. Thompson WR, Gordon NF, Pescatello LS. *ACSM's Guidelines for Exercise Testing and Prescription.* 8th ed. Philadelphia: Lippincott, Williams & Wilkins; 2010.

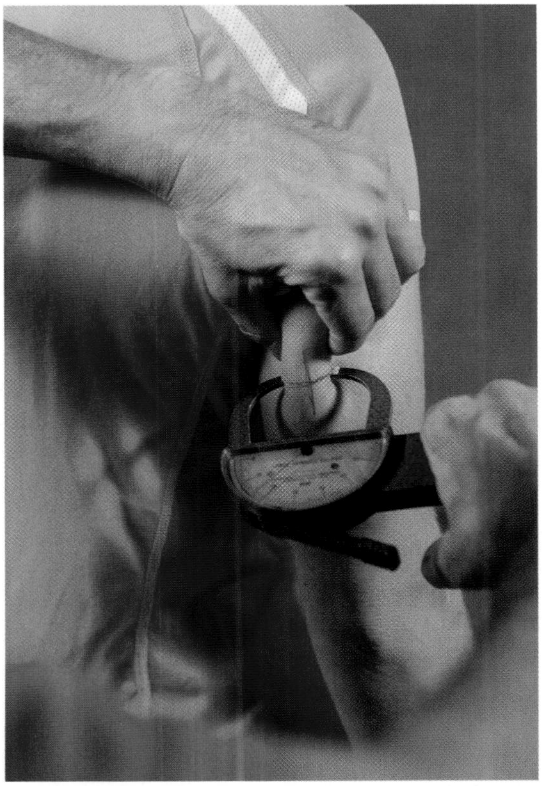

Figure 11-4. Triceps skinfold measurement. Vertical fold posterior midline of upper arm halfway between acromion process and olecranon process.

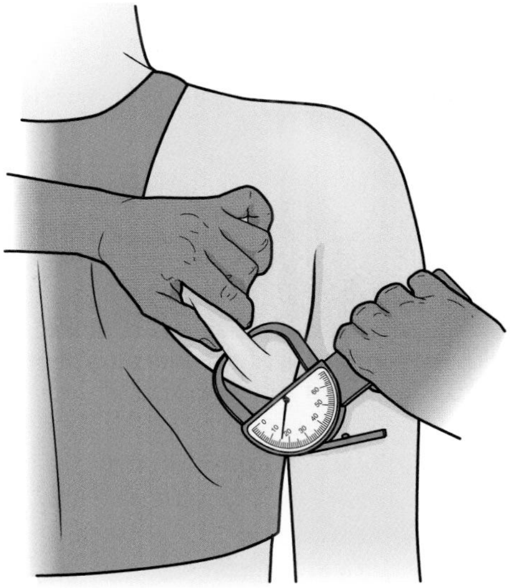

Figure 11-5. Subscapular skinfold measurement. Horizontal fold 2 cm from the undermost tip of the inferior angle of the scapula.

different sources that measure bone and soft tissue mass simultaneously (Fig. 11-15). At the conclusion of the study, the participant receives a printout of regional body fat distribution and overall muscle mass and fat mass characterization, such as that provided in Figure 11-16.

DXA is particularly appealing for athletes because it is quick and requires minimal preparation (unlike many of the other body composition assessment methods, it is not affected by water fluctuations). However, DXA scanning may not be accurate for especially lean athletes with a very high muscle mass. For example, DXA scanning in one study of very lean athletes estimated a negative amount of torso fat, which clearly is inaccurate and impossible.[9]

While DXA is reasonably accurate with a margin of error of 2% to 3%, 2 individuals should not undergo DXA scanning repeatedly due to the radiation (though small), as well as the inability of DXA scanning to detect

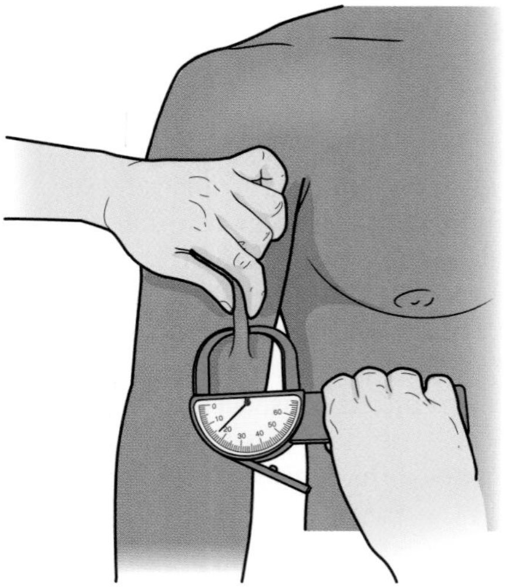

Figure 11-6. Bicep skinfold measurement. Vertical fold anterior midline of upper arm over the mid-belly of bicep.

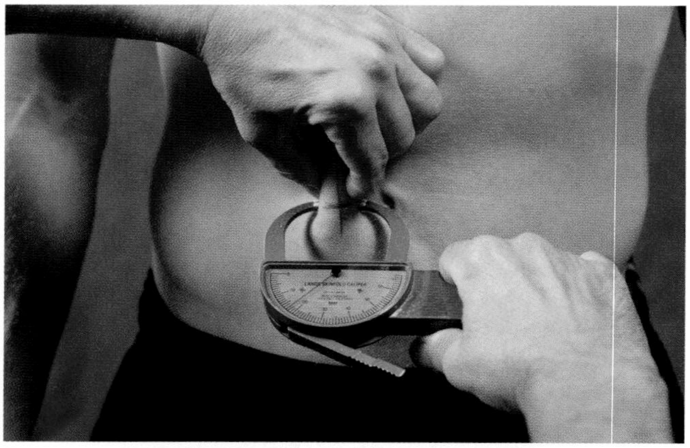

Figure 11-7. Abdominal skinfold measurement. Vertical fold 2 cm to the right of the umbilicus.

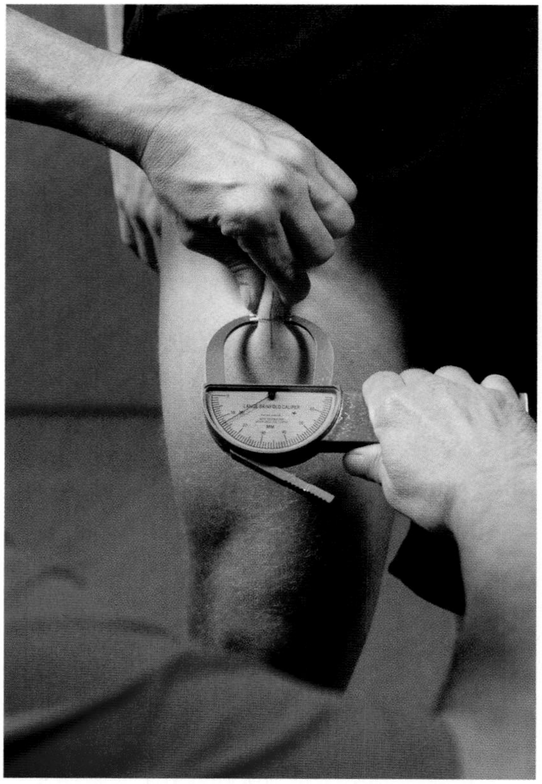

Figure 11-8. Anterior thigh skinfold measurement. Horizontal fold at midpoint of distance between inguinal fold and anterior surface of patella.

small changes in body composition over time.[2] The high cost and availability of the machine also limit the clinical use of DXA.

Near-Infrared Interactance. Developed by the U.S. Department of Agriculture to measure the fat content of beef and pork following slaughter, **near-infrared interactance** records the optical densities of skin, fat, and lean tissue as an infrared light probe is reflected off bone and back to the probe (Fig. 11-17). The method has been adapted for use in humans to predict body fat percentages. The data collected is entered into a prediction equation based on the athlete's height, weight, frame size, and level of activity. This method is not widely used due to its high rate of error and its sensitivity to probe pressure, skin color, and hydration status.

Box 11-5. Estimating Body Composition From Skinfold Measurements: The Jackson-Pollock Equations

Numerous prediction equations aim to translate the sum of skinfold measurements into an estimate of body composition. While the initial equations were based on the sum of all seven measurements, the following equations for men and women include just three measurement sites to facilitate practicality of measurement without sacrificing validity.

For men:[23]

Body density (BD) = $1.109380 - 8.267 \times 10^{-4}$ (sum of chest, abdomen, and thigh (mm)) + 1.6×10^{-6} (sum of chest, abdomen, and thigh (mm))^2 – 2.574×10^{-4} (age (yrs))

For women:[24]

Body density (BD) = $1.0994921 - 9.929 \times 10^{-4}$ (sum of triceps, suprailiac, thigh (mm)) + 2.3×10^{-6} (sum of triceps, suprailiac, thigh (mm))^2 – 1.392×10^{-4} (age)

% Body fat = [4.95/BD – 4.5] × 100

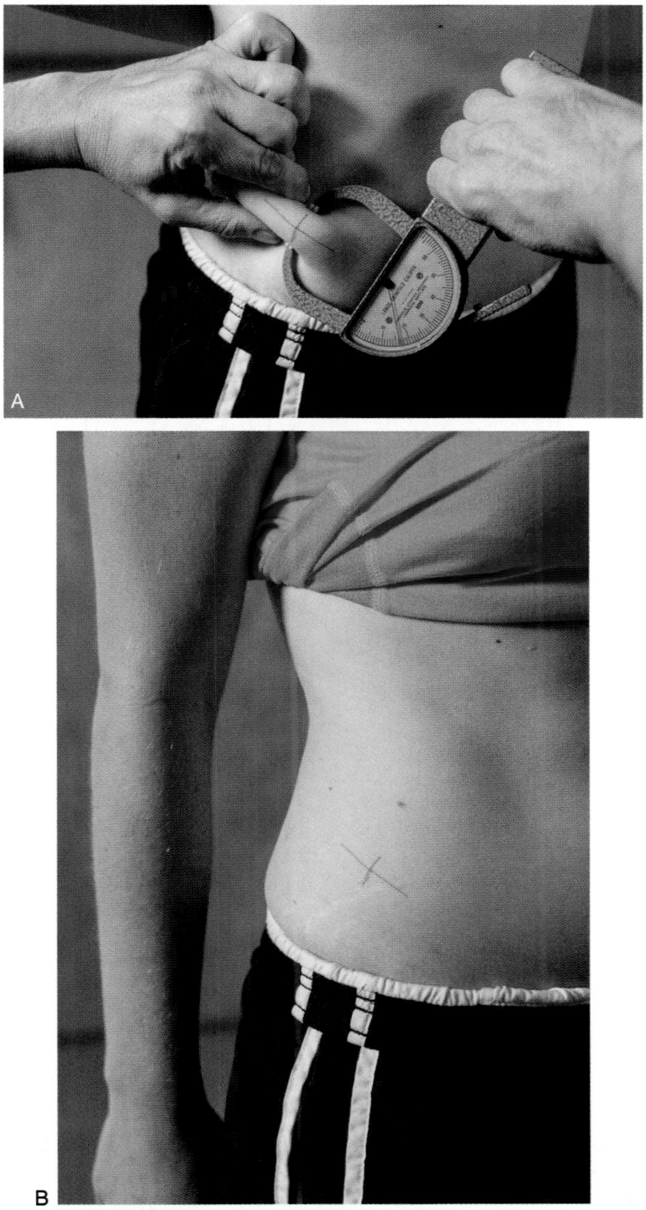

Figure 11-9. A. Supraspinale skinfold measurement. B. Vertical fold at the intersection of the line from the underarm to the anterior iliac spine and from the top of the iliac crest to the umbilicus.

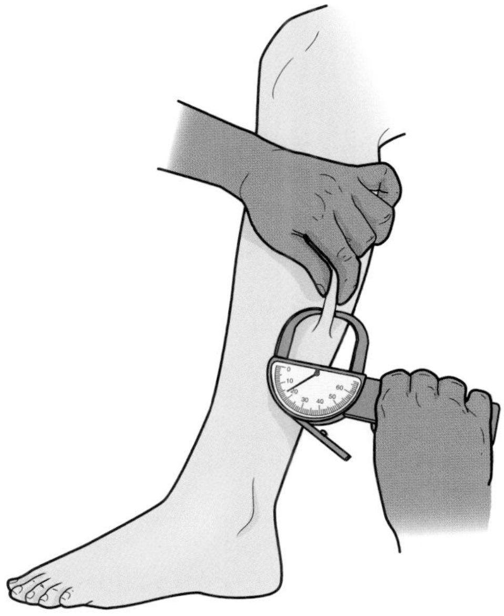

Figure 11-10. Calf skinfold measurement. Midline of medial aspect of calf muscle at the level of greatest girth.

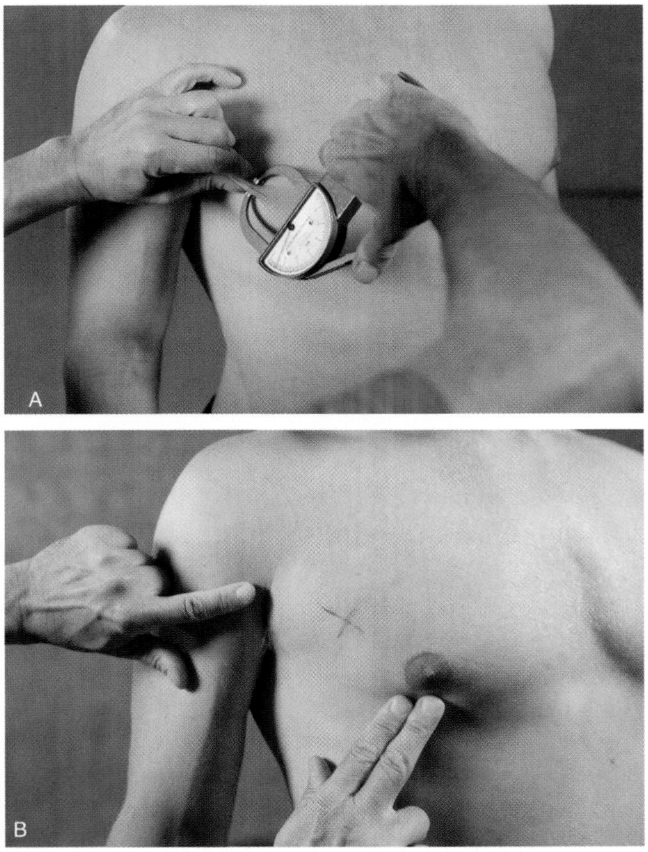

Figure 11-11. A. Chest skinfold. Not routinely measured as part of the seven-site assessment, but is frequently used in the three-site method to estimate body density in men. B. Men: one-half the distance between anterior axillary fold and nipple; women: one-third the distance between anterior axillary fold and nipple.

Three-Dimensional Photonic Scanning. Emerging as a popular and relatively new method of measuring body composition, **three-dimensional photonic scanning** uses a low-power laser light and digital cameras to rapidly produce a 3-D digital model of the human body, which is then used to approximate lean and fat mass (Fig. 11-18). For accurate assessment, participants must wear tight-fitting clothing. This may be a limiting factor with use for overweight or body-conscious participants, though the requirement is unlikely to impede assessment of most athletes. This method is limited by access to equipment and limited research evaluating its precision and validity.

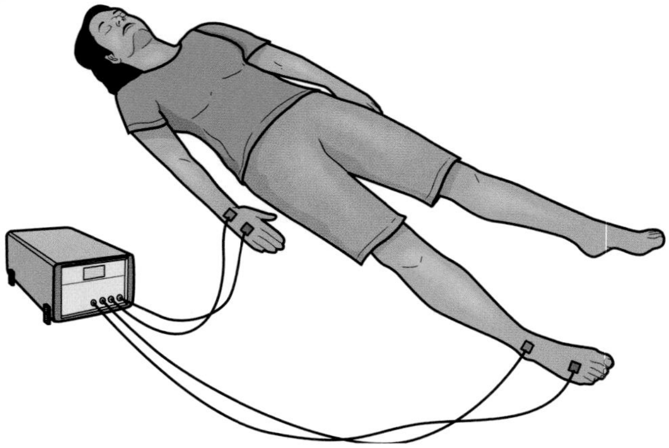

Figure 11-12. Bioelectrical impedance analysis.

Box 11-6. Prerequisites for Accurate Assessment of Body Composition Based on BIA

- BIA is an indirect measurement of body composition. As such, it relies on predictive equations to estimate fat mass and lean mass. To attain accurate readings, the appropriate validated predictive equation should be selected based on the client's gender, age, and body type.
- Fluid imbalances such as dehydration and overhydration may skew results. For accurate measurements, athletes must be well-hydrated. To assure appropriate hydration, the following protocol has been established for accurate measurement of BIA:
  - No alcohol 24 to 48 hours before assessment
  - Avoid intense exercise 6 to 12 hours before assessment
  - Avoid eating or drinking 4 hours before the assessment (especially coffee, tea, soda, or other caffeine-containing beverages)
  - Empty bladder 30 minutes before assessment
  - Avoid diuretics 7 days before assessment, if possible. Clients should not withhold prescribed medications for purpose of preparation for BIA measurement.

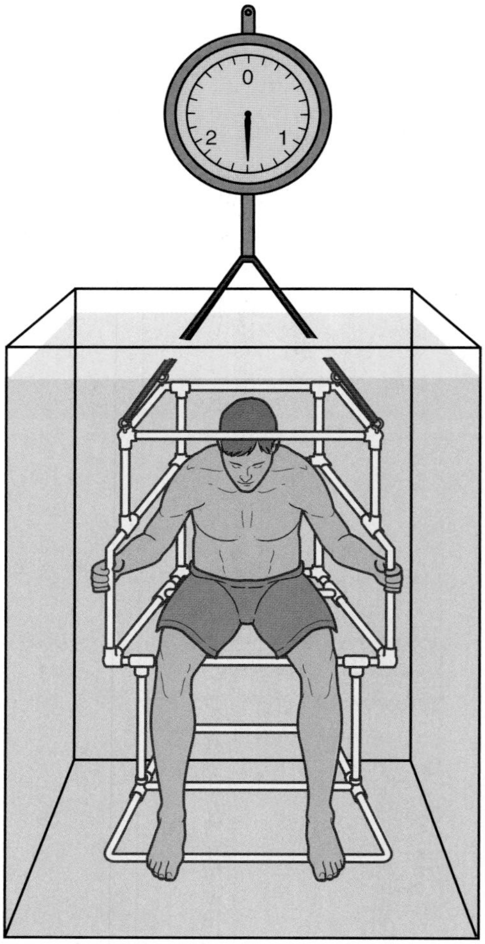

Figure 11-13. Hydrostatic weighing.

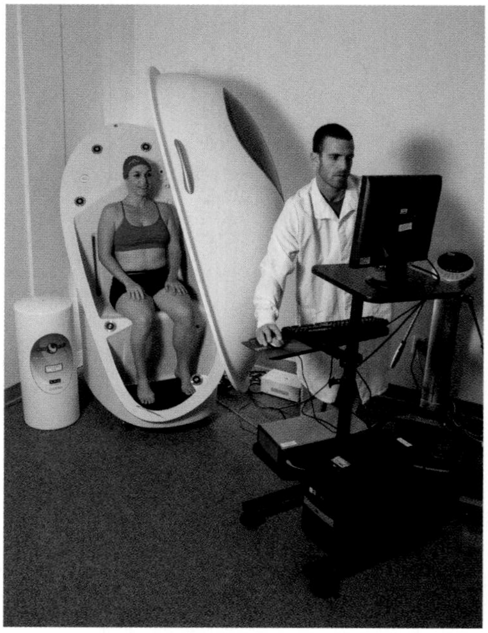

Figure 11-14. The BodPod.

Ultrasound. Ultrasound is a fairly inexpensive, portable, and safe radiological method for collecting body composition information (Fig. 11-19). With this method, an ultrasound probe is passed over the same anatomical sites that are used for estimating body composition with skinfold calipers. When the ultrasound waves penetrate tissue, the wave reflections vary for fat mass, lean mass, and bone. The high-resolution ultrasound image allows the technician to measure the subcutaneous fat tissue, similar as to what is done with skinfold calipers. This information can be entered into a regression equation to estimate body fat percentage or the site measurements can be used individually as a baseline or to monitor changes in response to a training program. As an emerging method for the assessment of body composition, standard protocols for using ultrasound to estimate total body fat composition are not yet available. However, given this method's

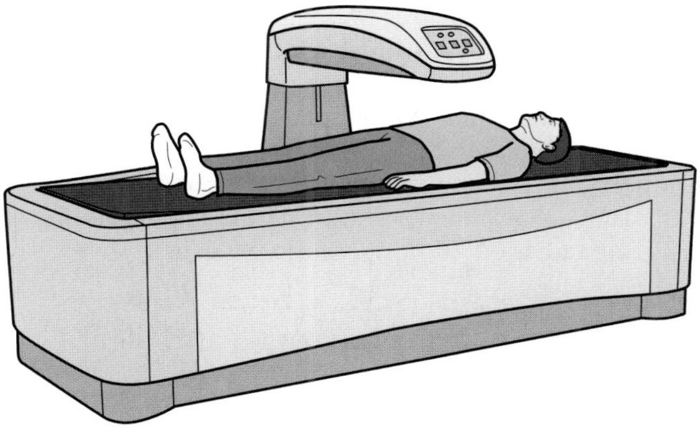

Figure 11-15. DXA scan.

accuracy and the trend toward more user-friendly and portable ultrasound methods, this research method may ultimately become widely used in practice.

Reference Methods

Reference methods for measuring body composition are of interest to health professionals primarily to understand the methods by which the field and research tests are based and compared.

Multi-Component Models. The recommended reference method for estimation of body composition is the **multi-component model**, which has a margin of error within 1% to 2%.[2] Multi-component models are not a measurement technique, but rather a way of assessing

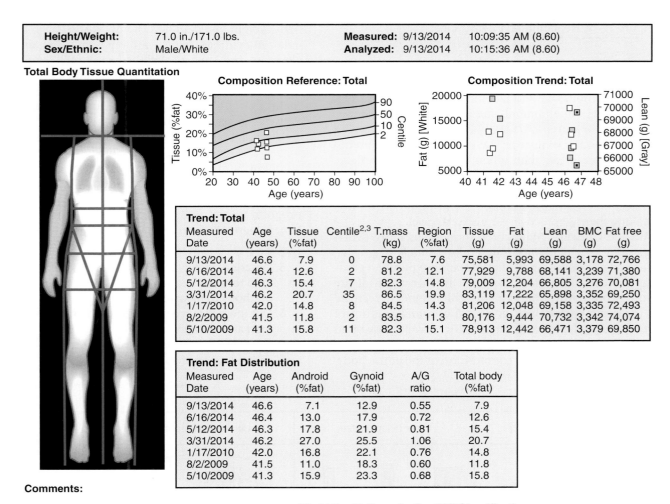

Height/Weight:	71.0 in./171.0 lbs.	**Measured:** 9/13/2014	10:09:35 AM (8.60)
Sex/Ethnic:	Male/White	**Analyzed:** 9/13/2014	10:15:36 AM (8.60)

Total Body Tissue Quantitation

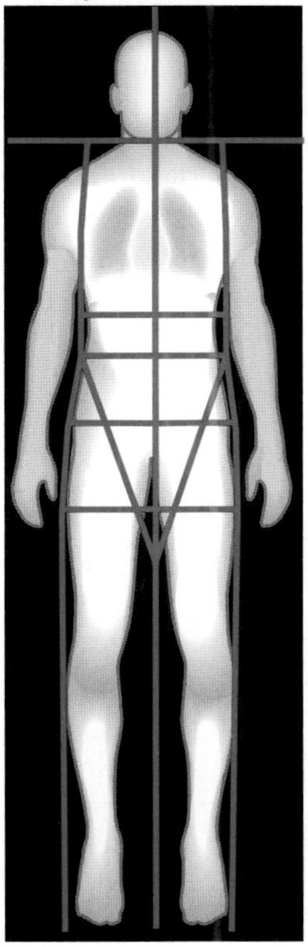

Composition Reference: Total

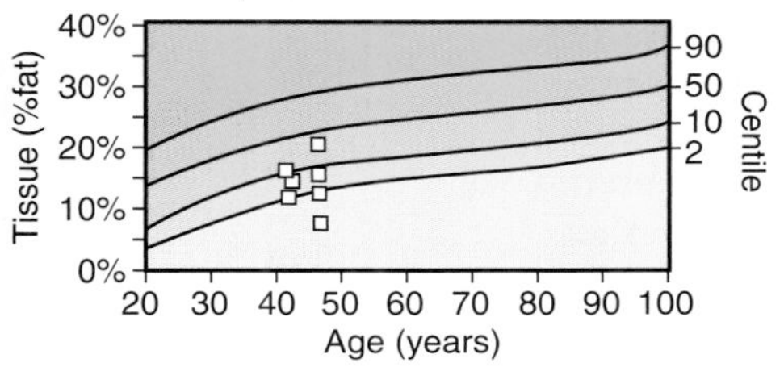

Composition Trend: Total

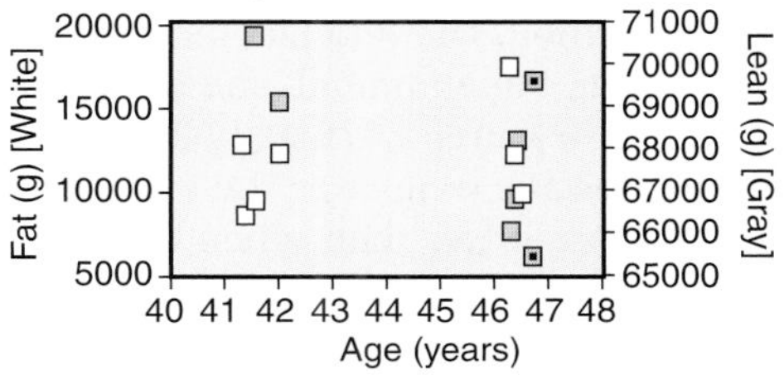

Trend: Total

Measured Date	Age (years)	Tissue (%fat)	Centile[2,3]	T.mass (kg)	Region (%fat)	Tissue (g)	Fat (g)	Lean (g)	BMC (g)	Fat free (g)
9/13/2014	46.6	7.9	0	78.8	7.6	75,581	5,993	69,588	3,178	72,766
6/16/2014	46.4	12.6	2	81.2	12.1	77,929	9,788	68,141	3,239	71,380
5/12/2014	46.3	15.4	7	82.3	14.8	79,009	12,204	66,805	3,276	70,081
3/31/2014	46.2	20.7	35	86.5	19.9	83,119	17,222	65,898	3,352	69,250
1/17/2010	42.0	14.8	8	84.5	14.3	81,206	12,048	69,158	3,335	72,493
8/2/2009	41.5	11.8	2	83.5	11.3	80,176	9,444	70,732	3,342	74,074
5/10/2009	41.3	15.8	11	82.3	15.1	78,913	12,442	66,471	3,379	69,850

Trend: Fat Distribution

Measured Date	Age (years)	Android (%fat)	Gynoid (%fat)	A/G ratio	Total body (%fat)
9/13/2014	46.6	7.1	12.9	0.55	7.9
6/16/2014	46.4	13.0	17.9	0.72	12.6
5/12/2014	46.3	17.8	21.9	0.81	15.4
3/31/2014	46.2	27.0	25.5	1.06	20.7
1/17/2010	42.0	16.8	22.1	0.76	14.8
8/2/2009	41.5	11.0	18.3	0.60	11.8
5/10/2009	41.3	15.9	23.3	0.68	15.8

Comments:

World Health Organization BMI Classification

Body Mass Index (BMI) = 23.8

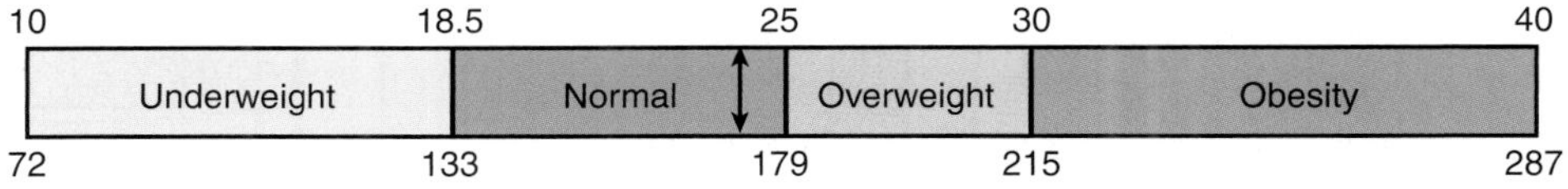

Weight (lbs.) for height = 71.0 in.

Figure 11-16. A DXA report.

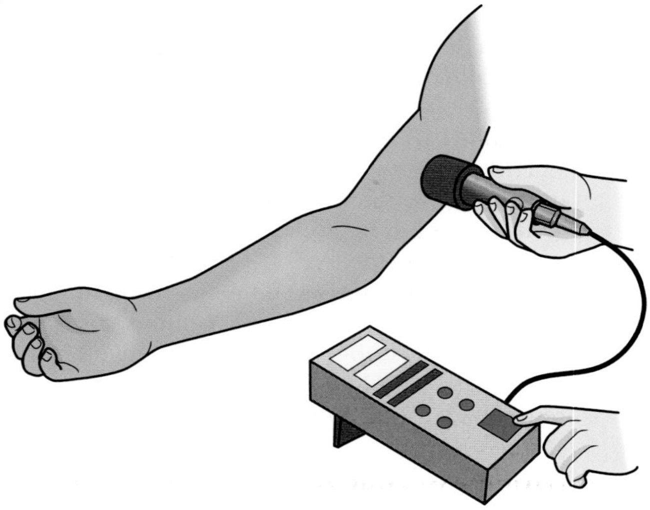

Figure 11-17. Near infrared interactance.

body composition based on other measurement techniques. The four-component equation is the leading reference method. The variables include body volume, total body water, bone mineral, and body mass. The components are measured with methods such as DXA scanning and hydrostatic weighing. The technical errors from the methods are lower than when the individual methods are used as the sole source for estimating body composition. While multi-component models have a high level of accuracy, they are expensive and time consuming, making them impractical for everyday use.

MRI and CT Scan. Magnetic resonance imaging (MRI) scanning is a highly accurate and extremely expensive method of gaining detailed information typically regarding the composition of a specific area or organ of the human body. MRI utilizes a powerful magnet to recreate a three-dimensional image in a substantial amount of detail, which far exceeds that produced from ultrasound or x-ray computed tomography (CT) scanning. While it can be used to assess the composition of the entire body, such an extensive degree of imaging is impractical. Further, evaluation of MRI measurements requires highly trained and skilled professionals, further limiting its widespread adoption. MRI does not generate an ionizing radiation. Similar to MRI, CT scans also provide high resolution internal images. Though less costly than MRI, CT scans are expensive and impose a large amount of ionizing radiation, limiting their practicality.

Body Composition Monitoring and Ideal Body Weight

Most body composition assessment methods preclude frequent monitoring due to a relatively high margin of error and generally slow changes in body composition. As a proxy, health professionals can calculate an ideal body weight based on body composition goals. This calculation assumes that the athlete retains or gains muscle mass and that all weight lost comes from fat. In order for this to be a true assumption, athletes must engage in a strength or resistance training program to maintain muscle mass. The equation to calculate ideal body weight is highlighted in Box 11-7.

Ultimately, providing body composition assessment for recreational, competitive, and elite athletes can play an important role in identifying baseline characteristics and providing a basis for goal setting. The athlete can then make modifications to both a fitness and nutrition program to improve body composition and ultimately benefit performance and health.

SPEED BUMP

5. **Describe the advantages and disadvantages of the field tests, laboratory methods, and reference methods to measure body composition.**
6. **Outline reference norms for body fat levels for men and women.**
7. **Describe the importance of body composition for various types of sports.**

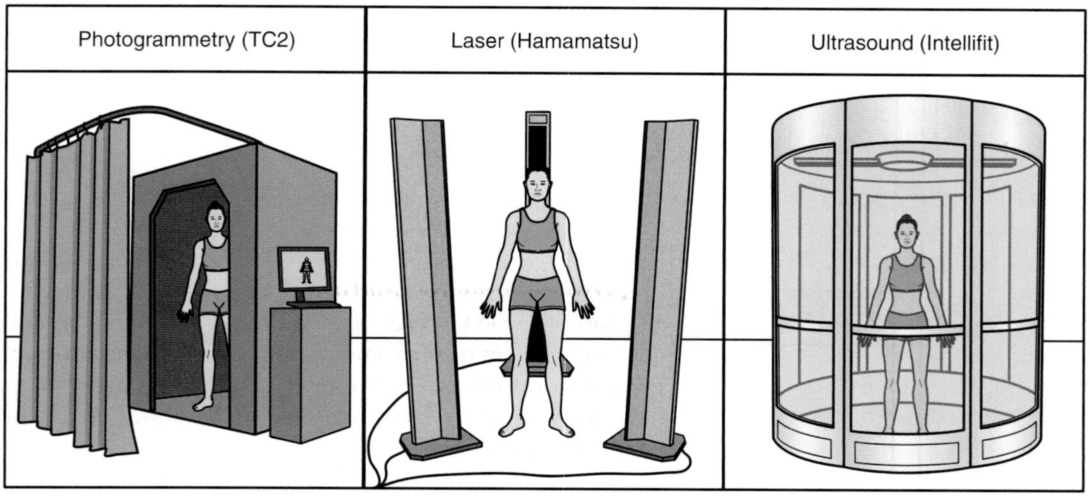

Figure 11-18. 3-D photonic scanning.

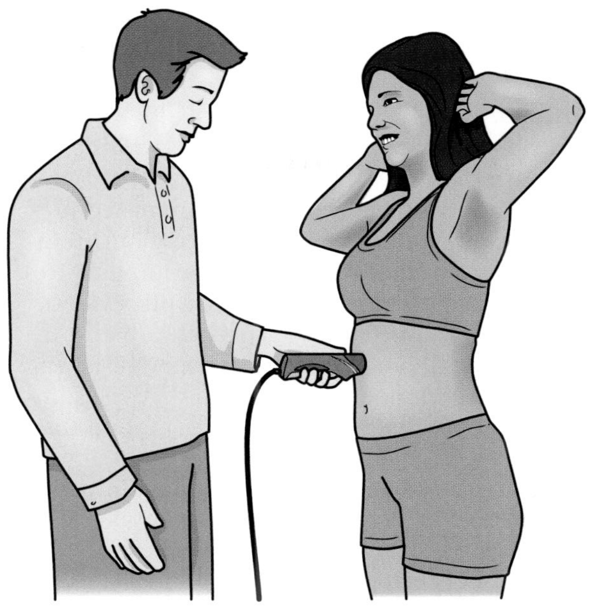

Figure 11-19. Ultrasound to measure body composition.

NUTRITION ASSESSMENT

An evaluation of a client's typical nutrition habits provides useful information as the athlete endeavors to achieve body composition and fitness goals. Many athletes recognize the importance of nutrition in optimizing performance and overall health, and would like to improve their nutritional status. However, contrary to the common belief that athletes are well-informed about nutrition, the baseline nutritional knowledge among athletes—and many of the health professionals who provide them with nutrition information—is relatively low (see Myths and Misconceptions). Health professionals can provide a valuable service to athletes by understanding the fundamentals of sports nutrition and effectively translating that information into practical strategies while staying within the health professional's scope of practice. One way to do this is through the appropriate use of nutritional assessment tools and nutrition coaching.

Nutrition assessment has historically been defined as the evaluation of an individual's nutritional status and unique nutritional needs, and has been the domain of the registered dietitian. However, nutrition assessment tools can be utilized by many health professionals to help clients best understand their nutritional behaviors without providing an individualized assessment of nutritional status or crossing outside professional scope of practice and potentially causing harm to the client or exposing the health professional to unanticipated legal liability. Health professionals who are very interested in providing detailed and individualized nutrition assessment and recommendations may consider pursuing credentials as registered dietitians and, potentially, **certified specialists in sports dietetics** (Box 11-8 highlights the requisite training for each).

The Commission on Dietetic Registration provides a link to the legislation dictating nutrition-related scope of practice for each state (www.cdrnet.org). While rules vary by state, it is generally accepted that it is within the scope of practice of the allied health professional to use government tools and guidelines, published position papers, and research studies and published texts to provide clients with nutrition information. The tools outlined below are contained within these domains. Each is described in turn, along with an explanation of their potential use for allied health professionals.

Box 11-7. Calculating Ideal Body Weight Based on Body Composition

Athletes can estimate ideal body weight based on a percentage of desired body fat. Then, instead of frequently monitoring body composition, the athlete can aim for a body weight goal. Once that goal is achieved, body composition can be reassessed to see how well actual body composition approximates the goal body composition. In order for this equation to be accurate, an athlete needs to engage in a regular resistance training program to retain muscle mass during weight loss. This assumes that the athlete is trying to lose weight and would like to retain an equal amount of lean mass.

Ideal body weight (IBW) = lean body weight/(1 – desired body fat percentage (decimal)) *Example.* A hockey player recently had a body composition assessment completed. He weighed 165 pounds of which 15% was body fat and 85% was lean mass. His desired body fat is 12%. How much weight will he need to lose to achieve this goal, assuming that all weight lost comes from fat?

IBW = 140.25/(1 – .12) = 159 pounds

Estimating Caloric Needs

The health professional can help a client determine estimated caloric needs and compare the estimated needs with the approximate calories that the client consumes in a typical day based on the dietary log. Determination of **resting energy expenditure** (REE), or the number of calories needed to fuel vital functions, is most accurately determined in the laboratory with **indirect calorimetry**. Indirect calorimetry is a noninvasive study that estimates energy needs based on the use of oxygen and production of carbon dioxide. Because this method is expensive and impractical for most people, indirect calorimetry is infrequently used in practice. Instead, several equations are

Myths and Misconceptions

Athletes are Natural Nutrition Experts

The Myth

Athletes know a lot about nutrition.

The Logic

By the very nature of their impressive physical feats and lean physiques, athletes certainly know how to strategically fuel for optimal performance.

The Science

As articulately stated in a *New York Times* article by researcher David Nieman, a professor of health and exercise science at Appalachian State University, in reference to vegan ultramarathoner Scott Jurek and whether athletes should become vegan: "He's a great guy—opinionated, sure, but he's been very successful as a racer, so he can have opinions. But runners always think they have inside information on nutrition. They don't. It's my duty as a scientist to separate out the hype from what's been validated."

Nieman continues, "What we know is that when it comes to endurance performance, it's all about the fuel, primarily carbohydrates, and you can get sufficient carbohydrates whether you're a vegetarian or a meat eater—unless you follow a really goofy diet, which some people do. It's possible to eat a lousy vegetarian diet, just as you as can eat a lousy meat-based diet."

While it is true that athletes are interested in nutrition and often are the ones setting nutrition trends, they do not always make nutrition choices that are in alignment with solid scientific evidence.

For example, one study of coaches, athletic trainers, strength and conditioning specialists, and NCAA Division I, II, and III athletes that was published in the *Journal of Athletic Training* found that 91% of athletes, 64% of coaches, 29% of athletic trainers, and 17% of strength and conditioning specialists had inadequate nutrition knowledge.[25] Topics assessed included micronutrients and macronutrients, supplements and performance, weight management and eating disorders, and hydration. The authors concluded that athletes and coaches especially had low levels of nutrition knowledge and that nutrition programming should be integrated into the curriculum for athletic trainers and strength and conditioning specialists given the frequency with which athletes rely on them for nutrition information.[25]

available to determine calorie needs. The most commonly used equations are highlighted in Box 11-9. Based on a systematic review of several methods to estimate energy needs, the Mifflin-St. Jeor equation is the most accurate estimation of REE for the majority of adults.[10]

Once the REE is calculated, the value should be multiplied by an activity factor to account for the individual's level of daily exercise. The end result is an estimate of the client's total daily needs, with a margin of error of about 10%.[10]

Attaining a Diet History

Attaining a diet history not only provides the health professional with baseline nutritional information about the client's typical eating habits, it also provides clients with insight into their own behaviors that they may not have considered previously. The health professional and client can use the information obtained from a diet history to better understand the types of foods eaten and the factors that influence intake, assess the quality of a client's nutritional habits, and evaluate how well the client's typical eating habits compare with an ideal diet. In some cases, the health professional may initiate the process of attaining a diet history and recognize that, to best meet the client's needs, referral to a registered dietitian is necessary. Situations in which referral clearly is indicated are included in Box 11-10.

Several commonly used tools to attain a diet history include the **24-hour recall**, **food frequency questionnaire**, and **food record**. These tools are best used in combination with an exercise and training log when working with active clients.

24-Hour Recall

The 24-hour recall is a method of gaining information about a client's eating habits by asking for detailed information about the foods and drinks the client consumed in the 24 hours prior to the consultation. While this method is not the most accurate method of obtaining nutrition information, it provides the health professional with insight into a client's typical eating patterns, including types of foods and drinks consumed, snacking, and meal-skipping, and time of day in which most food is consumed.

Food Frequency Questionnaire

The food frequency questionnaire is a multi-paged list of different foods or food types and the client is asked to indicate how often each of the foods is consumed on a daily, weekly, or monthly basis. This method is frequently used in population-based research studies, such as the National Health and Nutrition Examination Survey (NHANES) to characterize typical intake. While it provides useful information into typical eating patterns, it can be overbearing for a health professional to use effectively in practice due to the large amount of information obtained.

Box 11-8. The Path to Becoming a Registered Dietitian and Certified Specialist in Sports Dietetics

HOW TO BECOME A REGISTERED DIETITIAN

Required qualifications to become a registered dietitian from the Commission on Dietetic Registration (www.cdrnet.org):

To take the certifying examination to become a registered dietitian, applicants must meet the following academic and supervised practice requirements:

Academic Requirements

- Minimum of bachelor's degree
- Completion of an accredited didactic program in dietetics. A listing of acceptable programs is available at www.eatright.org/becomeanRDorDTR

Supervised Practice Requirements

- Completion of accredited dietetic internship program which consists of a minimum of 1,200 hours of supervised practice, OR
- Completion of an accredited coordinated program through integration of didactic instruction with a minimum of 1,200 hours of supervised practice

HOW TO BECOME A BOARD-CERTIFIED SPECIALIST IN SPORTS DIETETICS

Required qualifications to become a certified specialist in sports dietetics from the Commission on Dietetic Registration (www.cdrnet.org):

- Current Registered Dietitian (RD) status
- Maintenance of the RD status for a minimum of 2 years
- Documentation of 1,500 hours of specialty practice experience as an RD
- Pass a written multiple choice exam

Box 11-9. Calculating Energy Needs

Several equations are used in practice to estimate resting energy expenditure (REE). The REE is then multiplied by an activity factor to approximate daily energy needs to maintain weight. The equations for the methods most commonly used in practice are included below.

Harris Benedict[26]

For men: REE = 66 + 13.7 × wt(kg) + 5 × ht(cm) – 6.8 × age (yrs)

For women: REE = 655 + 9.6 × wt(kg) +1.8 × ht(cm) – 4.7 × age

Mifflin St. Jeor[*,27]

For men: REE = 9.99 × wt (kg) + 6.25 × ht (cm) – 4.92 × age (yrs) + 5

For women: REE = 9.99 × wt (kg) + 6.25 × ht (cm) – 4.92 × age (yrs) – 161

Owen[28,29]

For men: REE = 879 + (10.2 × wt (kg))

For women: REE = 795 + (7.18 × wt (kg))

World Health Organization/Food and Agriculture Organization/United Nations University[30]

The REE should be multiplied by an activity factor of 1.6 – 2.4 for the following equations.

Gender and Age	Equation (BW in kg)
Males, 10–18 years	REE = (17.5 × BW) + 651
Males, 19–30 years	REE = (15.3 × BW) + 679
Males, 31–60 years	REE = (11.6 × BW) + 879
Females, 10–18 years	REE = (12.2 × BW) + 749
Females, 19–30 years	REE = (14.7 × BW) + 496
Females, 31–60 years	REE = (8.7 × BW) + 29

Dietary Reference Intakes[31]

For men: REE = 662 – 9.53 × age (yrs) + PA × (15.91 × wt (kg) + 539.6 × ht (meters))

For women: REE = 354 – 6.91 × age (yrs) + PA × (9.36 × wt (kg) + 726 × ht (meters))

PA = physical activity factor

Physical Activity Factor[6]

Unless otherwise included in the equation, the REE should be multiplied by an activity factor to estimate daily energy needs to maintain weight.

1.0–1.39 Sedentary, typical daily living activities (e.g., household tasks, walking to bus).

1.4–1.59 Low active, typical daily living activities plus 30–60 minutes of daily moderate activity (e.g., walking at 5–7 km/h).

1.6–1.89 Active, typical daily living activities plus 60 minutes of daily moderate activity.

1.9–2.5 Very active, typical daily activities plus at least 60 minutes of daily moderate activity plus an additional 60 minutes of vigorous activity or 120 minutes of moderate activity.

*most accurate[10]

Food Record

The food record is the most frequently used method of dietary assessment. To gain the most accurate nutrition information, a client should keep, at the minimum, a 3-day record including 1 weekend day and 2 "typical" weekdays. A "typical" day is one that most resembles the client's usual routine. The client should be instructed to record everything consumed—both food and beverages—down to the measurement in cups and ounces, if possible. While this is a tedious process, and the client may modify intake so as to avoid having to record an extra snack or second serving, the detailed and specific information improves the value of the food log. Clients who eat out frequently should investigate if the restaurant supplies nutrition information on request. A growing number of chains make this information readily available. In addition to tracking *what* they eat, it is also helpful for clients to record what *time* of day, *where* they were when eating, what kind of *mood*

Box 11-10. When to Refer to a Registered Dietitian

- Specific, individualized meal plans which fall outside the recommendations of the *Dietary Guidelines for Americans* or MyPlate.
- Chronic health problem or taking prescription medications, dietary supplements, or over-the-counter medications to control a chronic health problem. Examples include cardiovascular disease, hypertension, hyperlipidemia, diabetes, eating disorder, anemia, osteoporosis.
- Post-operative nutrition.
- Unexpected or unexplainable weight loss or weight gain.
- Nutrition-related situation which the allied health professional feels is outside his or her level of training or expertise.

they were in, and *how hungry* they were on a scale of 1 (ravenous) to 10 (completely full to the point of discomfort). This additional information will help to identify patterns of non-hunger-related eating and other opportunities to improve intake. A sample food record form is included in Box 11-11.

While health professionals may choose to use their own tools and forms to collect dietary information, the federal government provides resources at www.choosemyplate.gov that not only collect the essential information but also provide an assessment of the food intake based on how well it conforms to the *Dietary Guidelines for Americans*. For example, the online **SuperTracker** provides tools to estimate calorie needs and to track, analyze, and evaluate nutrition and physical activity (www.supertracker.usda.gov) (Fig. 11-20).

By using a government-endorsed tool such as the SuperTracker, the health professional provides a client with a valuable service but stays within the scope of practice of a health professional who is not a licensed nutritionist or registered dietitian. Those health professionals who choose to use their own forms or nutrient analysis databases or programs should avoid *diagnosing* vitamin or nutrient deficiencies, *prescribing* supplements or other nutritional regimens, or *advising* clients of a specific nutrition plan in response to data collected. Rather, the health professional can use the forms as a tool to help a client recognize areas of potential improvement or concerns based on the *Dietary Guidelines for Americans* or position statements such as the position of the American College of Sports Medicine and the American Dietetic Association (now known as the Academy of Nutrition and Dietetics) Position Statement on Nutrition and Athletic Performance.[6] (The position statement is available free of charge through the Academy of Nutrition and Dietetics website (www.eatright.org). The details of this position statement also are described in Chapters 7, 8, and 9).

Comparing Needs to Present Intake

The athlete's nutritional goals form the basis for comparing needs to present intake. If the client would like to follow a generally healthy eating plan that conforms to the DRIs and other general nutritional standards, the MyPlate recommendations and analysis available from www.supertracker.usda.gov provide excellent tools to help evaluate how a person's typical eating plan compares to the *Dietary Guidelines for Americans*. If the client would like to use a different eating plan as the standard, the athlete should compare the dietary recommendations from that eating plan with actual intake. The "ideal" eating plan should be healthy overall and an eating approach that the client will be able to follow. Health professionals should exercise caution when helping an

Box 11-11. A Sample Food Log

TIME	FOOD EATEN	AMOUNT	APPROX CALORIES	HUNGER RATING	EMOTIONS	OTHER ACTIVITIES

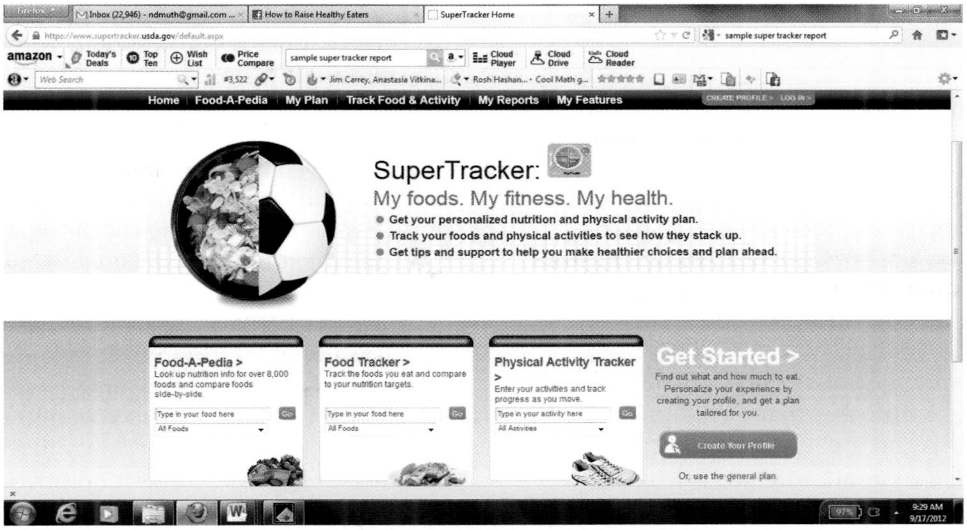
Home
Food-A-Pedia
My Plan
Track Food & Activity
My Reports
My Features
SuperTracker:
My foods. My fitness. My health.
Get your personalized nutrition and physical activity plan.
Track your foods and physical activities to see how they stack up.
Get tips and support to help you make healthier choices and plan ahead.
Food-A-Pedia >
Look up nutrition info for over 8,000 foods and compare foods side-by-side.
Food Tracker >
Track the foods you eat and compare to your nutrition targets.
Physical Activity Tracker >
Enter your activities and track progress as you move.
Get Started >
Find out what and how much to eat. Personalize your experience by creating your profile, and get a plan tailored for you.
Create Your Profile
Or, use the general plan.

Figure 11-20. The SuperTracker. *Source: USDA. Available at www.choosemyplate.gov/supertracker-tools/supertracker.html*

athlete to conform to a nongovernment-endorsed eating plan, as this may cross into the scope of a registered dietitian.

BODY COMPOSITION AND NUTRITION COACHING

Body composition and nutrition assessment tools help to form the basis upon which an athlete develops goals and accompanying actionable strategies to achieve those goals. In the case of an elite athlete, these assessments and strategies may be undertaken and developed by a multidisciplinary team of allied health professionals. For competitive or recreational athletes who do not have access to a multitude of experts, a single health professional such as an athletic trainer, personal trainer, sports coach or registered dietitian may help the athlete to set and achieve body composition and nutrition goals.

After completing the initial assessment and comparing estimated body composition and dietary habits with ideals, the health professional can adopt the role of coach to help the athlete set and achieve goals. In some cases, one of the most important steps the health professional can take to help the athlete is referral to a registered dietitian, physician, or specialist. For example, after body composition assessment and nutrition evaluation it may become clear that an athlete engaging in a weight-conscious sport may have an unsafely low body fat percentage and eating patterns that are alarming for disordered eating. This athlete is at increased risk for female athlete triad and other health complications and should be immediately referred to a physician and registered dietitian for evaluation. See Chapters 4, 9, and 15 for more information on the female athlete triad.

For those clients who do not require referral to another expert, the important next step after body composition and nutrition evaluation is to begin the coaching process. This includes assessing the athlete's readiness to change, goal setting (including development of an action plan), and ongoing health education and follow up.

SPEED BUMP

8. **Describe the common tools used to collect nutrition information.**
9. **Describe several benefits of providing nutrition and body composition coaching to clients.**
10. **List three actions related to nutrition coaching that are within the scope of practice of an allied health professional.**
11. **List three actions related to nutrition coaching that are outside the scope of practice of an allied health professional. Note the type of health professional best qualified to help the clients in those scenarios.**

Readiness to Change

Whether a client's goals are related to weight loss or muscle gain, optimal athletic performance, improved health status, or management of disease, athletes recognize that improvements in exercise and nutrition are essential to achieve success. The challenge is that making changes to long-standing, ingrained behaviors requires more than knowledge. It demands significant changes in the way a person lives, from how he or she responds to cues of hunger and fullness, to the mental self-talk that either supports or impedes a person's efforts to start or complete a workout. An exercise or nutrition program will not be successful without a behavioral assessment and plan to ensure that the client follows the agreed upon changes to activity and diet.

This can only happen if the client is psychologically ready to make changes.

Stages of Change

The **stages of change,** or transtheoretical model of behavior change, initially was described in an effort to increase the effectiveness of smoking cessation programs.[11] Over the years, this model has gained acceptance as a useful model of behavior change across many disciplines, including weight management. The model consists of several constructs, of which the stages of change is the most well-known.

The stages-of-change construct acknowledges that behavior change is a process that develops over time. The stages are based on a client's readiness to change and the anticipated or actual changes that are already in place. A client may progress through the stages linearly, waver between stages, or progress then relapse.

The *precontemplative stage* occurs when a person does not believe there is a problem and does not anticipate making any changes in the foreseeable future. This is a person who would benefit from educational information about the value of health behavior changes, but who would not be receptive to a fitness training or nutrition coaching program. Indications that a person is in the precontemplative stage include comments such as, "My doctor made me see you," "I don't understand why I am here," "I am not interested in making any changes," or "I don't think that changes in my nutrition will affect my sports performance." People in this stage may have unsuccessfully attempted changes in the past, do not believe they can successfully make changes, or do not believe that changes are necessary.

The *contemplative stage* occurs when a person believes that change is necessary and plans to take action within the next 6 months. A person in this stage believes that the benefits of change outweigh the drawbacks, but is acutely aware of the downsides of change and is not ready to commit to an intervention. This weighing of the pros and cons is commonly referred to as **decisional balance.** A person may remain in this stage for months to years. A prospective client in the contemplative stage may not be willing to commit to a program that is scheduled to begin soon, but may be receptive to receiving information about a program planned for the future. An athlete in this stage may state, "I want to improve my game, but I don't think I can spend any more time on this sport than I already do."

Motivational interviewing (MI) is particularly effective communication in this stage when most clients feel some ambivalence about change. MI is a collaborative communication strategy in which a coach uses listening skills including open-ended questions, reflections, affirmations, and summarizing to help a client identify his or her own strengths and motivation to change. MI generally follows a sequence of engaging, evoking, focusing, and planning.[33] Health professionals who will be doing a lot of coaching are advised to become very familiar with MI to achieve best results with clients.

The *preparation stage* occurs when a person intends to take action in the immediate future, typically within the next month. This person may have already made significant changes within the past year and may have plans to initiate change, such as joining a health club, discussing weight with a physician, training for a physical event such as a 5K, or seeking out the services of a fitness trainer or nutrition coach. A person in this stage is an ideal client and will benefit most from a well-designed program.

The *action stage* describes individuals who have made and maintained substantial lifestyle changes within the past 6 months. These individuals have overcome significant obstacles and barriers to change. An example may be a novice runner who recently began running three mornings per week with a friend with the goal to "get in shape." A client in the action stage is at highest risk for beginning a program but struggling to make a permanent change, as many fitness and nutrition programs are short-lived, with adherence progressively decreasing over the first several months after initiation.

The *maintenance stage* describes individuals who have committed to a significant behavioral change for longer than 6 months. At this stage, *relapses* occur less frequently, though they still occur at a rate greater than 7% until change has been maintained for 5 years. Individuals in maintenance have high self-efficacy that they can maintain the positive change and rely less frequently on *processes of change* (see below) than individuals in the earlier stages of change.

Processes of Change

The processes of change refer to the tools that people both knowingly and unknowingly use to progress through the stages of change. An awareness of these processes is useful for health professionals aiming to help ready someone to make a change and also to adhere to behavioral changes. While many processes exist, the following 10 have received the most support in studies of the model.[12]

1. *Consciousness raising* involves increasing awareness of the benefits of change and the potential harms of inaction. This is most useful for people in the precontemplative and contemplative stages of change.
2. *Dramatic relief* describes implementation of emotionally moving testimony, documentary, or role playing to increase motivation to make change.
3. *Self-reevaluation* prompts persons to envision themselves both with and without the unhealthy behavior. For example, a health professional may use this technique to help a college athlete who makes unhealthy food choices in the dorm cafeteria to envision herself overeating high-sugar, high-salt meals; how she feels afterwards; and how it affects her performance, and then envision herself choosing healthier options and the resulting benefits.

4. *Environmental reevaluation* prompts clients to consider how their behaviors affect the people around them. For example, this method may ask an athlete how he feels his behavior affects his teammates or his family members.
5. *Helping relationships* or *social support* greatly enhance success with behavior change. A health professional can help to improve social supports for a client through rapport building, follow-up calls and e-mails, and buddy systems.
6. *Contingency management* offers rewards for making planned behavioral changes. Contingency contracts, positive reinforcements, and group recognition all are powerful motivators for most people. Importantly, food rewards typically do more harm than good for children and for people trying to manage their weight.
7. *Social liberation* relies on the power of peer influence and changing societal norms and policies to induce behavioral change. Several research studies support that people are more likely to make healthful (or unhealthful) behavioral changes when they associate with peers who practice those behaviors.[13-16] More emerging evidence suggests that large-scale policy changes and changes to the built environment improve nutrition habits and support physical activity.[17-19]
8. *Self-liberation*, also known as willpower, employs making a commitment to change and acting on that commitment. A public assertion of this commitment (such as a declaration to family members or a Facebook post or Tweet) can help enhance adherence. However, an undue reliance on willpower to achieve lasting change can be counterproductive.
9. *Counterconditioning*, or behavioral substitution, refers to substitution of healthier behaviors for less healthy ones. For example, a person who always drinks a regular soda when he gets home from work might replace it with a glass of lemon water or unsweetened iced tea.
10. *Stimulus control*. A health professional can help clients reduce cues for undesirable behavior and increase cues for desirable behavior through stimulus control. For example, an allied health professional may advise an athlete striving to lose weight to keep junk food out of the pantry and stock up on fruits and vegetables, dissociate from friends and colleagues with destructive eating habits and attitudes, make an effort to spend more time with active and healthy individuals, and eat small well-planned meals throughout the day to avoid a starvation binge or stop at the closest vending machine or fast-food restaurant.

Goal Setting

Athletes can begin to tackle their most challenging health struggles with goal setting. "SMART" (specific, measurable, attainable, relevant, and time-bound) nutrition and physical activity goals help set the stage for success by transforming vague visions into a specific plan for a healthier lifestyle.

- *S—specific*. "What exactly do you hope to achieve?"
- *M—measurable*. "How will you know if you got there?"
- *A—attainable*. "Is this a goal you believe you can realistically achieve with a moderate amount of effort?"
- *R—relevant*. "When you achieve this goal, how will you feel?" Clients should choose a goal that is really meaningful to them so that they feel a sense of pride and accomplishment when they achieve the goal.
- *T—time-bound*. "When do you want to achieve this goal?" Encourage clients to set a specific date by which the goal will be realized.

Short-term *process-centered goals* can also be very effective to help a client celebrate smaller successes more frequently. Process-centered goals are the steps that lead to achieving an *outcome-centered goal*. For example, if a client has a goal to lose 5 pounds (an outcome-centered goal), smaller process-centered goals, such as replacing after-dinner pie with a piece of fruit or walking for 20 minutes every day, would help get him or her closer to the weight loss goal.

Health Education

An important function of a nutrition coach is to provide health education to clients, when appropriate. For adult learners, the most effective health education does not come from lectures, PowerPoint presentations, or study guides—the standard teaching fare in elementary, high school, and college classrooms. Adult learners are more likely to retain and act upon information when the information is presented in a way that is highly relevant, based on prior experiences, practical, and perceived to be important.[20] For example, while a child might memorize or learn something esoteric because the information is necessary to pass a test written by an authority figure, adult learners retain new information that is deemed by them (rather than an authority figure) to be important and useful for their daily lives.

A nutrition coach who understands the essentials of adult learning will experience increased success in helping clients learn, retain, and apply new information to their everyday lives. Box 11-12 highlights several tools a nutrition coach can use to provide health education for adult learners while staying within the scope of practice of an unlicensed nutrition expert. Importantly, the coach should be sensitive to how the sharing of information may be received by the client. Generally, the health professional should attain the client's permission before providing information or advice. Permission is generally attained in one of three ways: implied after the client asks the coach a specific question; explicit through the coach asking for permission; or, in cases when the client may benefit from information, but may not necessarily want to hear it, with a couching statement such as "I'm not sure if this will make a difference or not, but. . . " This autonomy-respecting language helps to support the client making a sustainable change.[33]

Arranging for Follow-Up

The context in which an allied health professional—who may come from fields as diverse as coaching, physical therapy, personal training, athletic training, massage therapy, or dietetics—helps an athlete improve nutrition or body composition varies considerably. As such, the most appropriate method to follow up with an athlete's nutrition and body composition goals, challenges, and successes also will vary. In any case, the allied health professional should regularly follow up or check in with the athlete to assess progress toward goals and provide continual information and reassurance to help the athlete be successful. This could be in the form of individual consultation and follow-up visits, ongoing workshops, electronic or online communication, or other modes of communication.

SPEED BUMP

12. Describe how understanding a client's readiness to change may impact nutrition recommendations.
13. Summarize adult learning theory and how it may be applied in body composition and nutrition coaching.
14. Outline a prototypical initial nutrition consultation.

Box 11-12. Tools for Nutrition Coaching

Many tools are readily accessible to help provide effective health and nutrition education to athletes while staying within the scope of practice of a health professional.

***Dietary Guidelines for Americans*:** Every 5 years, the USDA releases the federal government's best recommendations for how to eat a healthy diet. Generally more than 100 pages in length, the guidelines offer a great deal of information that can be parlayed into weekly e-mail tips, social media posts, client handouts, or any of a number of ways to provide clients with information in an easy-to-digest and remember format.

Food Diary: The food diary is more than a tool for a client to record intake. It also provides a client direct insight into eating behaviors. The mere act of maintaining a food log influences the dietary choices a person makes, making it a very effective strategy for inducing behavior change even in the absence of direct advice to the client.

Recipes: Athletes may struggle to consistently prepare healthy meals or develop new ways to meet their nutritional needs. Sharing recipes that are healthy and appropriate for the athlete offers a practical approach to making it easier for the client to achieve his or her nutrition or body composition goals.

Demonstrations and Cooking Demos: Hands-on demonstrations and brief cooking demos turn vague pieces of nutritional information into easy-to-remember and useful strategies to achieve goals. For example, telling a client to "eat carbohydrates and protein" after exercise for optimal recovery is forgettable. Providing several examples of healthy snacks that meet the recommended intakes is not only memorable, but also much more likely to influence future dietary choices.

Position Statements and Research Studies: Health professionals rely heavily on position statements and research studies which highlight what works and what does not in achieving nutrition or body composition goals. Athletes generally are very interested in the newest nutrition advances and findings. Sharing brief recaps of these studies helps athletes to stay informed, helps to counter the large amount of circulating nutrition misinformation, and increases the credibility of the allied health professional.

KEY POINTS SUMMARY

1. Health professionals with knowledge of nutrition and nutrition coaching provide a valuable asset to athletes and active adults who would like nutrition information but do not have access to or resources to afford individualized consultations with a registered dietitian. With this said, health professionals must practice within their scope of practice and initiate referrals to other health professionals, when appropriate. Being able to identify when referral is necessary and who would be most helpful to meet the client's needs is an important skill of a health professional.
2. The initial interview with a client includes time devoted to building rapport as well as time spent reviewing a client's health history and potential indications for referral. The initial interview is also a good time to discuss body composition and nutrition assessment tools and decide whether the use of specific tools will be beneficial for the client.
3. Body composition refers to a person's proportion of fat; lean tissue such as bone, muscle, and connective tissue; and water. Fat mass includes essential fat (about 3% to 5% for men and 12% to14% for women) and nonessential fat. Body composition is determined by modifiable factors such as physical activity and nutrition, and nonmodifiable factors such as gender, age, ethnicity, and somatotype. Athletes can train to maximize their genetically determined potential through strategic athletic training and nutrition.
4. Body composition plays an important role in athletic performance, especially for athletes who engage in gravitational, weight-based, and aesthetic sports. The body composition assessment can help to develop goals for target weight, evaluate effects of training and nutrition intake, develop a baseline from which to monitor progress of a nutrition and fitness program, and identify athletes who may be at increased health risk either due to too much body fat or not enough body fat.
5. Many methods are used in practice to monitor body composition. The most commonly used field methods include BMI, circumference, skinfold measurements, and BIA. Hydrostatic weighing and DXA scans are the most commonly used laboratory methods to monitor body composition. Manufacturers are currently developing products to bridge from the laboratory standards to methods that may be more feasible in practice. Two of these products include air displacement plethysmography, or the BodPod, and ultrasound techniques.
6. Body composition assessment is prone to error. Health professionals should be careful to follow protocols, undergo training, and interpret results cautiously. All results should be shared with the client as a range based on the method's margin of error rather than a precise number.
7. Indirect calorimetry is the most accurate method to estimate resting energy expenditure. Due to cost and convenience factors, it is rarely used in practice. Several equations are commonly used to estimate calorie needs. The most accurate of these methods is the Mifflin-St. Jeor equation.
8. Attaining a diet history is an important step to help athletes achieve nutrition and performance goals. The health professional and client can use the information obtained from a diet history to better understand the types of foods eaten and the factors that influence intake, assess the quality of a client's nutritional habits, and evaluate how well the client's typical eating habits compare with an ideal diet. In some cases, the health professional may initiate the process of assessing diet history and recognize that, to best meet the client's needs, referral to a registered dietitian is necessary.
9. Several tools are available to collect nutrition information including 24-hour recall, food frequency questionnaire, and food logs. The USDA offers an online tool, the SuperTracker, to track, analyze, and evaluate nutrition and physical activity.
10. After completing the initial assessment and comparing estimated body composition and dietary habits with ideals, the health professional can adopt the role of coach to help the athlete set and achieve goals. This includes assessing the athlete's readiness to change, goal setting (including development of an action plan), gaining proficiency in motivational interviewing, and ongoing health education and follow up.

PRACTICAL APPLICATIONS

1. Which of the following sport-specific attributes are MOST likely associated with endomorphs?
   A. Performance in gravitational sports
   B. Agility and speed
   C. Strength and lung capacity
   D. Leanness and quickness

2. An athlete with a body mass index of 26.3 is classified as ______________.
   A. normal weight
   B. overweight
   C. obese
   D. morbidly obese

3. Which of the following is NOT a means of measuring an individual's body-fat percentage?
   A. Hydrostatic weighing
   B. Skinfold measurements
   C. Bioelectrical impedance
   D. Body mass index
4. Which method of determining body composition is currently considered the premier method?
   A. Hydrostatic weighing
   B. Bioelectrical impedance analysis
   C. Duel energy x-ray absorptiometry
   D. Near-infrared interactance
5. Which method of body-composition assessment was initially developed to measure bone mineral content?
   A. Bioelectrical impedance
   B. Dual energy x-ray absorptiometry
   C. Air displacement plethysmography
   D. Near-infrared interactance
6. Air displacement plethysmography is a variation of which other method of body-composition assessment, in that it uses whole-body air displacement instead of water to measure body volume and density?
   A. Near-infrared interactance
   B. Body mass index
   C. Skinfold measurements
   D. Hydrostatic weighing
7. Bone, connective tissues, and internal organs are all included as part of a body's __________.
   A. essential fat
   B. nonessential fat
   C. lean tissue
   D. visceral tissue
8. A discussion designed to help an athlete weigh the pros and cons of making a behavioral change would be most effective during which stage of the transtheoretical model of behavioral change?
   A. Precontemplative
   B. Contemplative
   C. Action
   D. Maintenance
9. Which of the following is an element of SMART goal setting?
   A. Meaningful
   B. Action-oriented
   C. Relevant
   D. Simple
10. An athlete in which stage of the transtheoretical model of behavioral change is most likely to exhibit characteristics of having high levels of self-efficacy?
    A. Action
    B. Preparation
    C. Contemplative
    D. Maintenance

Case 1 Kate, the Marathon Runner

Kate is an experienced 22-year-old marathon runner. She has been training for the Boston Marathon. On your initial meeting with Kate she was 5′6″ and weighed 126 pounds. Now she is 114 pounds.

Body Composition and Nutrition Assessment

1. What is Kate's BMI? What does this mean?
2. If you were to conduct body composition assessment with Kate, what method would you choose? Why? Compare and contrast this method with another field method.
3. Kate tells you her doctor referred her to get a DXA scan. Explain how the DXA scan works. Why do you think her doctor referred her for this scan? What findings would you expect to see for Kate?
4. Using the Mifflin-St. Jeor equation, calculate Kate's approximate calorie needs.
5. Visit www.supertracker.usda.gov and enter Kate's age, height, weight, and physical activity to estimate daily calorie needs. This program uses the DRI method of calculating energy needs. State the result and compare it to the result obtained from the Mifflin-St. Jeor equation. Which method would you use?

Body Composition and Nutrition Coaching

1. You ask Kate to complete a dietary log through the MyPlate SuperTracker at www.supertracker.usda.gov. She provides you with the 2,400-calorie plan the SuperTracker produced. She also tells you that the program alerted her that she is underweight and asked her if she wanted a plan to maintain or gain weight. She tells you that she said "maintain weight" but asks you what you think.
   a. Print out a 2,400-calorie plan from SuperTracker. Explain why you agree or disagree whether or not this would be a good plan for Kate.
   b. Explain how you would respond to Kate's question about her weight.

Case 2 Susan, the Middle-Age Overweight Hiker

Susan is a 55-year-old overweight teacher who has struggled with obesity since childhood. After her best friend suffered a debilitating heart attack, she decided to change her lifestyle and achieve a healthier weight. As part of her fitness program, she is training to hike the Grand Canyon with her 17-year-old daughter and a guide. She is 5′2″ and weighed 180 pounds (BMI 32.9 kg/m2) at the onset of her training program, which she started about 2 months ago. Susan says that she has lost 10 pounds in the past 2 months and would like to make further changes to her fitness regimen and eating behaviors to continue to lose weight and keep it off.

While Susan has worked with you to improve her fitness and informally has asked nutrition questions, she says that she now would like to hire you to provide her with one health coaching session per week at least for the next month.

The Initial Consultation

1. Outline the approach you would take with Susan as part of the initial health coach consultation.
2. You complete a body composition assessment for Susan using BIA and find that she has a body fat percentage of 30% to 34%.
   a. Using the average of 32%, what is her current lean body weight?
   b. If Susan achieves her goal body composition of 28%, how much will she weigh (assuming all weight lost comes from fat)?

TRAIN YOURSELF

1. What is your BMI and BMI classification? Do you think that this accurately approximates your overall body composition?
2. Have you ever had a body composition assessment? If yes, describe your experience and thoughts. If not, would you want to have a body composition assessment? Which method do you find most appealing? Why?
3. Using the SuperTracker program at www.supertracker.usda.gov, do the following:
   a. Determine your daily calorie needs.
   b. Keep a 3-day food and activity log and enter your intake and activity into the SuperTracker program.
   c. Print out the analysis of your eating plan.
   d. How different is your typical intake from the SuperTracker recommendations?
   e. For 1 day, aim to follow the SuperTracker calorie and food group recommendations.
   Describe your experience.

REFERENCES

1. Lohman TG. *Advances in Body Composition Assessment.* Champaign, IL: Human Kinetics Publishers; 1992.
2. Ackland TR, Lohman TG, Sundgot-Borgen J, et al. Current status of body composition assessment in sport: review and position statement on behalf of the ad hoc research working group on body composition health and performance, under the auspices of the I.O.C. Medical Commission. *Sports Med.* March 1 2012;42(3):227-249.
3. Tran ZV, Weltman A. Generalized equation for predicting body density of women from girth measurements. *Med Sci Sports Exerc.* February 1989;21(1):101-104.
4. Tran ZV, Weltman A. Predicting body composition of men from girth measurements. *Hum Biol.* February 1988;60(1): 167-175.
5. National Heart Lung and Blood Institute. Clinical guidelines on the identification, evaluation, and treatment of overweight and obesity in adults the evidence report. [Preprinted June 1998]. Ed. Bethesda, MD: National Heart, Lung, and Blood Institute; 1998: http://purl.access.gpo.gov/GPO/LPS1019.
6. Rodriguez NR, Di Marco NM, Langley S. American College of Sports Medicine position stand. Nutrition and athletic performance. *Med Sci Sports Exerc.* March 2009;41(3):709-731.
7. Marfell-Jones MJ, Old T, Stewart AD, Carter L. *International Standards for Anthropometric Assessment.* Potchefstroom, South Africa: International Society for the Advancement of Kinanthropometry; 2006.
8. Sinning WE, Dolny DG, Little KD, et al. Validity of "generalized" equations for body composition analysis in male athletes. *Med Sci Sports Exerc.* February 1985;17(1):124-130.
9. Stewart AD, Hannan WJ. Prediction of fat and fat-free mass in male athletes using dual x-ray absorptiometry as the reference method. *J Sports Sci.* April 2000;18(4):263-274.
10. Frankenfield D, Roth-Yousey L, Compher C. Comparison of predictive equations for resting metabolic rate in healthy nonobese and obese adults: a systematic review. *J Am Diet Assoc.* May 2005;105(5):775-789.
11. Prochaska JO. *Systems of Psychotherapy: A Transtheoretical Analysis.* Homewood, IL: Dorsey Press; 1979.
12. Prochaska JO, Redding CA, Evers KE. The transtheoretical model and stages of change. In: Glanz K, Rimer BK, Lewis FM, Eds. *Health Behavior and Health Education.* 3rd ed. San Francisco: Jossey-Bass; 2002.
13. Cunningham SA, Vaquera E, Maturo CC, Narayan KM. Is there evidence that friends influence body weight? A systematic review of empirical research. *Soc Sci Med.* October 2012;75(7):1175-1183.
14. Howland M, Hunger JM, Mann T. Friends don't let friends eat cookies: effects of restrictive eating norms on consumption among friends. *Appetite.* October 2012;59(2):505-509.
15. Bond RM, Fariss CJ, Jones JJ, et al. A 61-million-person experiment in social influence and political mobilization. *Nature.* September 13 2012;489(7415):295-298.
16. Christakis NA, Fowler JH. The spread of obesity in a large social network over 32 years. *N Engl J Med.* July 26 2007; 357(4):370-379.
17. Gordon-Larsen P, Nelson MC, Page P, Popkin BM. Inequality in the built environment underlies key health disparities in physical activity and obesity. *Pediatrics.* February 2006; 117(2):417-424.
18. Sallis JF, Floyd MF, Rodriguez DA, Saelens BE. Role of built environments in physical activity, obesity, and cardiovascular disease. *Circulation.* February 7 2012;125(5):729-737.
19. Tester JM. The built environment: designing communities to promote physical activity in children. *Pediatrics.* June 2009;123(6):1591-1598.

20. Knowles MS, Swanson RA, Holton EF. *The Adult Learner, 7th Edition: The Definitive Classic in Adult Education and Human Resource*. Burlington, MA: Elsevier; 2011.
21. Klungland Torstveit M, Sundgot-Borgen J. Are under- and overweight female elite athletes thin and fat? A controlled study. *Med Sci Sports Exerc.* May 2012;44(5):949-957.
22. American College of Sports Medicine. Thompson WR, Gordon NF, Pescatello LS. *ACSM's Guidelines for Exercise Testing and Prescription*. 8th ed. Philadelphia: Lippincott, Williams & Wilkins; 2010.
23. Jackson AS, Pollock ML. Generalized equations for predicting body density of men. *Br J Nutr.* November 1978;40(3):497-504.
24. Jackson AS, Pollock ML, Ward A. Generalized equations for predicting body density of women. *Med Sci Sports Exerc.* 1980;12(3):175-181.
25. Torres-McGehee TM, Pritchett KL, Zippel D, Minton DM, Cellamare A, Sibilia M. Sports nutrition knowledge among collegiate athletes, coaches, athletic trainers, and strength and conditioning specialists. *J Athl Train.* March-April 2012;47(2):205-211.
26. Harris JA, Benedict FG. *A Biometric Study of Basal Metabolism in Man*. Washington, DC: Carnegie Institution of Washington; 1919.
27. Mifflin MD, St. Jeor ST, Hill LA, Scott BJ, Daugherty SA, Koh YO. A new predictive equation for resting energy expenditure in healthy individuals. *Am J Clin Nutr.* February 1990;51(2):241-247.
28. Owen OE, Holup JL, D'Alessio DA, et al. A reappraisal of the caloric requirements of men. *Am J Clin Nutr.* December 1987;46(6):875-885.
29. Owen OE, Kavle E, Owen RS, et al. A reappraisal of caloric requirements in healthy women. *Am J Clin Nutr.* July 1986;44(1):1-19.
30. Food and Agriculture Organization (FAO)/World Health Organization (WHO)/ United Nations University (UNU). Energy and protein requirements: report of a joint FAO/WHO/UNU expert consultation. *World Health Organization Technical Report Series.* 1985;724:1-206.
31. *Dietary Reference Intakes for Energy, Carbohydrate, Fiber, Fat, Fatty Acids, Cholesterol, Protein, and Amino Acids.* Washington, DC: Food and Nutrition Board, Institute of Medicine; 2005.
32. Torstveit MK, Sundgot-Borgen J. The female athlete triad: are elite athletes at increased risk? *Med Sci Sports Exerc.* February 2005;37(2):184-193.
33. Miller, W. & Rollnick, S. *Motivational Interviewing: Helping People Change.* New York: Guilford Press; 2013.

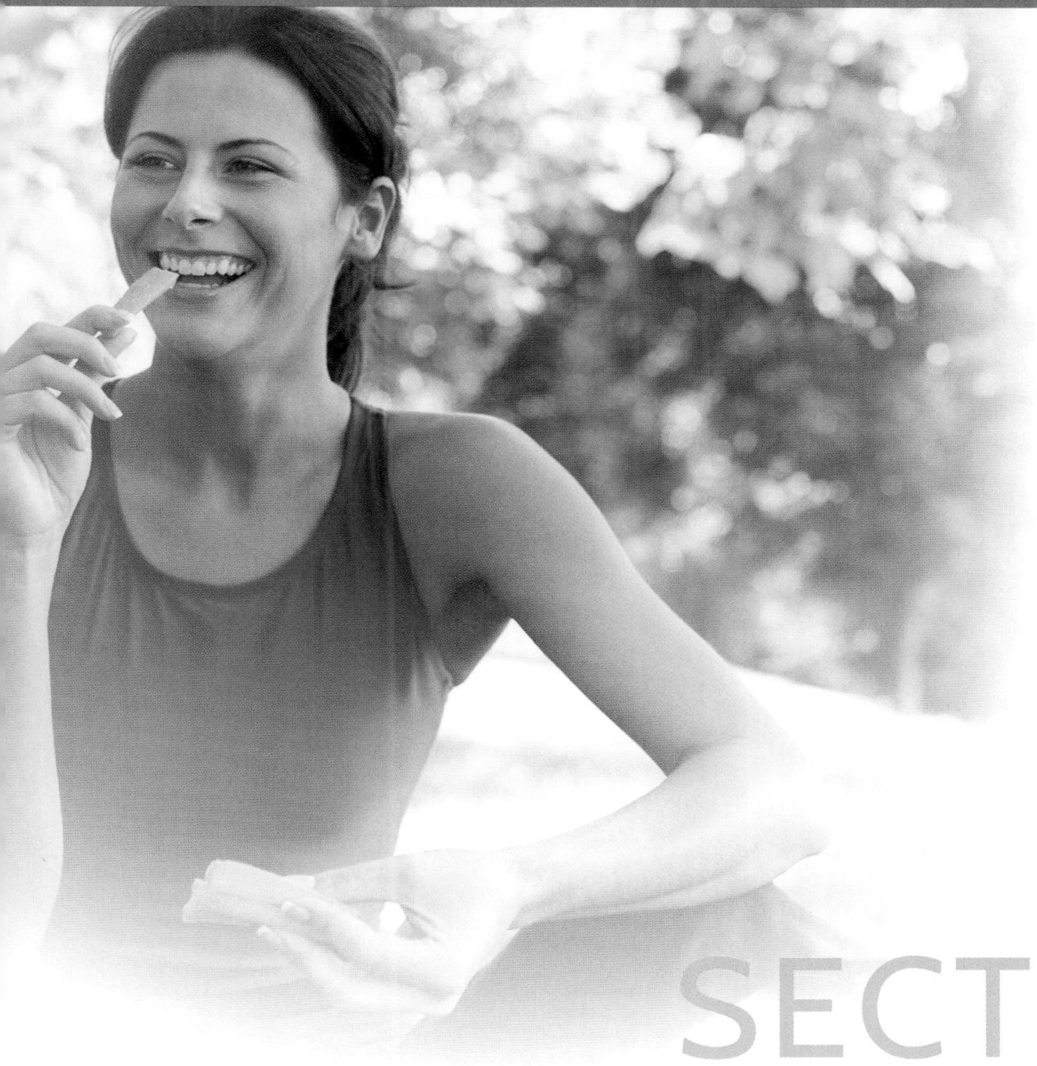

SECTION 4

Sports Nutrition for Special Populations

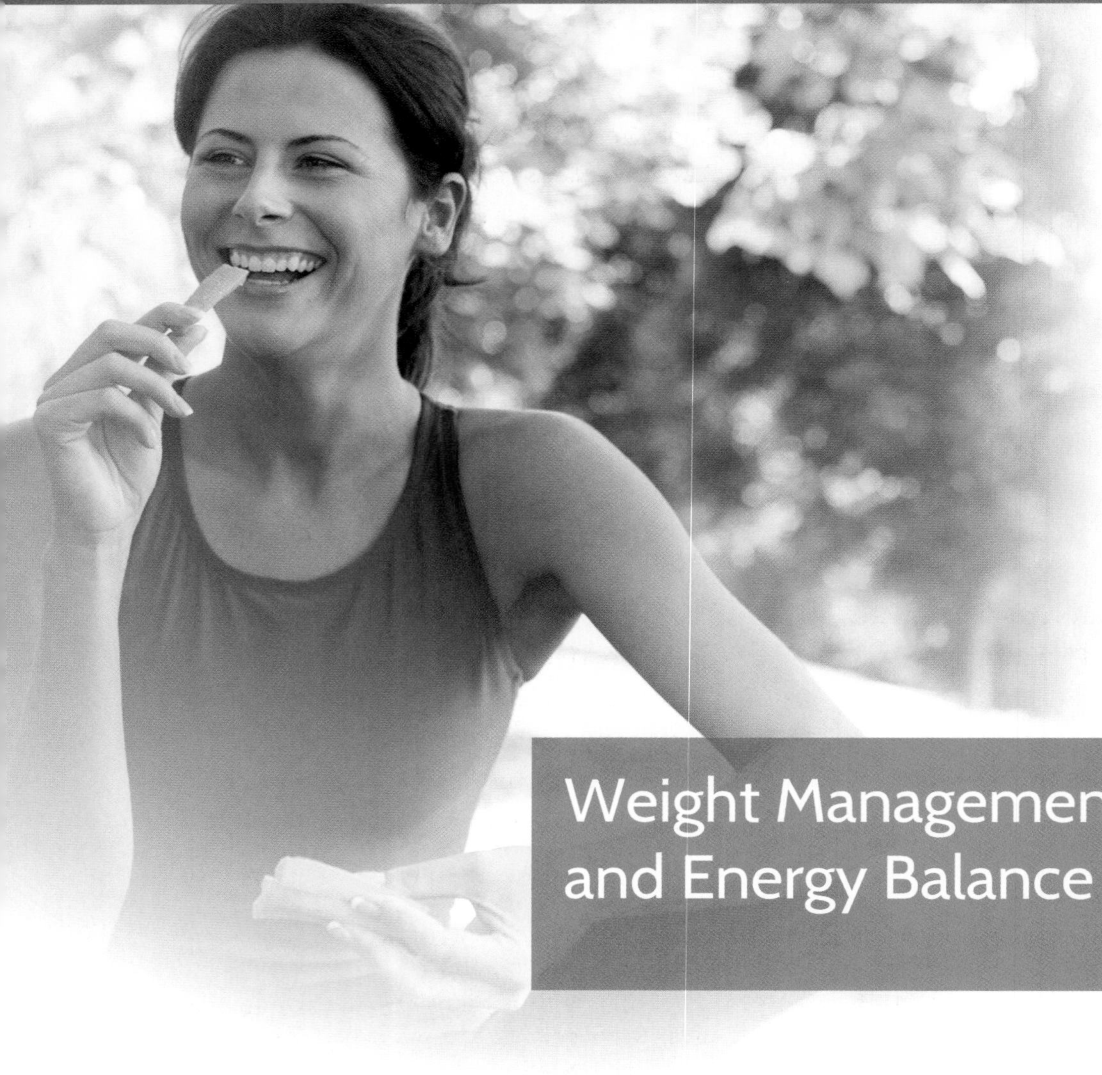

CHAPTER 12

Weight Management and Energy Balance

CHAPTER OUTLINE

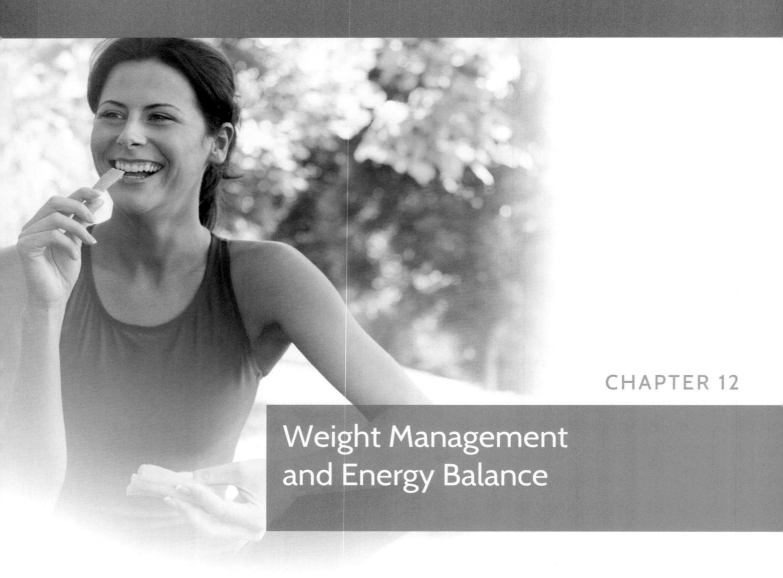

CHAPTER OUTLINE—cont'd

LEARNING OBJECTIVES

After studying this chapter the reader should be able to:

12.1 Describe the concept of energy balance.

12.2 List the factors that affect an individual's ability to maintain weight.

12.3 Describe how the determinants of energy balance change with aging.

12.4 List the major physical activity recommendations of the federal government's *Physical Activity Guidelines*.

12.5 Describe how the prevalence of obesity has changed over the past 20 years and list several reasons for the increase.

12.6 Explain how the hormones ghrelin, peptide YY, leptin, insulin, and adiponectin affect hunger and satiety.

12.7 List five health conditions that result from obesity.

12.8 Define and describe the term *metabolically healthy obesity*.

12.9 Provide a list of five tips to offer athletes who would like to gain weight or muscle mass.

12.10 Define what it means to adopt a healthy lifestyle.

12.11 Describe what factors increase the likelihood of sustained weight loss maintenance.

12.12 Provide a list of five tips to offer athletes who would like to lose weight or muscle mass.

KEY TERMS

adiponectin A hormone produced by fat cells; it increases insulin sensitivity and stimulates fat breakdown. Low levels may contribute to an increased risk for insulin resistance and diabetes.

android body type "Apple shaped"; body tends to carry excess fat around the abdomen.

caloric deficit The net expenditure of calories created when calories expended exceed calories consumed.

energy balance The relationship of calories consumed with calories expended.

energy expenditure The amount of calories burned by the body in a 24-hour period.

gastric bypass A weight-loss procedure in which a surgeon reduces the stomach to about the size of an egg and then reattaches it to the small intestine, thereby "bypassing" most of the stomach.

ghrelin The "hunger hormone"; a hormone released by the stomach in response to low energy levels in the body, which signals hunger.

gynoid body type "Pear shaped"; body tends to carry excess fat around the hips and thighs.

insulin A hormone secreted by the pancreas that is required for the transport of glucose from blood into tissues.

leptin A hormone produced by adipose tissue that suppresses appetite and increases energy expenditure; levels increase with increased fat storage. Obesity is associated with leptin resistance.

lifestyle changes Changes made to daily routines or habits; in this instance, changes are made to create a healthier lifestyle.

motivational interviewing A collaborative communication technique in which the client and coach work together to help the client develop a plan of action for behavior change.

negative energy balance When fewer calories are consumed than expended; leads to weight loss.

neutral energy balance When the number of calories consumed is equal to the number of calories expended.

peptide YY (PYY) An appetite suppressant released by the small intestine.

phytochemicals A variety of compounds found in plants that may have potential health benefits in humans.

positive energy balance When more calories are consumed than expended; leads to weight gain.

satiety A feeling of being fully satisfied, when there is no longer a desire to eat.

waist circumference Abdominal girth measured at the level of the umbilicus; values >40 inches (102 cm) in men and ≥35 inches (89 cm) in women are strong

CALCULATIONS

Body mass index = weight (kilograms)/ height (meters)^2

1 pound of fat = 3,500 calories

Desired body weight = Lean body weight/(1 – desired body fat percentage)

indicators of abdominal obesity and associated with an increased health risk.

waist-to-hip ratio (WHR) A measure for determining health risk due to the site of fat storage. Calculated by dividing the ratio of abdominal girth (waist measurement) by the hip measurement.

INTRODUCTION

"I get tired of people who say, 'It's simple, just eat less and move more,'" said Tara Parker-Pope, the creator and writer of "Well," a *New York Times* health blog and a woman with long-standing weight struggles. "We don't do dieters any favors by telling them that it's easy and simple."[1]

Parker-Pope's statement came in response to a highly personal piece she wrote for the *New York Times Magazine*, aptly titled "The Fat Trap."[2] The piece highlights the struggles of the millions of people attempting—mostly unsuccessfully—to lose and keep off significant amounts of weight. Parker-Pope tells the story of study participants who lost significant amounts of weight only to find themselves hungry, preoccupied with food, and hovering closer to their start weight only 1 year later. She describes her mother, a constant yo-yo dieter, who, as she was dying, was refused donation of her body to a local medical school due to her obesity. She highlights the plight of a formerly obese woman who maintains her 135-pound weight loss with a daily dose of 120 minutes of bicycle riding, water aerobics, and elliptical training.

Parker-Pope shows readers that weight loss is a long-term commitment, that obesity is not simply a reflection of a lack of "willpower," and that prevention of overweight and creating a healthier environment that does not reward unhealthy nutrition and activity behaviors may offer the best chance to improve the health of Americans. While written for the general population, the piece highlights many of the concepts health professionals must master to most effectively help athletes and the general population achieve their weight-management goals. These are the concepts discussed in detail in this chapter.

With about 25% of men and 40% of women on a diet at any given time,[3] 60 billion dollars spent each year on weight-loss products,[4] and the devastating health consequences resulting from excess weight and obesity, efforts to control weight and body size permeate the everyday lives of most Americans and most athletes. Even the minority of people who are satisfied with their current weight still may struggle to balance calories consumed with calories expended to avoid tipping the scale in either direction.

WEIGHT MANAGEMENT

The concept of weight plays an important role in the work of the health professional whose job is to help clients achieve optimal health and performance. In its Weight Management position statement, the Academy of Nutrition and Dietetics recommends that a discussion of weight management include:

- Prevention of weight gain
- Improvement in physical and emotional health
- Weight loss attained through changes in nutrition habits and physical activity
- Overall improvement in nutrition, exercise, and other behaviors.[5]

The definition may also be expanded to include gain in lean muscle mass through modified nutrition and physical activity.

ENERGY BALANCE

A person's success at controlling weight depends on the concept of **energy balance**, the relationship of calories consumed with calories expended (Fig. 12-1). When the number of "calories in" equals "calories out," a person is in **neutral energy balance**. When "calories in" is greater than "calories out," an individual is in **positive energy balance**. Positive energy balance is necessary during times of growth such as in infancy, childhood, and pregnancy. An athlete who is trying to gain muscle mass might also be in positive energy balance. With these exceptions, positive energy balance results in unnecessary weight gain. When "calories in" is less than "calories out," an individual is in **negative energy balance**. Negative energy balance is necessary for weight loss.

Calories consumed include all of the calories eaten in a 24-hour period. Determining this number depends mostly upon keeping a good record of food intake. Calorie, or energy, expenditure is generally more difficult to determine. This value includes not only the number of calories burned with structured exercise but also the calories necessary for physiological processes such as breathing, blood circulation, temperature regulation, food digestion and absorption, and the activities

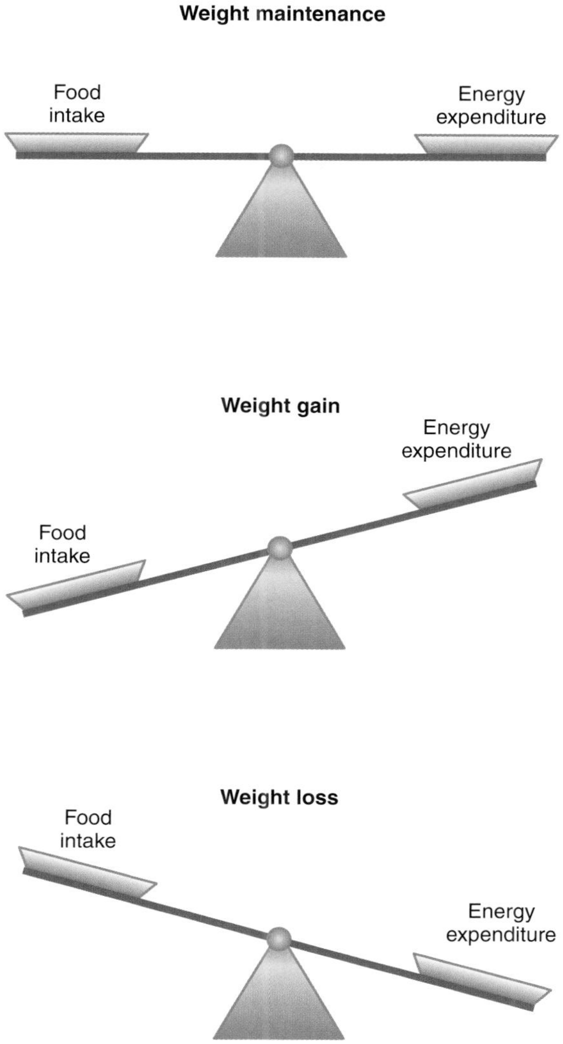

Figure 12-1. Energy balance.

of daily life. These factors are described in more detail in Chapter 11, along with various methods that health professionals may use to approximate an individual's daily caloric needs for weight maintenance and information on how to estimate a client's caloric expenditure.

While in the short term changes in caloric intake or expenditure are unlikely to cause significant changes in weight, chronic positive energy balance eventually contributes to overweight and obesity, while repeated negative energy balance leads to weight loss, and potentially, underweight. Mostly out of convenience and some scientific evidence that body mass index (BMI), a measure of height and weight (weight in kilograms divided by height in meters squared), provides a reasonably accurate estimate of body fatness,[6] health professionals use BMI to classify underweight, normal weight, overweight, and obesity (Table 12-1). However, if it is suspected that BMI has misclassified someone, for instance a bodybuilder who has gained muscle mass but is classified as overweight, the use of other methods to verify body composition is recommended. (For more information on BMI and other methods used to assess body composition, see Chapter 11.)

Table 12-1. BMI Classification of Weight

CLASSIFICATION	BMI
Underweight	<18.5 kg/m^2
Normal Weight	18.5–24.9 kg/m^2
Overweight	25–29.9 kg/m^2
Obesity	≥30 kg/m^2
Mild (Stage I)	30–34.9 kg/m^2
Moderate (Stage II)	35–39.9 kg/m^2
Severe/Morbid (Stage III)	>40 kg/m^2

SPEED BUMP

1. Describe the concept of energy balance.

NEUTRAL ENERGY BALANCE AND WEIGHT MAINTENANCE STRATEGIES FOR EXERCISE AND TRAINING

Neutral energy balance occurs when calories consumed equal calories expended. Neutral energy balance is essential to maintain current weight. Although the concept seems simple, many people struggle to maintain weight. This is exemplified by obesity trends: 30% of children are overweight or obese, while 67% of adults are overweight or obese.[7,8] That means that, over time, a lot of "normal" weight adolescents and teenagers become overweight adults. Whether due to a drop in metabolism or inattention to nutrition and physical activity, with each passing year, most people gain weight.

The National Health and Nutrition Examination Survey (NHANES) follow-up study found that among adults 25 to 44 years old, men gained about 3.4% of their body weight each 10-year interval; women gained 5.2% per 10 years.[9] This means that the typical normal-weight 6′0″ and 170-pound 25-year-old man would likely end up an overweight 182-pound 45-year-old. The average 120-pound 25-year-old woman can expect to weigh about 133 pounds by the time she is 45. Some research suggests that susceptibility to permanent weight gain seems to be highest during adolescence, pregnancy, and midlife in women and the period after marriage in men.[10] For most, weight gain does not end in middle age. A study conducted by the Centers for Disease Control and Prevention found that adults over age 60 were more likely to be obese than younger adults.[11] This may be due to a decades-long slow and steady loss of muscle mass and gain of fat, which translates to a decrease in the amount of calories burned. While this slowdown of metabolism can be responsible for weight gain, other contributors include: (1) lower levels of physical activity, (2) eating too many calories, (3) certain medications, and (4) unhealthy habits, such as lack of sleep and skipping breakfast. A study evaluating total energy expenditure (TEE)—the sum of calories burned from the basal metabolic rate (metabolism), the energy required to digest and absorb food, and physical activity—confirmed what most people already know: energy expenditure decreases with age.[12]

This reality is widely accepted and is even built in to formulas that estimate resting energy expenditure. While a small decrease in daily energy expenditure is probably inevitable, with a committed fitness program and eating low-calorie, nutrient-dense foods like vegetables and lean proteins, adults (i.e., anyone over 20 years old) can avoid the average weight gain due to the slowing of metabolism. No matter what age, the key to weight maintenance over time is to control caloric intake and emphasize exercise. Athletes, and most anyone interested in maintaining a healthy weight, should be encouraged to use feelings of hunger and fullness to help guide their intake.

Strength training and muscle building are essential to maintain metabolically active muscle mass, and regular cardiovascular physical activity is essential to maintain a high level of energy expenditure to help prevent increased fat mass. For optimal health, and for weight management, the U.S. Department of Health and Human Services' *Physical Activity Guidelines* recommend the following:[13]

- Children and adolescents should perform 60 minutes (1 hour) or more of physical activity daily. These activities should be fun, appropriate for their age, and varied.
- Adults should avoid inactivity. Some physical activity is better than none, and adults who participate in any amount of physical activity gain some health benefits.
- For substantial health benefits, adults should engage in at least 150 minutes (2 hours and 30 minutes) a week of moderate-intensity, or 75 minutes (1 hour and 15 minutes) a week of vigorous intensity aerobic physical activity, or an equivalent combination of moderate- and vigorous-intensity aerobic activity. Aerobic activity should be performed in episodes of at least 10 minutes, and preferably, it should be spread throughout the week.
- For additional and more extensive health benefits, adults should increase their aerobic physical activity to 300 minutes (5 hours) a week of moderate intensity, or 150 minutes a week of vigorous intensity aerobic physical activity, or an equivalent combination of moderate- and vigorous-intensity activity. Additional health benefits are gained by engaging in physical activity beyond this amount.
- Adults should also do muscle-strengthening activities that are moderate or high intensity and involve all major muscle groups on 2 or more days a week, as these activities provide additional health benefits.

SPEED BUMP

2. List the factors that affect a client's ability to maintain weight.

3. Describe how the determinants of energy balance change with aging.

4. List the major physical activity recommendations of the federal government's *Physical Activity Guidelines.*

POSITIVE ENERGY BALANCE

When more calories are consumed than expended, a person is in "positive energy balance" and will gain weight. During certain stages of life, such as infancy, childhood, and pregnancy, positive energy balance is essential for normal growth. However, chronic positive energy balance ultimately leads to overweight and obesity.

Overweight and Obesity

Overweight and obesity are worldwide health problems with about 1.4 billion people age 20 years or older being overweight and approximately 500 million of them obese.[14] About one-third of U.S. adults meet BMI criteria for obesity (BMI >30) and over two-thirds are overweight (BMI >25).[7] The rates of obesity vary by geographic region, with the highest prevalence in the Southeastern United States. A few states have fewer than one in five obese citizens, but for most states the numbers more commonly hover near 30%, according to data from the Centers for Disease Control and Prevention.[15] Figure 12-2 illustrates the surge in obesity levels over 20 years from 1990 to 2010, when obesity prevalence rates began to stabilize.

The obesity prevalence estimates rely exclusively on BMI to categorize weight. While not perfect, BMI is a well-established method of estimating body fatness. BMI is not a measure of body fat directly; however, BMI has been correlated to direct body fat measures such as underwater weighing and dual energy x-ray absorptiometry.[16,17] BMI may overestimate fat in muscular individuals, such as a football player who is "overweight" but not "overfat," and it may underestimate fat in others with normal weight but a high percentage of body fat compared to muscle, such as many elderly people (see Evaluating the Evidence). Still, it offers a good idea of whether or not to be concerned about a client's weight based on whether the client is categorized as underweight, normal, overweight, or obese.[6]

In adults, BMI ranges are set: any adult with a BMI greater than 25 is considered overweight and those with a BMI over 30 are considered obese. Children, however, are continually growing and experience growth spurts at certain ages; for example, a typical

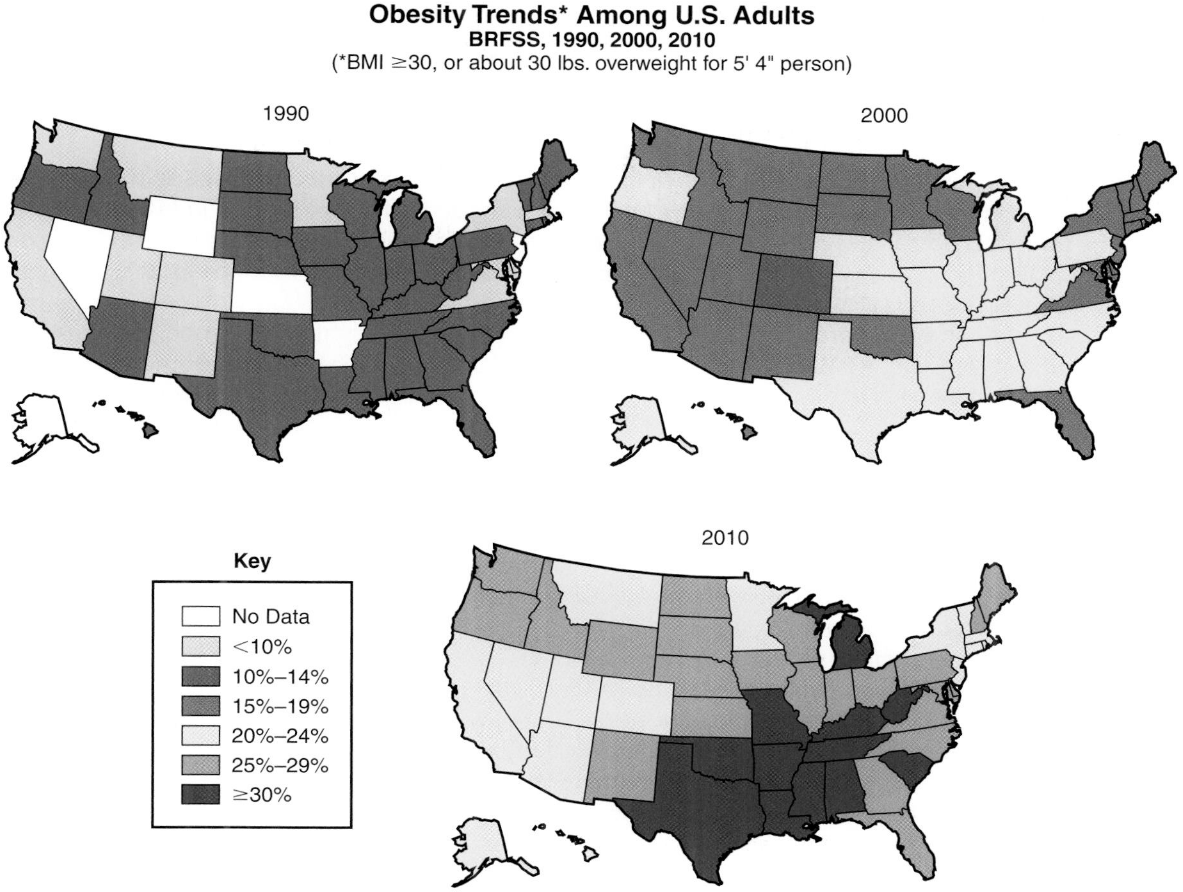

Figure 12-2. Obesity trends.

child will have a decrease in BMI around 4 years and then progressively increase throughout childhood. Thus, children's BMIs are plotted on an age- and gender-appropriate growth chart, and their BMI percentile is determined from that. For example, consider Dave, a 10-year-old male (his growth chart is shown in Fig. 12-3). He is 4′10″ and 110 pounds. His BMI is 23, which puts him in the 96th percentile. That means he weighs more than 96% of all children of the same age and gender, based on 1976 norms. (The BMI percentiles are based on the distribution of children's weights in 1976. Presently, considerably more than 5% of children have a BMI percentile >95%). According to these norms, Dave would be considered "obese."

Causes of Overweight and Obesity

While physiologically obesity results simply from longstanding positive energy balance in which more calories are consumed than are expended, many variables affect the equation. For example, obesity tends to run in families—partly due to genetic factors and a predisposition to store fat, and partly due to social factors and eating and activity habits. Genetic factors may also affect where body fat accumulates and subsequent health risks. **Waist circumference** and **waist-to-hip ratio** (WHR) measurements are simple ways to assess fat distribution. Many studies have reported fat storage primarily in the abdomen (**android**, or "apple shape") compared to fat storage in the hips and thighs (**gynoid**, or "pear shape"), which is characterized by a lower waist to hip ratio (WHR), contributes to significantly higher rates of hypertension, diabetes, elevated triglycerides, and coronary artery disease.[18] However, a large-scale and rigorous study of over 200,000 people in 17 countries found that BMI, waist circumference, and WHR are equally reliable in predicting cardiovascular disease risk, suggesting that carrying too much weight—regardless of where it is stored—negatively impacts heart health.[19]

The Physiology of Obesity

The human body is well equipped to recognize and respond when the body needs food for energy and sustenance (hunger) and when it has had enough (**satiety**). On the simplest level, a grumbling stomach signals it is time to eat; however, the physiology of hunger and satiety is intricate and complex. The hypothalamus part of the brain is in constant communication with the gastrointestinal system and the body's fat stores to regulate food intake. Two intestinal hormones are responsible for hunger and satiety signals. **Ghrelin,** also known as the hunger hormone, is released by the stomach when the stomach is empty. Ghrelin is responsible for stimulating

EVALUATING THE EVIDENCE

Is BMI a Good Measure of Fatness in Elite Athletes? A Look at the NFL

Professional football players are recognized for their massive body habitus and are often used as an example of "overweight" but not necessarily "overfat" athletes. Interested in the actual rates of BMI-defined overweight and obesity in the National Football League (NFL), researchers from the University of North Carolina carried out a study evaluating the BMIs of NFL players.[71] The researchers scoured the heights and weights of the football players as listed on the NFL website and calculated BMIs of 2,168 players.

Based on this study, an equal percentage of NFL players were of normal weight as were morbidly obese. The percentage of NFL players with a BMI of 30 or greater was more than double the percentage among 20- to 39-year-old men in a nationally representative sample. The study found that cornerback-defensive backs had the lowest mean BMI (26.8 [SD, 1.2]) and guards had the highest mean BMI (38.2 [SD, 2.1]).

Shortly after the study was released, the NFL issued a press release saying the study was irrelevant, mostly because it relied on BMI to classify obesity.

1. What are three strengths and three weaknesses of the study?
2. List three ways the authors might have strengthened the research design.
3. Explain why you agree or disagree with the following statement: "BMI is a good indicator of body fat percentage in football players."
4. Likely in response to the study described above, the NFL funded a study to evaluate the health risk profiles of players, which was published in the *Journal of the American Medical Association*. The authors concluded that "compared with a sample of healthy young-adult men, a sample of substantially larger NFL players had a lower prevalence of impaired fasting glucose, less reported smoking, a similar prevalence of dyslipidemia, and a higher prevalence of hypertension. Increased size measured by BMI was associated with increased CVD risk factors in this combined population."[72]

What do you make of these findings?

the neurons in the hypothalamus, which triggers the feeling of hunger. **Peptide YY** (PYY) is an appetite suppressant released by the small intestine whenever food is present in the gut. After a meal, ghrelin levels decrease and PYY increases. The increase in blood sugar that results after a meal triggers the pancreas to secrete **insulin**, which, among other functions, suppresses appetite.

Through this system, the body has mechanisms and processes to maintain a healthy weight. The hormone **leptin**, which is produced by adipose (fat) cells, is responsible for signaling feelings of satiety. However, a person who ignores the signals of satiety and continues to eat is bound to gain weight and fat stores. The chronically elevated insulin levels stimulate increased fat storage. This extra fat is metabolically active and also influences intake. When energy stored in fat is depleted, the leptin level decreases. The decrease in leptin signals to the brain to eat more (Fig. 12-4). It is worth noting that individuals above the 95th percentile actually have elevated leptin levels circulating in the blood. However, their body has built up a resistance to leptin, which continues the vicious cycle of eating and never feeling satisfied.[20]

Another hormone that plays an important role in weight control is **adiponectin**, which is produced by fat cells. Its major functions are to increase insulin sensitivity and stimulate fat breakdown. Overweight and obese people tend to have lower levels of adiponectin, which may contribute to an increased risk for insulin resistance and diabetes.

The hormonal interactions that determine hunger and satiety also affect a person's ability to successfully maintain weight loss. In a small study of 50 overweight and obese individuals, the participants lost a sizeable amount of weight on a very low-calorie diet. In response to the weight loss, levels of the hunger and satiety hormones adjusted in an intense effort to return to the baseline weight. Ghrelin levels surged to 20% above normal levels, leading to increased feelings of hunger, while PYY and leptin levels dropped, causing decreased feelings of satiety and slowing metabolism. Other hormones that affect hunger and metabolism also deviated from baseline levels. When the researchers followed up 1 year later, the hormone levels and the participants' subjective feelings of hunger were still elevated.[21] These persistent and counterproductive hormonal changes may help explain why it is so difficult for people who lose weight to maintain the weight loss, even with significant lifestyle changes.

Consequences of Obesity

Obesity affects every organ of the body, leading to serious complications including heart disease, hypertension, type 2 diabetes, respiratory disease, gallstones, osteoarthritis and other musculoskeletal disorders, social marginalization, discrimination, depression and other mental health disorders, and early death. Given its potentially devastating consequences, many researchers predict that obesity will be responsible for an

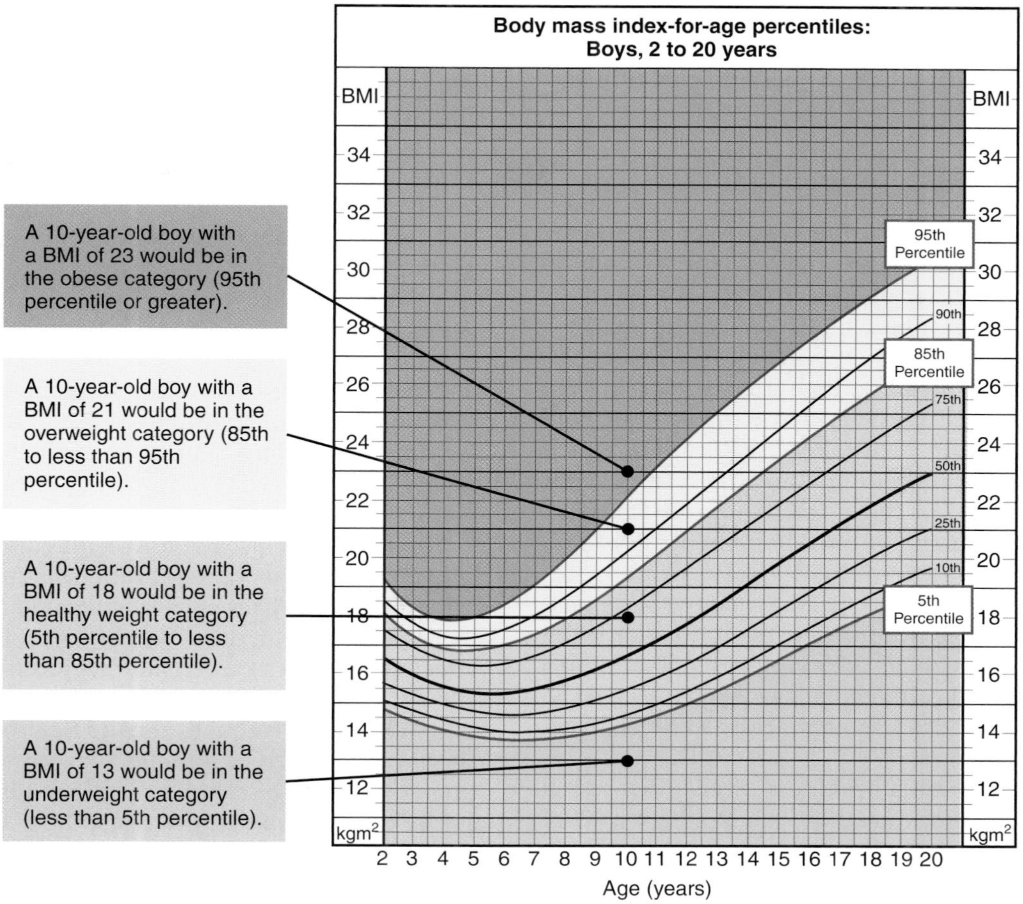

Figure 12-3. Dave's growth chart. *Adapted from Body Mass Index-for-Age Percentiles: Boys, 2 to 20 Years, Centers for Disease Control and Prevention.*

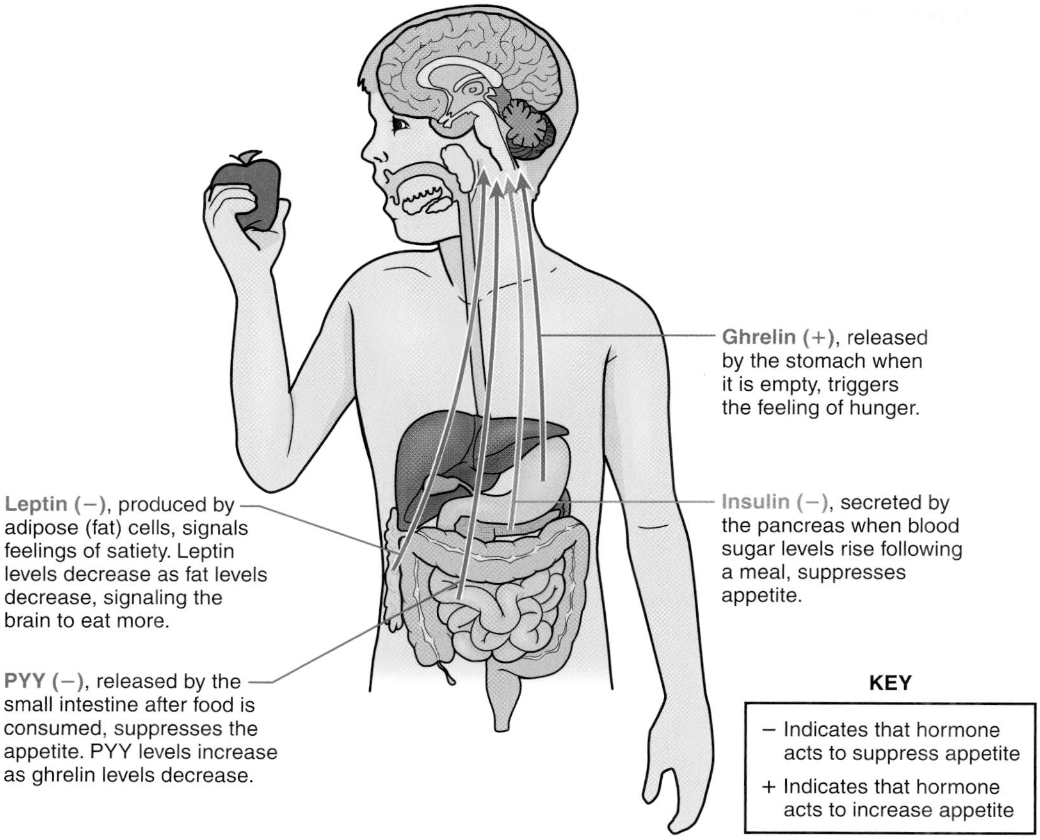

Figure 12-4. Hormonal control of appetite.

overall decrease in quality of life in the 21st century.[22,23] Obesity also contributes about $147 billion per year to health-care spending, which is about 9 cents of every health-care dollar.[24]

Obesity and Fitness

Despite the harmful health consequences associated with obesity, a number of studies have suggested that certain individuals appear to have a more benign or "metabolically healthy" obesity. This type of obesity is characterized by an absence of major cardiovascular risk factors often associated with excess weight including high blood pressure, high triglycerides, insulin resistance, impaired fasting glucose or diabetes, low HDL cholesterol, and high C-reactive protein, which is a marker of inflammation. In short-term studies it appeared as though these "metabolically healthy" obese individuals may not have increased risk of cardiovascular disease.[25-27] However, subsequent research, including a meta-analysis of peer-reviewed studies on the topic, found that even metabolically healthy obese individuals are at increased risk for all-cause mortality and cardiovascular events (though the risk is not increased for metabolically healthy overweight individuals).[76]

In studies that evaluated fitness levels, researchers found that obese individuals who attain a high level of fitness—even if they remain obese—seem to avert many of the harmful health consequences of carrying too much weight, at least in the short term.[28-31] Some studies have suggested "fat but fit" adults appear to be at no increased risk for cardiovascular disease or death compared to normal-weight and fit adults.[28,32] (The meta-analysis noted above was unable to analyze the role of physical activity due to inconsistent measurement criteria among studies.) In studies that have compared "fat but fit" adults with "unfat and unfit" adults, the heavier adults appear to be at decreased risk of death.[28,32] However, most obese adults are not fit. A study of 4,675 adults aged 20 to 49 found that only 9% of obese individuals who completed a submaximal exercise test had high fitness, whereas 17% of overweight and 30% of normal-weight individuals had high fitness.[33]

The epidemic of inactivity and poor fitness levels in the United States and other developed countries results from a variety of factors including the ready availability and promotion of high-calorie, low-nutrient-dense foods; emotional eating; and decreased daily physical activity. Most large-scale studies evaluating the relationship of weight and negative health outcomes do not rigorously evaluate or control for overall fitness level. As a result, when translating research into policy, the role of fitness in health is underemphasized in many policy recommendations and public health guidelines—even though fitness may be a more important marker of health than body size. Ultimately, a commitment to a regular exercise program will certainly improve fitness and thus mediate health risks—regardless of the amount of resulting weight loss.

Weight Gain and Athletes

While most people do not want to gain weight, some athletes and underweight individuals may need to gain weight for optimal performance and health. Many athletes strive to increase lean mass and strength. Adequate caloric consumption and strength training are essential to building muscle. Gains in lean mass may be most feasible for athletes during the off-season when overall caloric expenditure is lower and the athlete has more time to devote to strength training. During the heavy training season, athletes may have difficulty eating enough calories to gain weight and also have to balance high protein intake, which is essential for muscle building, with high carbohydrate intake, which is important for optimal endurance and peak performance for many sports.

The optimal approach to weight gain has not been as well studied as strategies for weight loss. A 1- to 2-pound weight gain per week created through a 500 to 1,000 calorie increase per day is probably safe and effective. Athletes can create this positive caloric balance by consuming higher-caloric foods, larger portion sizes, and more frequent meals. Health professionals should emphasize to athletes striving to gain weight that the quality of calories consumed is as important as the quantity of calories consumed. Lean proteins, nuts and legumes, fatty fish and other foods high in polyunsaturated fat, olive oil and other foods high in monounsaturated fat, and low-fat dairy products provide rich sources of calories and health benefit. Table 12-2 lists healthy, calorically dense snacks to promote weight gain.

SPEED BUMP

5. Describe how the prevalence of obesity has changed over the past 20 years and list several reasons for the increase.

6. Explain how the hormones ghrelin, peptide YY, leptin, insulin, and adiponectin affect hunger and satiety.

7. List five health conditions that result from obesity.

8. Define and describe the concept and scientific evidence related to *metabolically healthy obesity*.

9. Provide a list of five tips to offer athletes who would like to gain weight or muscle mass.

NEGATIVE ENERGY BALANCE

When fewer calories are consumed than are expended, an individual is in "negative energy balance" and will lose weight. This typically results from eating less (providing fewer "calories in") or increasing energy expenditure. Calorie intake may be decreased by a conscious effort to eat fewer calories or through decreased nutrient absorption (as occurs with some weight-loss medications and some health conditions).

Table 12-2. Healthy, Calorically Dense Snacks for Healthy Weight Gain

SNACK	PORTION SIZE	CALORIES
Dried fruit	¼ cup	80
Mixed nuts	1 oz	170
Granola	1 cup	600
Peanut butter sandwich	2 T. peanut butter 2 regular slices bread (52 g)	325
Fruit smoothie	16 oz	260
Avocado	1 cup cubes	240
Nonfat plain Greek yogurt	6 oz	100
Whole wheat pasta with olive oil	1 cup cooked pasta 1 T. olive oil	290
Tuna salad sandwich	3 oz tuna salad 2 regular slices bread (52 g)	300
Banana with peanut butter	1 medium 2 T. peanut butter	290
Part-skim mozzarella string cheese	1 oz	70

Source: http://ndb.nal.usda.gov/ndb/foods/list and www.choosemyplate.gov/SuperTracker/foodtracker.aspx

Increased calorie expenditure is most often achieved through increased physical activity or increased metabolic rate as a result of increased lean, highly metabolically active tissue. On rare occasions, increased energy expenditure may result from abnormal health conditions that cause a surge in metabolic rate, such as cancer, high fever, severe burns, or certain other ailments.

Fad diets have long tried to manipulate the components of the energy balance equation in creative ways to promote a negative energy balance, with limited degrees of short-term success. All fad diets promise big weight loss and all of them use negative energy balance to achieve results. However, most individuals find it challenging to maintain the eating pattern espoused by the fad diet in the long term and find that they regain any weight lost on the diet.

One popular, but ineffective, fad diet that claimed to create a negative energy balance while eating mass portions of a limited number of foods was the "negative calorie diet" or "catabolic diet" described in Myths and Misconceptions.

Myths and Misconceptions

Catabolic Foods Promote Weight Loss

The Myth

Certain "catabolic foods" promote weight loss. Catabolic foods are foods that purportedly require more calories to chew, digest, and absorb than are contained within the food itself.

The Logic

Some foods are so "low calorie" that it takes more energy to eat them than they contain, thus creating a negative energy balance and weight loss.

The Science

Proponents of catabolic diets encourage dieters to eat all the celery, grapefruit, apples, and other "negative calorie" foods they want, to ensure quick weight loss.

While it is true that metabolism is increased after eating—known as the thermic effect of food—this caloric expenditure is relatively small, and no study has ever demonstrated, regardless of the dietary composition of the food, that more calories are used to metabolize a food than the number of calories the food contains. Ultimately, there is *no* scientific research in support of a catabolic diet or the existence of any "negative calorie" foods.

That is not to say clients will not lose weight on a catabolic diet. While a client will not burn more calories eating a food than the number of calories the food contains, he or she can and should include low-calorie foods in a healthy eating plan to help keep weight-loss efforts on track.

Approaches to Weight Loss

While many people may have goals to lose a substantial amount of weight, even a 5% to 10% weight loss can improve health and decrease many of the risks associated with overweight and obesity.[34] There are four approaches to weight loss: **lifestyle changes**, which include eating less and exercising more; behavioral modification; medications; and surgery. All of the approaches attempt to manipulate calorie intake and calorie expenditure.

Lifestyle Changes: Nutrition and Exercise

To successfully lose a sizeable amount of weight, a client needs to be committed to significant long-term lifestyle changes. The goal is to create a **caloric deficit** so that fewer calories are eaten than are expended. With about 3,500 calories in a pound, a 500- to 1,000-calorie deficit each day through decreased food intake and increased physical activity leads to about a 1- to 2-pound weight loss per week (Box 12-1). By making relatively minor lifestyle changes such as drinking water rather than a 20-ounce bottle of soda (250 calories) and taking a 45-minute, 2.5-mile walk each day (about 250 calories), a client could lose a few pounds. But after a few weeks or months and several pounds later, continued weight loss becomes much more difficult. While predicting weight loss based on the equation of 3,500 calories per pound is useful early in weight loss, as an individual loses weight, metabolism (and thus energy expenditure) changes and the equation becomes less accurate and overpredicts weight loss.

A group of scientists at the National Institutes of Health developed a mathematical model to more accurately account for these metabolic changes. They approximate that for every 10-calorie decrease in intake, the average overweight adult will lose about 1 pound, with half of the weight lost by 1 year and 95% of the weight change by 3 years.[35] For example, a woman who decreased her daily caloric consumption from 2,200 calories to 2,000 calories would lose about 10 pounds by 1 year of the lowered caloric intake, and about 10 more pounds by the end of 3 years. If she had created a 500-kilocalorie deficit each day, she would lose 25 pounds in the first year and about 25 more pounds by the end of 3 years. Box 12-2 describes a weight-loss simulator based on this research.

The American Heart Association, American College of Cardiology, and the Obesity Society published a comprehensive guideline on the management of obesity, including nutritional considerations. Following are highlights from this report:

- Dietary approaches to weight loss may include (1) prescription of a 1,200–1,500 kcal/day for women and 1,500–1,800 kcal/day eating plan for men, with calorie level adjustments made based on body weight. [The dietary prescription should come from a physician or registered dietitian; diet prescription is outside the scope of most allied health professionals]; (2) prescription of an eating plan that will create a 500-750kcal/day energy deficit; or (3) prescription of an evidence-based eating plan that restricts certain food (such as high-carbohydrate foods, low-fiber foods, or high-fat foods) in order to create a caloric deficit.
- A comprehensive weight management program should include behavioral therapy in addition to dietary and activity changes. The best programs

Box 12-1. Doing the Math: 3,500 Calories Equals One Pound

A savvy client poses the following concern: "I keep seeing the number 3,500 kilocalories for a pound of fat. But if you convert pounds to grams (1,000 grams = 2.2 pounds), 454 grams = 1 pound and there are 9 calories per gram of fat, then 454 × 9 kilocalories = 4,086 kilocalories. This does not add up to 3,500 calories in a pound."

It is true that 1 pound of fat is 454 grams fat, but it is not stored as 100% lipid. Rather, it is approximately 90% lipid and 10% to 15% water. So, one pound of "fat" is approximately 400 grams of lipid × 9 calories/gram = 3,600 calories/pound. To make it simple, the value is commonly rounded to 3,500 calories per gram of fat. Of course, this equation supposes that weight loss is all fat and no muscle. In order for that to be the case, a client has to exercise (especially resistance training) to maintain muscle mass. Otherwise, about one-fourth of each pound lost will come from muscle.

What if a client is trying to gain muscle mass? The number of calories in a pound of muscle is remarkably similar to the number of calories in a pound of fat, but for different reasons. Muscle is made up of approximately 22% protein, 70% water, and 8% carbohydrates and fats. Therefore, 1 pound of muscle is approximately 100 grams of protein, or 400 calories from protein (454 g/pound × 0.22 = 100 grams × 4 kcals/gram). While this is a small number of calories, studies have shown that the additional energy necessary to build the small amount of carbohydrate and fat components of muscle and convert consumed protein into muscle (as fat cannot be converted into protein) requires about 8 calories per gram.[73] Because there are 454 grams in 1 pound, this turns out to be 3,600 calories (454 g × 8 kcal/gram = 3,632 kcal).

Box 12-2. A Weight-Loss Simulator

Scientists at the National Institutes of Health developed an online simulation to help determine how long and how much change in physical activity and caloric intake is necessary to achieve various weight-loss goals (for background on this simulation, see "A Mathematical Challenge to Obesity," by Claudia Dreifus, *New York Times*, May 14, 2012, available at www.nytimes.com/2012/05/15/science/a-mathematical-challenge-to-obesity.html). You can access the simulator at www.bwsimulator.niddk.nih.gov.

Based on this simulation, a 30-year-old female weighing 150 pounds (~68 kg) and measuring 5′4″ tall (~162.6 cm) who is classified in the "light work physical activity level, active leisure time physical activity level" could achieve a weight goal of 130 pounds (~59.1 kg) in 20 weeks (140 days).

The simulator divides weight change into two stages: weight change phase and weight maintenance phase. It shows that an individual needs to consume fewer calories to lose weight than to maintain weight loss. The calories are lower in the beginning to expedite the weight loss, and the calories during the maintenance phase are what are required to maintain the goal weight. If the maintenance calories were consumed the entire period, it would take longer to lose the desired amount of weight.

The scientists who developed this simulation are adamant that the commonly held belief that "there are 3,500 calories in a pound" is false. These scientists disagree because the data they have compiled indicate that the body changes as a person loses weight. They also found that "the fatter you get, the easier it is to gain weight. An extra 10 calories a day puts more weight onto an obese person than on a thinner one."

last at least 6 months and include a weight maintenance intervention afterwards. The weight loss maintenance intervention should include monthly or more frequent contact and an emphasis on physical activity, regular body weight monitoring, and consumption of a reduced-calorie diet.

- Adherence to a very low calorie diet (<800 kcal per day) results in significant weight loss and varying degrees of weight loss maintenance. However, this type of diet is contraindicated for certain populations and should only be followed under the supervision of a physician and/or registered dietitian due to the rapid weight loss and potential for complications.[77]

In its position statement on adult weight management, the Academy of Nutrition and Dietetics advises these additional considerations:[5]

- Consumption of a low-carbohydrate diet is associated with increased weight and fat loss compared to low-fat diets in the first 6 months, but these differences are not sustained at 1 year. Individuals with osteoporosis, kidney disease, or increased low-density lipoprotein should avoid diets with <35% of kilocalories from carbohydrate.
- A low-glycemic index diet is not recommended for weight loss or weight maintenance since evidence is insufficient to demonstrate its effectiveness. However, in order to maintain a healthy weight, one should consume complex carbohydrates, many of which are categorized as low-glycemic index foods, such as oatmeal, pumpernickel bread, grapefruits, strawberries and oranges, and plain yogurt.
- Attention to portion control results in decreased energy intake and weight loss.
- Total caloric intake should be distributed in four to five meals and snacks throughout the day, with greater consumption during the day compared with the evening.
- For individuals who have difficulty with selection and/or portion control, substituting one to two meals or snacks with meal replacement bars or drinks is a successful weight loss and weight maintenance strategy.

Since publication of these recommendations, it also has become clear that a change such as reducing or eliminating consumption of sugar-sweetened beverages such as sodas, sports drinks, and juices will reduce the prevalence of obesity and type 2 diabetes.[78]

The American College of Sports Medicine (ACSM) undertook a similar analysis to identify the factors most critical for weight loss, with similar recommendations. In regards to physical activity, the ACSM recommends that overweight and obese individuals gradually increase exercise duration to150 to 250 minutes per week of moderate intensity activity for improved health and to prevent weight regain.[36] For long-term weight loss, physical activity should exceed 250 minutes per week.[36] Resistance training does not enhance weight loss but helps to increase fat-free mass and preserve lean muscle mass during weight loss.[36]

Popular Diets

The best diet for weight loss is a source of contentious debate. From extremely low-fat diets and diets that severely limit carbohydrate intake, to meal replacements and strict calorie counting, each method has its followers. Every diet also has people who have failed to achieve their weight-loss goals.

A meta-analysis of 48 randomized controlled trials, the gold standard in research design, compared low-carbohydrate (Atkins, South Beach, Zone), moderate-macronutrient (Biggest Loser, Jenny Craig, Nutrisystem, Volumetrics, Weight Watchers), and low-fat (Ornish, Rosemary Conley) diets. The low-carbohydrate diets resulted in the greatest weight loss at 6 months (8.73 kg [19.2 lbs]), and the low-fat diets had the greatest weight loss at 12 months (7.25 kg [16 lbs]). However, the differences between the diets were marginal.[37] The moderate amount of weight lost reflects how people struggle to stick to rigid dietary restrictions, though it is worth noting that even a 5% to 10% weight loss confers significant health benefits.[38]

A study of 60,000 male and female participants of Jenny Craig, a commercial weight-loss program, found that those who followed the program for 1 year lost 16% of their body weight. But only 6.6% of the original dieters continued with the program for that long.[39] Another study found that people who replaced a meal each day with a 100- to 300-calorie substitute, such as a nutrition bar or formulated milk shake meal, maintained a substantial (8.4% ± 0.8%) weight loss at 4 years.[40] As Dansinger et al.[41] concluded after a 1-year randomized trial to assess the adherence rate and effectiveness of Atkins, Ornish, Weight Watchers, and the Zone diets, it does not matter what diet a person chooses as long as he or she can stick to it. However, this is a lot more difficult than it sounds.

The health professional can guide the client considering a new diet plan to critically evaluate whether or not a particular diet is a good choice. The client should be able to answer the following questions:

- *How does the diet cut calories?* In order for any diet to work, calories consumed need to be less than calories expended. Remember, it requires at least a 3,500-calorie deficit to lose 1 pound of fat. That is, if a client wants to lose about a pound per week, he or she needs to eat less and exercise more so that the net calorie balance is about 500 calories less per day than it is currently. Note that the rate of weight loss will slow over time.
- *What is the nutrient density of the diet?* The best diets will advocate at least nine servings daily of a variety of fruits and vegetables—low-calorie foods that provide most of the body's needed vitamins, minerals, and **phytochemicals**. Phytochemicals have been linked to decreasing the risk of infection and chronic diseases such as hypertension, stroke, and certain cancers.[42,43] Fiber-containing whole grains and calcium-rich low-fat dairy products should also be encouraged. If the diet relies primarily on a supplement to assure sufficient vitamins and minerals, it probably is not the healthiest choice.
- *Does the diet advocate exercise?* Nutrition is only one component in making a long-term lifestyle change. Exercise not only speeds weight loss by increasing caloric deficit, but is also essential in keeping the weight off.
- *Does it make sense?* Some diet plans make claims that oftentimes are based primarily on personal testimony. From promises to lose 10 or more pounds in the first 2 weeks of a diet, to the promotion of supplements that supposedly speed weight loss, diets are marketed as so easy and effective that they are irresistible—at first. But weight that is lost quickly is regained quickly. A client is most likely to be successful in losing weight and maintaining the weight loss if he or she aims for slow and steady weight loss with sustainable lifestyle changes.
- *Where is the evidence?* Research studies can be a rich source of information on the effectiveness and safety of different diets. When assessing research results, it is important to note the study limitations in addition to the results. For example, most of the diet research has been on obese middle-aged men and women. Thus, the results may not apply to younger people or those who are simply trying to lose 5 or 10 pounds but are not obese. Also, most diet studies were conducted over the course of 1 year or less. Therefore, the differences between the diets or the apparent benefits may not hold true for the long term.
- *Does it meet individual needs?* The client's health status and other individual factors must be considered when choosing a diet plan. If a client has a history of significant medical illness, such as (but not limited to) diabetes or heart disease, he or she should talk with his or her physician before starting a diet or exercise regimen.
- *How much does it cost?* While a client may initially be able to afford an expensive weight-loss program, he or she may not be able to sustain the cost for an extended period of time. Help him or her plan ahead and assess his or her readiness to change and commit to a program before making huge lifestyle adjustments and financial sacrifices.
- *What kind of social support does the client have?* Social support is key to successful weight loss. If a diet requires that a client eat a different food than the rest of the family, it is unlikely that he or she will be successful on the diet. If a client's family is not supportive and committed to helping him or her make the healthy change, he or she will probably struggle.
- *How easy is it to adhere to the diet?* Long-term adherence to a program (i.e., lifestyle change) is the most important factor for lifelong weight-loss success. It is not necessary to select a specific diet to achieve long-term weight loss; rather, individuals need to consume fewer calories from healthy food choices they like and are more likely to continue eating. Regardless of the weight-loss plan, most diets modestly reduce

body weight and cardiovascular risk factors, but people who adhere to the diet over the long term have greater weight loss and risk factor reductions.[41] The problem is that most dieters struggle to adhere to restrictive eating plans. A landmark study conducted by the National Institutes of Health found that most dieters had regained one-third to two-thirds of the weight lost within 1 year, and within 5 years dieters had regained almost all of the lost weight.[44] About one-third to two-thirds of dieters regain more weight than they initially lose.[45] This reiterates the key point: permanent lifestyle change is essential for successful weight loss and subsequent improved health.

Table 12-3 provides a summary of the strengths and weaknesses of some of the most popular and most studied diets.

Behavioral Management

Legendary football coach Vince Lombardi famously (and in the case of weight loss, incorrectly) said: "The difference between a successful person and others is not a lack of strength, not a lack of knowledge, but rather a lack of will." Dieters have long relied on willpower to adhere to short-term weight-loss plans. Consequently, when the pounds failed to melt away or were regained when the dieter resumed his or her normal eating and exercise patterns, many attributed the failure to a lack of willpower.

Long-term weight-loss success is more likely to occur by committing to permanent lifestyle changes including balanced and healthy nutrition choices (to control caloric intake), regular physical activity (to maximize caloric expenditure), and behavioral change (to facilitate adherence to nutrition and activity goals).

Of course, most people already know they should eat right and exercise. Following are several simple behavioral changes that may help clients turn knowledge into action and at the same time minimize reliance on willpower for weight-loss success.

- *Avoid tempting situations (also known as "stimulus control").* Clients may benefit from reducing cues for undesirable behaviors and increasing cues for desirable behaviors. For example, a client might remove junk food from the pantry and stock up on fruits and vegetables, dissociate from friends and colleagues with unhelpful eating and exercise habits and attitudes, make an effort to spend more time with active and healthy individuals, and eat small well-planned meals throughout the day to help avoid excessive eating or an unplanned stop at a vending machine or fast-food restaurant. To reduce psychological cues to eat

Table 12-3. An Overview of Several Popular Diets

DIET	STRENGTHS	WEAKNESSES
South Beach	Differentiates "good" and "bad" carbohydrates and fats Overall healthy after the first phase	Restrictive first phase Encourages too much initial weight loss Poorly studied
Atkins	Good short-term results Recipes simple to prepare	Nutritionally deficient (too much saturated fat, not enough fiber and fruits) Poor long-term adherence
Weight Watchers	Good variety of foods Behavioral support Lots of education Not too restrictive	Appeals to a specific audience Too costly for some Counselors not health professionals
NutriSystem	Food preparation easy to follow Serving sizes prepackaged	Requires prepackaged foods Expensive Not conducive to long-term adherence Has not been studied
Jenny Craig	Good nutritional value Behavioral support	Expensive Dependence on prepackaged food Counselors not health professionals Has not been studied
The Zone	Lower in saturated fat than Atkins Recipes simple to prepare Effective in short term	Poor long-term adherence Restricts many nutrient-dense foods

(such as boredom, habit, stress, or emotional distress), a client may restrict eating to the kitchen or dining room table.

- *Self-monitor.* One of the strongest predictors of successful and maintained lifestyle change is monitoring dietary intake.[46] While it can be tedious to keep a daily food log, this practice is highly effective. Clients may benefit from keeping a food log for at least 3 days including 1 weekend day. The log should list the type and amount of food eaten, complete with calories, time of intake, hunger ratings, emotions, and activities at the time of eating. Keeping a record of physical activity including activity, duration, and intensity is equally important. This exercise helps to identify strengths and weaknesses that otherwise might have gone unchecked and determine where formerly forbidden foods might fit in moderation.
- *Set SMART goals.* SMART (specific, measurable, achievable, results driven, and time bound) nutrition and physical activity goals help set the stage for weight-loss success by transforming vague visions of thinness into a specific plan for a healthier lifestyle. An example of a SMART goal might be: "I would like to lose 5 pounds in the next 2 months. I will do this by exercising for 30 minutes 3 days per week and limiting dessert to one time each week." A client can increase chances of success by posting visible reminders of the weight, dietary, or fitness goals.
- *Practice behavioral substitution.* Many people turn to food when bored or stressed. Encourage clients to tune into signs of hunger and fullness. One strategy might include asking themselves, "Am I hungry?" before opening the refrigerator or pantry door.
- *Retrain the brain—and taste buds.* If clients commit to eating a healthy, well-balanced diet that includes portion-controlled servings of a few of their favorite foods, deprivation and cravings are minimized. Over time the fat- and sugar-filled foods that were once so desirable may lose much of their allure.

Losing the Last 10 Pounds: A Marathon Analogy

Despite the most intensive physical activity regimen, nutrition changes, or behavioral rewiring, many people struggle to achieve their weight-loss goals, in large part because of the exceedingly difficult task of losing the last few pounds. A useful analogy when considering the challenges of trying to lose significant amounts of weight is to compare weight loss to competing in a marathon:

1. A marathon is 26.2 miles. An untrained and unprepared runner will "hit the wall" early on, most likely before the halfway mark, and will most likely fail to finish the race either because of mentally giving up or physically becoming injured. A novice runner who has trained well will be ready to quit around mile 20 when carbohydrate sources of energy are depleted and the fat becomes the primary energy source, when the ongoing stress and impact of running leads to muscle and joint pains, and when the race becomes very uncomfortable. But this person will endure and finish the race. A highly trained experienced marathoner will keep a steady pace throughout the long run and will finish the race at the top of the pack for age and gender. This performance is a direct result of a committed and well-designed physical training and mental toughness.

   Weight-loss application: Any client who is trying to lose significant amounts of weight has to practice persistence and patience. The client must have a realistic weight-loss plan with the full recognition that it takes time to lose weight. The lifestyle changes need to be ingrained and permanent—even a small deviance from the plan can derail weight loss and not only prevent future loss but also may lead to regaining the weight. This does not mean that a person trying to lose weight will never get to eat a piece of chocolate cake again. What it does mean is that chocolate cake needs to be built into the plan. Adopting a fad diet will not lead to long-term weight-loss success. For example, people who adopt very low-carbohydrate diets boast of significant early weight loss, but after a year's time, they are no better off than people who tried a different approach. The early weight loss was mostly water (and not fat) and the long-term outcome is dramatically slowed weight loss due to poor adherence to the eating plan. To permanently lose weight, an individual has to lose slowly and steadily through lifestyle changes that are maintained day in and day out, just as an athlete might train for a marathon by running 4 days per week for 18 weeks as he or she builds up to race day.
2. Our ancestors were capable of running long distances when hunting such animals as antelopes and gazelles. However, because we no longer have to hunt for our food, our bodies have to be trained, fed healthfully, and properly hydrated to run long distances such as marathons. To illustrate, in 2010 a Belgian man ran a marathon for every day of the year—365 marathons in as many days.

   Weight-loss application: The human body does not prefer to be on a diet. Everyone has a steady-state weight that the body tries very hard to maintain. When a person gains weight above that steady state, the body attempts to increase caloric expenditure. When a person loses a substantial amount of weight, the body attempts to gain weight to get back to the steady state. This is part of the reason why losing the last few pounds becomes increasingly difficult. While a client is trying to lose more weight, the body may resist by decreasing metabolism and increasing hunger. With permanent and effective nutrition and physical activity strategies, a client can achieve a new steady state. Following are tips to share with clients struggling to lose weight:

- *Change up the endurance routine.* The goal is to burn more calories. A client can do this without increasing the amount of time spent on cardiovascular exercise by increasing the intensity. Otherwise, the client will need to increase the amount of time committed to cardiovascular exercise, whether that's adding 15 or 20 minutes to a current routine or increasing the number of days per week.
- *Strength train at least twice per week.* Muscle mass is directly proportional to metabolism, and thus calories burned. People who have a large muscle mass burn more calories and can more easily lose weight when they control caloric intake than those who have low muscle masses. When a client loses considerable weight, about a quarter of the weight loss comes from muscle if strength training is not included in the workout routine. This helps explain why the last few pounds are so hard to lose. The metabolism has slowed down and, therefore, the client burns fewer calories at rest because every pound of lean muscle mass burns about 6 calories per day. While that may not sound like much, if a client lost 20 pounds of fat and kept all of his or her muscle mass, the 5 pounds of muscle mass kept (versus what might be lost without a resistance training program) would help him or her lose about 3 extra pounds. A client can maintain muscle mass while continuing to lose weight by committing to a resistance training routine.
- *Eat less.* To successfully lose weight, a client needs to make significant dietary changes. Assess the client's approximate daily caloric intake and then help the client devise strategies to cut an additional 250 calories per day (provided that will still keep the client at a healthy calorie level and not at risk for nutrient deficiencies). If the client eats 250 calories less per day and does not make any changes to his or her exercise regimen, he or she will lose those last 10 pounds over the course of the next 5 to 6 months.

Somewhere around 40% of women and 25% of men are trying to lose weight at any given time.[3] Some are successful initially, but most are unable to lose and keep off the weight. Losing weight is difficult. Keeping it off requires a constant effort. To achieve and maintain weight loss, a client must commit to making permanent changes. A client can slowly and steadily progress toward his or her goal with each of the small decisions he or she makes every day—such as taking the stairs instead of the elevator or going for the fresh apple instead of the apple pie. For many clients, being the first one done is not necessarily the goal, rather it is about having the strength, endurance, and mental toughness to successfully cross that finish line.

While health professionals may be well-versed in the nutrition, activity, and behavioral strategies necessary for successful weight loss, many may have difficulty translating information into an effective coaching approach. One approach that has gained increasing scientific support is **motivational interviewing** (see Communication Strategies).

Despite the highest quality intervention, superior motivation and desire, and implementation of agreed upon nutrition and physical activity improvements, many people will still struggle to achieve and maintain weight loss. In some of these cases, a client will desire medical or surgical weight-loss intervention. These forms of obesity therapy should always be initiated under the supervision of a physician, with the health professional taking a supportive role in close consultation with the treating doctor and bariatric team.

Pharmacological Approaches to Weight Loss

While pills are never a remedy for an unhealthy lifestyle, medications may be beneficial for obese clients and certain overweight clients with one or more weight-related disorders. Research suggests that overweight or obese people who eat healthfully, exercise regularly, and take a weight-loss medication lose more weight than those who use the drug alone or lifestyle treatment alone at 1 year.[47]

The two most well-studied weight-loss medications are sibutramine and orlistat. Sibutramine (Meridia) works by decreasing appetite. It costs approximately $100 per month, and on average leads to a 10-pound weight loss,[48] or 4% of body weight, after 1 year.[49] Sibutramine is available by prescription only. Orlistat (Xenical, Alli) blocks fat absorption. While orlistat was once available by prescription only, Alli may now be purchased over the counter. Weight loss is modest, about 6 pounds after 1 year,[48] and the cost reaches approximately $170 per month for the prescription version. The side effects are a significant impediment to continued use.

In 2012, lorcaserin and Qsymia became the first new FDA-approved weight-loss drugs in over 13 years. Lorcaserin (Belviq) binds to cell receptors in the brain, such as the hypothalamus, that help control appetite through satiety. Two clinical drug trials found that lorcaserin's weight-loss-promoting effects are modest—about 5.8% body weight in 1 year (participants in the placebo group lost 2.5%). But, a sizeable number of people taking the drug experienced these weight improvements—47% compared to just 23% in the placebo group.[49] Qsymia is the combination of two older medications: phentermine, an appetite suppressant and a stimulant,

COMMUNICATION STRATEGIES

Motivational Interviewing

Imagine that you have accepted a job as a health education coordinator for a large university-affiliated wellness center. One of your responsibilities includes providing individualized one-on-one health coaching to clients. While you thoroughly enjoy your work, you have become frustrated by the lack of progress in your overweight clients trying to lose weight.

Eager to learn the most effective coaching strategies to inspire permanent lifestyle change and subsequent weight loss, you decide to do some research on effective interviewing approaches. You find a review article that evaluates the role of a technique referred to as motivational interviewing in the treatment of obesity. Motivational interviewing is a collaborative communication technique in which the client and coach work together to help the client develop a plan of action for behavior change. Through open-ended questions, reflective listening, affirmations, and summarizing, the coach explores a client's ambivalence about change and helps the client to recognize his or her own strengths and motivation for change. [74] The coach provides information and education only when asked or provided permission by the client. This is in contrast to the traditional counseling technique in which the counselor provides advice and the client is supposed to listen and follow the counselor's advice.

The research article states that after reviewing and analyzing a total of 3,535 scientific articles, of which 11 were randomized controlled trials that included quantitative data analysis, the data confirmed that motivational interviewing leads to a significant improvement in body mass index in overweight and obese patients. The authors conclude that motivational interviewing enhances weight loss.[75] Impressed by the data, you prepare to practice motivational interviewing. You do more research on the technique and read that motivational interviewing is rooted in at least five basic components:

1. *Ask Open-Ended Questions.* Open-ended questions allow for deeper conversation and for the client to share his or her stories. Clients do most of the talking while the counselor listens and responds with reflective or summary statements. Sample questions might include, "What will be the biggest challenges in making this change?" or "Why is this time different?"
2. *Elicit "Change Talk."* This technique asks clients to identify reasons for wanting to change. This helps clients and counselors address discrepancies between what the client states he or she would like to do and what he or she actually does (e.g., the client states he or she would like to lose weight but then continues to eat a high-calorie diet). Sample questions might include, "What changes would you like to make?" or "How will your life be different from changes you make today?"
3. *Explore Importance and Confidence.* These questions help the client to articulate how important the desired change is to him or her and how confident he or she is that the goal will be achieved. Questions might include, "On a scale of 1 to 10, how confident are you that you can make this change?" and "Why did you choose [x] number, instead of [x-1] number?"
4. *Practice Reflective Listening and Summarizing.* Reflective listening involves carefully listening to the client and then guessing at the meaning of what the client said. For example, a coach might say, "You are highly motivated to change but think that it is going to be very difficult." This technique helps the client to identify the need for change, anticipated challenges, and how to overcome them. Summarizing statements are longer reflections, which may link different pieces of the conversation or provide a recap of a notable portion of the discussion.
5. *Affirm.* Affirming statements voice support and confidence in the client's commitment to behavior change. For example, "Your idea to take the stairs instead of the elevator will provide you with great health benefit and help you achieve your weight-loss goal. I have a lot of confidence that you are going to be successful."

Before using the technique with your clients, you ask a colleague to do a mock session with you so that you can get some practice and work out any major difficulties.

CLASSROOM EXERCISE

Together with a classmate, role play the client or the coach during a motivational interviewing session. Then switch roles.

1. What did you like best about this exercise?
2. What was the most challenging aspect of this exercise?
3. On a scale of 1–10, how likely are you to use this technique with your clients?
4. On a scale of 1–10, how confident are you that you will be able to successfully implement this technique? What could help you to feel more confident in your ability?

and topiramate, which is classically used to control seizures and headache. (Its physiological role in weight loss is unclear.) The combination appears to contribute to a 10% weight loss when combined with improved nutrition and exercise, and 62% of treated individuals lost 5% of body weight by 1 year compared to 20% in the placebo group.[49] In clinical trials, the drug also decreased blood pressure and diabetes risk, but it may increase heart rate and risk of birth defects when taken by pregnant women. Each of the FDA-approved weight-loss drugs carries significant potential side effects,[50] such as sleeplessness, and increased heart rate and blood pressure, which a client should discuss with a physician prior to beginning treatment.

In 2014 contrave, a combination of the antidepressant buproprion and naltrexone, a drug used to help treat alcohol and opiate dependence, was approved by the FDA.

Many non-FDA approved herbals and supplements claim to contribute to weight loss with varying degrees of safety and success (as described in Chapter 10). A medical professional should monitor any client who is considering taking a weight-loss medication.

Surgical Approaches to Weight Loss

When dietary, lifestyle, and pharmacological approaches aren't effective, some people may benefit from weight-loss surgery. According to 2001 National Institutes of Health Guidelines, ideal candidates are severely obese (BMI >40) or obese (BMI >35) with other high-risk conditions, such as diabetes, sleep apnea, or life-threatening cardiopulmonary problems; an "acceptable" operative risk determined by age, degree of obesity, and other pre-existing medical conditions; previously unsuccessful at weight loss with a program integrating diet, exercise, behavior modification, and psychological support; and carefully selected by a multidisciplinary team who have medical, surgical, psychiatric, and nutritional expertise.[51] Weight-loss surgery is not recommended for the overweight or mildly obese person who is trying to lose 20 or 30 pounds. Furthermore, only those patients who are committed to permanent lifestyle changes—including regular physical activity and a healthy diet—are considered good candidates for surgery.[51] Given advances in bariatric surgery over the past 25 years since publication of the NIH guidelines, scientists have urged the NIH to update the guidelines.[79] As of this writing, the NIH has not done so.

Gastric bypass, a procedure in which a surgeon reduces the stomach to approximately the size of an egg and then reattaches it to the small intestine, is the most common weight-loss surgery. During the surgery, most of the stomach and about 2 feet of the small intestine are stapled shut, or bypassed. This procedure leads to weight loss for two reasons. First, the small stomach pouch cannot hold very much food, so caloric intake is dramatically reduced. Second, the majority of nutrient absorption occurs in the small intestine; by bypassing 2 feet of the small intestine, fewer calories and nutrients are absorbed. On average, patients lose 62% of their excess body weight[52] and maintain a weight loss of about 16.1% during the 10-year period following surgery[53] in addition to achieving an improvement in a variety of other health indicators such as blood pressure, cholesterol, insulin sensitivity, and quality of sleep.[52,54] In fact, bariatric surgery is associated with drastic improvement in blood glucose levels in obese individuals with diabetes compared with medical management alone[55] and a reduced number of cardiovascular deaths and events such as heart attack and stroke.[56] One study of nearly 10,000 patients who had undergone gastric bypass surgery concluded that surgery significantly reduced mortality, especially from deaths related to diabetes, heart disease, and cancer.[57] Of course, surgery is never without risks. People who undergo bypass surgery are more likely to die from causes not related to disease.[57] One of every 200 people who has bypass surgery dies as a result of the procedure;[52] another 20 experience major morbidity such as infections, bleeding, nutritional deficiencies, blood clots, respiratory failure, and bowel obstruction.[58]

Weight Loss Maintenance

While there is some utility in imposing dietary or activity changes upon people or measuring the effect of a medication or surgical procedure, perhaps the most practical way to learn what works is to ask the people who have successfully lost, and kept off, large amounts of weight. The National Weight Control Registry (NWCR) (www.nwcr.ws), a database that tracks more than 5,000 people who have lost at least 30 pounds and maintained the loss for at least 1 year, has uncovered an abundance of tips to help people lose weight and keep it off. Results from several observational research studies further highlight what works and what does not. Following are 10 insights to share with clients:

1. *Control portions.* Successful "losers" control portions. In fact, research suggests portion control is the greatest predictor of successful weight loss.[59] Help clients control portions by teaching them to read nutrition labels, carefully measure out servings, eat only one helping, use smaller serving dishes, and resist the urge to "clean their plate."
2. *Be mindful.* Encourage clients to eat when hungry and stop when full. That means paying attention to everything they eat. Ask: Do you eat when you're bored, stressed, sad, tired, and sometimes even when you're full? Emotional eating can wreak havoc on a well-planned weight-management program. Clients should ask themselves "why" before heading to the pantry.
3. *Exercise.* Over 94% of participants in the National Weight Control Registry increased physical activity in order to lose weight.[54] In fact, many reported walking for at least 1 hour per day. And for those who kept the weight off, exercise was crucial. People who dropped their fitness

program regained weight.[60] This is mainly attributed to the reality that as people lose weight, a proportion of each pound comes from muscle. That slows down metabolism and makes it difficult to keep the weight off. While walking and other cardiovascular exercise is important for burning calories, a resistance training program preserves lean tissue and metabolic rate.

4. *Check the scale.* While it is not advisable to become obsessive about weight, people who maintain their weight loss keep tabs on the scale, weighing themselves at least once per week.[61] This way they are able to identify small weight increases in time to take appropriate corrective action.
5. *Eat breakfast.* Seventy-eight percent of NWCR participants eat breakfast daily; only 4% never do.[62] Research suggests that breakfast eaters weigh less and suffer from fewer chronic diseases than non-breakfast eaters.[63]
6. *Monitor intake.* One of the strongest predictors of successful and maintained lifestyle change is monitoring dietary intake.[46] While tedious, keeping a food log is a highly effective and proven strategy (the details of how to keep a food log are described in Chapter 11).
7. *Minimize screen time.* Screen time in front of the television, computer, smartphone, or tablet is usually spent: (1) being completely sedentary and thus expending minimal amounts of calories, and (2) eating. Successful NWCR "losers" watch less than 10 hours of television per week.[64]
8. *Do not cheat.* People who do not consistently give themselves a day or two off to cheat are 1.5 times more likely to maintain their weight loss.[65] Encourage clients to adopt a healthy lifestyle that they can stick with so they do not often feel compelling urges to unwittingly sabotage their weight-management success.
9. *Strengthen social support networks.* The healthiness of close peers significantly impacts a person's ability to lose weight and keep it off. A study of 12,000 people followed over 30 years concluded that "obesity appears to spread through social ties."[66] That is, obese people tend to have obese friends. Pairs of friends and siblings of the same sex seem to have the most profound effect. The study authors suspect the spread of obesity has to do with an individual's general perception of the social norms regarding the acceptability of obesity. The logic works like this: "If my best friend and my sister are both obese, and I love and admire them all the same, then maybe it's not so bad that I gain a few pounds." While this study was not conducted on participants in the National Weight Control Registry, the results are striking and worth including in this discussion of successful approaches to weight-loss maintenance. Clients can reverse this psychological phenomenon by spending time with peers who engage in healthful eating and activity habits. Or, clients can be the driving force for healthful changes by inviting friends to work out at the gym or go for a bike ride to stay or get fit.
10. *Encourage optimism.* Research suggests that people who are optimistic, that is, they have perceived control, positive expectations, empowerment, a fighting spirit, and lack of helplessness, are more successful at changing behaviors and losing weight.[46]

Beyond Individual Responsibility: Large-Scale Strategies to Combat the U.S. Weight Problem

While individuals are responsible for their behaviors, community- and policy-level factors can greatly influence eating and activity patterns. In 2012, the Institute of Medicine released "Accelerating Progress in Obesity Prevention: Solving the Weight of the Nation."[67] In the report, the authors outlined several goals that, if implemented collectively, would make significant strides in obesity prevention. The goals included:

1. Make physical activity an integral and routine part of daily life by enhancing the built environment; providing and supporting community programs designed to increase physical activity; adopting physical activity requirements for licensed child care providers; and providing support for the science and practice of physical activity.
2. Create food and beverage environments that ensure that healthy food and beverage options are the routine, easy choice by adopting policies and implementing practices that reduce overconsumption of sugar-sweetened beverages; increasing the availability of lower-calorie and healthier food and beverage choices for children in restaurants; utilizing strong nutritional standards for all foods and beverages sold or provided through the government and ensuring the healthy options are readily available; introducing, modifying, and utilizing health-promoting food and beverage retailing and distribution policies; and broadening the examination and development of U.S. agriculture policy and research to include implications for the American diet.
3. Transform messages about physical activity and nutrition by developing and supporting a sustained, targeted physical activity and nutrition social marketing program; implementing common standards for marketing food and beverages to children and adolescents; ensuring consistent nutrition labeling for the front of packages, retail store shelves, and menus and menu boards that encourage healthy choices; and adopting consistent nutrition education policies for federal programs with nutrition education components.
4. Expand the roles of health-care providers, insurers, and employers by providing standardized

care and advocating for healthy community environments; ensuring coverage of, access to, and incentive for routine obesity prevention, screening, diagnosis, and treatment; encouraging active living and healthy eating at work; and encouraging healthy weight gain during pregnancy and breastfeeding, and promoting breastfeeding-friendly environments.

5. Make schools a national focal point by requiring quality physical education and opportunities for physical activity at schools; ensuring strong nutritional standards for all foods and beverages sold or provided through schools; and ensuring food literacy, including skill development, in schools.

Chapter 5 describes potential large-scale strategies to put some of the recommendations into action. Health professionals entering the field at this time have an opportunity to shape their client interactions and communities to promote these ideals and create a healthier community where clients can live, work, and play.

Weight Loss and Athletes

Athletes across many sports and levels of competition strive to achieve weight-management goals. Like the general population, athletes benefit from making healthful nutrition and exercise changes to create a caloric deficit. However, unlike the general population, athletes experience other pressures, such as the need for appropriate nutrient intake to optimize performance, reliance on adequate hydration and fluid intake for performance as well as safety, and, in certain sports, requirements to achieve a particular weight or body composition to compete successfully. Competitive athletes with specific weight-management and performance goals may benefit from consultation with a registered dietitian who is a Certified Specialist in Sports Dietetics. This dietitian can provide the athlete an individualized nutrition plan to optimize nutrient needs for athletic performance while also creating a caloric deficit for safe weight loss. This consultation is especially important for athletes who seem overly concerned or attentive to body composition or weight and who may be at risk for an eating disorder. Eating disorders are discussed in more detail in Chapter 15.

Athletes who want to lose weight should lose no more than 1 to 2 pounds per week, not to exceed approximately 1.5% of body weight. Weight lost more rapidly may indicate dehydration or other unsafe weight-loss practices, such as self-deprivation, self-starvation, or disordered eating. These harmful practices negatively affect performance and health. Athletes in weight-conscious sports such as wrestling, boxing, dance, and gymnastics are at highest risk of adopting unsafe weight-loss practices. In response to the tragic deaths of three college wrestlers who died from complications of excessive weight loss while trying to reach a lower weight class, the National Federation of State High School Associations imposed strict regulations on weight loss in wrestlers. (These standards are described in Box 12-3).

Box 12-3. Weight-Loss Standards for Wrestlers

Already-lean wrestlers bundled in sweat suits, fleece hats, and winter coats jogging up and down the school halls panting and soaked in sweat, desperate to lose the last few ounces before the weekly weigh-in used to be an expected winter-season scenario in high schools across the country.

It was not until 2004, several years after the deaths of three collegiate wrestlers, that the National Collegiate Athletic Association and a year later the National Federation of State High School Associations, addressed unsafe weight practices among wrestlers. Now wrestlers must undergo a preseason evaluation to identify a safe weight and body fat percentage. If they weigh in at less than their minimal safe weight, they are automatically disqualified from competition.

The high school rules, which apply to 18,000 schools and approximately 13 million students in all 50 states and the District of Columbia, follow this procedure:

1. All wrestlers must undergo an initial assessment during which body composition is measured no longer than 6 weeks prior to the beginning of practice.
2. Male wrestlers must have at least 7% body fat; female wrestlers must have at least 12%. If at the initial assessment the athlete's body weight is less than the minimum, the athlete must receive medical clearance to participate. That athlete may not wrestle at a weight lower than the weight at initial assessment.
3. Prior to body fat measurement, athletes must have their urine checked. If the result is a specific gravity greater than 1.025 (a sign of dehydration), the athlete must wait 24 hours before being retested. Body fat percentage is measured with skinfold calipers by a trained and certified assessor.
4. The minimum wrestling weight corresponds to that weight at which the athlete would have either 7% or 12% body fat, for males or females, respectively. If this minimum weight is between two weight classes, the wrestler's minimum weight class will be the higher weight.
5. Athletes may not lose more than 1.5% of their weight per week.
6. The lowest weight class for wrestlers is 106 pounds (up from 103 pounds prior to the 2012-2013 season).

Unlike the well-researched and accepted guideline that an individual should lose no more than 1 to 2 pounds per week, body fat percentage loss is not as well studied and no official guidelines have been published. Most methods of measuring body fat (such as calipers and bioelectrical impedance analysis) are prone to measurement error, and detection of small changes in body fat percentage is just as likely due to this error as an actual change in body fat. Thus, it is best to wait 2 to 3 months to recheck body composition to see if a client has made progress.

Weight loss alone will not necessarily lead to large decreases in body fat, as weight loss without exercise will lead to decreases in lean mass as well. The most effective way to lose body fat is to eat a healthy, portion-controlled diet; engage in regular cardiovascular exercise; and develop a consistent resistance training program to build lean mass. Assuming a client engages in regular resistance training, and all the weight lost comes from the fat, the following formula predicts how much weight a client should lose in order to achieve an ideal body fat percentage:

Desired body weight = Lean body weight/ (1 – desired body fat percentage)

Desired body weight = how much the client will weigh when he or she achieves desired body fat percentage
Lean body weight = how many pounds of lean tissue the client currently has (to know this, the client needs to have had a body composition assessment)
Desired body fat percentage = the goal body fat percentage (in decimal form)

For example, Angela weighs 120 pounds and has 25% body fat (30 lbs fat, 90 lbs lean). Her goal is to have 20% body fat. How much weight will she need to lose (assuming all of the weight loss comes from fat)?

Desired body weight = 90/(1 – 0.20) = 113 pounds
So, she would need to lose 7 pounds to achieve her goal (120 – 113 = 7).

Ideal body fat percentage is different for men compared to women, as women require a higher body fat percentage in order to maintain menstruation and the ability to have children (see Chapter 11).

The National Athletic Trainers' Association recommends that the best time to strive to optimize weight and body composition is during the preparatory phase of sport conditioning, during the off-season.[68] During the competitive season focus should be on optimizing sport performance at the highest level of fitness.

Underweight and Health

Approximately 2% of Americans are underweight, defined as 15% to 20% or more below accepted weight standards, or as a BMI less than 18.5.[69] Underweight generally results from one or more of several potential scenarios, including: (1) inadequate intake to meet caloric needs; (2) excessive activity, which may occur with some athletes; (3) ineffective food absorption and digestion; (4) a disease that increases metabolic rate and energy needs, such as cancer or hyperthyroidism; and (5) psychological stress or depression.

Underweight is associated with increased morbidity and mortality compared to normal weight individuals.[70] Health professionals should consider referring an underweight client to a medical professional who can help to determine the underlying cause of underweight and whether medical or psychological intervention is necessary. After the initial evaluation, allied health professionals may offer several suggestions on how to healthfully gain weight (see Table 12-2). Concerns of underweight among older adults are described in Chapter 13, and concerns for clients with signs and symptoms of eating disorders are described in Chapter 15.

SPEED BUMP

10. Define what it means to adopt a healthy lifestyle.
11. Describe what factors increase the likelihood of sustained weight-loss maintenance.
12. Provide a list of five tips to offer athletes who would like to lose weight or muscle mass.

CHAPTER SUMMARY

Overall, many people, including the general population, recreational athletes, and collegiate and professional athletes, struggle to achieve or maintain an "ideal" weight. The health professional plays an important role in helping a client to identify effective strategies to optimize health and achieve healthy weight goals.

KEY POINTS SUMMARY

1. Energy balance is the relationship of calories consumed and calories expended. A positive energy balance occurs when more calories are consumed than expended. A negative energy balance occurs when more calories are expended than consumed. A neutral energy balance occurs when calories consumed equal calories expended.
2. Body Mass Index (BMI) is a measure of height and weight (weight in kilograms divided by height in meters squared), and provides an estimate of body fatness.
3. Any adult with a BMI greater than 25 is considered "overweight" and those with a BMI over 30 are considered "obese."
4. Factors affecting a client's ability to maintain his or her weight include a decline in metabolism, which often occurs with aging, and attention to nutrition and physical activity.

5. As metabolism decreases with aging, so do energy needs. Increasing energy expenditure through exercise and controlling caloric intake can help offset this decline in metabolism.
6. Strength training and muscle building are essential to maintain metabolically active muscle mass, and regular cardiovascular physical activity is essential to maintain a high level of energy expenditure and prevent increased fat mass. The U.S. Department of Health and Human Services provides *Physical Activity Guidelines* to achieve both.
7. Ghrelin, the "hunger hormone," signals hunger to the brain. Leptin, insulin, and peptide YY signal feelings of satiety and suppress appetite. Adiponectin is another hormone that plays a role in weight control. In obese individuals, leptin and insulin are elevated, and the cells in the body are no longer responsive to these hormones.
8. Obesity can lead to many serious health risk factors including heart disease, hypertension, type 2 diabetes, respiratory disease, gallstones, osteoarthritis and other musculoskeletal disorders, social marginalization, discrimination, depression and other mental health disorders, and early death.
9. Certain obese individuals appear to have a more metabolically healthy obesity, characterized by the lack of other cardiovascular risk factors often associated with excess weight. Some research suggests this may be due to these individuals maintaining a high level of fitness.
10. Safe rates of weight gain have not been rigorously studied, but 1 to 2 pounds per week with 500 to 1,000 additional calories per day from quality food sources is probably an acceptable rate.
11. There are four approaches to weight loss: lifestyle changes, behavioral modification, medications, and surgery.
12. The following factors help clients choose the diet that is right for them: How does the diet cut calories? What is the nutrient density of the diet? Does the diet advocate exercise? Does it make sense? Where is the evidence? Does it meet individual needs? How much does it cost? What kind of social support does the client have? How easy is it to adhere to the diet?
13. The following are 10 insights for successful weight loss maintenance: (1) control portions; (2) be mindful; (3) exercise; (4) check the scale; (5) eat breakfast; (6) monitor intake; (7) minimize screen time; (8) do not cheat; (9) strengthen support networks; (10) encourage optimism.
14. Competitive athletes may be under tremendous pressure to attain a particular weight. Those with specific weight management and performance goals may benefit from consultation with a registered dietitian who is a Certified Specialist in Sports Dietetics.
15. An underweight individual is defined as being 15% to 20% or more below accepted weight standards, or having a BMI less than 18.5.[69]

PRACTICAL APPLICATIONS

1. Jennifer is 5′7″ and weighs 190 pounds. What is her BMI?
   A. 19 kg/m^2
   B. 25 kg/m^2
   C. 30 kg/m^2
   D.35 kg/m^2

2. Over the past year, Cynthia has gained 15 pounds. Assuming this weight gain is the result of excess energy intake, how many total extra calories has Cynthia consumed beyond her body's average daily needs to create the added weight over the past year?
   A. 35,000 calories
   B. 46,500 calories
   C. 52,500 calories
   D. 60,000 calories

3. Christina is a 60-year-old woman who weighs 190 pounds (86 kg) and has an estimated body fat of 36%. Her goal is to reduce her body fat to 23%. What will her corresponding body weight be when she reaches her goal of 23% body fat, assuming all weight loss is from fat?
   A. 138 pounds
   B. 148 pounds
   C. 158 pounds
   D. 168 pounds

4. Follow-up assessments show that a female client with whom you have been working has lost 5 pounds (2.3 kg), but has seen little change in her body composition. Her current exercise routine consists of walking for 40 minutes, 4 days per week. What modification would be MOST important to improve body composition at this time?
   A. Add resistance training 2 to 3 days per week to maintain lean body mass and resting metabolic rate.
   B. Increase cardiorespiratory exercise intensity to increase caloric expenditure so that she will lose more weight.
   C. Decrease caloric intake by 200 kilocalories per day to facilitate greater fat loss.
   D. Increase protein consumption to maintain lean body mass while losing weight.

5. A client tells you in his initial interview that he would like to lose 40 pounds (18.2 kg) in 2 months. What is a more realistic timeframe for this weight to be lost safely and effectively?
   A. 10 weeks
   B. 14 weeks
   C. 17 weeks
   D. 20 weeks

6. A new client with whom you are working wants to lose 30 pounds (13.6 kg) in 20 weeks. She has already decreased her caloric intake from 2,000 to 1,500 kilocalories per day. At least how many additional kilocalories would she have to expend through exercise per week to meet her goal?
   A. 1,000 kilocalories per week
   B. 1,750 kilocalories per week
   C. 2,750 kilocalories per week
   D. 3,500 kilocalories per week
7. Which of the following statements is a SMART goal?
   A. "I will reach my goals by working 2 days per week with a personal trainer."
   B. "I will run a marathon in 14 weeks by running 2 miles (3.2 km) this week and increasing the mileage of my long run by 2 miles (3.2 km) each week."
   C. "I will decrease my blood pressure by losing 10% of my body weight."
   D. "I will lose 15 pounds (7 kg) in 3 months by lifting weights 2 days per week, taking three group exercise classes per week, and switching from regular to diet sodas."
8. You are working with a client who would like to lose 30 pounds (13.6 kg) in the next 20 weeks. What minimum daily caloric deficit would be needed to achieve this goal?
   A. 500
   B. 750
   C. 875
   D. 1,000
9. Which of the following is an example of an open-ended question?
   A. "What do you hope to achieve from an exercise program?"
   B. "Do you enjoy exercising?"
   C. "Are you more interested in weight training or flexibility training?"
   D. "Have you had success in previous exercise programs?"
10. During the initial interview, your client claims, "I want to lose all my excess weight within a month or two." Which of the following responses represents the most realistic approach for helping this client?
    A. Work with the client to determine activities that will best fit his or her objectives.
    B. Find out the client's preferences, exercise history, and motivational readiness for change.
    C. Structure appropriate exercise expectations at the beginning of your time together.
    D. Provide regular feedback that is specific and relevant to the client.

Case 1 Susan, the Middle-Age Overweight Hiker

Susan is a 55-year-old overweight teacher who is training to hike the Grand Canyon with her 17-year-old daughter and a guide. She is 5′2″ and 180 pounds (BMI 32.9 kg/m2) with a body fat percentage of 32%. She says that she would like to do the hike to spend time with her daughter and to begin a weight-loss program. She tells you that ultimately she would like to get down to her pre-wedding size of 130 pounds.

1. What questions would you ask Susan to better understand her goals and assess her likelihood of success?
2. Put together a weight-loss plan for Susan through increased physical activity and decreased caloric intake. Susan requires about 1,800 calories per day to maintain her current weight.
   a. How much of a caloric deficit does Susan need to create to meet her weight-loss goals? Provide examples of how she might meet this caloric deficit.
   b. How long would it take Susan to lose the desired amount of weight if she decreases her caloric intake by 300 calories per day?
   c. How long would it take Susan to lose the desired amount of weight if she decreases her caloric intake by 300 calories per day and increases her physical activity by 200 calories per day?
3. You do a body composition assessment and find that Susan has 30% body fat. Assuming that she engages in a consistent resistance-training program and all of the weight lost comes from fat, how much body fat will she have if she successfully loses 25 pounds?
4. What physiological changes will occur when Susan loses weight that will make it difficult for her to maintain the weight loss?
5. What advice would you provide Susan in her efforts to maintain her weight loss?

Case 2 Eric, the Recreational Bodybuilder

Eric is a 31-year-old competitive bodybuilder. He participates in bodybuilding competitions in the fall and trains the rest of the year. He is 5′11″ and weighs

184 pounds (14% fat, 86% lean muscle mass). He tells you that he would like to gain 5 pounds of muscle in the next 3 months.

1. What questions would you ask Eric to better understand his goals, and assess his likelihood of success in achieving his goal?
2. What would be some nutritional and exercise considerations to help Eric gain muscle mass (and not fat)?
3. If all of Eric's 5-pound increase is muscle, what will be his body fat percentage when he achieves his weight-gain goal?

TRAIN YOURSELF

1. What are your weight-management goals? (Lose, gain, maintain?) What efforts do you make each day to achieve these goals? What could you do differently?
2. Develop a short-term SMART goal to help you achieve your long-term goal described in the previous question.

REFERENCES

1. Nolan R. Behind the cover story: Tara Parker-Pope on weight loss. *The New York Times;* 2012.
2. Parker-Pope T. The fat trap. *The New York Times Magazine*. New York: *The New York Times*; 2011.
3. Kruger J, Galuska DA, Serdula MK, Jones DA. Attempting to lose weight: specific practices among U.S. adults. *Am J Prev Med*. June 2004;26(5):402-406.
4. MarketData Enterprises. The U.S. weight loss and diet control market. Tampa, FL: Marketdata Enterprises, 2011.
5. Seagle HM, Strain GW, Makris A, Reeves RS. Position of the American Dietetic Association: weight management. *J Am Diet Assoc.* February 2009;109(2):330-346.
6. Okorodudu DO, Jumean MF, Montori VM, et al. Diagnostic performance of body mass index to identify obesity as defined by body adiposity: a systematic review and meta-analysis. *Int J Obes (Lond)*. May 2010;34(5):791-799.
7. Ogden CL, Carroll MD, Kit BK, Flegal KM. Prevalence of childhood and adult obesity in the United States, 2011-2012. *JAMA*. February 2014, 311(8): 806-814.
8. Ogden CL, Carroll MD, Kit BK, Flegal KM. Prevalence of obesity and trends in body mass index among U.S. children and adolescents, 1999-2010. *JAMA*. February 1, 2012;307(5): 483-490.
9. Williamson DF. Descriptive epidemiology of body weight and weight change in U.S. adults. *Ann Intern Med*. October 1 1993;119(7 Pt 2):646-649.
10. Yanovski JA, Yanovski SZ, Sovik KN, Nguyen TT, O'Neil PM, Sebring NG. A prospective study of holiday weight gain. *N Engl J Med*. March 23 2000;342(12):861-867.
11. Flegal KM, Carroll MD, Kit BK, Ogden CL. Prevalence of obesity and trends in the distribution of body mass index among U.S. adults, 1999-2010. *JAMA*. January 20 2012.
12. Roberts SB, Dallal GE. Energy requirements and aging. *Public Health Nutr.* October 2005;8(7A):1028-1036.
13. *Physical Activity Guidelines*. Washington, DC: United States Department of Health and Human Services; 2008.
14. World Health Organization. Obesity and Overweight Fact Sheet No 311.Last updated March 2013. http://www.who.int/mediacentre/factsheets/fs311/en/. Accessed February 13, 2014.
15. Centers for Disease Control and Prevention. Overweight and obesity: Adult obesity facts. www.cdc.gov/obesity/data/adult.html. Accessed February 13, 2014.
16. Mei Z, Grummer-Strawn LM, Pietrobelli A, Goulding A, Goran MI, Dietz WH. Validity of body mass index compared with other body-composition screening indexes for the assessment of body fatness in children and adolescents. *Am J Clin Nutr.* 2002;7597-7985.
17. Garrow JS, Webster J. Quetelet's index (W/H2) as a measure of fatness. *Int J Obes*. 1985;9:147-153.
18. Manolopoulos KN, Karpe F, Frayn KN. Gluteofemoral body fat as a determinant of metabolic health. *Int J Obes (Lond)*. June 2010;34(6):949-959.
19. Wormser D, Kaptoge S, Di Angelantonio E, et al. Separate and combined associations of body-mass index and abdominal adiposity with cardiovascular disease: collaborative analysis of 58 prospective studies. *Lancet*. March 26 2011; 377(9771):1085-1095.
20. Myers MG Jr, Leibel RL, Seeley RJ, Schwartz MW. Obesity and leptin resistance: distinguishing cause from effect. *Trends Endocrinol Metab*. November 2010;21(11):643-651.
21. Sumithran P, Prendergast LA, Delbridge E, et al. Long-term persistence of hormonal adaptations to weight loss. *N Engl J Med*. October 27 2011;365(17):1597-1604.
22. Lakdawalla DN, Goldman DP, Shang B. The health and cost consequences of obesity among the future elderly. *Health Aff (Millwood)*. 2005;24 Suppl 2:W5R30-41.
23. Jia H, Lubetkin EI. The impact of obesity on health-related quality-of-life in the general adult U.S. population. *J Public Health (Oxf)*. June 2005;27(2):156-164.
24. Finkelstein EA, Trogdon JG, Cohen JW, Dietz W. Annual medical spending attributable to obesity: payer-and service-specific estimates. *Health Aff (Millwood)*. September-October 2009;28(5):w822-831.
25. Stefan N, Kantartzis K, Machann J, et al. Identification and characterization of metabolically benign obesity in humans. *Arch Intern Med*. August 11 2008;168(15):1609-1616.
26. Wildman RP, Muntner P, Reynolds K, et al. The obese without cardiometabolic risk factor clustering and the normal weight with cardiometabolic risk factor clustering: prevalence and correlates of 2 phenotypes among the U.S. population (NHANES 1999-2004). *Arch Intern Med*. August 11 2008;168(15):1617-1624.
27. Hamer M, Stamatakis E. Metabolically healthy obesity and risk of all-cause and cardiovascular disease mortality. *J Clin Endocrinol Metab*. April 16 2012.
28. McAuley PA, Blair SN. Obesity paradoxes. *J Sports Sci*. May 2011;29(8):773-782.
29. Lee CD, Blair SN, Jackson AS. Cardiorespiratory fitness, body composition, and all-cause and cardiovascular disease mortality in men. *Am J Clin Nutr*. March 1999;69(3): 373-380.
30. McAuley PA, Kokkinos PF, Oliveira RB, Emerson BT, Myers JN. Obesity paradox and cardiorespiratory fitness in 12,417 male veterans aged 40 to 70 years. *Mayo Clin Proc*. February 2010;85(2):115-121.
31. Wei M, Kampert JB, Barlow CE, et al. Relationship between low cardiorespiratory fitness and mortality in normal-weight, overweight, and obese men. *JAMA*. October 27 1999;282(16):1547-1553.
32. McAuley PA, Smith NS, Emerson BT, Myers JN. The obesity paradox and cardiorespiratory fitness. *J Obes*. 2012;2012: 951582.
33. Duncan GE. The "fit but fat" concept revisited: population-based estimates using NHANES. *Int J Behav Nutr Phys Act*. 2010;7:47.

34. *Clinical Guidelines on Identification, Evaluation, and Treatment of Overweight and Obesity in Adults: The Evidence Report.* Rockland, MD: U.S. Department of Health and Human Services;1998.
35. Hall KD, Sacks G, Chandramohan D, et al. Quantification of the effect of energy imbalance on bodyweight. *Lancet.* August 27 2011;378(9793):826-837.
36. Donnelly JE, Blair SN, Jakicic JM, Manore MM, Rankin JW, Smith BK. American College of Sports Medicine Position Stand. Appropriate physical activity intervention strategies for weight loss and prevention of weight regain for adults. *Med Sci Sports Exerc.* February 2009;41(2):459-471.
37. Johnston BC, Kanters S, Bandayrel K, et al. Comparison of weight loss among named programs in overweight and obese adults. *JAMA*. September 3, 2014; 312(9): 923-933.
38. *Clinical Guidelines on Identification, Evaluation, and Treatment of Overweight and Obesity in Adults: The Evidence Report.* Rockland, MD: U.S. Department of Health and Human Services;1998.
39. Finley CE, Barlow CE, Greenway FL, Rock CL, Rolls BJ, Blair SN. Retention rates and weight loss in a commercial weight loss program. *Int J Obes (Lond).* February 2007;31(2): 292-298.
40. Flechtner-Mors M, Ditschuneit HH, Johnson TD, Suchard MA, Adler G. Metabolic and weight loss effects of long-term dietary intervention in obese patients: four-year results. *Obes Res.* August 2000;8(5):399-402.
41. Dansinger ML, Gleason JA, Griffith JL, Selker HP, Schaefer EJ. Comparison of the Atkins, Ornish, Weight Watchers, and Zone diets for weight loss and heart disease risk reduction: a randomized trial. *JAMA.* January 5 2005;293(1):43-53.
42. Liu RH. Health benefits of fruit and vegetables are from additive and synergistic combinations of phytochemicals. *Am J Clin Nutr.* 2003;78(suppl):517S-520S.
43. Boeing H, Bechthold A, Bub A, et al. Critical review: vegetables and fruit in the prevention of chronic diseases. *Eur J Nutr.* 2012;51:637-663.
44. Methods for voluntary weight loss and control. NIH Technology Assessment Conference Panel. *Ann Intern Med.* June 1 1992;116(11):942-949.
45. Mann T, Tomiyama AJ, Westling E, Lew AM, Samuels B, Chatman J. Medicare's search for effective obesity treatments: diets are not the answer. *Am Psychol.* April 2007; 62(3):220-233.
46. Tinker LF, Rosal MC, Young AF, et al. Predictors of dietary change and maintenance in the Women's Health Initiative Dietary Modification Trial. *J Am Diet Assoc.* July 2007; 107(7):1155-1166.
47. Wadden TA, Berkowitz RI, Womble LG, et al. Randomized trial of lifestyle modification and pharmacotherapy for obesity. *N Engl J Med.* November 17 2005;353(20): 2111-2120.
48. Li Z, Maglione M, Tu W, et al. Meta-analysis: pharmacologic treatment of obesity. *Ann Intern Med.* April 5 2005; 142(7):532-546.
49. Hiatt WR, Thomas A, Goldfine AB. What cost weight loss? *Circulation.* March 6 2012;125(9):1171-1177.
50. Weight-control Information Network (WIN), National Institute of Diabetes and Digestive and Kidney Diseases (NIDDK). *Prescription medications for the treatment of obesity 2010.* http://win.niddk.nih.gov/publications/prescription.htm. Accessed April 14, 2013.
51. NIH conference. Gastrointestinal surgery for severe obesity. Consensus Development Conference Panel. *Ann Intern Med.* December 15 1991;115(12):956-961.
52. Buchwald H, Avidor Y, Braunwald E, et al. Bariatric surgery: a systematic review and meta-analysis. *JAMA.* October 13 2004;292(14):1724-1737.
53. Sjostrom L, Lindroos AK, Peltonen M, et al. Lifestyle, diabetes, and cardiovascular risk factors 10 years after bariatric surgery. *N Engl J Med.* December 23 2004;351(26):2683-2693.
54. Poirier P, Cornier MA, Mazzone T, et al. Bariatric surgery and cardiovascular risk factors: a scientific statement from the American Heart Association. *Circulation.* April 19 2011; 123(15):1683-1701.
55. Schauer PR, Kashyap SR, Wolski K, et al. Bariatric surgery versus intensive medical therapy in obese patients with diabetes. *N Engl J Med.* April 26 2012;366(17):1567-1576.
56. Sjostrom L, Peltonen M, Jacobson P, et al. Bariatric surgery and long-term cardiovascular events. *JAMA.* January 4 2012;307(1):56-65.
57. Adams TD, Gress RE, Smith SC, et al. Long-term mortality after gastric bypass surgery. *N Engl J Med.* August 23 2007; 357(8):753-761.
58. Steinbrook R. Surgery for severe obesity. *N Engl J Med.* March 11 2004;350(11):1075-1079.
59. Logue EE, Jarjoura DG, Sutton KS, Smucker WD, Baughman KR, Capers CF. Longitudinal relationship between elapsed time in the action stages of change and weight loss. *Obes Res.* September 2004;12(9):1499-1508.
60. Catenacci VA, Ogden LG, Stuht J, et al. Physical activity patterns in the National Weight Control Registry. *Obesity (Silver Spring).* January 2008;16(1):153-161.
61. Butryn ML, Phelan S, Hill JO, Wing RR. Consistent self-monitoring of weight: a key component of successful weight loss maintenance. *Obesity (Silver Spring).* December 2007;15(12):3091-3096.
62. Wyatt HR, Grunwald GK, Mosca CL, Klem ML, Wing RR, Hill JO. Long-term weight loss and breakfast in subjects in the National Weight Control Registry. *Obes Res.* February 2002;10(2):78-82.
63. Timlin MT, Pereira MA. Breakfast frequency and quality in the etiology of adult obesity and chronic diseases. *Nutr Rev.* June 2007;65(6 Pt 1):268-281.
64. Raynor DA, Phelan S, Hill JO, Wing RR. Television viewing and long-term weight maintenance: results from the National Weight Control Registry. *Obesity (Silver Spring).* October 2006;14(10):1816-1824.
65. Gorin AA, Phelan S, Wing RR, Hill JO. Promoting long-term weight control: does dieting consistency matter? *Int J Obes Relat Metab Disord.* February 2004;28(2):278-281.
66. Christakis NA, Fowler JH. The spread of obesity in a large social network over 32 years. *N Engl J Med.* July 26 2007; 357(4):370-379.
67. *Accelerating Progress in Obesity Prevention: Solving the Weight of the Nation.* Washington, DC: Institute of Medicine; 2012.
68. Turocy PS, DePalma BF, Horswill CA, et al. National Athletic Trainers' Association position statement: safe weight loss and maintenance practices in sport and exercise. *J Athl Train.* 2011;46(3):322-336.
69. Fryar CD, Ogden CL. Prevalence of underweight among adults: United States, 2003-2006. www.cdc.gov/nchs/data/hestat/underweight/underweight_adults.htm 2009. Accessed June 3, 2012.
70. Flegal KM, Graubard BI, Williamson DF, Gail MH. Excess deaths associated with underweight, overweight, and obesity. *JAMA.* April 20 2005;293(15):1861-1867.
71. Harp JB, Hecht L. Obesity in the National Football League. *JAMA.* March 2 2005;293(9):1061-1062.
72. Tucker AM, Vogel RA, Lincoln AE, et al. Prevalence of cardiovascular disease risk factors among National Football League players. *JAMA.* May 27 2009;301(20):2111-2119.
73. Forbes GB, Brown MR, Welle SL, Lipinski BA. Deliberate overfeeding in women and men: energy cost and composition of the weight gain. *Br J Nutr.* July 1986;56(1):1-9.
74. Miller WR, Rollnick S. *Motivational Interviewing: HelpingPeople Change.* 3rd ed. NY: Guilford Press; 2013.
75. Armstrong MJ, Mottershead TA, Ronksley PE, Sigal RJ, Campbell TS, Hemmelgarn BR. Motivational interviewing to improve weight loss in overweight and/or obese patients: a systematic review and meta-analysis of randomized controlled trials. *Obes Rev.* September 2011;12(9):709-723.

76. Kramer, C.K., Zinman, B., Retnakaran, R. Are metabolically healthy overweight and obesity benign conditions?: A systematic review and meta-analysis. *Ann Intern Med.* December 3, 2013;159(11):758–69.
77. Jensen MD, Ryan DH, Apovian CM, et al. AHA/ACC/TOS guidelines for the management of overweight and obesity in adults: a report of the American College of Cardiology/American Heart Association Task Force on Practice Guidelines and the Obesity Society. *Circulation.* 2013. Available at www.lipid.org/sites/default/files/ManagementOverweightObesity.pdf
78. Hu FB. Resolved: there is sufficient scientific evidence that decreasing sugar-sweetened beverage consumption will reduce the prevalence of obesity and obesity-related diseases. *Obes Rev.* 2013; 14(8): 606-619.
79. Pomp, A. Safety of bariatric surgery. *The Lancet Diabetes & Endocrinology.* 2014; 2, 2, 98-100.

CHAPTER 13

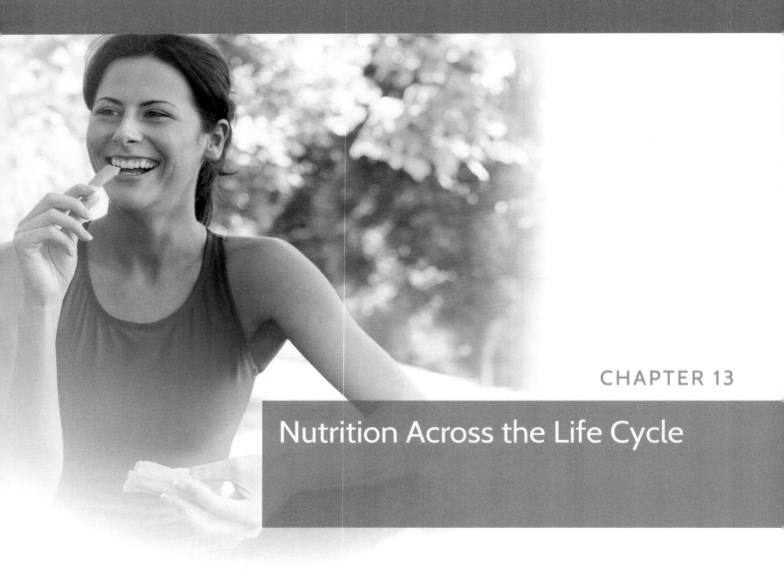

Nutrition Across the Life Cycle

CHAPTER OUTLINE

CHAPTER OUTLINE–cont'd

LEARNING OBJECTIVES

After studying this chapter, the reader should be able to:

13.1 List at least three special considerations when working with youth athletes.
13.2 Describe the role of sports and energy drinks in a youth athlete and a typical child's hydration regimen.
13.3 List the nutrients that require increased intake during pregnancy and lactation. Among those, describe which ones are most likely to be suboptimal in pregnant and lactating athletes.
13.4 Explain why and how much caloric needs change during pregnancy and lactation.
13.5 List several nutrition considerations when working with older adults.
13.6 Describe several unique nutritional needs for master athletes.

KEY TERMS

bone age A determination of the maturation of the bones in relation to chronological age used as a marker to assess further growth potential; assessed by x-ray.
empty calories Calories that provide little to no nutritional value; also referred to as SoFAS (solid fats and added sugar) in the *Dietary Guidelines for Americans*.
energy drinks Beverages containing caffeine or other supplements in addition to carbohydrates; potential risks outweigh benefits in children.
epiphyses Growth plates; closure signifies the cessation of further linear growth.
iron deficiency A type of anemia caused by inadequate intake of iron that leads to decreased oxygen-carrying capacity due to decreased production of iron-requiring, oxygen-carrying hemoglobin.
iron depletion A state of decreased body stores of iron but normal levels of iron in the red blood cells; if not corrected, progresses to iron-deficiency anemia.
master athletes Adult competitive athletes ranging in age from 30 to over 85 years.
nutrient density An indicator of nutritional value of a food based on the levels of vitamins and minerals compared with the number of calories.
older adult Defined by the Older Americans Act as a person older than 60 years.
peak growth velocity The period in early adolescence in which a child experiences the fastest rate of growth.
pregnancy-induced anemia The low red blood cell count that occurs during pregnancy due to increased blood volume and lag in increased red blood cell production; a normal phenomenon.
sarcopenia "Muscle wasting" or a decrease in muscle mass and strength.
sarcopenic obesity Decline in skeletal muscle and strength combined with excess body fat, which is common during older adulthood.
sports drinks Beverages containing carbohydrates, protein, or electrolytes.
successful aging Maintenance of low disease risk and cognitive and physical function.

INTRODUCTION

Elite athletes range from the teenaged Olympian to the centenarian challenging the limits of the human body. Consider the following examples:

- First introduced to the sport at the age of 2, and competitive before age 7, legendary golfer Tiger Woods achieved high levels of athletic success throughout high school, college, and his professional career. Other elite athletes such as decorated swimmer Michael Phelps and NBA star Lebron James experienced similar successes throughout childhood and adolescence.
- Olympic marathon runners Paula Radcliffe and Kara Goucher trained strenuously together throughout their pregnancies. Radcliffe previously won the New York City Marathon just 10 months after giving birth to her first child. Goucher went on to place 11th in the marathon in the 2012 Summer Olympics, despite a season off and less than 2 years after the birth of her daughter.
- Fauja Singh of London drew attention when he became the first centenarian to finish a marathon. At 100 years old he completed the 26.2-mile 2011 Toronto course in slightly over 8 hours to earn his place in the Guinness Book of World Records. This marked his eighth marathon; the first of which he ran at 89 years old. Eighty-year-old Ed Whitlock finished the same marathon in 3:15:54—a Boston-marathon qualifying time for someone half his age.

Though competitive and recreational athletes may not achieve the same level of physical performance as these elite athletes, at all life stages physical activity, exercise, and sports play a major role in optimizing health and quality of life. As is the case for healthy and active adults, optimal nutrition and optimal fitness are closely related for athletes across the lifespan. However, a well-balanced eating plan to fuel activity and maintain or improve fitness extends beyond universal dietary recommendations. That is especially the case for active children and adolescents, pregnant and breastfeeding women, and older adults.

YOUTH ATHLETES

Over 7,500,000 adolescents participate in high school sports,[1] and millions more elementary-school aged children engage in organized sports. Active children have unique nutritional and fitness needs to maintain health and optimize sports performance.

Nutrition Considerations for Active Children and Adolescents

Nutritional intake for active children must be adequate to supply the calories and nutrients needed for basic physiological functions, to fuel exercise, and to provide for growth and maturation.

Growth

After about 2 years of age until puberty, children tend to follow a constant genetically determined percentile curve on the growth chart (Figs. 13-1 and 13-2). Growth occurs at a rate of about 2.5 inches per year throughout childhood until early adolescence when preteens achieve a **peak growth velocity** of about 4 inches per year. The growth spurt starts at about 9 to 10 years in girls and peaks around 11.5 to 12 years. Peak growth velocity typically occurs about 1.5 years before menarche; at the time of first menarche a female is within 1 to 2 inches of adult height. The male growth spurt generally starts at 11 and peaks around 13.5 years. Growth continues into mid-adolescence for females and well into late adolescence for most males. Closure of the **epiphyses**, or growth plates, marks the end of linear growth. When necessary, a child or adolescent's future growth potential can be evaluated with an x-ray of the epiphyses of the wrist and interpretation by a radiologist to determine **bone age**. Notably, adolescents whose parents were "late bloomers" may show a decrease in growth rate in early adolescence, which may not peak until 16 years. One can predict a child's adult height based on the height of a child's mother and father. A female will grow to be about the (height of the mother (inches)) plus (father (inches) – 5 inches) divided by two (plus or minus 10%). A male will grow to be about the (height of the mother (inches) plus 5 inches) plus father (inches)) divided by two (plus or minus 10 percent).

Many environmental factors influence whether a child achieves full genetic growth potential. For example, while moderate levels of physical activity benefit growth, intensive physical training during childhood can negatively impact growth. Athletes who are most affected are those who engage in intensive training more than 18 hours per week and who restrict or limit calories, such as gymnasts.[2] In fact, though other sports such as swimming, rowing, wrestling, track and field, and tennis demand prolonged hours of intense training, research suggests that the growth potential for gymnasts is most compromised, especially for male gymnasts.[2] Elite youth athletes are not the only children at risk for growth delays. Research suggests that overweight females who go through puberty early due to the effects of excess weight may also be at risk for decreased adult height,[3] though the same does not appear to be true for boys.[4]

Measured height and weight parameters can be used to calculate a child's body mass index (BMI), which can then be plotted on a BMI growth chart to assess whether a child is underweight, normal weight, overweight, or obese. In adults, BMI ranges are set: any adult with a BMI greater than 25 is considered overweight and those with a BMI over 30 are considered obese. Because children are continually growing and experience spurts at certain ages (e.g., a typical child

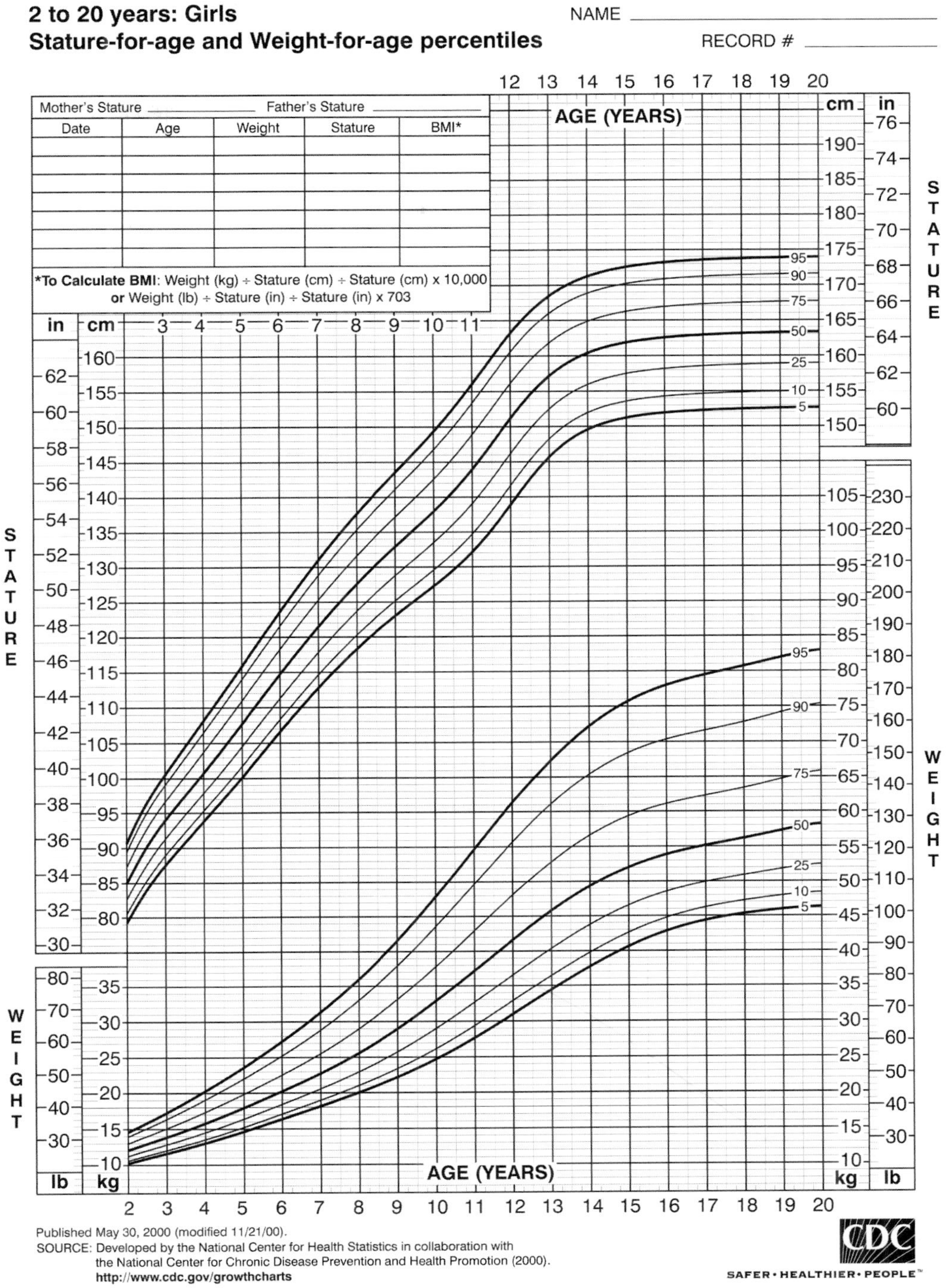

Figure 13-1. Girls, 2–20 years growth chart. *Source: Developed by the National Center for Health Statistics in collaboration with the National Center for Chronic Disease Prevention and Health Promotion (2000).*

will have a decrease in BMI around 4 years and then progressively increase throughout childhood), BMI is plotted on an age- and gender-appropriate growth chart. A BMI below 10% is underweight, 10% to 84% is normal weight, 85% to 94% is overweight, and greater than 95% is obese. Even if a child is considered to have a normal BMI, a rapid change in trajectory across percentile lines is cause for alarm and may trigger further investigation into the cause of the change. The BMI curves for females and males ages 2 to 20 are included in Figures 13-3 and 13-4.

Low BMI in children and adolescents can be due to genetic factors and a predisposition to be small or, especially in preadolescent and adolescent girls (but certainly not limited to them), a restriction of calories. This can happen on the part of the child in response to perceived increased weight. Or, it can occur accidentally in some cases, such as in very active children who do not eat enough to support physical demands. A child identified as underweight would benefit from referral to the pediatrician for further evaluation.

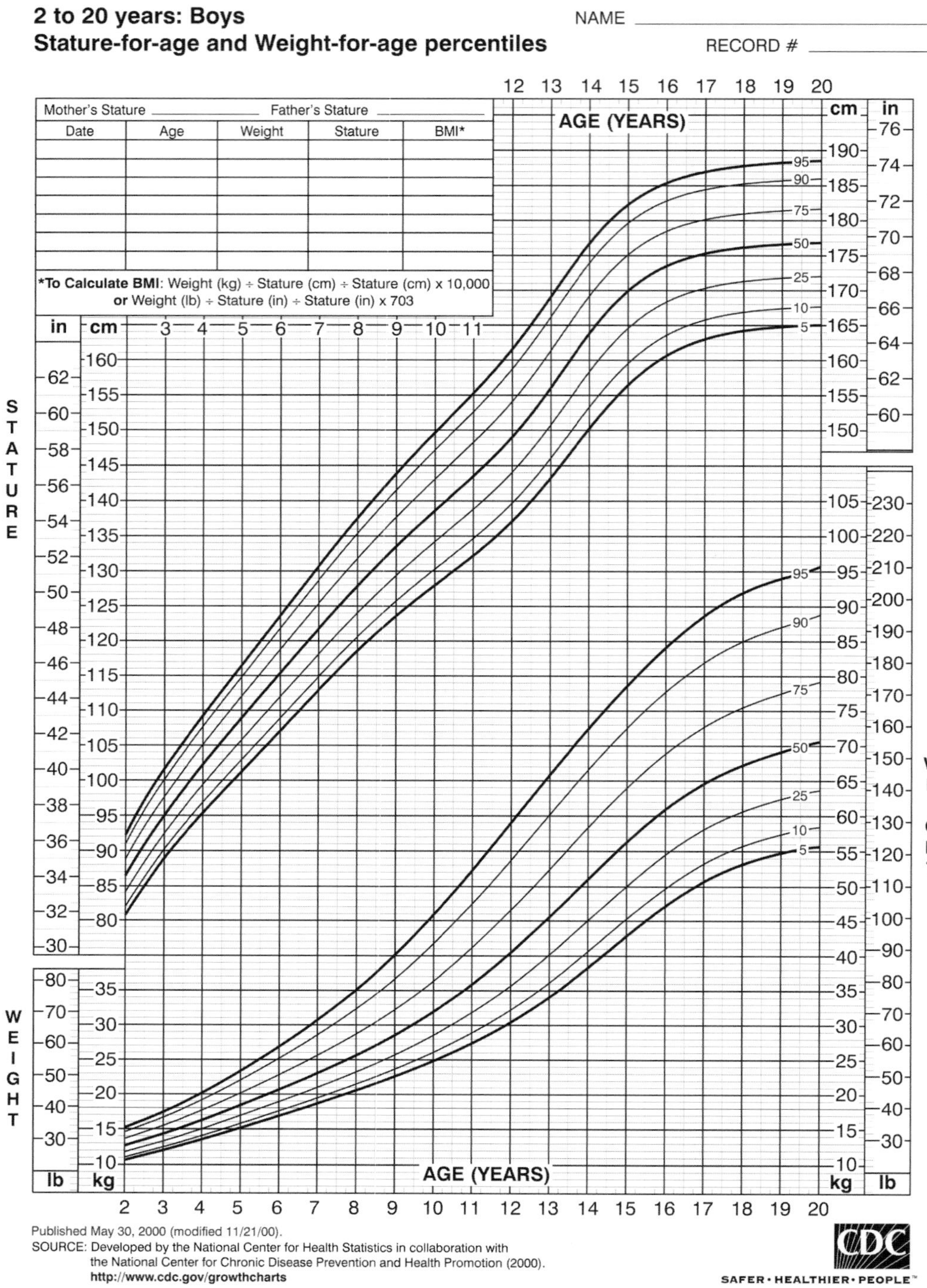

Figure 13-2. Boys, 2–20 years growth chart. *Source: Developed by the National Center for Health Statistics in collaboration with the National Center for Chronic Disease Prevention and Health Promotion (2000).*

A disproportionate number of children have a BMI greater than the 85th percentile. (The percentile norms are based on the distribution of children in 1976, when only 15% of children exceeded the 85th percentile. Now over one-third of children are classified as overweight or obese.[5]) Resulting from poor nutrition habits and low levels of physical activity, childhood overweight and obesity negatively affect nearly every organ of the body, causing complications as varied as asthma and sleep apnea to gallstones, liver dysfunction, bone fractures, and infertility in girls.[6] Many complications of obesity that are common in adults—such as impaired fasting glucose and type 2 diabetes, high blood pressure, abnormal cholesterol, and metabolic syndrome—are present in obese children.[7] In fact, a study of severely obese 2- to 18-year-olds in the Netherlands found that two-thirds of the children already had at least one of the following cardiovascular risk factors: high blood pressure, high LDL or "bad" cholesterol, low HDL or "good" cholesterol, high total cholesterol, high triglycerides, high fasting blood sugar, or type 2 diabetes.[8] These findings are on track with

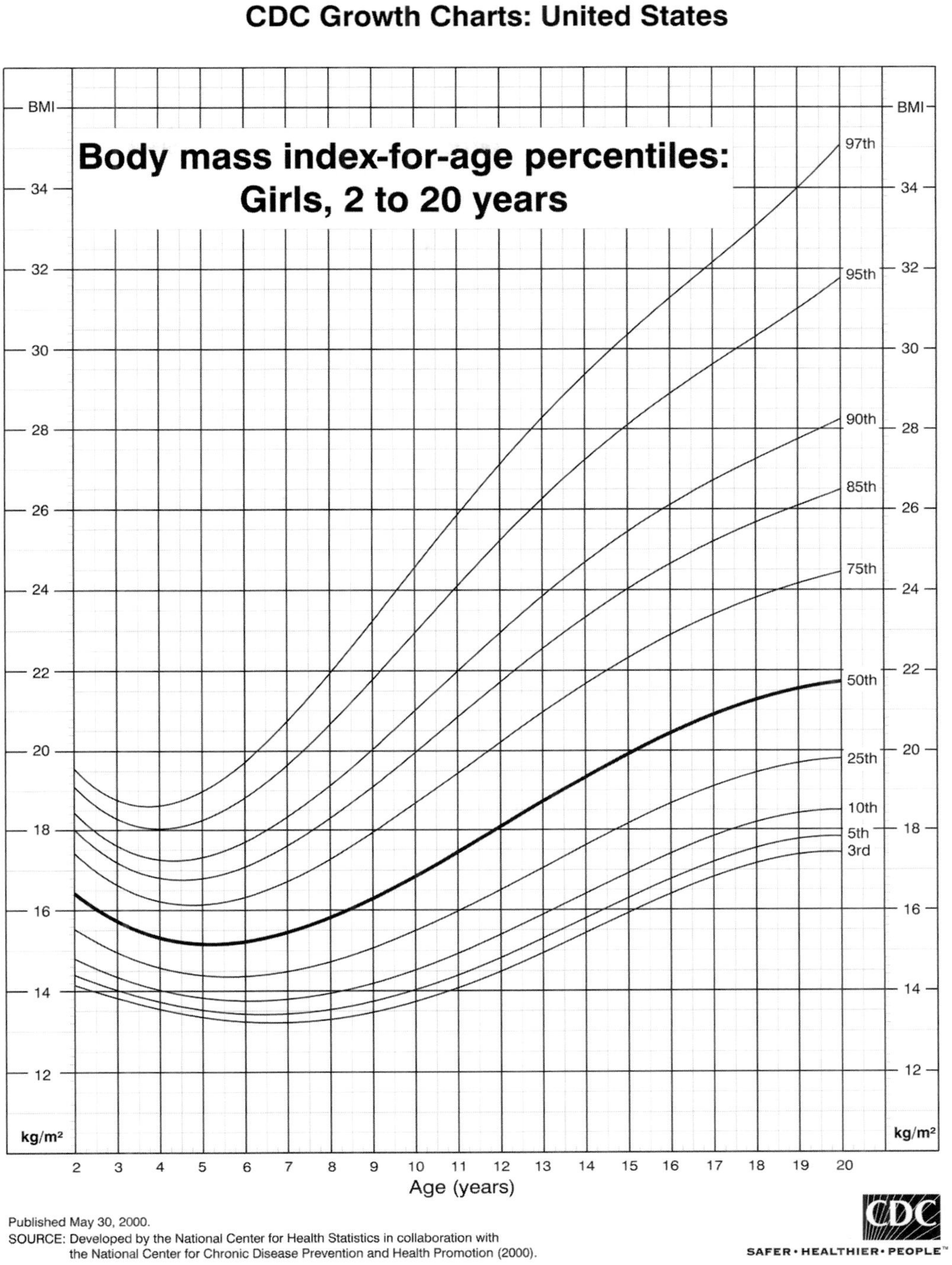

Figure 13-3. Girls, 2–20 years BMI chart. *Source: Developed by the National Center for Health Statistics in collaboration with the National Center for Chronic Disease Prevention and Health Promotion (2000).*

U.S. data from the National Health and Nutrition Examination Survey (NHANES) showing that about half of overweight teens and two-thirds of obese teens have at least one risk factor for cardiovascular disease. For nearly 25% of the American teens surveyed, including those at a normal weight, that risk factor is increased fasting glucose or type 2 diabetes.[9] If current trends continue, researchers predict that the average boy born in the year 2000 has a 33% chance of developing diabetes in his lifetime, while the average girl has a 39% chance.[10]

In addition to the severe health consequences from obesity, an obese child is more likely to be teased, bullied, and socially isolated than normal-weight peers. A review spanning over 130 research articles evaluating the association of childhood obesity with mental health and wellness found that obese children have increased rates of depression and anxiety, low self-esteem, body dissatisfaction, disordered eating, unhealthy weight control practices, counterproductive dietary restraint, and emotional distress.[11] The authors propose that weight-based stigmatization and teasing along with preoccupation with

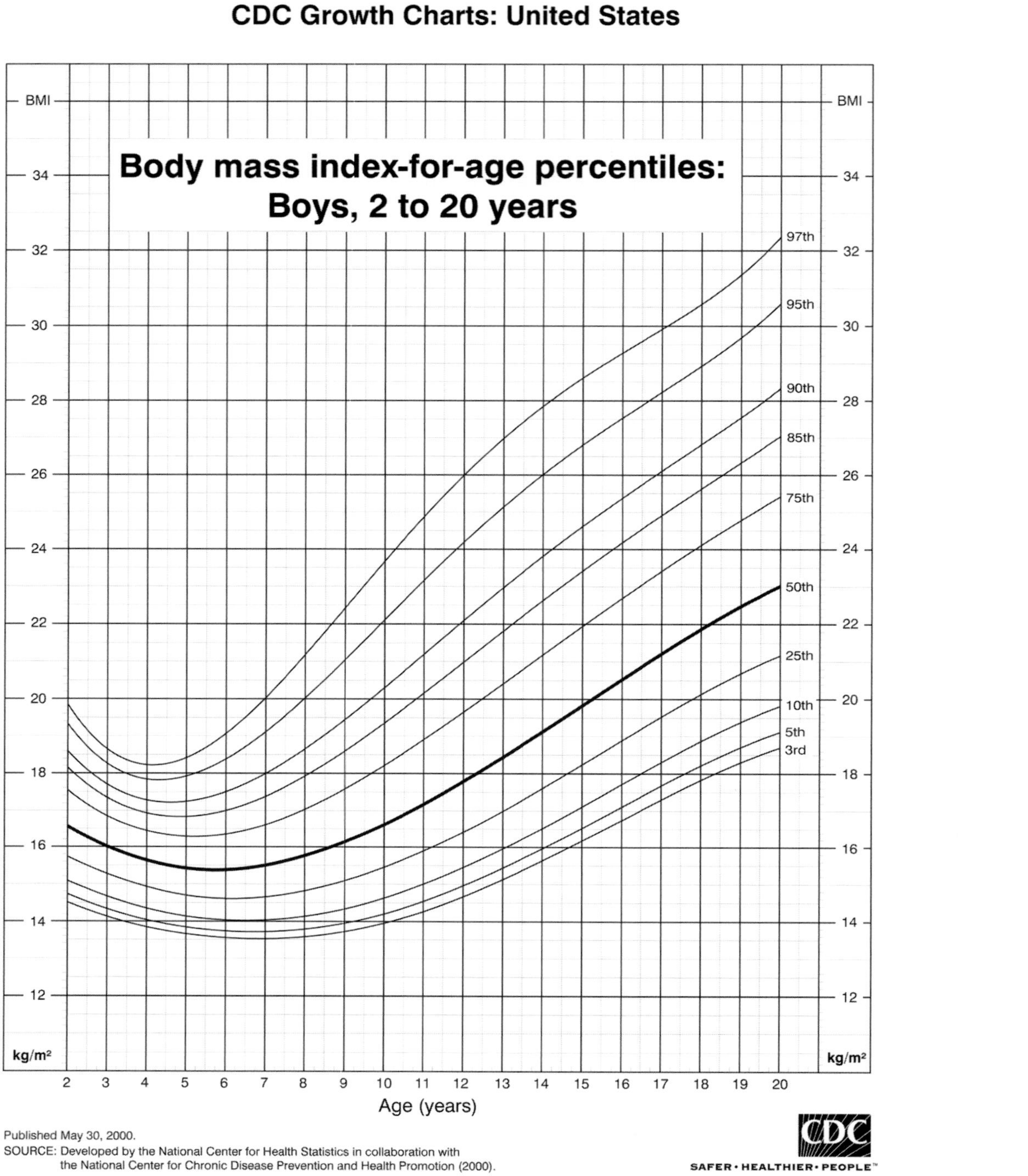

Figure 13-4. Boys, 2–20 years BMI chart. *Source: Developed by the National Center for Health Statistics in collaboration with the National Center for Chronic Disease Prevention and Health Promotion (2000).*

weight and size serve as the major mediators in the development of these mental health concern.[11]

Health professionals who work with youth athletes may consider including outreach to children who are not currently active but who may find sports and athletic participation enjoyable and beneficial. More information on childhood obesity and how to help solve the epidemic of childhood obesity is included in Communication Strategies.

While BMI is a commonly used method of approximating body composition, as with adults, health professionals may consider direct measurement of body composition with bioelectrical impedance analysis or skinfold measurements. Skinfold measurement is the method commonly employed by school districts to measure body composition as part of their fitness assessment, though schools have the option to use other methods instead (highlighted in Box 13-1). If these methods are used, norms for children are available at www.fitnessgram.net. For more information on body composition assessment, see Chapter 11.

COMMUNICATION STRATEGIES

Childhood Obesity

It is well known that the United States faces a childhood obesity epidemic. In fact, 81% of respondents in a poll on the topic considered childhood obesity a serious problem; two-thirds believed the problem is getting worse (cited in Hassink et al., 2011).

A Surge in Childhood Obesity–and Now Stabilization?

Obesity prevalence among children has increased from 5% in the 1960s to about 17% currently. [5] Black girls and boys (24%), Hispanic boys (23%),[5] and children from lower-income communities with little access to healthy foods and physical activity opportunities suffer the highest rates.[71] Following the rapid increases in rates of obesity over the past 30 years, the latest estimates have shown stabilization for all age groups except for teenage males, who continue to gain. [5] The stabilization may be due at least in part to the increased attention and awareness surrounding obesity, including initiatives such as the Let's Move campaign. Still, despite the widespread attention, obesity rates have not yet decreased for children or adults,[5,72] though some studies, such as one of Massachusetts children, show some promise with a substantial decrease in rates of obesity for boys and girls. Notably, the decrease was substantially smaller for the low-income children.[73]

As with adults, behavior-based weight loss and subsequent weight maintenance prove to be extremely challenging for children. In fact, obesity in childhood, especially among older children and those with the highest BMIs, is likely to persist into adulthood.[74] Social marginalization, type 2 diabetes, cardiovascular disease, and myriad other morbidities are real threats for overweight children during childhood and into adulthood.[7]

Making Changes

Alarmed by these sobering statistics, stakeholders–including health professionals from a variety of disciplines–have responded with the development of numerous policies, programs, and interventions aimed to prevent childhood obesity. A Cochrane Review highlighted several areas which may help to prevent childhood obesity, especially for children ages 6 to 12 years.[75] Many of these areas are perfectly suited targets of interventions and programs that could be designed by health professionals.

The specific recommendations provided in the review include:

- School curriculum that includes healthy eating, physical activity, and body image
- Increased sessions for physical activity and the development of fundamental movement skills throughout the school week
- Improvements in nutritional quality of the food supply in schools
- Environments and cultural practices that support children eating healthier foods and being active throughout each day
- Support for teachers and other staff to implement health promotion strategies and activities (e.g., professional development, capacity-building activities)
- Parent support and home activities that encourage children to be more active, eat more nutritious foods, and spend less time in screen-based activities

While it is not easy to attain a healthier weight, with the right tools and support, children are more successful than their adult counterparts. By improving nutrition habits and increasing physical activity, many children can avert the harmful consequences of obesity to achieve and maintain a healthy weight. But the intervention must begin as soon as possible. The earlier a child is identified as overweight or obese and lifestyle changes are initiated, the more likely the child will achieve a healthier weight and enter adulthood without the burden of obesity.[76]

Prompt

You have decided that you would like to take a more active role in your community in addressing the epidemic of childhood obesity. Choose one of the recommendations to prevent childhood obesity that is outlined in the Cochrane Review.

1. Describe how you might offer your services or develop a program to address that particular recommendation.
2. Detail your approach to identifying stakeholders and reaching out to them for their involvement.
3. Describe several ways in which effective communication would be necessary for your proposed program to be successful.

Box 13-1. The Presidential Youth Fitness Program

In response to prompting by the White House 2010 Task Force on Childhood Obesity to make fitness assessment more health-based, fun, and educational for students, in 2012 the President's Council on Physical Fitness, Sports, and Nutrition updated fitness standards for students.

A measure of school-aged fitness, the voluntary fitness tests have been administered to students every year since 1966. Previously, students completed a battery of fitness tests and performance was measured against age- and gender-determined norms. In 2012, the Fitnessgram was adopted. The Fitnessgram is a tool developed by researchers at the Cooper Institute in Dallas, Texas, that evaluates performance based on health-based standards. It includes assessment in the four categories of fitness: cardiovascular fitness, muscular strength and endurance, flexibility, and body composition. The recommended method for assessing body composition is with skinfold calipers, but body mass index and bioelectrical impedance analysis are included as alternatives.

Instead of performance being compared to standardized norms, students are classified one of three ways based on established age- and gender-appropriate criteria: Healthy Fitness Zone, Needs Improvement—Some Risk, or Needs Improvement—High Risk. Students who score Healthy Fitness Zone in five out of six tests receive a Presidential Award of Fitness. Those who do not score in the healthy zone receive information and tools to improve fitness and incorporate more physical activity into their daily routines.

The hope is that the new classification system will be easier for students and their parents to understand, and hopefully help to motivate children to increase their level of physical activity and physical fitness. The Fitnessgram assessment standards are also accompanied by a computer program that schools can use to monitor and track progress for individual students as well as by school. More information is available at www.presidentalyouthfitnessprogram.org and www.fitnessgram.net.

General Nutrition Recommendations for Children and Adolescents

The *Dietary Guidelines for Americans* (www.dietaryguidelines.gov) recommend that, similar to adults, children eat a diet rich in fruits, vegetables, whole grains, low-fat and nonfat dairy products, beans, fish, and lean meat.[12] Specifically, the guidelines and joint recommendations from the American Heart Association and the American Academy of Pediatrics[13] recommend that families choose:

- Mostly whole grains as opposed to refined sugars. Brown bread, brown rice, and brown pasta provide more nutrients than the more heavily processed white versions. Cereal should be high in fiber and low in sugar.
- Ample nutrient-dense dark green and orange vegetables, such as broccoli and carrots, rather than disproportionate amounts of starchy vegetables, such as white potatoes and corn, which contain fewer vitamins and minerals. A general rule of thumb is, the more colorful the vegetable, the more nutrients it contains.
- A variety of fruits, preferably from whole food sources, as opposed to fruit juices. While the dietary guidelines still consider 100% juice as a serving of fruit, the sugar in juice usually outweighs the benefit from the fruit. Even though the sugar in 100% juice is fructose—a natural fruit sugar—it takes about three apples to make an 8-ounce glass of juice. That is more apple than a child would typically eat in a day and the juice does not contain the healthy fiber found in the skin. Children should limit juice to no more than 4 ounces per day.
- Oils in moderation, with an emphasis on mono- or polyunsaturated fats instead of trans or saturated fats. While fats are calorie dense, some fats are heart healthy, particularly polyunsaturated fats such as the omega-3 fatty acids contained in salmon, tuna, walnuts, and a variety of fortified products (such as milk and eggs) and other foods.
- Low-fat or nonfat milk products in contrast to regular whole milk products. Starting at the age of 2 (and the age of 1 for children already overweight), all children should consume 2%, 1%, or, preferably, skim milk. The higher-fat milk contains more calories, saturated fat, and no additional nutritional value.
- Lean meat and bean products instead of higher-fat meats, such as regular (75% to 80% lean) ground beef or chicken with the skin. Lean meats include the white meat from chicken (breast and wings) and the leanest red meats (typically round or loin).

Table 13-1 provides a summary of the dietary guidelines for children.

A wide gap exists between nutrition recommendations for children and what children eat. Compared to the recent past, children and adolescents eat breakfast less often, eat away from home more often, consume a greater proportion of calories from snacks, eat more fried and nutrient-poor foods, consume greater portion sizes, eat fewer fruits and vegetables, ingest excess sodium, drink more sweetened beverages, and

Table 13-1. **Nutrition Needs for Children and Adolescents**

	1-3 YEARS	4-8 YEARS	9-13 YEARS	14-18 YEARS
Calories[a]				
Female	900–1,000	1,200	1,400–1,600	1,800
Male	900–1,200	1,200–1,400	1,600–2,000	2,000–2,400
Milk/dairy	2 cups	2.5 cups	3 cups	3 cups
Lean meat/ beans/nuts/eggs				6 oz
Female	2 oz	3 oz	5 oz	5 oz
Male	3 oz	4 oz	6 oz	6 oz
Fruits	1 cup	1.5 cups	1.5 cups	
Female				1.5 cups
Male				2 cups
Vegetables		1.5 cups		
Female	1 cup		2 cups	2.5 cups
Male	1.5 cups		2.5 cups	3 cups
Grains	3 oz			
Female		4 oz	5 oz	6 oz
Male		5 oz	6 oz	7 oz

a. Estimated calorie needs are based on a sedentary lifestyle. Increased physical activity will require additional calories: by 0–200 kcal/d if moderately physically active and by 200–400 kcal/d if very physically active.

Source: Table adapted from Appendix 6, Appendix 7, and Appendix 8 of the *Dietary Guidelines for Americans* (2010); www.healthierus.gov/dietaryguidelines.

consume fewer dairy products.[14,15] As a result, children and especially adolescents consume smaller amounts of many nutrients, such as calcium and potassium, than the recommended values.[15]

Children and their parents benefit from tips on how to make healthy choices to support athletic performance. However, more so than the information, families benefit from strategies that support them in teaching their children how to eat healthfully (Box 13-2).

Youth Sports Nutrition

Youth athletes push themselves physically and mentally to achieve impressive levels of athletic performance. The high training loads create unique nutritional demands. Children are not just "little adults" and the rules of adult sports nutrition do not necessarily apply to them.

Energy Needs

A highly active youth athlete requires first and foremost an adequate number of calories to fuel not only the strenuous exercise regimen but also to provide for optimal growth and development. Athletes involved in endurance sports, aesthetic sports like gymnastics and cheerleading, and weight-class sports are at highest risk of not consuming adequate calories. Typical energy needs for children and adolescents are presented in Table 13-2. Note that the calorie recommendations are based on the needs of a sedentary child. Moderately active children need up to 200 additional calories per day, while very active children need 200 to 400 calories more than the basic recommendations.[16] The additional calories should come from nutrient-dense whole grains, lean proteins, fruits, and vegetables.

The USDA's Supertracker program (available at www.supertracker.usda.gov) provides users with an individualized meal plan that can be used to help athletes consume an optimally healthy diet including all of the essential nutrients, such as iron and calcium, which are deficient in many preteens and teens. This individualized plan will be appropriate for most children, though athletes who exercise more than 1 to 2 hours per day may have higher calorie needs and should pay attention to their internal feelings of hunger and fullness to guide their intake and inform their meal and snack choices.

Box 13-2. Strategies to Help Teach Families How to Implement the Dietary Guidelines

Most parents know *what* their children should eat, but the challenge frequently arises in understanding *how* to make that happen. The following strategies are adapted from recommendations provided by the American Academy of Pediatrics and the American Heart Association.[13]

- Practice what is referred to as the *division of responsibility*. That is, parents choose what foods are available in the home and when the food can be eaten. Children choose of the food that is offered, *what* they will eat, and *how much*. With this approach, the parent has control over nutrient quality and snack and meal times while the child feels a sense of control in choosing what to eat from the food offered and also is able to use internal feelings of hunger and fullness in deciding how much to eat.
- Arrange for family meals. While the schedules for families of youth athletes can often be very busy and sometimes chaotic, committing to scheduling family meals as frequently as possible provides many benefits in determining the health and nutrition of a child's food intake and provides an opportunity to strengthen the family bond.
- Teach children about food and healthful nutrition by engaging them in choosing food at the grocery store, preparing meals, and possibly through a family garden, even if it is only a few herbs on a window sill.
- Be a source of quality nutrition information and actively counteract nutrition misinformation in the media and through other sources. Teach children and adolescents how to critically evaluate advertisements and avoid purchases based exclusively on marketing or packaging tactics.
- Discuss nutrition preferences and goals with other adults who provide food to the children such as other family members, babysitters, carpool participants, after-school program leaders, and coaches.
- Serve as role models and lead by example.
- Promote and participate in regular daily physical activity.

Table 13-2. Calorie Needs

The limit for **empty calories** is based on estimated calorie needs by age/gender group. Physical activity increases calorie needs, so those who are more physically active need more total calories and have a larger limit for empty calories. The chart gives a general guide.

AGE AND GENDER	ESTIMATED CALORIES FOR THOSE WHO ARE NOT PHYSICALLY ACTIVE	
	Total Daily Calorie Needs[a]	**Daily Limit for Empty Calories**
Children 2–3 yrs	1,000	135[b]
Children 4–8 yrs	1,200–1,400	120
Girls 9–13 yrs	1,600	120
Boys 9–13 yrs	1,800	160
Girls 14–18 yrs	1,800	160
Boys 14–18 yrs	2,200	265
Females 19–30 yrs	2,000	260
Males 19–30 yrs	2,400	330
Females 31–50 yrs	1,800	160
Males 31–50 yrs	2,200	265
Females 51+ yrs	1,600	120
Males 51+ yrs	2,000	260

a. These amounts are appropriate for individuals who get less than 30 minutes of moderate physical activity most days. Those who are more active need more total calories and have a higher limit for empty calories. To find your personal total calorie needs and empty calories limit, enter your information into My Daily Food Plan.

b. The limit for empty calories is higher for children 2 and 3 years old than it is for some older children, because younger children have lower nutrient needs and smaller recommended intakes from the basic food groups.

Source: Reproduced from www.choosemyplate.gov/weight-management-calories/calories/empty-calories-amount.html.

Macronutrient Considerations

Carbohydrates. While adults are advised to consume a carbohydrate-rich food within 30 minutes of finishing exercise for optimal recovery and to increase overall protein intake to help rebuild muscles, nutrient needs for children are less clear. The recommended dietary allowance of carbohydrates for most children is 130 grams per day.[17] Ideally, athletes will meet their needs from a diet rich in whole grains like cereals, rice, pasta, fruits, and vegetables, and limited in simple sugars. This recommended carbohydrate amount is based on the body's needs to provide glucose for brain development and does not include the needs for active children to replenish glucose stores. Children metabolize sugars differently than adults and it is not yet clear if and how much more carbohydrates youth athletes need for optimal performance.[18] Likewise, it is not well understood if children involved in long-distance endurance events benefit from carbohydrate loading the same way adults do. Generally, most youth athletes will do well eating a healthy, nutrient-dense diet that contains at least 50% of calories from carbohydrates.[18]

Protein. Children and adolescents experience periods of rapid growth, during which sufficient protein intake is essential to support the maintenance and development of lean body mass and other tissues. The protein needs of children and adolescents are shown in Table 13-3. Some evidence suggests that very active children may have somewhat increased needs. For example, a study of 14-year-old male soccer players demonstrated that active adolescents require more protein than their inactive counterparts.[19] However, most athletes spontaneously increase their caloric and protein intake to meet these needs.[20]

Fat. Dietary fat intake provides energy for growth and a source of the essential fatty acids: linoleic and linolenic acids. Fat needs for youth athletes likely parallel needs of inactive children, though limited research is available to evaluate whether modifications of fat intake influence athletic performance in youth athletes. No minimal amount of fat is essential for adequate nutrition, other than that which contains adequate essential fatty acids to meet minimal needs and which is necessary to ensure adequate protein, calcium, magnesium, iron, zinc, chromium, vitamin B12, and fat-soluble vitamin (A, D, E, K) intake. Given its high caloric density (9 calories per gram compared to 4 calories per gram for carbohydrates and protein), manipulation of fat intake provides a strategy to increase or decrease caloric intake, depending on the athlete's needs.

Table 13-3. Protein Needs of Children and Adolescents[17]

AGE	PROTEIN (GRAMS/KG/DAY)
1–3 years	1.05
4–13 years	0.95
14–18 years	0.85

Micronutrient Considerations

Micronutrients serve similar functions in youth athletes as they do in adult athletes (discussed in detail in Chapter 4). Physical activity does not seem to substantially increase needs for vitamins or minerals, other than those minerals lost in large amounts in sweat, such as sodium and chloride. An athlete's nutritional needs for these minerals beyond the DRI are based heavily on extent of physical activity, amount of sweat lost, and individual factors such as the concentration of electrolytes in sweat (which tend to be lower in concentration in children and adolescents than in adults). Unlike their sedentary counterparts, the majority of youth athletes obtain sufficient amounts of vitamins and minerals from their diets with two notable exceptions: calcium and iron.[20]

Sufficient calcium intake is essential for optimal bone density and is especially important in adolescence and early adulthood when peak bone density is attained. Despite its importance, the average calcium intake for adolescent females is half of the recommended 1,200 milligrams per day.[21] Low calcium intake during adolescence contributes to suboptimal bone mineralization and increased future risk for stress fractures and osteoporosis.[22]

Iron plays a central role in the production of hemoglobin, the molecule in the red blood cell that transports oxygen from the lungs to the working cells. It is also an important component of myoglobin, the molecule that stores oxygen in the muscle. Many biochemical reactions, including many of those involved in energy metabolism, require iron.

Iron consumed in the diet is used to meet current needs or stored as ferritin. Inadequate iron intake in the diet in combination with iron losses from urine, sweat, stool, gastrointestinal bleeding, and hemolysis resulting from intense exercise can deplete iron stores and leave an athlete at risk for iron deficiency. Female athletes are at further increased risk due to blood losses with menstruation.

While **iron deficiency** is not common, depleted iron stores (as measured by low serum ferritin levels) is common, occurring in up to half of female adolescent athletes.[23,24] Endurance runners, swimmers, gymnasts, volleyball players, basketball players, and tennis players of both genders are at highest risk.[23,24] While the effects of **iron depletion** on performance may not be as pronounced as that of iron deficiency, athletes should take care to meet the RDA for iron of 18 milligrams per day. Many adolescents, especially females, do not achieve this level of intake and will benefit from nutritional coaching to improve consumption of iron-rich foods such as red meat, egg yolks, dark green leafy vegetables, oysters, clams, beans, and iron-enriched grains. Excellent sources of iron and the amount of iron contained in a typical serving are shown in Chapter 4. Youth athletes may also consider an evaluation by a physician to test for iron depletion or deficiency and, when advised by a physician, take iron supplementation.[18]

A table of the DRIs for micronutrients is shown in Chapter 4.

Hydration

Driven to excel, many youth athletes push through sports practices and games to the point of exhaustion. While this physical exertion can benefit cardiovascular fitness, a developing competitive spirit, and a child's enjoyment of the game, without appropriate attention to hydration, youth athletes can suffer serious consequences, especially when exercising in the heat.

It is commonly taught that children have a more difficult time regulating body temperature than adults, especially in extreme environments like a hot and humid summer day. Consequently, children are taught to pay careful attention to consuming sufficient fluids. Frequently **sports drinks**, **energy drinks**, and other flavored beverages are the youth athlete's drink of choice. In one study, over 50% of adolescents used sports drinks and 42% used energy drinks in the 2 weeks preceding the survey.[25] While in some cases sports drinks (but not energy drinks) may provide benefits to youth athletes, in other cases the reliance on sweetened beverages does little more than negate the health benefits of exercise and contribute to the worldwide problem of childhood obesity (see Evaluating the Evidence).

In an effort to avoid confusion and guide pediatricians, coaches, parents, and youth fitness professionals, the American Academy of Pediatrics (AAP) has published two important articles related to optimal hydration for youth athletes: one, a policy statement on heat stress and exercise,[26] and the other, a clinical report on sports drinks and energy drinks for children and adolescents.[27] Following is a brief recap of the major conclusions and recommendations from these reports:

1. Contrary to previous thinking, children do *not* have less effective ability to regulate body temperature and tolerate high levels of physical exertion when exercising in the heat compared to their adult counterparts *as long as they maintain appropriate hydration*. This conclusion is a major departure from the previous caution that children innately have a poor ability to regulate body temperature.

EVALUATING THE EVIDENCE

When Do Sports Drinks Benefit Youth Athletes?

The American Academy of Pediatrics published a clinical report titled, "Sports Drinks and Energy Drinks for Children and Adolescents: Are They Appropriate?"[27] (The full text of the article is available free of charge at www.pediatrics.aappublications.org). Table 13-4 is based on the information contained within the report.

In deciding whether or not to implement findings from research studies, health professionals need to critically evaluate the research and decide whether or not the findings apply to individual clients.

1. Based on the benefits and risks noted in Table 13-4, which children do you think are most likely to benefit from sports drinks? Which children are most likely to be harmed by sports drinks?
2. In what situations do you think that the benefits of sports drinks outweigh the risks?
3. What information would you provide a mother who asks you whether or not she should encourage her child to drink a sports drink?
4. Will this information change your practice in working with youth athletes? Why or why not?

Table 13-4. The Benefits and Risks of Sports Drinks

BENEFITS OF SPORTS DRINKS	RISKS OF SPORTS DRINKS
Rehydrate and replenish carbohydrates, electrolytes, and water lost during exercise	Dental erosion
Contribute to improved athletic performance before, during, or after intensive exercise	Excess calories/contribution to childhood obesity
	Use tied with use of energy drinks
	Displace water and milk

2. Proper hydration is essential for optimal health and athletic performance. Thirst is generally a good guide in determining intake. A more precise method of monitoring hydration status is to weigh the child before and after exercise. The goal is to avoid weight loss. If weighing is not possible, the AAP suggests that consumption of 100 to 250 milliliters (approximately 3–8 oz) every 20 minutes for 9- to 12-year-olds and up to 1.0 to 1.5 liters (approximately 34–50 oz) per hour for adolescents is sufficient to avoid dehydration, as long as the athlete's prehydration status is good. Fluid needs may differ based on heat and humidity, diet, medications, and illness or chronic health conditions.
3. Most children and adolescents can safely participate in outdoor sports and other physically challenging endeavors in a variety of climates, including warm to hot conditions. However, in addition to ensuring adequate hydration, coaches, parents, and other supervising adults need to ensure the children are allowed sufficient recovery between workouts, same-day training sessions, or rounds of sports competition; that they wear appropriate clothing, uniforms, and protective equipment (when necessary) so as to not retain excessive heat; and that the adults consider the child's fitness level and gradually (rather than abruptly) increase exercise exertion.
4. Sports drinks play a role in ensuring appropriate hydration and nutrition for optimal performance in combination with water during intense and prolonged exercise lasting more than 1 hour or multiple strenuous workouts in a single day (more on this in Box 13-3). However, consumption of sports drinks for the average child engaged in routine physical activity or in place of water in the lunchroom or at home can lead to excessive calorie intake and increased risk of overweight and dental problems. This has become an especially widespread problem as sports drinks have replaced soda in school vending machines and cafeterias.
5. Energy drinks—beverages containing caffeine or other supplements in addition to carbohydrates—should be avoided. While caffeine may provide performance benefits for adults, its effects have not been well studied in children. Furthermore, it is difficult to know the true caffeine content for many drinks. Some may contain as much as 500 milligrams, which is equivalent to about 14 cans of soda. A lethal dose of caffeine is somewhere around 100 to 200 milligrams per pound of body weight (thus, the impact of caffeine is most significant for younger and lighter children), but caffeine toxicity can occur at much smaller doses. The guidelines suggest that parents, coaches, and schools should not offer or allow children to drink energy drinks. Energy drinks pose potential health risks due

Box 13-3. Tips for Coaches: Optimizing Nutrition and Hydration for Preseason 'Two-A-Days'[26,77]

Preseason training for many sports often consists of two practices in one day. The sport in which this practice is most likely to lead to problems is youth football. The major concern is heat-related illness and dehydration due to the high heat and humidity during this time of year and the intense exercise.

Here are a few tips from the American Academy of Pediatrics, the American College of Sports Medicine, and the Academy of Nutrition and Dietetics:

- Coaches, trainers, and athletes themselves need to be well informed of the risks and hydration needs of working out in a hot, humid environment.
- When athletes engage in vigorous physical activity in hot environments, trained personnel who can identify and treat heat-related illness need to be easily accessible.
- Athletes need the opportunity to safely adapt to the intensity and heat through acclimatization, a process that usually takes about 10 to 14 days of gradually increasing intensity, heat, and equipment use.
- Fluid should be readily accessible and athletes should be sure to stay well hydrated during activity. When repeated practices are held in the same day or during very intense or prolonged exercise, athletes should have access to sports drinks that are high in sodium (most sports drinks do not contain a high enough concentration of sodium for optimal electrolyte replenishment when there is a high rate of sweat loss).
- Exercise intensity should be modified during very hot or humid days.
- Athletes should limit or avoid exercise if they are currently ill or have recently suffered a febrile, diarrheal, or vomiting illness, as risk of dehydration is high.
- At least 2 hours or more are scheduled between two-a-day practices in hot or humid weather to allow for sufficient recovery and rehydration.
- For serious athletes, consumption of a high-carbohydrate snack (approximately 0.5 g/lb body weight) within 30 minutes of exercise and then every 2 hours for 4 to 6 hours will help to replenish glycogen stores.

mostly to their stimulant (caffeine) content and are never safe for children.

Working With Youth Athletes

Children and adolescents face unique nutritional challenges due to periods of rapid bone growth, other maturational changes associated with the onset of puberty, a dependence on adults to ensure their well-being, and emerging independence as adolescents. Adapting to these changes may be most pronounced for youth athletes, especially those who engage in intensive training or weight-conscious sports. Ultimately, any health professional who works with children or adolescent athletes should become knowledgeable about the unique considerations for this population and avoid treating children and adolescents as if they are little adults.

SPEED BUMP

1. **List at least three special considerations when working with youth athletes.**
2. **Describe the role of sports and energy drinks in a youth athlete and a typical child's hydration regimen.**

NUTRITION FOR ACTIVE PREGNANT AND LACTATING WOMEN

The American College of Obstetricians and Gynecologists advises pregnant women to become or remain active during pregnancy.[28] Pregnant women already engaging in intensive activity such as running may continue to do so throughout pregnancy.[29] While beginning an intensive exercise program during pregnancy probably is not advisable, starting a low- to moderate-intensity program or maintaining an exercise regimen throughout pregnancy and up until the birth of a child is generally considered to be safe and advantageous to both mother and developing infant. This is especially the case as a growing number of women struggle with excessive weight gain during pregnancy. General recommendations and considerations related to exercise during pregnancy are shown in Box 13-4.

As with all athletes, optimal nutrition is essential to fuel optimal performance. For pregnant women, it is especially critical to provide both mother and infant the necessary calories and nutrients needed for growth and development. As a lactating woman returns to exercise after giving birth to a child, attention to nutrition and

Box 13-4. Exercise During Pregnancy

Exercise during pregnancy provides numerous benefits to both expectant mothers and their fetuses. For the mothers, exercise improves fitness, prevents urinary incontinence and back pain, and lessens swelling and constipation. It improves energy, mood, and sleep; promotes muscle strength and endurance; helps to prevent risk of gestational diabetes; and promotes a faster labor.[29,78] Furthermore, women who are more active during pregnancy are more likely to continue their commitment to physical activity once their infants are born.[78] Infants of exercising mothers tolerate the stress of labor better and are more alert and less irritable immediately after delivery. Exercise is not associated with decreased birth weight or preterm delivery.[78]

Health professionals who work with pregnant women should encourage them to discuss their physical activity regimen and goals with their obstetrician. Few absolute contraindications to exercise during pregnancy exist; however, women at high risk of complications should be identified early and managed appropriately by their obstetrician. Most sports can be continued during pregnancy, but downhill skiing, contact sports (e.g., hockey, basketball, and soccer), sports with increased risk of falling (e.g., gymnastics, water skiing, mountain biking, and horseback riding), and scuba diving are specifically discouraged by the American College of Obstetricians and Gynecologists.[29]

EXERCISE RECOMMENDATIONS

Exercise recommendations for women during pregnancy are based on the woman's pre-pregnancy exercise regimen and gestational age, as shown in Table 13-5.

All pregnant women should use their own feelings of comfort in guiding exercise during pregnancy. Likewise, exercise should be terminated immediately if a woman develops vaginal bleeding, dizziness or feeling faint, increased shortness of breath, chest pain, headache, muscle weakness, calf pain or swelling, uterine contractions, decreased fetal movement, or leakage of fluid.[29]

NUTRITION AND HYDRATION CONSIDERATIONS WHEN EXERCISING DURING PREGNANCY

Pregnancy increases nutritional and fluid demands. Further, women at risk of becoming overheated during exercise, in particular those exercising at a very high intensity or in hot and humid environments, are at increased risk of fetal distress. To avoid negative effects of exercise, pregnant women should:

- Pay particular attention to hydration status and ensure appropriate fluid intake.
- Consume increased calories to support physical activity in addition to fetal growth. Avoid prolonged periods of exercise without carbohydrate intake.
- Avoid exercise in hot, humid weather or when ill with a fever.

Box 13-4. Exercise During Pregnancy—cont'd

Table 13-5. Exercise Recommendations During Pregnancy[28,78]

GESTATIONAL AGE	FREQUENCY	INTENSITY (RPE)[a]	TIME	TYPE
Previously Sedentary, Overweight, or Obese				
1–6 weeks	Most, if not all (at least 3–5 days per week)	12–15	Approx 30 min moderate or 60 min light most days	Aerobic, large muscle groups (e.g., stationary cycling, swim, walk, jog)
6–26 weeks		15–16	Approx 45 min moderate or 90 min light most days	
27–40 weeks		13–14	Approx 30 min moderate or 60 min light most days	
Throughout	1–2 days	1–2 sets	8–10 exercises	Muscular strengthening
Previously Healthy and Active				
1–6 weeks	4–6 days per week	13–15	Approx 45 min moderate or 30 min moderate-vigorous most days	Aerobic, large muscle groups (e.g., stationary cycling, swim, walk, jog)
6–26 weeks		15–16	Approx 60 min moderate-vigorous or 40 min vigorous most days	
27–40 weeks		14–15	Approx 30 min moderate-vigorous most days	
Throughout	1–2 days	15–20 repetitions	8–10 exercises	Muscular strengthening; avoid free weights, do not lie on back

a. RPE = rating of perceived exertion. This is a scale to monitor intensity based on the exerciser's perception of intensity. The scale ranges from 6–20, 6 = no exertion, 13–14 = somewhat hard, 15–16 = hard, 17–18 = very hard, 19 = extremely hard, 20 = maximal exertion.

hydration is necessary to support continued breastfeeding and a smooth transition back into a regular, and sometimes intensive, fitness training regimen.

Nutrition for Pregnancy

Good nutrition habits during pregnancy optimize maternal health and reduce the risk for some birth defects, suboptimal fetal growth and development, and chronic health problems in the developing child.[30]

The key components of a health-promoting lifestyle during pregnancy include:

- *Appropriate physical activity.* Pregnant women should aim to incorporate at least 30 minutes or more of moderate-intensity physical activity appropriate for pregnancy on most, if not all, days of the week.[30]
- *Consumption of a variety of foods and calories in accordance with the* Dietary Guidelines for Americans. The USDA's MyPlate and SuperTracker websites offer specialized guidance for optimal nutrition for pregnant and lactating women (www.choosemyplate.gov and www.supertracker.usda.gov). In general, women do not have increased caloric needs until the second trimester, at which time needs increase by about 300 calories per day. The typical woman needs an additional 450 calories above baseline in the third trimester.[30] Notably, caloric needs vary considerably among women, with one

study finding a range of 25 calories to 800 calories more than pre-pregnancy.[31]

- *Appropriate and timely vitamin and mineral intake or supplementation.* Pregnant women need 600 μg of folic acid daily from fortified foods or supplements in addition to food forms of folate from a varied diet.[30] Folic acid reduces the risk of neural tube defects if taken prior to conception through the sixth week of pregnancy and may reduce birth defects if taken later in pregnancy. Many pregnant women suffer from iron-deficiency anemia and may benefit from iron supplementation. The DRIs for pregnancy and lactation are included in Chapter 4. Vitamins and minerals that are needed in larger quantities during pregnancy and lactation are highlighted in Table 13-6. A woman considering pregnancy should consult with her primary care physician prior to becoming pregnant to discuss vitamin and mineral supplement needs. If this is not possible, a visit as soon as pregnancy is suspected or confirmed is advisable.
- *Avoidance of alcohol and tobacco.* The Centers for Disease Control and Prevention urges pregnant women not to drink alcohol any time during pregnancy. Alcohol passes readily through the placenta and can cause a variety of problems to an exposed fetus including learning disabilities; low IQ; poor judgment; problems with the heart, kidney, or bones; and many others. Risks of smoking during pregnancy include abnormal implantation of the placenta, prematurity, miscarriage, certain birth defects (such as some heart defects and cleft lip/palate), and sudden infant death syndrome.[32]
- *Safe food handling.* Pregnant women and their fetuses are at higher risk of developing food-borne illness and should take extra precautions to prevent consumption of contaminated foods by avoiding:
  - Soft cheeses not made with pasteurized milk
  - Deli meats, unless they have been reheated to steaming hot
  - Raw or unpasteurized milk or milk products, raw eggs, raw or undercooked meat, unpasteurized juice, raw sprouts, and raw or undercooked fish
  - Cat litter boxes
  - Handling pets when preparing foods
  - Shark, swordfish, king mackerel, or tilefish. Pregnant women can safely consume 12 ounces or less of fish or shellfish per week,

Table 13-6. Nutrient Needs That Increase During Pregnancy and Lactation, Females 19–50 years

NUTRIENT	NONPREGNANT	PREGNANCY	LACTATION
Carbohydrate (g/d)	130	175	210
Fiber (g/d)	25	28	29
Linoleic acid (g/d)	12	13	13
Linolenic acid (g/d)	1.1	1.4	1.3
Protein (g/d)	46	71[a]	71
Vitamin A (ug/d)	700	770	1,300
Vitamin D (ug/d)	(5)[b]	(5)	(5)
Vitamin E (mg/d)	15	15	19
Vitamin K (ug/d)	(90)	(90)	(90)
Thiamin (mg/dl)	1.1	1.4	1.4
Riboflavin (mg/d)	1.1	1.4	1.6
Niacin (mg/d)	14	18	17
Pantothenic acid (mg/d)	5	6	7
Biotin (ug/d)	30	30	35
Vitamin B_6 (mg/d)	1.3	1.9	2.0
Folate (ug/d)	400	600	500
Vitamin B_{12} (ug/d)	2.4	2.6	2.8
Vitamin C (mg/d)	75	85	120
Choline (mg/d)	425	450	550
Sodium (g/d)	(1.5)	(1.5)	(1.5)

Table 13-6. Nutrient Needs That Increase During Pregnancy and Lactation, Females 19–50 years–cont'd

NUTRIENT	NONPREGNANT	PREGNANCY	LACTATION
Potassium (g/d)	4.7	4.7	5.1
Chloride (mg/d)	(2.3)	(2.3)	(2.3)
Calcium (mg/d)	(1,000)	(1,000)	(1,000)
Phosphorus (mg/d)	(700)	(700)	(700)
Magnesium (mg/d)	310/320	350–360	310/320
Iron (mg/d)	18	27	9
Zinc (mg/d)	8	11	12
Selenium (ug/d)	55	60	70
Iodine (ug/d)	150	220	290
Copper (ug/d)	900	1000	1300
Manganese (mg/d)	1.8	2.0	2.6
Fluoride (mg/d)	(3)	(3)	(3)
Chromium (ug/d)	25	30	35
Molybdenum (ug/d)	45	50	50
Total water (L/D)	2.7	3	3.8

a. Increased protein needs during pregnancy are only for the second half of pregnancy. Needs are the same as nonpregnant women in the first half.
b. ( ) indicates that needs do not change during pregnancy or lactation.

provided that it is low in mercury, such as shrimp, canned light tuna, salmon, pollock, and catfish. Consumption of albacore tuna should be limited to 6 ounces or less per week.

Physiology of Pregnancy and Changes in Nutritional Needs

From implantation, a pregnant woman's body adapts to meet the demands of the developing embryo and create the most favorable environment for a growing baby. In fact, the function of nearly every organ system of the body is affected by the pregnancy. The cardiovascular system responds by working more efficiently and pumping out more blood per beat to better supply tissues with oxygen. Blood volume also increases drastically during pregnancy. This causes the normal phenomena of **pregnancy-induced anemia** because the increase in red blood cell production is not as rapid or complete as the increase in blood volume. The rapid blood volume increase that usually occurs near the end of the first trimester is also responsible for the lightheadedness and dizziness that some women may experience. Blood levels return to normal near the end of the second trimester.

In an effort to rid the developing fetus of carbon dioxide and provide the pregnant woman with sufficient oxygen to add tissue mass to the uterus and breasts, the pregnant woman breathes more deeply and increases her respiratory rate slightly. The kidneys must work harder to excrete fetal and maternal waste. With the growing uterus applying pressure on the bladder, the pregnant woman needs to urinate more frequently. The gastrointestinal system undergoes the most noticeable pregnancy-induced changes. These include increased appetite, nausea and vomiting, decreased motility and slowing of digestion, changes in sense of taste, increased nutrient absorption, heartburn-causing reflux, and constipation.

Many of the physiological changes associated with pregnancy are due to a hormonal influx, with many different hormones secreted throughout gestation. At conception, the embryo begins producing human chorionic gonadotropin. This hormone is thought to be largely responsible for the early pregnancy changes such as a missed period, morning sickness, and tender breasts. Near the end of the first trimester, the placenta begins taking over hormone production. Progesterone, which is at its highest levels in the early months of pregnancy, causes relaxation of smooth muscles and is responsible for the stretching of the uterus as well as many of the changes to the gastrointestinal system. It also induces maternal fat deposition. Estrogen, which rises sharply near the end of pregnancy, promotes the growth and function of the uterus and is responsible for fluid retention and swelling often experienced in the third trimester. Hormonal changes also help maintain nutrient flow to the fetus and promote mammary development, which later becomes important for breastfeeding.

Beginning by about the fourth month of pregnancy, maternal metabolism increases until it is 15% to 20% above baseline by time of delivery.[33] This leads to increased hunger and caloric intake. Metabolism returns to nonpregnant levels by 1 week postpartum if the new mother does not breastfeed. The increase in caloric intake is essential during pregnancy to meet all of the changing needs of the various organ systems as well as to provide adequate fuel and nutrition to the developing fetus. Conscientious nutritional choices during the 40 weeks of pregnancy help the woman's body function optimally to meet the increasing demands of pregnancy and prepare for the birth of a strong and healthy baby.

General Nutrition Considerations

Pregnant women, especially those with unique nutritional needs, such as competitive athletes or those with underlying medical conditions, may benefit from consultation with a registered dietitian or other qualified professional to develop an individualized nutritional care plan. But the fulfilling task of sharing nutrition information with pregnant women is not limited to licensed nutritionists. In fact, health professionals from a range of disciplines can help assure that pregnant clients are aware of the major nutritional considerations during pregnancy.

A first question that many women will ask is: "How much weight should I gain?" The Institute of Medicine (IOM) weight gain recommendations are shown in Table 13-7. Too little weight gain often leads to low birth weight, while too much is associated with macrosomia, or excessive birth weight greater than about 9 pounds. Excessive gestational weight gain is also associated with childhood obesity in the infant (Box 13-5). Of total weight gain, the fetus weighs about 7 to 8 pounds, the placenta and amniotic fluid 3 to 4 pounds, tissue fluid 5 to 6 pounds, enlargement of the uterus 2 to 3 pounds, and maternal fat stores 5 to 8 pounds. An obstetrician will provide further information about healthful weight gain as well as an individualized assessment of each woman's situation.

Table 13-7. Pregnancy Weight Gain Recommendations[87]

PREPREGNANCY BMI	RECOMMENDED WEIGHT GAIN
Underweight (BMI <18.5)	28–40 pounds (12.7–18.2 kg)
Normal weight (BMI 18.5–24.9)	25–35 pounds (11.4–15.9 kg)
Overweight (BMI 25–29.9)	15–25 pounds (6.8–11.4 kg)
Obese (BMI >30)	11–20 pounds (5–9.1kg)

While it is often said that a pregnant woman is "eating for two," energy needs during pregnancy increase by an average 300 calories per day from nonpregnant needs throughout the second and third trimesters[29] (see Myths and Misconceptions). Importantly, it is not only the quantity of calories that must be increased, it is also the *quality* of the foods that are eaten. While an occasional ice cream dessert or extra serving of a calorie-dense side dish can be part of a healthful eating plan when consumed in moderation, an overall balanced, nutrient-dense, and healthy diet will assure adequate intake of nutrients that are vital for a healthy pregnancy and growing baby.

A healthy nutrition plan in pregnancy begins with eating small, frequent meals. Three meals are best replaced by five small meals per day including breakfast, lunch, an afternoon snack, dinner, and a bedtime snack. Pregnant women should avoid fasting (longer than 13 hours) and never skip breakfast due to a risk of ketosis, an increased acidity of the blood that can lead to a heightened increased risk of preterm delivery. Importantly, dieting is never healthy during pregnancy.

Myths and Misconceptions

Pregnant Women Need to "Eat for Two"

The Myth

Pregnant women need to nearly double their nutritional intake—after all, they are eating for two!

The Logic

Nutritional needs during pregnancy increase substantially to support the growth and development of a growing fetus. Metabolic rate increases, hunger increases, and micronutrient needs increase. All of these increases should require a pronounced increase in caloric needs. Active women who are expending large amounts of energy from exercise need to compensate with large caloric intakes in order to also support a growing fetus.

The Science

It is true that metabolic rate and caloric needs increase with pregnancy. While the extent of increase varies substantially among women, the typical increased need is minimal in the first trimester and from 300–450 calories thereafter.[33] That is equivalent to a glass of milk and a peanut butter sandwich. This increase is only about 15% more than pre-pregnancy caloric needs. Women who are very physically active during pregnancy should be careful to monitor weight to ensure appropriate weight gain, but many women overcompensate during pregnancy, consuming many more calories than the body needs for appropriate growth and development.

Box 13-5. Childhood Obesity That Begins at Conception

A growing body of research points to the role of the prenatal environment on later health outcomes for children, especially when it comes to the propensity to gain weight. A retrospective study of 10,000 babies found that risk of overweight by age seven was 48% higher for babies whose mothers had excessive pregnancy weight gain, even after accounting for numerous potential confounders.[79] Other studies found similar results for preschoolers[80] and adolescents.[81]

The authors of these studies suggest several potential explanations for the relationship between excess pregnancy weight gain and childhood obesity, but none are certain. To start, it may just be that mothers who gain too much weight during pregnancy share the same obesity-promoting genetic make-up and dietary and activity preferences as their children. While certainly this plays some role, the relationship between too much pregnancy weight gain and childhood obesity holds even for mothers who started pregnancy underweight or at a normal weight. In fact, the effects of excessive weight gain are most pronounced for underweight mothers. It probably has a lot to do with blood sugar, which tends to be elevated in women who gain too much weight, whether or not they end up developing gestational diabetes. Glucose passes the placenta but insulin does not. When the fetus experiences the elevated blood sugar, the pancreas must secrete more insulin to normalize blood sugar levels. Insulin itself is a growth factor, causing a fetus to be larger. It also may initiate a hormonal cascade which leads to increased appetite and weight gain in childhood, adolescence, and adulthood.

TAKING ACTION

Both an expecting mother and her developing baby can benefit from lifestyle changes the mother makes during pregnancy.

Curb Excessive Weight Gain

Perhaps the most important action a pregnant woman can take is to optimize her nutrition and physical activity to avoid excessive weight gain. A pregnant woman needs about 300 extra calories to support a developing baby—a little less in the first trimester and more in the third. An expecting mother should let hunger be her guide in determining how much to eat, but she should also keep an eye on the scale to prevent excessive weight gain. If she is gaining too little or too much, she should pay careful attention to her nutrition and physical activity habits.

The research to date is insufficient to guide obstetricians and expecting women with proven strategies to prevent excessive weight gain.[82] Women may be most likely to gain an appropriate amount of weight by following the basic principles for weight management for the general population: balance calories in with calories out. This comes from a well thought-out nutrition and activity plan.

Food Choices

For optimal maternal health and growth of the baby, the federal government recommends an individualized Daily Food Plan for Moms (check out www.choosemyplate.gov or www.supertracker.usda.gov). The following general guidelines should set the stage for a healthy pregnancy and appropriate weight gain:

- Eat five small meals per day including breakfast, lunch, an afternoon snack, dinner, and a bedtime snack.
- Focus on fruits, vegetables, whole grains, and high-calcium foods to meet micronutrient (vitamin and mineral) needs. Most obstetricians also recommend a prenatal vitamin with folic acid.
- Meet increased protein needs through a varied diet high in nutrient-dense foods and lean proteins.
- Eat low-mercury fatty fish twice per week. Some research suggests that fish oils (omega-3s) may enhance pregnancy duration and improve the baby's later cognitive, visual, and cardiovascular development.
- Leave a little room to satisfy cravings, but try to limit "empty" calories (food without much nutritional value).

Physical Activity

The American College of Obstetricians and Gynecologists (ACOG) recommends that otherwise healthy pregnant women engage in at least 30 minutes of moderate-intensity exercise on most if not all days of the week.[83] To expound on these guidelines, ACOG endorsed clarification presented by Zavorksy and Longo which was published simultaneously in the journals *Sports Medicine*[84] and *Obstetrics and Gynecology*[85].

A woman who is physically active during her pregnancy may improve the cardiovascular health of her baby as well as improve her own health and well-being. According to one study, babies of mothers who were physically active had lower heart rates and greater heart rate variability at 36 weeks' gestation[86].

While mass efforts are underway to shape the nutrition and activity behaviors of school-age children, the most successful interventions to optimize maternal and child health may be the ones that start at conception.

While an abundance of fruits, vegetables, whole grains, and high-calcium foods are key throughout pregnancy, other nutrition recommendations are best understood in the context of the stage of fetal growth and development, which by convention is divided into pregnancy trimesters and postpartum lactation.

The First Trimester (Weeks 0–12)

Hormonal changes in early pregnancy cause nausea, vomiting, fatigue, stress, and other discomforts in the first trimester for many pregnant women. For the baby, the first trimester is the most critical period for future health. It marks the time of implantation, organ development, and rapid growth. It is when good nutrition is paramount and, for many, especially for those women plagued by relentless morning sickness, nearly impossible. Weight gain may be nonexistent or up to about 1 pound per month in the first trimester.

Assuring Adequate Nutrient Intake: The Best Foods and the Prenatal Vitamin as Insurance. While maintaining optimal nutrition through healthful food choices such as fruits, vegetables, dairy products, and whole grains is ideal, when this is not guaranteed, the CDC advocates that the most important goal for a future mother early in the first trimester (and ideally long before conception) is to take a prenatal vitamin every day (see www.cdc.gov/ncbddd/folicacid for more information). Among a variety of other nutrients, a prenatal vitamin should contain at least 400 mcg of folic acid. Adequate folic acid intake prevents about 60% of neural tube defects like spina bifida and anencephaly, which are devastating neurological abnormalities that result from an improperly formed spinal cord.[34] The vitamin prevents the defects if initiated by the first several weeks of pregnancy, as the neural tube closes within 3 weeks of conception. Generous consumption of dark green, leafy vegetables; fortified cereals; and fruits like oranges and strawberries may provide enough folate, but a prenatal vitamin eliminates the guesswork and assures sufficient intake. While a fairly simple and inexpensive insurance policy against severe neurological defects, according to CDC data only 40% of women of child-bearing age take the supplement (www.cdc.gov/folicacid). Importantly, vegans should also consider a vitamin B_{12} supplement or ensure adequate intake through fortified foods, as a deficiency in this vitamin can also contribute to neural tube defects.

Iron is another important component of the prenatal vitamin. The Centers for Disease Control and Prevention recommend that all pregnant women take a low-dose iron supplement containing 30 milligrams per day, as many women have difficulty maintaining iron stores during pregnancy.[35] Though it has not been well-established that all women need an iron supplement, supplementation is generally not associated with health risks and it helps women to maintain iron stores during pregnancy. Very athletic women, especially those who engage in extensive endurance training during pregnancy, may be at highest risk for iron deficiency. Pregnant women should aim to get the recommended 27 milligrams of iron per day from food sources and supplementation, in consultation with their physician. Excellent food sources of iron include lean red meat, fish, poultry, beans, dried fruits, and iron-fortified cereals. Consumption of vitamin C with iron increases iron absorption. The vitamin C can be in the form of food or a supplement.

Calcium intake is also important throughout pregnancy. The developing fetus builds its bones through available calcium in the maternal bloodstream. In the fetus, calcium is also used to conduct nerve impulses and build a strong heart and muscles. Similar to other nutrients, the fetus receives access to circulating nutrients first. If calcium intake is not adequate, maternal bone strength is at risk. Because calcium absorption is increased during pregnancy, calcium needs in pregnant women are similar to nonpregnant women—about 1,000 to 1,200 milligrams per day—the equivalent of about three to four glasses of milk per day. Adequate calcium intake may also help prevent pregnancy-induced high blood pressure and preeclampsia.[36] Sufficient calcium intake is best gained through food sources such as dairy products, fortified foods and juices, and cooked spinach or broccoli. However, if necessary, a calcium supplement may also help to meet needs. Vitamin D intake is also important as it aids in calcium absorption.

Prenatal vitamins also provide other vitamins and minerals important in early pregnancy. However, the vitamin should act more as "insurance" than as the primary source of nutrition. In some cases it is also possible to have too much of a good thing. For instance, consumption of greater than 10,000 IU of vitamin A in early pregnancy can cause birth defects. Health professionals should encourage pregnant women to discuss supplement needs with their obstetrician.

Substances Potentially Harmful in the First Trimester. A precaution throughout pregnancy and especially during the first trimester when the baby's organs develop is to avoid alcohol consumption. Certainly, many women do not know that they are pregnant from the first day of conception and may have had a glass of wine or beer early in the pregnancy. Most research suggests that this will not cause serious birth defects, and in fact, in the first 2 weeks following conception, many defects are "all or none," meaning that the fetus will either miscarry or develop normally.[37] However, risks increase substantially depending upon the amount of alcohol consumed, and no safe level of alcohol consumption during pregnancy has been established. Because alcohol-induced problems such as mental retardation, learning disabilities, and fetal alcohol syndrome and its associated birth defects are entirely preventable with abstinence, and it is unknown at what amount of alcohol intake damage occurs, alcohol should be avoided entirely throughout pregnancy.[38]

Caffeine is also a potentially dangerous substance during pregnancy, particularly at high doses. Caffeine readily crosses the placenta (which develops at the end of the first trimester) and can affect fetal heart rate and breathing. Caffeine is hypothesized to cause an increase in risk of miscarriage, sudden infant death syndrome, low birth weight, and possibly congenital anomalies or birth defects at very high doses. However, a Cochrane Review evaluating the available randomized controlled trials determined that there is insufficient high-quality research to determine whether or not caffeine has an effect on pregnancy outcome.[39] A subsequent observational study of 60,000 pregnancies over a period of 10 years found no link between caffeine and preterm birth, but it did find a link between caffeine intake and decreased birth weight. A child expected to weigh about 8 pounds who was exposed to caffeine weighed three-quarters of an ounce to an ounce less in birth weight for each 100 milligrams of average daily caffeine intake from all sources by the mother.[40] While the research is inconclusive and no one fully understands the true risks of caffeine consumption, most experts recommend limiting caffeine consumption to no more than two cups of coffee or six cans of soda per day (200 mg).[41]

The Second Trimester (Weeks 13–26)

Often known as the "honeymoon" of pregnancy, many women feel better and develop somewhat of a voracious appetite during the second trimester. While this is true for many women, it is not uncommon for the first trimester symptoms such as morning sickness and fatigue to long outlast the crossover from week 12 to week 13. For the majority of women who do experience relief, the second trimester provides an opportune time to commit or recommit to an exercise program. By week 20, most women will become visibly pregnant.

Second trimester weight gain is about 1 pound per week, though actual gain varies considerably among women. This is a period of rapid fetal growth leading to increased maternal nutritional needs of about 300 calories per day. Protein is especially important to help in the development and growth of the fetus' vital organs. In fact, protein needs increase from about 46 grams pre-pregnancy to about 70 grams during pregnancy.[17] The second trimester also may be a good time for women to increase omega-3 fatty acid intake either from foods (such as salmon or other fatty fishes) or a DHA supplement. Research suggests that fish oils may enhance pregnancy duration and improve the baby's later cognitive, visual, and cardiovascular development, and reduce allergic disease.[42]

Pregnant women are encouraged to meet increased nutritional needs through a varied diet high in nutrient-dense foods such as fruits, vegetables, whole grains, and lean proteins. Food cravings can also manifest during this time. Many believe that cravings may signify a nutrient deficiency. For example, craving meat may function to increase iron intake, whereas craving non-food substances such as dirt and paper may be a sign of generalized malnutrition that needs medical attention. More typical cravings may be for ice cream or fast food. While these indulgences are acceptable in moderation, pregnant women are encouraged to meet increased caloric needs through healthful foods and also be aware that energy needs do not increase that substantially during pregnancy. Excess calories consumed beyond those needed will be readily stored as fat.

The Third Trimester (Weeks 27–40)

The nutritional needs of the fetus are most pronounced during the third trimester. Approximately 50% to 70% of the calories required by the fetus are derived from glucose, 20% from protein, and the remaining from fat. In order to maximize glucose availability to the fetus, the maternal energy source is primarily fat.[33] During this trimester it is especially important to consume carbohydrates regularly throughout the day to provide an adequate supply of glucose to the fetus. Weight gain is about 1 pound per week. By the end of the third trimester, total weight gain should be in accordance with the IOM recommendations shown in Table 13-6.

Nutrition for Lactation

Prior to a child's birth, most women will decide whether they plan to breastfeed. Breastfeeding provides optimal nutrition and health protection for the first 6 months of life. From 6 to 12 months, breastfeeding combined with the gradual introduction of solid foods is optimal. Breastfeeding is nature's perfect source of nutrition for a newborn, providing the ideal nutrient mix, increased protection against a variety of infections, increased bonding, higher IQ, stronger bones, and many other benefits.[43] All mothers who are motivated and capable to breastfeed are highly encouraged to do so, not only for the significant benefits to the child, but also for maternal benefits, which include accelerated postpartum weight loss, decreased risk of breast and ovarian cancer, increased bonding, and decreased cost, among other maternal benefits.[43]

Women who breastfeed require approximately 500 additional calories per day for weight maintenance.[43] Thus, breastfeeding generally quickens postpartum weight loss. Health professionals can help women return to pre-pregnancy weight by reinforcing the positive nutrition changes made during pregnancy, such as increased fruit, vegetable, and whole-grain consumption. Referral to a registered dietitian may be warranted if the woman requests or requires more extensive nutritional intervention such as meal planning. Also, health professionals should facilitate entry or re-entry into a regular physical-activity program.

Special Considerations for Pregnant and Lactating Athletes

Recommendations for optimal nutrition during pregnancy and lactation generally apply to athletes. To date, no organizations have published position statements or practice guidelines specifically related to nutrition for pregnant and lactating athletes. However, several considerations are worthy of special mention, as athletes may be at higher risk for inadequate intakes or other potential undesirable outcomes.

- *Energy intake*. Endurance athletes and other athletes who expend large amounts of energy during training should pay particular attention to energy intake and ensure appropriate weight gain. Athletes who engage in aesthetic sports or who may otherwise consider energy restriction should be advised against dieting or caloric restriction. Athletes who have concerns about ensuring adequate caloric intake should seek consultation from a nutrition professional who will help to develop a healthful nutrition plan during pregnancy.
- *Nutrient intake*. Female athletes are at increased risk of certain nutritional deficiencies compared to the general population, especially calcium and iron. Pregnant women also are at increased risk of inadequate calcium and iron intake, vitamin B_{12} in vegans, and folic acid. Due to the "double risk," pregnant athletes should pay particularly careful attention to meet needs for calcium and iron, as well as other nutrients of special importance during pregnancy.
- *Caffeine and supplements*. Because the effects of many ergogenic supplements on a developing fetus are unknown, pregnant athletes should avoid taking supplements, other than the standard vitamins mentioned above, in the quantities recommended by the CDC or a personal obstetrician. Large doses of caffeine, while potentially beneficial for athletic performance, may be detrimental to a developing fetus. Lactating women should also pay careful attention to supplement intake as some pass into breast milk and may induce undesirable effects in the infant.
- *Breast milk production*. A lactating athlete faces unique challenges in maintaining breastfeeding in the midst of a strenuous training program. In order to maintain adequate milk supply, the athlete should pay special attention to hydration status and ensuring appropriate water and other liquid intake during training as well as throughout the day. While each woman will find a solution that works best with her schedule, frequent breastfeeding or pumping also supports continued milk production. Athletes who will engage in a prolonged training workout or competition will benefit from breastfeeding and pumping immediately prior to exercise to minimize risk of engorgement and leakage during training.

SPEED BUMP

3. List the nutrients that require increased intake during pregnancy and lactation. Among those, describe which ones are most likely to be suboptimal in pregnant and lactating athletes.

4. Explain why and how much caloric needs change during pregnancy and lactation.

NUTRITION IN AGING

Optimal nutrition choices are important for **successful aging**, which Rowe and Kahn initially defined as "the ability to maintain a low risk of disease, high mental and physical function, and active engagement in life."[44] While nearly 80% of older adults have one chronic disease or disability and half have at least two (www.cdc.gov/aging), attention to nutrition and activity and avoidance of smoking play a significant role in staving off illness and disease and keeping older adults healthy, independent, and in their homes. In fact, older adults who eat a diet high in vegetables, fruits, whole grains, poultry, fish, and low-fat dairy products have increased quality and quantity of life.[45] Eating patterns such as the DASH diet and Mediterranean diet are particularly beneficial for older adults.[46]

Nutrition for Older Adults

One in eight Americans is an **older adult**, defined by the Older Americans Act as a person older than 60 years.[47] The main goal for older adults, based on *Healthy People 2020* is to "improve the health, function and quality of life."[48] Two major ways to help achieve that objective include physical activity and attention to healthful nutrition.

An ideal eating pattern for older adults closely resembles an ideal eating pattern for the general adult population with a few notable exceptions and considerations, which are depicted in the My Plate for Older Adults icon developed by Tuft University's Jean Mayer USDA Human Nutrition Research Center on Aging.[49] As demonstrated in the icon, on the whole, older adults need to pay particular attention to fluid intake, affordable and easy-to-prepare food, and physical activity. The DRIs provide nutrient recommendations for older adults in categories from 51 to 70 years and greater than 70 years, though actual needs may vary considerably among individuals. The DRIs are shown in Chapter 4.

A study that assessed the nutritional intake of older adults and various physical and mental health outcomes found that older adults who ate a diet high in vegetables, fruits, whole grains, poultry, fish, and low-fat dairy products had superior nutritional status, quality of life, and longevity.[45] Unfortunately, many potential barriers may impede an older adult's ability to achieve dietary goals. These barriers include use of multiple medications, each with varying nutritional interactions and restrictions and diet-altering side effects; economic hardships; changes in mental functioning; physiological changes in smell, taste, chewing, swallowing, digestion, and absorption; and social isolation. A health professional who helps an older adult develop a physical activity program or improve nutritional intake must take these factors into consideration when providing information and making recommendations. These challenges are most pronounced in individuals older than 85 years.

Calorie Needs

Energy needs decrease with age.[50] Basal metabolic rate, which accounts for about 50% to 70% of total energy expenditure, is thought to decrease about 1% to 2% per decade after age 20 such that daily energy expenditure decreases about 150 calories per decade.[50] The decline is probably due in large part to decreased physical activity and subsequent decreased muscle mass (which is highly metabolically active) and increased fat mass (which is relatively metabolically inactive). Some studies have also found that, even when controlling for fat-free mass, basal metabolic rate is 5% lower in older adults compared with younger adults.[50] It is not clear why, but some researchers speculate that it may be due to an unavoidable loss of very metabolically active organ tissue or a decreased metabolic rate within muscle tissues. Decline seems to be most rapid after age 40 in men and 50 in women.[50] Though declining muscle mass is expected with advancing age, older adults who maintain a strenuous physical activity regimen that includes some resistance training may be able to maintain muscle mass and minimize the decrease in metabolic rate.

Caloric intake and appetite decrease with age; however, many older adults are overweight or obese because the age-related decrease in physical activity and metabolic rate is often more pronounced than reduced caloric intake. This scenario leads to a positive energy balance and weight gain.

Micronutrient Needs

Though caloric needs decrease with age, many nutrient needs stay the same or increase.[17, 51-54] Thus, in order to consume appropriate amounts of needed nutrients without exceeding calorie needs, older adults need to increase the **nutrient density** of their diets, eating more lower-calorie nutrient-packed foods like fruits and vegetables and eating fewer foods that contain very little nutrition and a large number of calories, such as many desserts and snacks. Many older adults suffer from inadequate nutrient intake, especially calcium; zinc; iron; vitamins A, D, E, and K; potassium; B vitamins; and fiber.[55,56] Older adults are at particularly high risk of vitamin B_{12} insufficiency or deficiency.[57]

Macronutrient Needs

The typical older adult requires a minimum of approximately 130 grams per day of carbohydrates.[17] Active older adults may have increased needs. High-fiber fruits, vegetables, and whole grains are an excellent source of carbohydrates for older adults. These foods are high in nutrients and the fiber provides additional benefits of improved glycemic control, gastric motility, and reduced LDL cholesterol. The recommended fiber intake is 30 grams for men and 21 grams for women over age 50.[17]

Protein needs for most older adults are similar to that of the general population—about 0.8 grams per kilogram of body weight.[17] Very active older adults probably have increased needs. While protein intake may play some role in attenuating **sarcopenia,** "muscle wasting," or a decrease in muscle mass and strength—the research to date is inconclusive. It affects up to 40% of adults older than 60 years, and 50% of those older than75 years.[58] While multiple factors contribute to sarcopenia, the most pronounced is decreased physical activity and poor nutrition.[59] Sarcopenia is associated with the increased burden of chronic disease, increased frailty, functional dependence, and death.[41] Sarcopenia can be offset with a physical activity regimen.

The Academy of Nutrition and Dietetics (AND) suggests that intake "moderately greater" than the RDA may enhance protein anabolism and reduce age-related decrease in muscle mass.[46] Other experts advise an intake of 1.0 to 1.6 grams per kilogram per day for healthy older adults.[60] Some evidence suggests that a protein intake of approximately 30 grams per meal is ideal for optimal muscle synthesis.[61]

Essential fatty acid needs for older adults mirror that of younger adults. Otherwise, fat intake should be based on individual needs and weight-management goals.

Fluids and Hydration

The risk of dehydration is pronounced in older adults, especially those older than 85 years or living in institutionalized settings. Many factors compromise hydration status in older adults. The sensation of thirst decreases with age. The kidneys become less effective at concentrating urine, leading to unnecessary water loss in urine. Medication side effects and interactions interfere with appropriate hydration. Consequently, unless prompted, many older adults may not achieve the adequate intake for fluids, an amount intended to replace normal daily losses and prevent dehydration. Provision of sufficient fluids is especially critical for exercising older adults who have additional exercise-related fluid losses.

Body Composition

Sarcopenic obesity, the decline in skeletal muscle and strength combined with excess body fat, is common during older adulthood.[59,60,62] This combination increases disability, morbidity, and mortality.[59] Health professionals working with older adults should screen for sarcopenic obesity and develop programs to improve muscle mass and weight status. The AND advises using multiple assessment methods when measuring body composition in older adults, including current weight and weight change, waist-to-hip ratio and waist circumference, BMI, and body composition.[46] The history of weight change is particularly important, as studies suggest that older adults who had gained more than 20 pounds, lost more than 10 pounds, weight cycled, or unintentionally lost more than 5% to 10% of body weight over 3 to 5 years had decreased physical function.[46] A multidisciplinary team of health professionals including, at the minimum, a nutrition specialist, exercise professional, and physician should work closely together when developing a weight-management program for an older adult.

Physical Activity and Older Adults

The benefits of physical activity in older adults are pronounced: decreased risk of chronic and degenerative disease, improved heart health, better cognitive function, decreased obesity, decreased risk of fracture, improved sleep quality, and overall increased mood and quality of life.[46] Regular physical activity can also benefit nutritional status by improving caloric and nutrient intake.[63] Progressive resistance training decreases risk of sarcopenia and improves protein efficiency.[64] To achieve these benefits, the U.S. Department of Health and Human Services' *Physical Activity Guidelines for Americans* (www.health.gov/paguidelines) recommend that older adults:

- Engage in at least 150 minutes per week of moderate-intensity, or 75 minutes per week of vigorous-intensity physical activity, or an equivalent combination of moderate- and vigorous-intensity physical activity. Aerobic exercise episodes should occur in bouts of at least 10 minutes spread throughout the week. For additional benefits, adults should increase aerobic exercise to 300 minutes per week of moderate intensity or 150 minutes per week of vigorous intensity. If these goals are not possible due to health limitations, older adults should engage in as much activity as abilities and conditions allow.
- Do muscle-strengthening exercises that are moderate or high intensity and involve all major muscle groups on 2 or more days a week.
- Do exercises that help to maintain or improve balance, if at risk of falling.
- Engage in activity with an appropriate level of effort to match level of fitness.

Despite these recommendations, only 5% of adults engage in 30 minutes of physical activity per day, with rates even lower among the oldest adults.[12]

Special Considerations for Master Athletes

Master athletes refer to competitive athletes ranging from about 30 to 85 years, though most of the special considerations for master athletes described below relate to the older masters, aged 60 and older. Compared to their sedentary peers, master athletes experience a variety of health benefits from their sport participation including increased muscle mass, improved physical and cognitive functioning, and decreased risk of chronic illness, falls, and early death.[46] However, compared to their younger counterparts, master athletes also face unique fitness and nutritional challenges. For optimal fitness and nutrition, master athletes need to be more conscientious and strategic in developing training regimens and nutrition programs to offset the reality that athletic performance declines with age across all sports.[65]

Nutritional factors play an important role in offsetting an age-related fitness decline. One study of master swimmers ("young" masters defined as 30 to 60 years, while "older" masters were 61 to 85 years) attributed performance decline to an increase in the energy cost of swimming as well as a decrease in available metabolic power.[65,66] A follow-up study found that the energy cost of swimming increased by about 0.75% per year.[66] Another study of strength training in cyclists found that the deficit in metabolic power may be overcome with an intensive strength-training program. In this study, nine master endurance athletes with an average age of 51.5 years and eight young endurance athletes with an average age of 25.6 years engaged in a 3-week quadriceps strength training program. After the 3 weeks, the master athletes had a substantial improvement in strength and cycling efficiency. In fact, the improvement was so pronounced that it negated all previous differences in strength and efficiency among the master and younger athletes.[67]

Taken together, these studies help to highlight the importance of nutrition in ensuring a high level of athletic performance for older athletes. First, sufficient caloric intake is essential to provide a high level of energy availability to meet the increased age-related energy demands of strenuous exercise. Furthermore, optimal protein intake provides the amino acids necessary to induce muscle protein hypertrophy in response to resistance training. Some studies suggest that older adult athletes may require a protein intake of 1.6 grams per kilogram per day to optimize the hypertrophic response to resistance training.[64]

When master athletes optimize nutritional intake and engage in an exercise program that includes resistance training, they end up with higher caloric intake and lower weight and leaner body composition than their inactive peers. As one author noted, this is an example of a phenomena of "eat more, weigh less."[68]

Overall, active older adults require increased calories, protein, fluids, and micronutrients compared to their age-matched peers. When athletes meet these needs, performance benefits.[62] Studies of master athletes suggest that most follow an appropriate eating plan, though many still do not attain the recommended levels of vitamin D, vitamin E, folic acid, calcium, magnesium, and zinc.[69]

Ultimately, the general sports nutrition principles that apply to younger athletes also apply to older adults, though modifications may be necessary based on the individual athlete's health status, motivation and cognitive function, and access to resources. For older adults, the benefits of physical activity in combination with healthful and strategic nutrition extend far beyond improvement in athletic performance to increased quality and quantity of life.

SPEED BUMP

5. List several nutrition considerations when working with older adults.

6. Describe several unique nutritional needs for master athletes.

CHAPTER SUMMARY

Health professions who work with active children, pregnant and lactating women, and older adults are well advised to gain familiarity with the unique nutritional needs of these special populations.

KEY POINTS SUMMARY

1. Children have unique nutritional needs. One major consideration is that, unlike adults, children undergo periods of rapid growth and development. To achieve their full growth potential, many environmental factors must be optimized, including appropriate nutrition, physical activity, maintenance of a healthy weight, and adequate sleep.
2. Allied health professionals, parents, and pediatricians can monitor a child's growth through the use of growth charts. Growth charts can also be used to monitor BMI to ensure a child is at a normal weight for height, or to rapidly identify a child who is at risk for too little or too much weight gain and growth.
3. Youth athletes who engage in intensive physical training more than 18 hours per week, restrict caloric intake, or participate in weight-conscious sports are at highest risk of impaired growth.
4. There is currently a worldwide epidemic of childhood obesity due primarily to decreases in physical activity and poor nutrition habits. The health consequences of childhood obesity are severe. The treatment includes increased physical activity and improved nutrition intake to more closely align with the *Dietary Guidelines for Americans* for children and adolescents. These are two areas where health professionals can work closely with children and their parents and make a substantial impact.
5. Youth athletes are not just "little adults." Youth athletes require sufficient calories and protein to support growth and maturation as well as athletic performance. Children are more susceptible than adults to heat illness in the face of dehydration, thus, adequate hydration takes on critical importance, especially for athletes exercising in the heat and humidity.
6. Sports drinks provide benefit to youth athletes engaging in prolonged activity or who participate in multiple practices or competitions in 1 day. However, sports drinks are not appropriate for routine hydration. Energy drinks are never safe or recommended for children.
7. The benefits of physical activity during pregnancy outweigh the risks for most women. Women already engaged in a vigorous exercise regimen prior to pregnancy often may continue throughout pregnancy, depending on how they feel and the recommendation of their obstetrician.
8. Optimal nutrition during pregnancy is essential to support the growth and development of the mother and fetus as well as athletic performance. Needs for most nutrients increase during pregnancy. Caloric needs increase by about 300 calories per day, though the amount differs considerably among women. Women should aim to meet increased caloric needs through healthful and nutrient-dense foods. Women may also benefit from a prenatal vitamin containing folic acid and iron. The use of supplementation and nutritional needs should be discussed with an obstetrician.
9. Normal weight women are advised to gain 25 to 35 pounds throughout pregnancy, with the majority of weight gain in the late-second and third trimesters. Underweight women should gain 28 to 40 pounds, overweight women 15 to 20 pounds, and obese women 11 to 20 pounds. Many women gain too much weight during pregnancy. Elite athletes may be at risk for not gaining enough weight. Importantly, dieting is not safe during pregnancy.

10. A healthy eating plan during pregnancy includes: small, frequent meals; avoiding fasting (longer than 13 hours); daily breakfast; and an abundance of whole grains, fruits, vegetables, and foods high in calcium and iron.
11. Increased nutritional needs extend beyond pregnancy for breastfeeding mothers. Calorie needs increase by about 500 calories per day beyond baseline. Nutrient needs are also increased compared to baseline and pregnancy.
12. Pregnant and lactating female athletes should avoid high intakes of caffeine beyond about 200 milligrams per day. Supplement use other than a prenatal vitamin and nutritional supplementation advised by a physician is strongly discouraged.
13. Physical activity and healthful nutrition play key roles in successful aging. While calorie needs decrease for older adults, due in large part to loss of muscle mass (sarcopenia) and basal metabolic rate, nutrient needs increase or stay the same. Thus, older adults require a more nutrient-dense eating plan than their younger counterparts.
14. The Tufts MyPlate for Older Adults icon provides nutrition guidance specifically for older adults. It emphasizes nutrient-dense foods that are easy to prepare, convenient, affordable, low in sodium, and easy to chew and digest. It also includes recommendations for physical activity and attention to adequate hydration.
15. Master athletes benefit from optimal nutritional intake to offset age-related declines in performance. Attention to calorie and protein intake in combination with resistance training may help minimize decreases in lean muscle mass.

PRACTICAL APPLICATIONS

1. Jacqueline and Jonathan are 10-year-old identical twins. Which of the following statements is most accurate about the twins' rate of growth throughout their teenage years?
   A. Jacqueline will reach her maximum growth height before Jonathan.
   B. Jonathan will reach his maximum growth height before Jacqueline.
   C. Jacqueline's growth spurt will start in about 3.5 years.
   D. Jonathan's growth spurt has most likely already begun.

2. Which of the following types of high-level, elite athletes is at the highest risk for suffering from growth delays?
   A. Female rowers
   B. Male wrestlers
   C. Male gymnasts
   D. Female track and field athletes

3. Which of the following youth groups has shown a continued increase in the rate of obesity, while other groups have shown stabilization in the obesity rate in recent years?
   A. Adolescent females
   B. Preadolescent males
   C. Teenage females
   D. Teenage males

4. Ryder is a moderately active child who participates in physical activities such as soccer, gymnastics, and skateboarding most days of the week. How many additional daily calories does Ryder need to consume above those recommended for sedentary children to maintain his active lifestyle?
   A. 50 calories
   B. 100 calories
   C. 150 calories
   D. 200 calories

5. Which of the following statements is true regarding optimum hydration in youth athletes?
   A. Children innately have a poor ability to regulate body temperature.
   B. Thirst is generally a good guide in determining fluid intake.
   C. Sports drinks for the average child engaged in routine physical activity are recommended.
   D. Energy drinks are appropriate for children older than 12 years of age.

6. Dianne is nearing the end of her first trimester of her first pregnancy. She often feels lightheaded and dizzy and is concerned that these symptoms could be abnormal. Her physician assures her that what she is experiencing is the result of a normal pregnancy-related condition called ________________.
   A. pregnancy-induced anemia
   B. gestational syncope
   C. pregnancy-associated hypotension
   D. gestational blood reduction

7. Samantha is newly pregnant and has concerns about the amount of caffeine she consumes. She enjoys drinking two cups of coffee in the morning and two caffeine-containing diet sodas in the afternoon. Which of the following responses would be an appropriate recommendation for Samantha as she continues through her pregnancy?
   A. Maintain current caffeine consumption, but do not increase it by any amount.
   B. Do not worry about caffeine consumption because the evidence suggests it has no effect on pregnancy outcomes.
   C. Reduce current consumption by one cup of coffee.
   D. Limit coffee intake to two cups and replace sodas with noncaffeinated beverages.

8. Charlene is a new mother who has chosen to breastfeed her infant. She is also an avid runner and after her 6-week postpartum doctor's visit she was cleared to start pursuing her running program more vigorously. Excluding the amount needed to fuel her running endeavors, approximately how many additional daily calories does Charlene need to consume in order to maintain her weight and provide adequate breast milk for her baby?
   A. 300 calories
   B. 400 calories
   C. 500 calories
   D. 600 calories
9. Which of the following statements is true regarding older adults and weight gain?
   A. Both caloric intake and appetite increase with age.
   B. Age-related decreases in physical activity and metabolic rate are often the cause of added weight.
   C. Increased body weight in old age is associated with a higher metabolic rate.
   D. Maintaining an exercise program prevents age-related metabolic-rate reductions.
10. Which of the following responses represents the term used to describe the decline in skeletal muscle and strength combined with excess body fat common during older adulthood?
   A. Geriatric morphology
   B. Age-related atrophy
   C. Sarcopenic obesity
   D. Older adult adiposity

Case 1 Brian, the High School Basketball Player

Brian is a 15-year-old high school basketball player. He is 6'2" and 180 pounds. He would like to play college basketball.

1. Brian asks you if you think that he is going to grow any taller.
   a. What information would you need to answer this question?
   b. Seeing an opportunity to provide health education, you offer Brian several suggestions on how to optimize his growth potential. What do you tell him?
2. Brian shares that he is excited to graduate from high school in 2 years and go to college away from home. He asks what you think are the three most important pieces of nutrition information for a college athlete that he should remember when he is on his own. What do you tell him?

Case 2 Kate, the Marathon Runner

Kate is an experienced 22-year-old marathon runner who recently achieved her goal of qualifying for the Boston Marathon. Over the course of her training she struggled with disordered eating and weight loss and adopted a vegetarian diet. Her current BMI is 19. She shares that she interested in becoming pregnant in the next several months and asks how this might affect her training and nutritional needs.

1. Describe how nutritional needs change during pregnancy. How do these changes differ for athletes?
2. Kate shares that she is very nervous about becoming pregnant and gaining weight. She expresses doubts that she will ever get her body "back."
   a. How much weight should Kate gain during her pregnancy?
   b. How do you respond to Kate's concern?

Case 3 Adele, the Active Octogenarian

Adele is an 85-year-old woman who recently moved to a retirement community to start fresh after her husband died. She has maintained her 3-day per week exercise regimen for the past 10 months. She especially enjoys meeting her friends for water aerobics and going to breakfast afterwards. Adele shares that she is having difficulty eating healthfully because she doesn't feel like cooking for just herself and often finds herself snacking on processed foods or not eating at all.

1. What unique nutritional challenges do older adults face?
2. Compare and contrast MyPlate for Older Adults with MyPlate for the general population.
3. What tips might you provide Adele to help improve her nutrition? Relate at least one tip to her physical activity regimen.

TRAIN YOURSELF

Choose one period of time in your life when you either had special nutritional needs or challenges or anticipate that you will have special nutritional needs or challenges (e.g., as an overweight child, a teenager who subsisted on a poorly balanced diet, a competitive athlete engaging in large amounts of activity and a sporadic schedule, during pregnancy, as a parent attempting to feed children a healthy and balanced diet, or as an older adult with limited resources available to prepare meals).

1. Identify your selected life stage and explain why you chose this life stage.
2. Outline three to four major nutritional and/or physical activity considerations or challenges you experienced or might anticipate experiencing during this life stage. For each consideration, list one to two strategies you would use to try to optimize nutrition and physical activity during this period of time. Try to integrate the knowledge that you have gained from this chapter for the life stage that you selected.
3. How does the process of imagining yourself in this particular situation affect the type of information and advice you might provide your clients?

REFERENCES

1. *2011-2012 High School Athletes Participation Survey*: National Federation of State High School Associations; 2012.
2. Georgopoulos NA, Roupas ND, Theodoropoulou A, Tsekouras A, Vagenakis AG, Markou KB. The influence of intensive physical training on growth and pubertal development in athletes. *Ann NY Acad Sci.* September 2010; 1205:39-44.
3. Biro FM, McMahon RP, Striegel-Moore R, et al. Impact of timing of pubertal maturation on growth in black and white female adolescents: the National Heart, Lung, and Blood Institute Growth and Health Study. *J Pediatr.* 2001;138(5):636-643.
4. Vizmanos B, Marti-Henneberg C, Cliville R, Moreno A, Fernandez-Ballart J. Age of pubertal onset affects the intensity and duration of pubertal growth peak but not final height. *Am J Hum Biol.* 2001;13(3):409-416.
5. Ogden CL, Carroll MD, Kit BK, Flegal KM. Prevalence of childhood and adult obesity in the United States, 2011-2012. *JAMA.* February 2014; 311(8): 806-814.
6. Barlow SE. Expert committee recommendations regarding the prevention, assessment, and treatment of child and adolescent overweight and obesity: summary report. *Pediatrics.* December 2007;120 Suppl 4:S164-192.
7. Friedemann C, Heneghan C, Mahtani K, Thompson M, Perera R, Ward A. Cardiovascular disease risk in healthy children and its association with body mass index: a systematic review and meta-analysis. *Br Med J.* 2012;345:e4759.
8. Van Emmerik NM, Renders CM, Van de Veer M, et al. High cardiovascular risk in severely obese young children and adolescents. *Arch Dis Child.* 2012;2012 July 23(epub ahead of print).
9. May AL, Kuklina EV, Yoon PW. Prevalence of cardiovascular disease risk factors among US adolescents, 1999-2008. *Pediatrics.* June 2012;129(6):1035-1041.
10. Narayan KM, Boyle JP, Thompson TJ, Sorensen SW, Williamson DF. Lifetime risk for diabetes mellitus in the United States. *JAMA.* October 8 2003;290(14):1884-1890.
11. Russell-Mayhew S, McVey G, Bardick A, Ireland A. Mental health, wellness, and childhood overweight/obesity. *J Obes.* 2012;2012:281801.
12. U.S. Department of Agriculture. *2010 Dietary Guidelines for Americans Backgrounder, History and Process.* Washington, DC: U.S. Dept. of Agriculture; 2010: http://purl.fdlp.gov/GPO/gpo4085.
13. Gidding SS, Dennison BA, Birch LL, et al. Dietary recommendations for children and adolescents: a guide for practitioners. *Pediatrics.* February 2006;117(2):544-559.
14. Dwyer JT, Butte NF, Deming DM, Siega-Riz AM, Reidy KC. Feeding Infants and Toddlers Study 2008: progress, continuing concerns, and implications. *J Am Diet Assoc.* December 2010;110(12 Suppl):S60-S67.
15. French SA, Story M, Neumark-Sztainer D, Fulkerson JA, Hannan P. Fast food restaurant use among adolescents: associations with nutrient intake, food choices and behavioral and psychosocial variables. *Int J Obes Relat Metab Disord.* December 2001;25(12):1823-1833.
16. U.S. Department of Agriculture, Center for Nutrition Policy and Promotion. *Dietary Guidelines for Americans 2010.* www.cnpp.usda.gov/DGAs2010-PolicyDocument.htm. Accessed March 17, 2013.
17. *Dietary Reference Intakes for Energy, Carbohydrate, Fiber, Fat, Fatty Acids, Cholesterol, Protein, and Amino Acids.* Washington, DC: Food and Nutrition Board, Institute of Medicine; 2005.
18. Nemet D, Eliakim A. Pediatric sports nutrition: an update. *Curr Opin Clin Nutr Metab Care.* May 2009;12(3):304-309.
19. Boisseau N, Vermorel M, Rance M, Duche P, Patureau-Mirand P. Protein requirements in male adolescent soccer players. *Eur J Appl Physiol.* May 2007;100(1):27-33.
20. Petrie HJ, Stover EA, Horswill CA. Nutritional concerns for the child and adolescent competitor. *Nutrition.* July-August 2004;20(7-8):620-631.
21. Winzenberg T, Shaw K, Fryer J, Jones G. Effects of calcium supplementation on bone density in healthy children: meta-analysis of randomised controlled trials. *Br Med J.* October 14 2006;333(7572):775.
22. Eliakim A, Beyth Y. Exercise training, menstrual irregularities and bone development in children and adolescents. *J Pediatr Adolesc Gynecol.* August 2003;16(4):201-206.
23. Dubnov G, Constantini NW. Prevalence of iron depletion and anemia in top-level basketball players. *Int J Sport Nutr Exerc Metab.* February 2004;14(1):30-37.
24. Beals KA. Eating behaviors, nutritional status, and menstrual function in elite female adolescent volleyball players. *J Am Diet Assoc.* September 2002;102(9):1293-1296.
25. O'Dea JA. Consumption of nutritional supplements among adolescents: usage and perceived benefits. *Health Educ Res.* February 2003;18(1):98-107.
26. Bergeron MF, Devore C, Rice SG. Policy statement: climatic heat stress and exercising children and adolescents. *Pediatrics.* September 2011;128(3):e741-747.
27. Schneider MB, Benjamin HJ, and the Committee on Nutrition and the Council on Sports Medicine & Fitness. Sports drinks and energy drinks for children and adolescents: are they appropriate? *Pediatrics.* June 2011;127(6):1182-1189.
28. Zavorsky GS, Longo LD. Exercise guidelines in pregnancy: new perspectives. *Sports Med.* May 1 2011;41(5):345-360.
29. American College of Obstetricians and Gynecologists. *FAQ 119: Exercise During Pregnancy. www.acog.org/~/media/For%20Patients/faq119.pdf?dmc=1&ts=20140214T0159593449* Accessed February 13, 2014.
30. Kaiser L, Allen LH. Position of the American Dietetic Association: nutrition and lifestyle for a healthy pregnancy outcome. *J Am Diet Assoc.* March 2008;108(3):553-561.
31. Pitkin RM. Energy in pregnancy. *Am J Clin Nutr.* April 1999; 69(4):583.
32. Centers for Disease Control and Prevention. Pregnancy. www.cdc.gov/pregnancy/. Accessed March 17, 2013.
33. King JC. Physiology of pregnancy and nutrient metabolism. *Am J Clin Nutr.* May 2000;71(5 Suppl):1218S-1225S.

34. Blencowe H, Cousens S, Modell B, Lawn J. Folic acid to reduce neonatal mortality from neural tube disorders. *Int J Epidemiol.* April 2010;39 Suppl 1:i110-121.
35. Centers for Disease Control and Prevention. Recommendations to prevent and control iron deficiency in the United States. Centers for Disease Control and Prevention. *MMWR Recomm Rep.* April 3 1998;47(RR-3):1-29.
36. Buppasiri P, Lumbiganon P, Thinkhamrop J, Ngamjarus C, Laopaiboon M. Calcium supplementation (other than for preventing or treating hypertension) for improving pregnancy and infant outcomes. *Cochrane Database of Systematic Reviews.* 2011(10):CD007079.
37. Foltran F, Gregori D, Franchin L, Verduci E, Giovannini M. Effect of alcohol consumption in prenatal life, childhood, and adolescence on child development. *Nutr Rev.* November 2011;69(11):642-659.
38. American Academy of Pediatrics. Committee on Substance Abuse and Committee on Children With Disabilities. Fetal alcohol syndrome and alcohol-related neurodevelopmental disorders. *Pediatrics.* August 2000;106(2 Pt 1):358-361.
39. Jahanfar S, Jaafar SH. Effects of restricted caffeine intake by mother on fetal, neonatal and pregnancy outcome. *Cochrane Database of Systematic Reviews.* 2013(2): Art. No.: CD006965. DOI: 10.1002/14651858.CD006965.pub3.
40. Sengpiel, V, Elind, E, Bacelis, J, et al. Maternal caffeine intake during pregnancy is associated with birth weight but not gestational length: results from a large prospective observational cohort study. *BMC Med.* 2013;11:43 doi: 10.1186/1741-7015-11-42.
41. American College of Obstetricians and Gynecologists, Committee on Obstetric Practice. *Moderate Caffeine Consumption During Pregnancy.* www.acog.org/Resources_And_Publications/Committee_Opinions/Committee_on_Obstetric_Practice/Moderate_Caffeine_Consumption_During_Pregnancy. Accessed February 13, 2014.
42. Larque E, Gil-Sanchez A, Prieto-Sanchez MT, Koletzko B. Omega 3 fatty acids, gestation and pregnancy outcomes. *Br J Nutr.* June 2012;107 Suppl 2:S77-84.
43. American Academy of Pediatrics. Breastfeeding and the use of human milk. *Pediatrics.* 2012;129(3):e827-e841.
44. Rowe JW, Kahn RL. Successful aging. *Aging (Milano).* April 1998;10(2):142-144.
45. Anderson AL, Harris TB, Tylavsky FA, et al. Dietary patterns and survival of older adults. *J Am Diet Assoc.* January 2011;111(1):84-91.
46. Bernstein M, Munoz N. Position of the Academy of Nutrition and Dietetics: food and nutrition for older adults: promoting health and wellness. *J Acad Nutr Diet.* August 2012;112(8): 1255-1277.
47. U.S. Department of Health and Human Services, Administration on Aging. Older Americans Act. www.aoa.gov/AOA_programs/OAA/index.aspx. Accessed February 13, 2014.
48. U.S. Department of Health and Human Services. *Healthy People 2020, Older Adults.* www.healthypeople.gov/2020/topicsobjectives2020/overview.aspx?topicId=31. Accessed March 17, 2013.
49. Tufts University. Tufts University Nutrition Scientists Unveil MyPlate for Older Adults. http://now.tufts.edu/news-releases/tufts-university-nutrition-scientists-unveil-. Accessed May 7, 2013.
50. Roberts SB, Dallal GE. Energy requirements and aging. *Public Health Nutr.* October 2005;8(7A):1028-1036.
51. National Research Council. *Dietary Reference Rntakes for Water, Potassium, Sodium, Chloride, and Sulfate.* Washington, DC: National Academies Press; 2005.
52. Institute of Medicine. *Dietary Reference Intakes for Calcium and Vitamin D.* Washington, DC: National Academies Press; 2011.
53. Bandura A. Social cognitive theory: an agentic perspective. *Annu Rev Psychol.* 2001;52:1-26.
54. Centers for Disease Control and Prevention. Trends in intake of energy and macronutrients—United States, 1971-2000. *MMWR Morb Mortal Wkly Rep.* February 6 2004;53(4):80-82.
55. Bachman JL, Reedy J, Subar AF, Krebs-Smith SM. Sources of food group intakes among the U.S. population, 2001-2002. *J Am Diet Assoc.* May 2008;108(5):804-814.
56. Lichtenstein AH, Rasmussen H, Yu WW, Epstein SR, Russell RM. Modified MyPyramid for older adults. *J Nutr.* January 2008;138(1):5-11.
57. Allen L. How common is vitamin B12 deficiency? *Am J Clin Nutr.* 2009;89(2):712s-716s.
58. Kim JS, Wilson JM, Lee SR. Dietary implications on mechanisms of sarcopenia: roles of protein, amino acids and antioxidants. *J Nutr Biochem.* January 2010;21(1):1-13.
59. Zamboni M, Mazzali G, Fantin F, Rossi A, Di Francesco V. Sarcopenic obesity: a new category of obesity in the elderly. *Nutr Metab Cardiovasc Dis.* June 2008;18(5):388-395.
60. Houston DK, Nicklas BJ, Ding J, et al. Dietary protein intake is associated with lean mass change in older, community-dwelling adults: the Health, Aging, and Body Composition (Health ABC) Study. *Am J Clin Nutr.* January 2008;87(1):150-155.
61. Symons TB, Sheffield-Moore M, Wolfe RR, Paddon-Jones D. A moderate serving of high-quality protein maximally stimulates skeletal muscle protein synthesis in young and elderly subjects. *J Am Diet Assoc.* September 2009;109(9): 1582-1586.
62. Stenholm S, Harris TB, Rantanen T, Visser M, Kritchevsky SB, Ferrucci L. Sarcopenic obesity: definition, cause and consequences. *Curr Opin Clin Nutr Metab Care.* November 2008;11(6):693-700.
63. Rivlin RS. Keeping the young-elderly healthy: is it too late to improve our health through nutrition? *Am J Clin Nutr.* November 2007;86(5):1572S-1576S.
64. Evans WJ. Protein nutrition, exercise and aging. *J Am Coll Nutr.* December 2004;23(6 Suppl):601S-609S.
65. Zamparo P, Gatta G, di Prampero PE. The determinants of performance in master swimmers: an analysis of master world records. *Eur J Appl Physiol.* February 1 2012.
66. Zamparo P, Dall'ora A, Toneatto A, Cortesi M, Gatta G. The determinants of performance in master swimmers: a cross-sectional study on the age-related changes in propelling efficiency, hydrodynamic position and energy cost of front crawl. *Eur J Appl Physiol.* March 17 2012.
67. Louis J, Hausswirth C, Easthope C, Brisswalter J. Strength training improves cycling efficiency in master endurance athletes. *Eur J Appl Physiol.* February 2012;112(2):631-640.
68. Rosenbloom C, Bahns M. What can we learn about diet and physical activity from master athletes? *Hol Nurse Prac.* 2006;20(4):161-166.
69. Beshgetoor D, Nichols JF. Dietary intake and supplement use in female master cyclists and runners. *Int J Sport Nutr Exerc Metab.* June 2003;13(2):166-172.
70. Ogden CL, Carroll MD, Kit BK, Flegal KM. Prevalence of obesity and trends in body mass index among US children and adolescents, 1999-2010. *JAMA.* February 1 2012;307(5): 483-490.
71. Centers for Disease Control and Prevention. Trends in the prevalence of extreme obesity among US preschool-aged children living in low-income families. *JAMA.* 2012; 308(24): 2563-2565.
72. Ogden CL, Carroll MD, Kit BK, Flegal KM. Prevalence of obesity and trends in body mass index among US children and adolescents, 1999-2010. *JAMA.* February 1, 2012;307(5): 483-490.
73. Wen X, Gillman MW, Rifas-Shiman SL, Sherry B, Kleinman K, Taveras EM. Decreasing prevalence of obesity among young children in Massachusetts from 2004 to 2008. *Pediatrics.* May 2012;129(5):823-831.

74. Whitaker RC, Wright JA, Pepe MS, Seidel KD, Dietz WH. Predicting obesity in young adulthood from childhood and parental obesity. *N Engl J Med.* September 25 1997;337(13): 869-873.
75. Waters E, de Silva-Sanigorski A, Hall BJ, et al. Interventions for preventing obesity in children. *Cochrane Database of Systematic Reviews.* 2011(12):CD001871.
76. Freedman DS, Khan LK, Serdula MK, Dietz WH, Srinivasan SR, Berenson GS. The relation of childhood BMI to adult adiposity: the Bogalusa Heart Study. *Pediatrics.* January 2005; 115(1):22-27.
77. Rodriguez NR, Di Marco NM, Langley S. American College of Sports Medicine position stand. Nutrition and athletic performance. *Med Sci Sports Exerc.* March 2009;41(3):709-731.
78. Nascimento SL, Surita FG, Cecatti JG. Physical exercise during pregnancy: a systematic review. *Curr Opin Obstet Gynecol.* September 25 2012.
79. Wrotniak BH, Shults J, Butts S, Stettler N. Gestational weight gain and risk of overweight in the offspring at age 7 y in a multicenter, multiethnic cohort study. *Am J Clin Nutr.* June 2008;87(6):1818-1824.
80. Oken E, Taveras EM, Kleinman KP, Rich-Edwards JW, Gillman MW. Gestational weight gain and child adiposity at age 3 years. *Am J Obstet Gynecol.* April 2007;196(4):322 e321-328.
81. Oken E, Rifas-Shiman SL, Field AE, Frazier AL, Gillman MW. Maternal gestational weight gain and offspring weight in adolescence. *Obstet Gynecol.* November 2008;112(5): 999-1006.
82. Gardner B, Wardle J, Poston L, Croker H. Changing diet and physical activity to reduce gestational weight gain: a meta-analysis. *Obes Rev.* July 2011;12(7):e602-620.
83. ACOG committee opinion. Exercise during pregnancy and the postpartum period. Number 267, January 2002. American College of Obstetricians and Gynecologists. *Int J Gynaecol Obstet.* April 2002;77(1):79-81.
84. Zavorsky GS, Longo LD. Exercise guidelines in pregnancy: new perspectives. *Sports Med.* May 1 2011;41(5):345-360.
85. Zavorsky GS, Longo LD. Adding strength training, exercise intensity, and caloric expenditure to exercise guidelines in pregnancy. *Obstet Gynecol.* June 2011;117(6):1399-1402.
86. May LE, Glaros A, Yeh HW, Clapp JF, 3rd, Gustafson KM. Aerobic exercise during pregnancy influences fetal cardiac autonomic control of heart rate and heart rate variability. *Early Hum Dev.* April 2010;86(4):213-217.
87. Rasmussen KM, Yaktine AL, Institute of Medicine (U.S.). Committee to Reexamine IOM Pregnancy Weight Guidelines. Weight gain during pregnancy reexamining the guidelines. Washington, DC: National Academies Press; 2009: http://VB3LK7EB4T.search.serialssolutions.com/?V=1.0&L=VB3LK7EB4T&S=JCs&C=TC0000445755&T=marc.

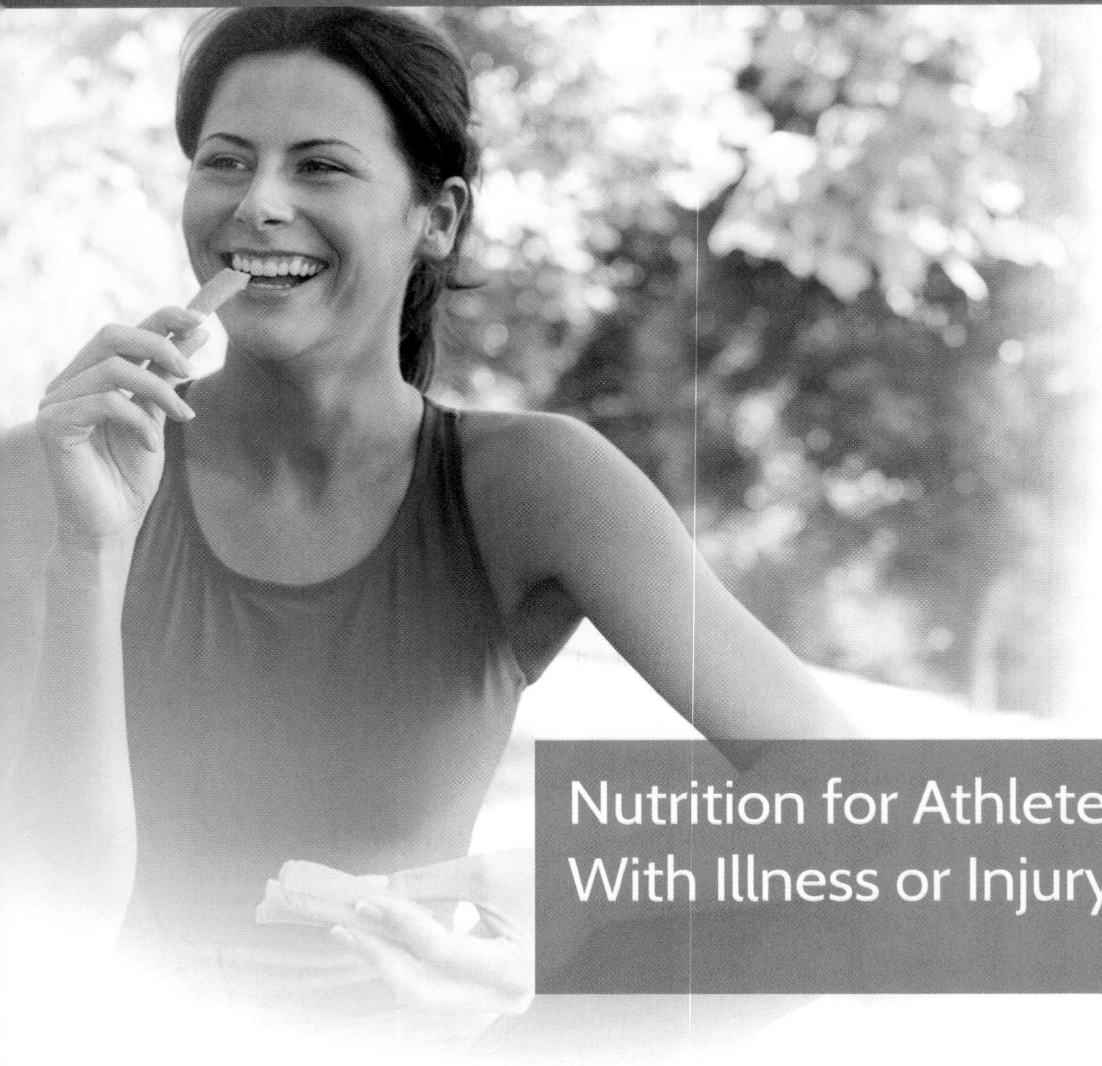

CHAPTER 14

Nutrition for Athletes With Illness or Injury

CHAPTER OUTLINE

LEARNING OBJECTIVES

After studying this chapter, the reader should be able to:

14.1 Describe nutritional factors that influence risk of acute illness.

14.2 Describe nutritional factors that mediate recovery from acute illness or injury.

14.3 List and describe several chronic diseases that may afflict athletes and the general nutritional principles to consider for each disease.

14.4 Describe the role of the health professional in the nutritional management of clients who suffer from chronic illness.

KEY TERMS

acute illness Sudden onset of a time-limited ailment.

bone remodeling The continual process of bone resorption and bone formation.

DASH eating plan Dietary Approaches to Stop Hypertension; an eating plan that is high in fruits and vegetables and low in sodium; it has been found to reduce blood pressure in people with hypertension as well as provide countless other benefits.

exercise immunology The study of the effects of exercise on the immune response.

exercise-related transient abdominal pain (ETAP) Abdominal pain of uncertain etiology that occurs during physical exercise; more common in novice athletes and individuals who have rapidly increased exercise intensity or duration.

flavonoid Antioxidant found naturally in many fruits and vegetables.

functional foods Defined by the Academy of Nutrition and Dietetics as any whole, fortified, enriched, or enhanced food that has a potentially beneficial effect on human health beyond basic nutrition.

immunonutritional support The use of nutrient intake or supplementation to attenuate immune changes and inflammation following intensive exercise or injury.

insulin resistance The cells respond inefficiently or ineffectively to insulin.

medical nutrition therapy Nutritional assessment, one-on-one counseling, and therapy intended to treat a specific illness or disease; should only be administered by a registered dietitian.

open window of impaired immunity A period of time lasting 3 to 72 hours in which athletes who engage in intensive training are at particularly increased risk of infection.

osteopenia A condition in which bone density is lower than normal; a precursor to osteoporosis.

osteoporosis Weakening of the bones, which can lead to bone fracture of the hip, spine, and other skeletal sites.

probiotics Bacteria that can be consumed in foods or supplements that help the body maintain a healthy balance of gut organisms.

quercetin A flavonoid that may help to protect from illness and enhance healing from injury.

INTRODUCTION

Sixty-three-year-old marathoner Colon Terrell of Raleigh, North Carolina, seemed an unlikely victim of heart disease. Despite being a former marathoner and living a relatively healthy lifestyle, Terrell suffered a severe myocardial infarction in February 2009. Doctors reported a 95% to 100% blockage in several of his coronary arteries, resulting in open heart bypass surgery. Just 3.5 years after his catastrophic illness, Terrell completed a 3,275-mile trek across the United States from the Cape Hatteras lighthouse in North Carolina to the Santa Monica Pier in California to celebrate his survival and to raise awareness and funds to fight heart disease.

Athletes often pride themselves on their focus and attention to good health. While it is true that athletes and active individuals benefit from a strengthened immune system and decreased risk for many acute and chronic illnesses, even the most elite athlete will at some point suffer from an acute illness or injury and its impact and implications on physical training and nutrition (see Myths and Misconceptions). In the most devastating situations, an athlete may suffer a catastrophic event or receive a diagnosis of a life-altering chronic illness requiring significant changes to nutrition and activity patterns. A health professional can be an important source of information and support to help athletes prevent, manage, and overcome these life events.

NUTRITION FOR ATHLETES WITH ACUTE ILLNESS OR INJURY

An athlete who suffers from an unexpected illness or injury will require change to nutrition patterns to meet new nutritional needs and promote healing.

Myths and Misconceptions

An Athlete Who Looks Healthy Is Healthy

The Myth
An athlete who looks healthy is healthy.

The Logic
Athletes develop fit bodies in response to the intense physical training and attention to nutrition required to excel in a sport. It seems logical that this high level of fitness would translate into a high level of health. Therefore, these fit bodies must be immune to chronic disease and illness, especially diseases such as cardiovascular disease, hypertension, and diabetes, which are heavily associated with lifestyle factors.

The Science
It is hard to tell from the outside how healthy a person's body is on the inside. Some of the leanest and most fit appearing female endurance athletes suffer from the female athlete triad (disordered eating, amenorrhea, and osteoporosis). Other athletes who have high caloric needs to maintain weight during training may choose unhealthy foods to meet those calorie needs, thus increasing levels of LDL cholesterol and increasing risk for cardiovascular disease. Still other athletes have overcome the odds and excelled at a sport despite a chronic disease such as type 1 diabetes or inflammatory bowel disease. Ultimately, a person's level of health cannot be determined solely from outward appearance or fitness regimen. This is evidenced by the opening case story of Colon Terrell, an apparently fit and healthy marathon-running man in his sixties who, without warning, suffered a life-threatening heart attack.

Acute Illness

Acute illness is defined as the sudden onset of a time-limited ailment such as a viral or bacterial infection. Athletes who engage in very high-intensity exercise are at increased risk of mild infections, while athletes who engage in moderate-intensity exercise are afforded a protective effect against common illnesses.[1] This difference is based on the effects of exercise on the immune response.

Acute Illness and the Immune Response

The growing interest in understanding the relationship between exercise, illness, and immune function led to the formation of a relatively new scientific field—**exercise immunology**—and the publication of over 2,000 research articles on the topic. In an effort to summarize the literature and provide guidance to exercise professionals, the International Society of Exercise and Immunology published a comprehensive two-part position statement. The major conclusions of these papers[2,3] and other pertinent research, including their nutritional implications, are highlighted here.

The existing research is inconclusive as to whether exercise-induced changes in immune function affect disease susceptibility or severity. However, levels of immune cells—namely, B cells, T cells, and immunoglobulin A (IgA)—decline in athletes engaging in long periods of intensified training, thus potentially increasing susceptibility to acute infection. Athletes are most likely to maintain immune health by starting a program of low to moderate intensity and volume and gradually increasing training volume and loads, including cross training, ensuring sufficient rest and recovery, and staying attuned to signs of overtraining. These signs include irritability and lack of concentration, fatigue, increased and poorly healing injuries, frequent upper respiratory illnesses, difficulty sleeping, poor appetite, increased resting heart rate, and menstrual irregularities in women. Periods of training in which risk of illness is particularly high include intensive training weeks, the taper prior to competition, and during competition.[2]

Elite athletes experience an **open window of impaired immunity** that lasts between 3 and 72 hours. It is the period of time following a strenuous workout (such as a marathon, ultramarathon, or very heavy training) in which susceptibility to illness is highest due to a suppression of immune cells.

When an athlete becomes ill, careful attention should be paid to when to return to exercise and to what extent. Due to the increased risk of dehydration, athletes suffering from an acute illness accompanied by fever should refrain from exercise until the fever has defervesced (been reduced). Otherwise, no strict criteria exist, though it may be prudent for athletes suffering a minor illness to decrease the intensity of training and avoid very strenuous exercise.

Nutritional Implications

Active individuals involved in moderate-intensity exercise do not benefit from nutritional supplementation to reduce susceptibility to illness.[2] After all, moderate-intensity exercise is associated with enhanced immune function. A well-balanced and varied diet is sufficient to promote optimal immune function. On the other hand, competitive and elite athletes engaging in intensive physical training may benefit from nutritional strategies to boost immune function during periods of increased physical stress. Likewise, athletes who have suffered an injury may benefit from an enhanced immune response to quicken recovery and return to play (discussed later in this chapter). The use of nutrients to attenuate immune changes and inflammation following intensive exercise or injury is referred to as **immunonutritional support**. The understanding of the impact of nutrients on immune function is in its infancy. To date only two nutrition interventions have received scientific support: carbohydrate intake and intake of the flavonoid **quercetin**.[1] Carbohydrates help to lessen the immune response to strenuous exercise by decreasing blood levels of stress hormones and cytokines. Quercetin is a **flavonoid** found naturally in fruits, vegetables, and some grains. It is also readily available as a supplement (the form in which it has been studied most as it relates to exercise and immune function).

Notably, the expert committee of the International Society of Exercise and Immunology does not believe that sufficient evidence exists to support the common teaching that vitamin C protects from acute illness.[1] However, this is a topic of ongoing and intensive evaluation (see Evaluating the Evidence). The scientific understanding of the role of many supplements such as branched chain amino acids (BCAAs), probiotics, and bovine colostrum in the immune response is limited. It is possible that as research evolves many of those supplements considered to not be helpful may ultimately be found to enhance the immune response. Athletes at high risk of compromised immune function or who have suffered a recent injury or undergone surgery should discuss the use of supplements to promote healing with their physician or sports dietitian who can help the athlete to weigh the evidence and research, benefits, and harms.

EVALUATING THE EVIDENCE

Can Vitamin C Supplementation Prevent and Treat the Common Cold?

One study of ultraendurance triathletes found that 60% took vitamin and mineral supplements. The most commonly used supplement was vitamin C, which was consumed by 97.5% of supplement users. The reason the athletes most often cited for taking the supplement was to prevent cold symptoms.[1]

Ever since vitamin C was first isolated in the 1930s, people have believed that it may be effective in the prevention or treatment of respiratory viral infections. This view was supported in the 1970s when Nobel Laureate Linus Pauling supported these conclusions based on a series of randomized trials. Vitamin C supplements are widely available and promoted as important in the prevention and treatment of wintertime colds. But do they work?

Researchers at the Cochrane Review set out to answer this question.[2] The abstract of the article presenting their conclusions follows:

Background: Vitamin C (ascorbic acid) in preventing and treating the common cold has been a subject of controversy for 60 years.
Objectives: To discover whether oral doses of 0.2 grams per day or more of vitamin C reduce the incidence, duration, or severity of the common cold when used as continuous prophylaxis (regularly every day) or as therapy after onset of symptoms.
Search strategy: We searched the Cochrane Central Register of Controlled Trials (CENTRAL) (The Cochrane Library 2010, issue 1) which contains the Acute Respiratory Infections Group's Specialised Register, MEDLINE (2006 to February 2010) and EMBASE (2006 to February 2010).
Selection criteria: We excluded trials if a dose less than 0.2 grams per day of vitamin C was used, or if there was no placebo comparison. We did not restrict to randomised controlled trials (RCTs).
Data collection and analysis: Two reviewers independently extracted data. "Incidence" of colds during prophylaxis was assessed as the proportion of participants experiencing one or more colds during the study period. "Duration" was the mean days of illness of cold episodes.
Main results: Twenty-nine trial comparisons involving 11,306 participants contributed to the meta-analysis on the risk ratio (RR) of developing a cold while taking prophylactic (preventive) vitamin C. In the general community trials, involving 10,708 participants, the pooled RR was 0.97 (95% confidence interval (CI) 0.94 to 1.00). Five

Continued

EVALUATING THE EVIDENCE–cont'd

trials involving a total of 598 marathon runners, skiers, and soldiers on subarctic exercises yielded a pooled RR of 0.48 (95% CI 0.35 to 0.64).[a]

Twenty-nine trial comparisons examined the effect of prophylactic vitamin C on common cold duration (9,649 episodes). In adults, the duration of colds was reduced by 8% (3% to 12%), and in children by 13% (6% to 21%). The severity of colds was significantly reduced in the prophylaxis trials.

Seven trial comparisons examined the effect of therapeutic vitamin C (3,249 episodes). No consistent differences from the placebo group were seen in the duration or severity of colds.

Authors' conclusions: The failure of vitamin C supplementation to reduce the incidence of colds in the general population indicates that routine prophylaxis is not justified. Vitamin C could be useful for people exposed to brief periods of severe physical exercise. While the prophylaxis trials have consistently shown that vitamin C reduces the duration and alleviates the symptoms of colds, this was not replicated in the few therapeutic trials that have been carried out. Further therapeutic RCTs are warranted.

1. Based on this systematic review, do you feel that the triathletes are justified in taking the vitamin C supplements? Explain why or why not.
2. How would you describe the findings of this review to a recreational athlete who asked you if he or she should take vitamin C to prevent a cold?
3. Research is constantly evolving. Likely many further studies evaluating the relationship of vitamin C in the prevention and treatment of colds in athletes have been conducted since the publication of this trial.
   a. Using www.pubmed.gov, find the abstract of another scientific article addressing this topic. Include its citation here.
   b. Describe the findings of this study and how they might be relevant to clients with whom you work.

a. The authors of this study used the measure relative risk (RR) to determine the role of vitamin C supplementation in reducing the incidence of colds in the population. Relative risk describes the ratio of the probability of an event happening in the intervention group versus a control group. For this study, the relative risk is the ratio of the probability of a participant given vitamin C supplementation to catch a cold versus a participant not given vitamin C supplementation. An RR of 1 means there is no difference in risk between the intervention and control group. An RR of less than 1 means that the event is less likely to occur in the intervention group than the control group. An RR of greater than 1 means that the event is more likely to occur in the intervention group than the control group. The 95% confidence interval (CI) helps to indicate the reliability of a measure. If the CI contains the value "1," there is not a statistically significant difference between the two groups.

Injury

Athletes are at high risk for musculoskeletal and other exercise- or sport-induced injuries. While athletes employ a variety of tactics to hasten healing such as ice, massage, and acupuncture, one often overlooked variable is the role of nutrition in healing.

Certainly, nutritional needs change for an injured athlete. As physical activity level diminishes, caloric and macronutrient needs also decrease, though they remain elevated above sedentary rates due to increased energy and protein required to support healing. Injuries that require immobilization lead to muscle protein atrophy, regardless of the amount of protein consumed in the diet. This is due to the resistance of immobilized muscle to the anabolic effects of amino acids and other nutrients. There is some evidence that intake of the branched chain amino acids, in particular leucine, may help to offset the immobilization-induced muscle atrophy.[4,5] Regardless of whether or not it prevents muscle atrophy, sufficient protein intake is essential to promote wound and fracture healing, if present.

Several investigators have evaluated a potential role of creatine supplementation in the attenuation of immobility-associated muscle loss with equivocal results. One study measured the concentration of GLUT4 protein content during immobilization in athletes who were and were not supplemented with creatine. GLUT4 is the insulin-dependent glucose transporter. Increased concentrations promote increased muscle glycogen storage. The authors found that GLUT4 protein content decreased less in the supplemented group compared to placebo and was upregulated during rehabilitation.[6] Similarly, another study found that supplementation during 2 weeks of lower-limb casting provided no improvement in muscle strength after the cast was removed; however, strength improved more during rehabilitation in the participants who had used creatine supplementation.[7] Yet another study found no effect of supplementation after total knee arthroplasty in individuals with osteoarthritis.[8] In contrast, a study of upper extremity immobilization in otherwise healthy young men found that creatine supplementation preserved muscle mass and strength.[9] In all, this is an area of interesting research without conclusive findings to be applied in practice.

The role of the essential fatty acids in promotion of healing after injury is a topic of active research. Omega-3 fatty acids are well known to possess potent anti-inflammatory effects, theoretically lending a role in improved healing after injury or with illness. They may also play a role in reducing immobilization-associated muscle atrophy, though the research supporting this is mixed and so far has been limited to studies in rodents[10,11] and sarcopenia (loss of muscle and function related to aging) in the elderly.[12] Recent evidence suggests that omega-6 fatty acids—found in high amounts in flaxseed, canola, and soybean oils and green leaves—may also provide anti-inflammatory benefits,[13] though their role in healing after injury or illness is unknown.

Several micronutrients such as vitamins E and C, glutamine, and N-3 PUFAs (fish oil) have been hypothesized to play a role in reducing the inflammatory response that can result from illness and acute injury; however, compelling scientific evidence supporting the majority of the nutritional interventions is lacking. Ultimately, while a nutrient-dense and varied diet is recommended to ensure adequate intake of the vitamins and minerals necessary for healing, supplementation is generally not necessary.[14]

SPEED BUMP

1. **Describe nutritional factors that influence risk of acute illness and strategies athletes should use to maintain immune health.**
2. **Describe nutritional factors that are thought to mediate recovery from acute illness or injury.**

NUTRITION FOR ATHLETES WITH CHRONIC DISEASE

Health professionals can be a trusted source of nutrition information for athletes who are concerned about, at risk for, or who have a chronic illness (see Communication Strategies). With the rapid increase in chronic diseases among Americans, a growing number of athletes also face these conditions. While it is essential that health professionals are aware of general nutrition recommendations for the treatment and prevention of the most common illnesses, it is clearly outside the scope of practice of most health professionals to provide nutrition advice or recommendations on how to use nutrition to manage these conditions. This is known as **medical nutrition therapy** and is the domain of the registered dietitian.

COMMUNICATION STRATEGIES

Promoting Health Literacy

Clients often rely on information shared by health professionals to make decisions about their health. However, miscommunication and misunderstanding frequently interfere with health communication. A report of the Institute of Medicine noted that adults with lower levels of health literacy have less knowledge about their medical condition and treatment, worse health status, less understanding and use of preventive services, and higher rates of hospitalization.[1] Adults who are older, less educated, poor, minorities, and non-native English speakers tend to have the lowest levels of health literacy.[1]

The Centers for Disease Control and Prevention recommend the following 10 tips to improve health literacy:[2]

1. Do not assume understanding. Pilot test health education materials with the target audience prior to widespread dissemination.
2. Know your audience. Develop materials based on what you learn. A one-size-fits-all approach is not effective.
3. Engage the target audience in the development and implementation of health education materials. Ask for feedback on communication effectiveness and ease of understanding.
4. Evaluate whether or not your target audience has been able to effectively learn and apply the shared information. Ask the audience to restate or demonstrate what they have learned.
5. Aim for simplicity. Limit teaching sessions or materials to no more than three to four main messages. Give only the necessary information, unless the client asks for further details.
6. Provide a list of resources for further information.
7. Collaborate with other health professionals and community members who know and understand the target audience well.
8. Avoid jargon. Consider the client's culture and language, and speak at the appropriate level.

Continued

COMMUNICATION STRATEGIES—cont'd

9. Evaluate your environment. How comfortable and welcoming is the setting? How conducive is it to understanding clear health messages?
10. Make improved health literacy a personal and professional priority.

Identify a topic related to health literacy of interest to you (e.g., how to identify credible websites, understanding nutrition or supplement labels, effective use of social media to share health information, choosing a health professional, choosing healthy foods while grocery shopping). Following the 10 steps outlined by the CDC above, put together a brief handout, blog post, demonstration, or other format of your choice to provide health education on your chosen topic.

Gastrointestinal Disorders

Over 33 million people visit a physician with the chief complaint of gastrointestinal (GI) symptoms each year.[1] Though most athletes have at some point during training or competition experienced GI distress, a sizeable subgroup of these individuals suffer from a chronic, potentially debilitating gastrointestinal disorder such as gastroesophageal reflux disease (GERD) and other upper GI tract anomalies, irritable bowel syndrome (IBS), celiac disease, and inflammatory bowel disease (IBD). In these cases, attention to appropriate nutrition for training and competition not only improves performance but also helps mitigate symptoms such as heartburn, diarrhea, constipation, and crampy or colicky abdominal pain.

Upper GI Disorders and Gastroesophageal Reflux Disease (GERD)

Upper GI complaints are exceedingly common in athletes, especially athletes who engage in intense activity and anaerobic sports. The most common chronic upper GI disorder is GERD, but shorter-lived ailments such as nausea, vomiting, gastritis, peptic ulcers, GI bleeding, and **exercise-related transient abdominal pain** (ETAP)—a condition especially prevalent in novice athletes and those increasing the intensity of their training—are also common.[15] Upper GI symptoms likely result from a combination of mechanical stressors, reduced blood flow to the GI system, and neuroendocrine-induced changes such as relaxation of the lower esophageal sphincter and excess acid production in the stomach.[15] Frequent use of nonsteroidal anti-inflammatory drugs (NSAIDs) also contributes to GI symptoms, especially gastritis (Box 14-1).

GERD results from stomach acids being transferred into the esophagus due to relaxation of the sphincter that separates the esophagus from the highly acidic stomach contents. Characteristic signs of GERD include chest pain that worsens after lying down, difficulty swallowing, coughing and wheezing, and regurgitation of sour tasting food. Athletes, people who are obese, and those who smoke experience a greater risk of developing the aggravating disease. Typically, smoking, alcohol, coffee and other caffeinated beverages, chocolate, citrus fruits, and fatty foods exacerbate GERD. Treatment includes avoiding the foods mentioned above, use of over-the-counter antacids, eating smaller meals, sitting upright for 2 to 3 hours after a meal, and engaging in exercise if weight loss is needed.[16]

Athletes suffering from upper GI symptoms may start with dietary and lifestyle changes to reduce symptoms, including alteration in pre- and during-exercise fluid and nutrition intake, consistent training, and avoidance of foods that make symptoms worse, and avoiding eating within 3 hours of bedtime. Importantly, individuals with upper GI symptoms or GERD should seek medical treatment promptly if they experience unexplained weight loss, difficulty swallowing, or if the symptoms return multiple times per week, are not relieved by over-the-counter antacids, or cause them to wake up at night.[17] Athletes should discuss these and any other concerning symptoms with their physician, who may undertake further evaluation and testing to understand the underlying disease process.

Irritable Bowel Syndrome

The most prevalent gastrointestinal disorder is irritable bowel syndrome (IBS), a poorly understood disorder of the large intestine that causes recurrent abdominal pain, bloating, discomfort, and changes in the frequency and consistency of bowel movements. Young women are most often the victims of IBS, though it can be diagnosed in both genders at any age. While the pathology of IBS is unknown, many experts believe that it is a manifestation of a hypersensitive GI tract that is easily pained and stimulated, causing excess bloating, gas, and cramping after minor assaults, such as the physical burden of digesting a large and bulky meal.

IBS is called a syndrome rather than a disease because a cluster of symptoms that typically occur together defines the disorder. For instance, in order to diagnose someone as having IBS, he or she must have pain or discomfort 3 days per month for the past 3 months and two of the following three symptoms: relief of pain with

Box 14-1. Exploring the Role of Prophylactic Ibuprofen With Exercise: Does It Help or Hurt?

Many competitive endurance athletes use ibuprofen and nonsteroidal anti-inflammatory drugs (NSAIDs). Despite their widespread use, NSAIDs may do athletes more harm than good, especially when the drugs become a regular part of an athlete's routine.

NSAIDs work by inhibiting the production of prostaglandins. Prostaglandins are chemicals made by the kidneys in response to stress and inflammation and are at least partly responsible for the swelling and pain associated with strenuous exercise. Prostaglandins also play an important role in maintaining blood flow to the kidneys during exercise. Athletes take NSAIDs before a race in hopes of blocking prostaglandin production and thus preventing subsequent muscle pain and soreness. Several researchers have attempted to prove the validity of this reasoning with equivocal results.[1] For example, in one study ibuprofen taken before and after exercise lessened muscle damage.[2] In another, ibuprofen taken before 45 minutes of downhill running and every 6 hours for the 3 days following exercise had no effect on inflammation or muscle soreness.[3] Overall, it is not clear whether or not NSAIDs help decrease pain during and after exercise. Researchers do agree that NSAID use does not improve athletic performance.[1]

NSAID use before exercise may increase exercise-related health risks. By blocking prostaglandin function, blood flow to the kidneys during exercise is lessened and the kidneys may not be able to function optimally. Some researchers postulate that NSAID use leads to decreased free water clearance by the kidneys, contributing to asymptomatic hyponatremia (low blood salt concentration) during prolonged endurance events. For example, an observational study of 330 athletes in the 2004 New Zealand Ironman Triathlon found that the six athletes who became hyponatremic had all used NSAIDs before the race. NSAID use was also associated with worse kidney function immediately following the race.[4] Another study found that NSAID use increased the risk and severity of exercise-induced GI disturbances, including small intestinal injury and gut barrier dysfunction.[5]

Nieman et al.[38] evaluated the role of NSAIDs on race time, perceived exertion during the race, delayed onset muscle soreness, and markers of inflammation in ultramarathoners participating in the 160-kilometer Western States Endurance Run. Researchers divided runners into two groups: one group of 29 runners took 600 milligrams of ibuprofen the day before the race and 1,200 milligrams the day of the race; the other group of 25 controls avoided ibuprofen and all other medications. Notably, the runners who used NSAIDs had elevated markers of inflammation after the race. There was no significant difference in race times, perceived exertion, or muscle soreness. Another important risk from NSAID use during a grueling endurance event is that the analgesic may mask the pain from a serious injury.

Long-term use of NSAIDs may cause several adverse effects. To start, blocking the natural inflammatory response to exercise interferes with collagen synthesis. Collagen provides strength to connective tissues including muscles, tendons, and ligaments. When collagen production is compromised, athletes become more prone to musculoskeletal injury and experience delayed healing following an injury. Further, chronic NSAID use can lead to harmful effects throughout the body including increased gastrointestinal distress and ulceration, blood thinning and risk of bleeding, cardiovascular disease and stroke, depressed immune response, and electrolyte imbalances. These risks are worth noting, as a sizeable percentage of athletes have come to routinely rely on NSAIDs.

Ultimately, NSAIDs may play an important role in helping to relieve the pain and swelling after an acute injury or intense physical exertion, but the risks of their use as prophylactic pain mediators outweigh the benefits. Athletes considering prophylactic NSAID use should first discuss the risks and benefits with their doctor.

defecation, looser or more frequent stools, and harder or less frequent stools.[18] Symptoms are often worsened by large meals; some medicines; emotional upsets; and certain foods such as milk products, chocolate, alcohol, caffeine, carbonated drinks, and fatty foods. High-fiber foods like broccoli, apples, and whole grain breads can make IBS better by softening the stool and relieving constipation. Research suggests (but has not proven) that probiotics—live microbial organisms in some foodstuffs such as yogurt—may help with IBS[18,19] (Box 14-2). While it is unclear what specifically causes the illness, for many people minimizing stress through regular exercise is an effective component to a treatment plan.[20]

Celiac Disease

Nearly 1% of the population suffers from celiac disease; for unknown reasons the prevalence appears to be increasing slightly.[21] Celiac disease is characterized by an autoimmune rejection of gluten-containing foods. Gluten is a protein compound made up of two proteins called gliadin and glutenin that is found joined with starch in the grains wheat, rye, and barley. For people

Box 14-2. Probiotics

Functional foods are defined by the Academy of Nutrition and Dietetics as any whole, fortified, enriched, or enhanced food that has a potentially beneficial effect on human health beyond basic nutrition.[1] **Probiotics** qualify as functional foods when they meet specific criteria; namely, they must be living, ingested in ample amounts, and capable of colonizing the intestinal tract. When these criteria are met, the organisms help keep a healthy balance of the gut organisms. Probiotics from the *lactic acid bacteria (LAB)* family also can convert sugars like lactose and other carbohydrates into lactic acid. These two functions help explain why a fair number of studies have supported the claim that probiotics offer benefits for the treatment of rotavirus diarrhea, lactose intolerance, and antibiotic-associated diarrhea.[2-4] Acting through various partly understood mechanisms, which may include a strengthened intestinal wall and readied immune system, probiotics also may *possibly* provide beneficial effects in irritable bowel syndrome (IBS), Crohn's disease, cholesterol metabolism, cancer prevention, diverticulitis, allergies, obesity, urogenital infections, and other ailments, though, importantly, the research is inconclusive at best.[2]

While probiotics potentially offer substantial benefits for those plagued with rotavirus diarrhea or prone to stomach pains following dairy consumption, to provide benefit probiotics must be consumed daily to adequately colonize the gut and confer health benefits.[3] It is unclear how many bacteria must be consumed to achieve a health benefit, though the number undoubtedly is high as the bacteria have to stay alive through the harsh conditions of the GI system with its low stomach pH, bile salts, and digestive enzymes. Food manufacturers are not required to disclose the number, viability, nor type of bacteria.

Most probiotics on the market contain one or more organisms from the LAB family. This family of microorganisms includes *L. acidophilus, L. rhamnosus, L. casei, L. gasseri, B. bifidum,* and *B. animalis* (which Dannon cleverly renamed and trademarked bifidus regularis). LAB are thought to offer various health benefits including improved intestinal tract health, enhanced immune function, improved lactose intolerance, and decreased risk of some cancers.[3]

Currently, much uncertainty surrounds the efficacy of probiotics in promoting gastrointestinal health. Until a more robust body of scientific evidence is available, individuals should decide for themselves whether or not they experience improvement in their symptoms with regular probiotic consumption. Meanwhile, clients should keep the following considerations in mind before using probiotics:

1. Not all probiotics are created equal. Only microorganisms that can colonize the human gut are capable of providing benefit.
2. Food manufacturers are not required to use accepted nomenclature for the bacteria in a product, thus some companies have created their own official-sounding unscientific names such as bifidus regularis and l. casei defensis. These names may overstate the probiotic benefits.
3. While probiotics could provide myriad health benefits, to date sufficient research exists only to support its effects in the treatment of rotavirus diarrhea, lactose intolerance, and antibiotic-associated diarrhea. Much of the research conducted to date has been funded by the very companies poised to profit from the findings.
4. Probiotics must be alive and consumed in sufficient quantity on a daily basis to exert their beneficial effects.
5. Probiotics carry no approved health claims. They are regulated as foods, not drugs, and do not require ingredient testing or proof of potency. And, at times, promises are made that are not backed by quality research nor FDA approval.

with celiac disease, when the body is exposed to gliadin, the "toxic" component of gluten for people with celiac disease, it goes into immunological overdrive. The gastrointestinal system becomes inflamed and pathological changes to the small intestine, the body's main site for nutrient absorption, ensue. When the gut is unable to absorb nutrients, common symptoms like vitamin deficiency, anemia, weight loss, and diarrhea occur. Other symptoms include abdominal pain and distention, and in some cases neurological dysfunction. Celiac disease is very difficult to diagnose and, though it begins in childhood, many people do not learn that they have the disease until well into adulthood. The longer a person suffers from undiagnosed and untreated celiac disease, the more likely he or she is to develop complications such as other autoimmune disorders, osteoporosis, infertility, neurological problems, and, in rare cases, cancer.[21] This is why it is very important for anyone who suffers from the symptoms of celiac disease to see a physician immediately for evaluation. Celiac disease can be diagnosed with laboratory testing and biopsy of the small intestine. The only definitive treatment for the disease is strict avoidance of gluten-containing foods.

Many people who do not have celiac disease describe complaints of gluten-intolerance and may benefit from a gluten-free diet. See Chapter 16 for detailed information on gluten-free diets.

Inflammatory Bowel Disease

Not to be confused with irritable bowel syndrome, inflammatory bowel disease (IBD) consists of two separate disorders—Crohn's disease and ulcerative colitis—that cause severe damage and inflammation to the gastrointestinal tract. Unlike IBS, which although uncomfortable is not life-threatening, at its worst IBD can lead to severe disability and ultimately death.

Crohn's Disease. Crohn's disease can cause inflammation to any part of the GI tract from the mouth to the anus, although damage is usually done to the ileum, the lower portion of the small intestine. Like many other GI disorders, it is not well understood what causes Crohn's disease, though it is thought to be at least partly genetically inherited. Similar to celiac disease, some exposure causes the body's immune system to attack the lining of the GI tract. The difference is that with Crohn's disease the trigger is unknown. Some speculate that perhaps a type of bacteria, food, or protein causes the immune reaction. The consequences of this inflammation can be severe, leading to malnutrition, intestinal blockage, and ulcers that tunnel through to other areas such as the anus, bladder, vagina, and skin. The ulcers can easily become badly infected. Other signs of Crohn's disease include abdominal pain, bloody diarrhea, rectal bleeding, weight loss, fever, and extra-intestinal symptoms like mouth sores and inflammation of the eye.[22]

Ulcerative Colitis. Ulcerative colitis also is characterized by inflammation of the GI tract, but unlike Crohn's disease, ulcerative colitis is limited to the rectum and colon. Ulcers form in areas where inflammation has destroyed the cells. The ulcers then bleed and pus, causing bloody, mucousy diarrhea. Like many other GI disorders, anemia, fatigue, weight loss, and decreased appetite are other symptoms of ulcerative colitis. Joint pain and skin lesions are other somewhat more specific symptoms. Ulcerative colitis is usually diagnosed in people between the ages of 15 to 30 and less often 50 to 70, though it can begin at any age. Five percent of people with ulcerative colitis develop colon cancer.[22]

Nutritional Care for IBD. While nutrition is never the sole treatment for IBD, nutritional choices play an important role in the management of the diseases. During acute illness or for those with more severe disease, aggressive nutritional therapy, such as tube or intravenous feeding, may be indicated. During periods of remission, nutritional management is focused on preventing severe nutritional deficiency, which can result from malabsorption, insufficient caloric intake, increased nutrient losses from the gut, and drug-nutrient interactions. Encouraging a high-calorie diet with a particular emphasis on calcium (dairy products), vitamin D (fortified dairy products), folate (dark leafy greens, fortified grains, strawberries), vitamin B_{12} (lean beef and other meat products), and zinc (seafood, spinach) intake are important in the nutritional management for people with IBD.[22] Athletes with IBD require a multidisciplinary management team to include a gastroenterologist, primary care physician, registered dietitian, exercise professional, and other appropriate health professionals.

Clearly, nutrition plays an important role in the disease process of many gastrointestinal illnesses. While the culprit foods and the antidotes may be obvious for some diseases, in other cases it may take some investigative work to figure out what foods help and which hurt. When symptoms flare, GI-disease sufferers and the health professionals involved in their care should seize the opportunity to better understand their illness. What symptoms do they have? When do the symptoms occur? What did they eat during the day? What foods always make them feel bad? What foods always make them feel better? This quick exercise may help to uncover the individual nutrition choices that can help alleviate many gastrointestinal ailments.

Cardiovascular Disease

Cardiovascular disease, defined as any disease of the heart or blood vessels, is the leading killer of American men and women, responsible for one in three deaths.[23] Heart disease is any condition affecting the heart muscle itself, the valves of the heart, or the blood vessels that supply the heart (coronary arteries). Vessel disease, or vascular disease, includes conditions such as hypertension and atherosclerosis. Atherosclerosis of the coronary arteries is the main culprit behind angina (chest pain) and myocardial infarction (MI), the medical term for heart attack.

Atherosclerosis

While usually not deadly until middle age and beyond, atherosclerosis begins to develop in childhood.[24] *Fatty streaks*, or oxidized cholesterol and lipid particles that accumulate deep in the arterial wall, reveal the earliest stages of atherosclerosis (Fig. 14-1). Most Americans develop fatty streaks by their teenage years.[24] Because fatty streaks do not obstruct blood flow, no signs or symptoms of cardiovascular disease are evident—yet. Over time, a cholesterol plaque, which may become susceptible to rupture, develops in the artery. An advanced lesion, or *complicated plaque*, develops as the fibrous plaque continues to progress and becomes calcified. Many times the first sign of heart disease is an MI in which a clot breaks off of a lesion and completely obstructs blood flow.[25] High blood cholesterol levels—in particular, low-density lipoprotein (LDL)—and cholesterol's susceptibility to oxidation are main culprits in the development of atherosclerosis.

Hypertension

Hypertension is defined as having a systolic blood pressure (SBP) greater than or equal to 140 mmHg, a diastolic blood pressure (DBP) greater than or equal to 90 mmHg, and/or being on antihypertensive medication. According to these criteria, approximately

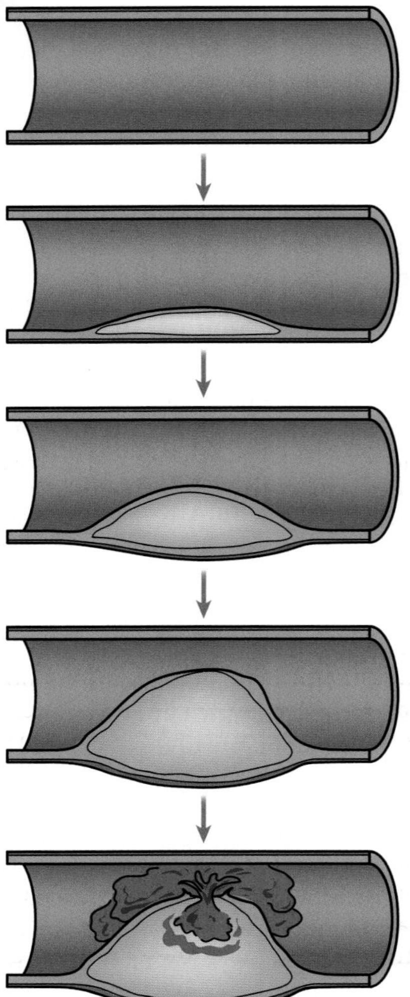

Figure 14-1. The progression of atherosclerosis. Poor diet contributes to early development and progression of atherosclerosis, with the development of foam cells during adolescence for many people.

76 million adults in the United States have hypertension.[23] Millions more are prehypertensive, with a blood pressure greater than 120/80 mmHg.[23] Hypertension is the leading cause of stroke in the United States and a major contributor to cardiovascular morbidity and mortality.[23]

While prescription medications are highly effective in reducing blood pressure, nutrition and physical activity are also important in the treatment and prevention of hypertension. Multiple studies have shown that the **DASH eating plan** combined with decreased salt intake can substantially reduce blood pressure levels and potentially make blood-pressure medications unnecessary.[26] The DASH eating plan, while developed to reduce blood pressure, is an overall healthy eating plan that can be adopted by anyone regardless of whether he or she has elevated blood pressure. Some studies suggest that the DASH eating plan may also reduce coronary heart disease risk by lowering total cholesterol and LDL cholesterol in addition to lowering blood pressure.[26] The eating plan is low in saturated fat, cholesterol, and total fat. The DASH eating plan is described in detail in Chapter 5.

Minimizing Cardiovascular Risk

While many athletes are very physically fit, and exercise is protective against heart disease, some athletes may still be at high risk for cardiovascular disease. For instance, sudden cardiac arrest may be the first indication of an underlying cardiovascular disease in previously asymptomatic athletes. This is the most likely cause of a marathoner who suddenly dies during or at the end of a race, or a football player who collapses on the field. Previously sedentary older adults or individuals with cardiovascular risk factors may experience a life-threatening cardiovascular event during or after an exercise bout.

Athletes can minimize their risk of cardiovascular disease by striving to achieve what the American Heart Association (AHA) terms "ideal cardiovascular health," which consists of seven components of optimal heart health. Of note, 3.3% of people across all ages meet this ideal. The seven components of optimal heart health include:

1. Has never been told by a doctor, nurse, or other health professional that he or she has high blood pressure.
2. Has a self-reported BMI less than 25 kg/m^2.
3. Has never been told by a doctor, nurse, or other health professional that he or she has high cholesterol.
4. Has not smoked at least 100 cigarettes in his or her lifetime, or reported smoking 100 cigarettes in his or her lifetime but not currently smoking.
5. Has never been told by a doctor that he or she has diabetes.
6. Participates in more than 150 minutes per week of moderate physical activity or more than 75 minutes of vigorous physical activity per week.
7. Consumes five or more servings of fruits and vegetables per day.[27]

Health professionals can get more information and help clients identify their risk profile by using the AHA ideal cardiovascular health metrics available at http://mylifecheck.heart.org/.

As demonstrated by the AHA metrics, maintaining a high level of physical activity and following a heart-healthy diet can help athletes to minimize their overall risk of future cardiovascular disease. Studies have shown that following these basic dietary recommendations leads to beneficial changes in cardiovascular risk profile.[23] The Mediterranean diet and the DASH eating plan, both discussed in detail in Chapter 5, are two examples of effective ideal eating plans for cardiovascular disease prevention. Still, very few Americans eat healthfully, engage in regular physical activity, maintain a healthy weight, and do not smoke.[23]

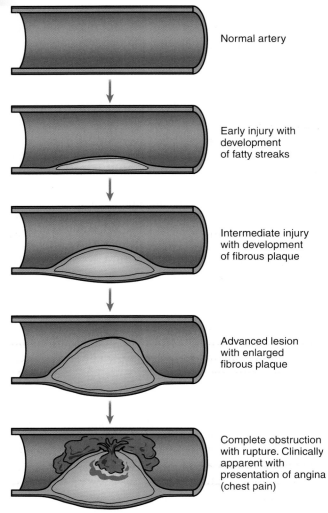

Athletes may believe that following a heart-healthy diet is not important due to their high levels of activity and energy expenditure. This is not the case, as risk factors for cardiovascular disease may develop even in the face of healthful activity. Furthermore, management of cardiovascular risk factors during young- and middle-adulthood may portend very low risk in older age. One study found that individuals with optimal risk factor levels at age 50 have a very low lifetime risk of developing heart disease (5.2% risk in men and 8.2% risk in women versus a 68.9% risk in men and a 50.2% risk in women who have ≥2 risk factors).[28] However, only 3.2% of men and 4.5% of women in the study accomplished this feat.[28] It is never too early for athletes to start their heart disease prevention lifestyle change.

Diabetes Mellitus

Diabetes mellitus is a condition that results from abnormal regulation of blood glucose. An estimated 25 million people in the United States have diabetes, with more than 6 million undiagnosed cases.[23] An additional 81.5 million adults have prediabetes, or elevated fasting glucose.[23]

Diabetes mellitus can be classified into three types: type 1 diabetes, type 2 diabetes, and gestational diabetes. Gestational diabetes occurs exclusively during pregnancy and increases the woman's risk of future development of type 2 diabetes. It is discussed in more detail in Chapter 13.

Type 1 Diabetes

Type 1 diabetes results from the inability of the pancreas to secrete insulin, the hormone that allows the cells to take up glucose from the bloodstream. Without a ready supply of glucose entering the cell, the cell becomes starved of energy and relies on the production of energy from muscle proteins and fat through gluconeogenesis. The process contributes to muscular weakness and atrophy from the catabolism of muscle protein and the formation of ketone bodies, which are byproducts of fat metabolism. An accumulation of ketone bodies can incite diabetic ketoacidosis, characterized by an acidification of the blood and life-threatening complications.

Meanwhile, sensing the deprivation of glucose, the liver inappropriately responds by releasing more glucose into the bloodstream, further increasing serum glucose levels. This hyperglycemia can overwhelm the body and cause spillage of serum glucose into urine, known as glycosuria. Glycosuria is the reason for increased urination, which is often a presenting sign of type 1 diabetes. Other common presenting symptoms include increased thirst and appetite.

Type 1 diabetes accounts for only about 5% of cases of diabetes[23] and is a genetic dysfunction that cannot be prevented. Type 1 diabetes usually presents in childhood or adolescence. Uncontrolled type 1 diabetes progresses rapidly into diabetic ketoacidosis, which requires immediate medical management. Treatment with exogenous insulin is essential. The specific nutritional management of type 1 diabetes, in particular the titration of carbohydrate intake and insulin dosing, is beyond the scope of this text.

Type 2 Diabetes

Type 2 diabetes results from the cells' decreased ability to respond to insulin. It is characterized by **insulin resistance** rather than insulin deficiency. With insulin resistance, the pancreas functions appropriately but the body's cells do not respond normally to insulin. Initially, the pancreas can overcome insulin resistance by secreting more insulin. When the pancreas is no longer able to maintain glucose levels in a normal range, the person is said to have prediabetes (a fasting blood glucose >100 mg/dL). When glucose levels rise high enough (a fasting blood glucose of >126 mg/dL or a 2-hour postprandial glucose of >200 mg/dL), the individual meets diagnostic criteria for type 2 diabetes.

Ninety-five percent of people with diabetes have type 2 diabetes.[23] Historically, type 2 diabetes occurred only in adults; however, with the epidemic of childhood obesity, an increasing number of children are diagnosed with the disease. Treatment for type 2 diabetes is targeted at increasing insulin sensitivity. In severe cases, the overburdened pancreas may eventually cease production of insulin, causing a person with type 2 diabetes to become insulin dependent. People at highest risk of developing type 2 diabetes have a positive family history as well as other cardiovascular risk factors such as high blood pressure, high cholesterol, obesity, and a sedentary lifestyle.

The hyperglycemia characteristic of untreated or poorly controlled type 1 and type 2 diabetes can cause a variety of serious health consequences including retinopathy, which can lead to blindness; nephropathy, which can lead to end-stage renal disease; and neuropathy, which is loss of sensation, usually in the extremities. People with diabetes are also at high risk for heart attack and stroke, limb amputation, and periodontal gum disease.

The latest research has put exercise and healthful nutrition at the forefront in the prevention, control, and treatment of type 2 diabetes.[29] Exercise works through at least two pathways to decrease diabetes symptoms. First, exercise activates insulin-independent glucose transporters and increases insulin sensitivity in the insulin-dependent GLUT4 transporters. Thus, more glucose is passed from the bloodstream into the cells. Second, exercise helps to decrease risk of cardiovascular disease by decreasing blood pressure, cholesterol levels, and body fat. The loss of body fat also helps to improve insulin sensitivity. In addition, because insulin stimulates appetite, improved insulin sensitivity prompts the pancreas to secrete less insulin, which leads to a decreased appetite and further weight loss.

Given the growing medical burden of type 2 diabetes treatment and the increasing recognition of the important role that exercise plays in treating diabetes, more people with diabetes are seeking out the services of health professionals who can help clients implement effective lifestyle programs. Exercise considerations for recreational exercisers and athletes with diabetes are highlighted in Box 14-3.

Nutrition Recommendations

In most cases, the nutrition recommendations for individuals with diabetes closely resemble the *Dietary Guidelines for Americans*. However, it is especially important for people with diabetes to maintain a relatively stable blood sugar level throughout the day. To do this, clients should: (1) balance nutrition intake with exercise and insulin or other medications, and (2) consume five to six equally sized small meals. All individuals with diabetes who have not already had a comprehensive nutrition consultation prior to beginning an exercise program should be referred to a registered dietitian or certified diabetes educator (CDE) for an evaluation and nutrition teaching. While nutrition therapy for people with diabetes is best initiated and managed by a registered dietitian or CDE, an understanding of appropriate nutrition for people with diabetes will help the health professional to identify potential complications and reinforce the nutrition education and teaching initially provided by other health professionals.

Osteoporosis

Osteoporosis is a severe weakening of the bones, which can lead to fracture of the hip, spine, and other skeletal sites (Fig. 14-2). Osteoporosis is diagnosed by a physician when bone density is greater than 2.5 standard deviations below the mean for age and gender. **Osteopenia** is the less severe precursor to osteoporosis. It is diagnosed when bone density is between –1 and –2.4 standard deviations below the mean for age and gender.

Characterized by low bone density and diminished bone strength, osteoporosis is responsible for more than 1.5 million fractures, including 300,000 hip fractures each year.[30] Hip fracture, the most serious consequence of osteoporosis, leads to hospital admission, serious disability, and a 10% to 20% increased mortality.[31] Osteoporosis most often affects elderly women, although it can occur in men and younger women. In fact, very physically active women and women who try to lose weight by restricting intake are at substantially increased risk of osteoporosis. The surgeon general estimates that more than half of Americans will have osteopenia or osteoporosis by 2020.[30]

Accelerated bone loss in older age and a low peak bone mass from suboptimal bone growth in childhood, adolescence, and young adulthood equally contribute to

Box 14-3. Exercise Considerations for Clients With Diabetes

Individuals with diabetes can participate and excel in fitness activities and sports. However, people with diabetes, especially those with type 1 diabetes, need to carefully monitor blood sugar levels and be well-informed of the effects of exercise on blood sugar control. The target blood glucose range is 100 to 250 mg/dL.

Prior to beginning an exercise program, a client with diabetes should undergo an evaluation by his or her physician. The physician should note whether any specific precautions or limitations are necessary. Ideally, the client will authorize the physician, allied health professional, and registered dietitian or certified diabetes educator to communicate and develop an optimal plan of care.

At the onset of each exercise session, the client should check his or her blood glucose level. If the level is less than 100 mg/dL, the client will benefit from a 15- to 40-gram carbohydrate load prior to beginning exercise to avoid hypoglycemia. Symptoms of hypoglycemia include blurred vision, confusion, loss of consciousness, and dizziness. It is rare for people with type 2 diabetes to have low blood sugar, but common for people with type 1 diabetes who have to titrate insulin dosages with meals and exercise. If the pre-exercise blood sugar level is below 250 mg/dL, the client should check for urine ketones and monitor for symptoms of hyperglycemia such as excessive urination and thirst, weight loss, and blurred vision. If the client is asymptomatic and ketones are negative, initiating exercise is safe. If they are positive, the client should discuss with his or her physician an appropriate management plan. A client with diabetes should always have insulin on hand in the case of hyperglycemia.

Monitoring blood glucose during exercise is important, especially for an individual with diabetes who is new to exercise; who has recently made changes in the intensity, duration, or type of activity; or who has a new diagnosis of diabetes. Exercisers with diabetes should also be sure to have a carbohydrate snack on hand in the case of a blood sugar level below 100 mg/dL. Athletes with diabetes need to regularly consume carbohydrate drinks and snacks during prolonged exercise bouts, not only to optimize athletic performance, but most importantly, to avoid symptoms of hypoglycemia.

The effects of exercise on blood sugar can persist for several hours after exercise is stopped. Consequently, the risk of exercise-induced hypoglycemia remains high. For this reason, athletes with diabetes should also check blood sugar 2 to 3 hours after exercise.

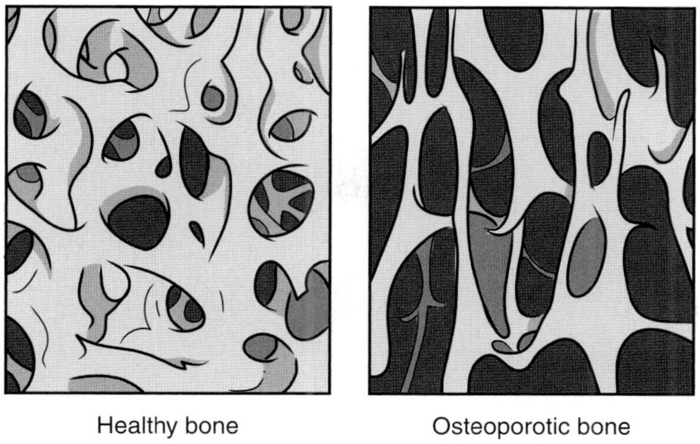

Figure 14-2. Osteoporosis and weak bones. Osteoporosis causes bone to become weak, porous, and susceptible to fracture.

the development of osteoporosis.[32] Bone is living tissue made mostly of collagen and calcium phosphate. Bone is constantly undergoing **bone remodeling**, wherein old bone is removed (resorption) and new bone is added (formation). During childhood and adolescence, bone formation predominates and new bone is added more rapidly than old bone is resorbed. After approximately age 30, peak bone mass is attained. After that time, the equation shifts and the rate of bone resorption exceeds bone formation. Postmenopausal women who no longer benefit from the bone-protecting effects of estrogen experience the highest rates of bone resorption. While bone density can never exceed the peak bone density attained in young adulthood, with attention to nutrition and lifestyle factors, the rate of bone resorption can be slowed.

Health professionals can play a key role in helping clients build and maintain strong bones and avoid osteoporosis and bone fracture with the following evidence-based recommendations.

Five Steps to Optimal Bone Health

1. Start with good nutrition. This means more than meeting calcium and vitamin D recommendations, although a deficiency in either nutrient probably precludes optimal bone health.[33] An overall healthy and balanced diet with adequate calories and appropriate nutrients provides a solid foundation for all body tissues, including bone. Clients should also be sure to get enough vitamin K[34] and potentially vitamin C, as these vitamins may further help decrease fracture risk.[35]
2. Maintain an overall healthy lifestyle. Eating disorders, smoking, and depression contribute to bone weakening and increased risk of osteoporosis.[32] While weight loss in those who are overweight or obese is important for overall health, lighter people tend to be at increased risk for osteoporosis. Research suggests, however, that individuals who lose weight primarily through exercise (versus calorie restriction) do not have reduction in bone mineral density at clinically important fracture sites such as the hip.[36]
3. Engage in weight-bearing physical activity. Exercise early in life leads to a higher peak bone mass. Exercise in the later years likely slows the decline in bone mineral density and increases muscle mass and strength more than twofold in frail persons. Additional benefits include improved function, delayed loss of independence, and improved quality of life. Importantly, elderly individuals who engage in regular physical activity are less likely to fall.[32]
4. Aim to prevent falls. Without a fall, even brittle bones are unlikely to break. Muscle strengthening, balance training, a regular Tai Chi program, removal of home hazards such as rugs and clutter, elimination of psychiatric medications when possible, and use of a multidisciplinary program to assess risk factors for falls all contribute to a substantial reduction of falls,[37] which translates into a reduction in debilitating fractures.
5. Encourage clients to visit their doctor regularly, especially those clients with risk factors for osteoporosis. Risk factors include female gender, increased age, estrogen deficiency (postmenopausal or amenorrheic), white race, low weight and body mass index, family history of osteoporosis, smoking, and history of prior fracture.[32] A physician can order a dual-energy x-ray absorptiometry (DXA) bone scan to confirm or rule out a diagnosis of osteoporosis. Also, several medications are available for the treatment and prevention of the bone disease.

SPEED BUMP

3. List and describe several chronic diseases that may afflict athletes and the general nutritional principles to consider for each disease.

4. Describe the role of the health professional in the nutritional management of clients who suffer from chronic illness.

CHAPTER SUMMARY

Athletes may suffer from a variety of injuries and illness. The health professional can work as part of a multidisciplinary team to help the athlete adopt nutrition and activity practices most effective in supporting recovery and return to play.

KEY POINTS SUMMARY

1. Athletes who engage in very high-intensity exercise are at increased risk of mild infections, while athletes who engage in moderate-intensity exercise are afforded a protective effect against common illnesses. Periods of particularly increased risk of infection include intensive training weeks, the taper prior to competition, and during competition. Athletes can reduce risk of illness by gradually increasing program intensity and volume, including cross training in their training program, and allowing sufficient time for rest and recovery.
2. Research to date does not support supplementation to decrease risk of illness in athletes. However, attention to carbohydrate intake helps to reduce the immune response. There is limited evidence that quercetin supplementation may provide benefit. Athletes should discuss nutritional supplementation with a registered dietitian or physician.
3. Athletes should refrain from exercise when they have a fever due to increased risk of dehydration. Otherwise, no strict criteria exist, though it may be prudent for athletes suffering a minor illness to decrease the intensity of training and avoid very strenuous exercise.
4. Injured athletes have decreased calorie and protein needs compared with needs during periods of intense activity, but increased needs compared with baseline in order to support healing. Muscle atrophy occurs with immobilization. There is some evidence that intake of the branched chain amino acids, in particular leucine, may help to offset this immobilization-induced muscle atrophy. There is growing interest in possible roles for creatine and omega-3 fatty acid supplementation in protecting against immobilization-induced atrophy and improving wound healing.
5. While it is essential that health professionals are aware of general nutrition recommendations for the treatment and prevention of most common illnesses, it is clearly outside the scope of practice of the non-registered dietitian allied health professional to provide nutrition advice or recommendations on how to use nutrition to help treat these conditions.
6. Gastrointestinal discomforts are the most common ailments experienced by athletes. While many of these symptoms may be short-lived, some athletes suffer from chronic GI disease such as GERD, IBS, celiac disease, and IBD. Many of these illnesses can be managed at least in part with changes in nutritional habits.
7. Cardiovascular disease is the leading killer of American men and women. Signs and symptoms of cardiovascular disease develop in childhood. While exercise is protective, athletes still may experience risks of cardiovascular disease and should aim to adopt a healthful eating plan to minimize risk. A person with "ideal cardiovascular health" does not smoke; is of normal weight; has total cholesterol less than 200 mg/dL, blood pressure less than120/80, and fasting plasma glucose less than 100 mg/dL; participates in moderate-intensity exercise at least 150 minutes per week or vigorous-intensity exercise 75 minutes per week; and follows a healthy diet. A healthy diet includes at least 4.5 cups of fruits and vegetables per day, at least two 3.5-ounce servings of fish per week, less than or equal to 1,500 milligrams per day of sodium, fewer than or equal to 450 kilocalories per week from sugar-sweetened beverages, and at least three servings of whole grains per day.
8. Type 1 and type 2 diabetes are very different manifestations of a similar disease process, characterized by dysfunction in insulin production and/or utilization. Health professionals who work with clients who have diabetes should understand the basic nutrition and exercise principles underlying diabetes care and work closely with a physician and registered dietitian in order to provide the best care for the client. Three major nutritional considerations when working with clients with diabetes include balancing nutrition intake with exercise and/or insulin; consuming several small meals throughout the day in an effort to maintain relatively stable blood sugar levels; and monitoring blood glucose before, during, and after exercise, being sure to have a carbohydrate snack on hand in the case of hypoglycemia.
9. Athletes at highest risk for osteoporosis are females who are estrogen-deficient (postmenopausal or amenorrheic), have a family history of osteoporosis, have very low body mass index, or have a history of a prior fracture. Attention to minimizing risk factors and consuming recommended amounts of vitamin D, calcium, vitamin K, and vitamin C will help to reduce risk. Weight-bearing physical activity also helps to reduce risk. Clients with risk factors for osteoporosis may benefit from an evaluation by a physician who may consider a DXA bone scan to determine bone mineral density.

PRACTICAL APPLICATIONS

1. After a bout of very strenuous exercise training, what is the typical maximum amount of time that an athlete's immune system could experience weakened function?
   A. 12 hours
   B. 24 hours
   C. 48 hours
   D. 72 hours
2. Which of the following substances have been shown by research-supported evidence to act as effective nutrition interventions in exercise immunology?
   A. Quercetin and vitamin A
   B. Vitamin E and probiotics
   C. Carbohydrate and quercetin
   D. Multivitamin supplement and glutamine
3. Which of the following gastrointestinal disorders when untreated is MOST likely to lead to severe disability and ultimately death?
   A. Gastroesophageal reflux disease (GERD)
   B. Exercise-related transient abdominal pain (ETAP)
   C. Celiac disease
   D. Inflammatory bowel disease (IBD)
4. Which of the following cardiovascular events is often reported as the first indication of an underlying cardiovascular disease in previously asymptomatic athletes?
   A. Sudden cardiac arrest
   B. Heart murmur
   C. Myocardial infarction
   D. Aortic aneurism
5. For exercisers with type 1 diabetes, what is the amount of blood glucose considered too low to begin a workout session to avoid hypoglycemia?
   A. 80 mg/dL
   B. 90 mg/dL
   C. 100 mg/dL
   D. 110 mg/dL
6. Jonathan has type 2 diabetes and has made efforts to change his lifestyle to improve his health. According to his physician, Jonathan has experienced many positive health changes due to his exercise program and diet modifications, including weight loss. Which of the following is the most likely positive adaptation due to his lifestyle changes?
   A. Increased insulin resistance
   B. Decreased insulin resistance
   C. Increased protein in the urine
   D. Decreased use of blood fats for energy
7. Women who have not yet transitioned through menopause are protected from bone loss from which hormone?
   A. Progesterone
   B. Estrogen
   C. Testosterone
   D. Androstenedione
8. Which of the following persons would have the highest risk for developing osteoporosis?
   A. A woman who has repeatedly lost weight and regained it through dietary restriction and fasting.
   B. A 60-year-old man who is overweight and sedentary.
   C. A middle-aged woman who has lost weight primarily through exercise.
   D. A physically active man who has a low body mass index (BMI).
9. Which analgesic drug has been associated with kidney dysfunction and hyponatremia in endurance-trained athletes?
   A. Acetaminophen
   B. Codeine
   C. Furosemide
   D. Ibuprofen
10. Which of the following statements is true regarding probiotics?
    A. Probiotics manufacturers are required to use accepted nomenclature for the bacteria in a product.
    B. Probiotics have been proven to be effective in the clinical treatment of diarrhea and lactose intolerance.
    C. Probiotics must be alive and consumed in sufficient quantity on a daily basis to exert their beneficial effects.
    D. Probiotics are regulated as drugs and require ingredient testing or proof of potency.

Case 1 Scott, the Professional Triathlete

Scott is a 29-year-old professional triathlete. He is due to run the Kona Ironman in the coming month and is very concerned that his intensive training regimen will leave him susceptible to injury or illness.

1. What precautions should Scott take to minimize his risk of injury and illness?
2. What nutritional factors may be helpful for Scott to protect against injury and illness?
3. If Scott does get injured, what nutritional strategies may help to promote healing?

Case 2 Susan, the Middle-Age Overweight Hiker

Susan is a 55-year-old overweight teacher who has struggled with obesity since childhood. After her best friend suffered a debilitating heart attack, she decided to change her lifestyle and achieve a healthier weight. She has been following her training program and doing very well. Recently, another friend was diagnosed with type 2 diabetes. Susan has become very anxious about her health and even more committed to achieving her weight loss goals.

1. Susan says that she recently visited her physician for her annual exam. He ordered a series of blood tests and told her she had high cholesterol, prediabetes, and increased risk for heart disease. What further information would you like to know to understand her risk?
2. Susan asks you what is considered to be an ideal eating plan to prevent cardiovascular disease and diabetes?
3. Susan asks for three things that she can do to prevent disease. What might you tell her?

TRAIN YOURSELF

1. Choose an acute or chronic illness or injury for which you believe you are at highest risk. Describe why you feel that you are at risk. Explain what nutritional or exercise considerations are important to help minimize that risk.
2. Highlight three aspects from this chapter that were of most interest and relevance to you. Explain why. Will you change the way you train or eat based on what you learned?

REFERENCES

1. Harris MD. Infectious disease in athletes. *Curr Sports Med Rep.* March-April 2011;10(2):84-89.
2. Walsh NP, Gleeson M, Pyne DB, et al. Position statement. Part two: maintaining immune health. *Exerc Immunol Rev.* 2011;17:64-103.
3. Walsh NP, Gleeson M, Shephard RJ, et al. Position statement. Part one: immune function and exercise. *Exerc Immunol Rev.* 2011;17:6-63.
4. Haegens A, Schols AM, van Essen AL, van Loon LJ, Langen RC. Leucine induces myofibrillar protein accretion in cultured skeletal muscle through mTOR dependent and independent control of myosin heavy chain mRNA levels. *Mol Nutr Food Res.* May 2012;56(5):741-752.
5. Baptista IL, Leal ML, Artioli GG, et al. Leucine attenuates skeletal muscle wasting via inhibition of ubiquitin ligases. *Muscle Nerve.* June 2010;41(6):800-808.
6. Op't Eijnde B, Urso B, Richter EA, Greenhaff PL, Hespel P. Effect of oral creatine supplementation on human muscle GLUT4 protein content after immobilization. *Diabetes.* January 2001;50(1):18-23.
7. Hespel P, Op't Eijnde B, Van Leemputte M, et al. Oral creatine supplementation facilitates the rehabilitation of disuse atrophy and alters the expression of muscle myogenic factors in humans. *J Physiol.* October 15 2001;536(Pt 2):625-633.
8. Roy BD, de Beer J, Harvey D, Tarnopolsky MA. Creatine monohydrate supplementation does not improve functional recovery after total knee arthroplasty. *Arch Phys Med Rehabil.* July 2005;86(7):1293-1298.
9. Johnston AP, Burke DG, MacNeil LG, Candow DG. Effect of creatine supplementation during cast-induced immobilization on the preservation of muscle mass, strength, and endurance. *J Strength Cond Res.* January 2009;23(1):116-120.
10. You JS, Park MN, Song W, Lee YS. Dietary fish oil alleviates soleus atrophy during immobilization in association with Akt signaling to p70s6k and E3 ubiquitin ligases in rats. *Appl Physiol Nutr Metab.* June 2010;35(3):310-318.
11. You JS, Park MN, Lee YS. Dietary fish oil inhibits the early stage of recovery of atrophied soleus muscle in rats via Akt-p70s6k signaling and PGF2alpha. *J Nutr Biochem.* October 2010;21(10):929-934.
12. Smith GI, Atherton P, Reeds DN, et al. Dietary omega-3 fatty acid supplementation increases the rate of muscle protein synthesis in older adults: a randomized controlled trial. *Am J Clin Nutr.* February 2011;93(2):402-412.
13. Harris WS, Mozaffarian D, Rimm E, et al. Omega-6 fatty acids and risk for cardiovascular disease: a science advisory from the American Heart Association Nutrition Subcommittee of the Council on Nutrition, Physical Activity, and Metabolism; Council on Cardiovascular Nursing; and Council on Epidemiology and Prevention. *Circulation.* February 17 2009;119(6):902-907.
14. Tipton KD. Nutrition for acute exercise-induced injuries. *Ann Nutr Metab.* 2010;57 Suppl 2:43-53.
15. Waterman JJ, Kapur R. Upper gastrointestinal issues in athletes. *Curr Sports Med Rep.* March-April 2012;11(2):99-104.
16. Kahrilas PJ. Clinical practice. Gastroesophageal reflux disease. *N Engl J Med.* October 16 2008;359(16):1700-1707.
17. Kahrilas PJ, Shaheen NJ, Vaezi MF, et al. American Gastroenterological Association Medical Position Statement on the management of gastroesophageal reflux disease. *Gastroenterology.* October 2008;135(4):1383-1391, 1391 e1381-1385.
18. Mayer EA. Clinical practice. Irritable bowel syndrome. *N Engl J Med.* April 17 2008;358(16):1692-1699.
19. Hoveyda N, Heneghan C, Mahtani KR, Perera R, Roberts N, Glasziou P. A systematic review and meta-analysis: probiotics in the treatment of irritable bowel syndrome. *BMC Gastroenterol.* 2009;9:15.
20. Henningsen P, Zipfel S, Herzog W. Management of functional somatic syndromes. *Lancet.* March 17 2007;369(9565): 946-955.
21. Armstrong MJ, Hegade VS, Robins G. Advances in coeliac disease. *Curr Opin Gastroenterol.* March 2012;28(2):104-112.
22. Abraham C, Cho JH. Inflammatory bowel disease. *N Engl J Med.* November 19 2009;361(21):2066-2078.
23. Roger VL, Go AS, Lloyd-Jones DM, et al. Heart disease and stroke statistics—2012 update: a report from the American Heart Association. *Circulation.* January 3 2012; 125(1):e2-e220.
24. McGill HC, Jr., McMahan CA, Herderick EE, Malcom GT, Tracy RE, Strong JP. Origin of atherosclerosis in childhood and adolescence. *Am J Clin Nutr.* November 2000;72 (5 Suppl):1307S-1315S.
25. Fuster V, Moreno PR, Fayad ZA, Corti R, Badimon JJ. Atherothrombosis and high-risk plaque: part I: evolving concepts. *J Am Coll Cardiol.* September 20 2005;46(6): 937-954.

26. Champagne CM. Dietary interventions on blood pressure: the Dietary Approaches to Stop Hypertension (DASH) trials. *Nutr Rev.* February 2006;64(2 Pt 2):S53-56.
27. Fang, J., Yang, Q., Hong, Y, & Loutstalot, F. Status of cardiovascular health among adult Americans in the 50 states and the District of Columbia, 2009. *J Am Heart Assoc.* 2012; 1: doi: 10.1161/JAHA.112.005371.
28. Lloyd-Jones DM, Leip EP, Larson MG, et al. Prediction of lifetime risk for cardiovascular disease by risk factor burden at 50 years of age. *Circulation.* February 14 2006;113(6): 791-798.
29. Ismail-Beigi F. Clinical practice. Glycemic management of type 2 diabetes mellitus. *N Engl J Med.* April 5 2012;366 (14):1319-1327.
30. U.S. Public Health Service. The Surgeon General's report on bone health and osteoporosis, what it means to you. Washington, DC: U.S. Dept. of Health and Human Services, Office of the Surgeon General; 2004: http://purl.fdlp.gov/GPO/gpo5936.
31. Sambrook P, Cooper C. Osteoporosis. *Lancet.* June 17 2006; 367(9527):2010-2018.
32. Osteoporosis prevention, diagnosis, and therapy. *JAMA.* February 14 2001;285(6):785-795.
33. Avenell A, Gillespie WJ, Gillespie LD, O'Connell D. Vitamin D and vitamin D analogues for preventing fractures associated with involutional and post-menopausal osteoporosis. *Cochrane Database of Systematic Reviews.* 2009(2):CD000227.
34. Cockayne S, Adamson J, Lanham-New S, Shearer MJ, Gilbody S, Torgerson DJ. Vitamin K and the prevention of fractures: systematic review and meta-analysis of randomized controlled trials. *Arch Intern Med.* June 26 2006; 166(12):1256-1261.
35. Levis S, Lagari VS. The role of diet in osteoporosis prevention and management. *Curr Osteoporos Rep.* September 22 2012.
36. Villareal DT, Fontana L, Weiss EP, et al. Bone mineral density response to caloric restriction-induced weight loss or exercise-induced weight loss: a randomized controlled trial. *Arch Intern Med.* December 11-25 2006;166(22):2502-2510.
37. Gillespie LD, Robertson MC, Gillespie WJ, et al. Interventions for preventing falls in older people living in the community. *Cochrane Database of Systematic Reviews.* 2012;9: CD007146.
38. Nieman, D.C., Henson, D.A., Dumke, C.L., et al. Ibuprofen use, endotoxemia, inflammation, and plasma cytokines during ultramarathon competition. *Brain Behav Immun.* 2006;20(6): 578-584.

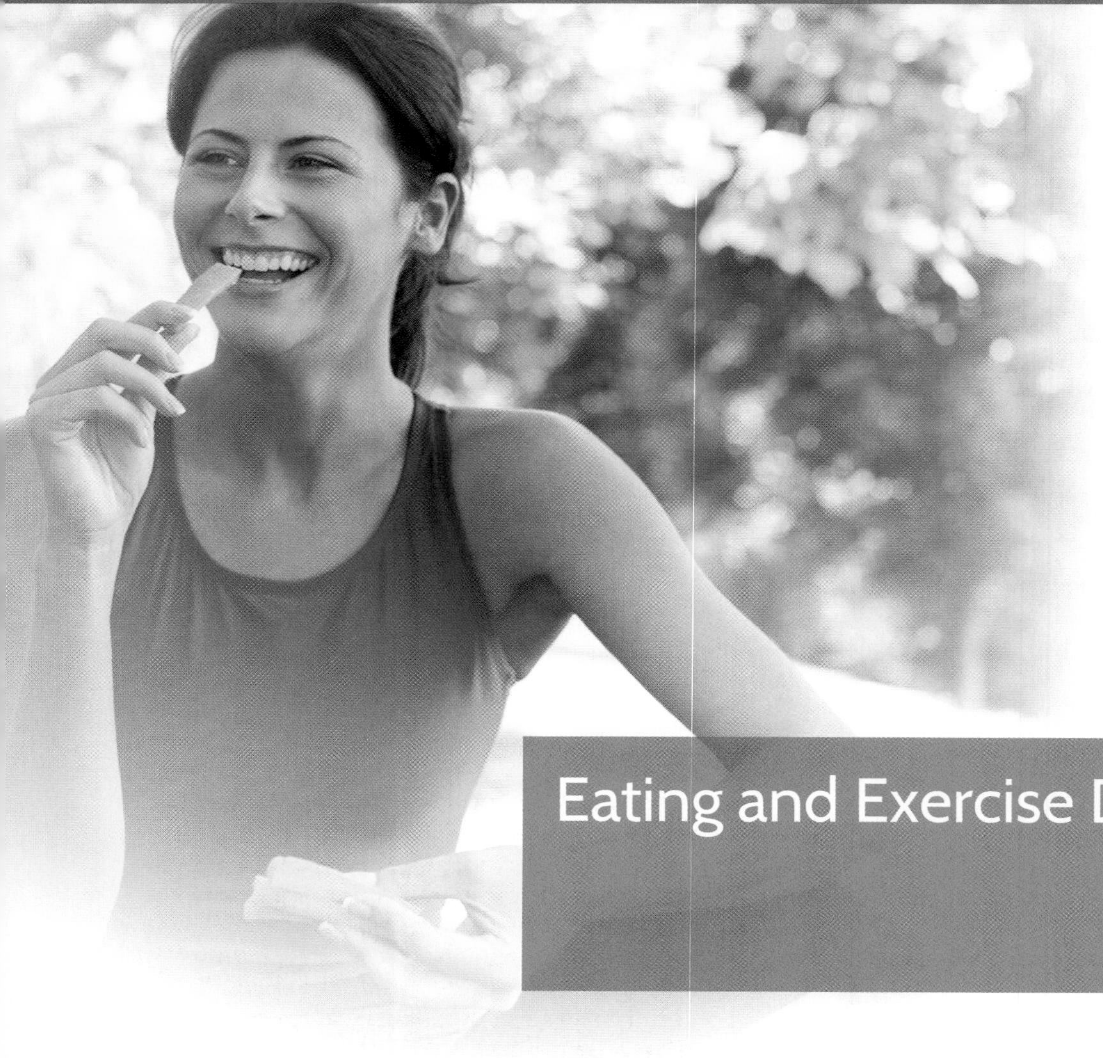

CHAPTER 15

Eating and Exercise Disorders

CHAPTER OUTLINE

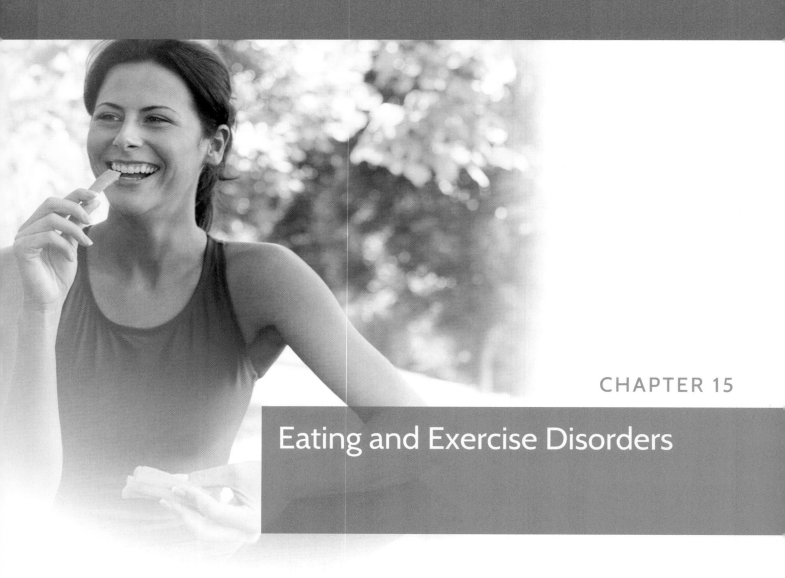

CHAPTER OUTLINE—cont'd

LEARNING OBJECTIVES

After studying this chapter, the reader should be able to:

15.1 Define and describe the signs and symptoms of the major eating disorders.
15.2 Define the major exercise disorders.
15.3 Define the female athlete triad and its consequences on health and performance.
15.4 Identify risk factors for developing an eating or exercise disorder.
15.5 Describe strategies to prevent eating and exercise disorders in high-risk populations.
15.6 Develop a sensitive and effective approach to confronting clients with a suspected eating or exercise disorder.

KEY TERMS

active dehydration Dehydration resulting from increasing exercise and heat exposure.

adipositas athletica A term describing athletes who try to gain body fat to increase insulation or increase body energy stores.[35]

amenorrhea A condition defined by at least 3 months without a menstrual period.

anorexia athletica A sport-induced subclinical eating disorder.

anorexia nervosa An eating disorder characterized by caloric restriction leading to significantly low body weight, intense fear of gaining weight or becoming fat, and preoccupation with the body or inability or refusal to recognize the harm of extremely thin body size.

atypical anorexia nervosa A condition in which all of the criteria for anorexia nervosa are met, except that, despite significant weight loss, the individual's weight is within or above the normal range.

avoidant/restrictive eating disorder A condition in which an individual restricts or limits food intake, but does not meet the criteria for other eating disorders.

binge eating Excessive eating in a discrete period of time (e.g., within any 2-hour period).

binge-eating disorder A condition characterized by repeated overconsumption of large amounts of food in a short period of time.

binge-eating/purging type of anorexia nervosa A subtype of anorexia nervosa; during the last 3 months, the individual has engaged in recurrent episodes of binge eating or purging behavior.

body dysmorphic disorder A disorder in which an individual develops persistent and obtrusive thoughts and preoccupations with an imagined or slight defect in appearance.

bulimia nervosa An eating disorder characterized by regular episodes of overeating and binge eating, which is then compensated with unhealthy weight-loss strategies including vomiting, excessive exercise, or laxative abuse.

continuance Continuing to exercise despite knowing that this activity is creating or worsening physical, psychological, and/or interpersonal problems.[17]

disordered eating Eating patterns that are considered to be irregular, especially when compared to a normal, healthy individual of the same culture.

diuretic Any substance that acts to decrease the amount of water in the body through increased urination.

eating disorder not elsewhere specified Eating disorders that do not meet the strict diagnostic criteria to be classified as more specific disorders.

enemas Procedures used to flush out the colon and rectum using liquid applied through the anus.

energy availability The energy available in the body to fuel physical activity and energy-requiring body functions. Determined by the relationship between the calories consumed in the diet and the calories expended in physical activity.

exercise dependence A condition in which a person is preoccupied with exercise and training to the extent that the person engages in excessive levels of exercise, resulting in negative physiological and psychological consequences.[16]

feeding or eating disorders not elsewhere classified Eating disorders that do not meet the strict diagnostic criteria to be classified as more specific disorders.

female athlete triad A condition in which disordered eating and low energy availability lead to abnormal menstruation and decreased bone mineralization with eventual development of amenorrhea and osteoporosis.

food addiction A controversial concept; may occur in certain individuals in which consumption of highly palatable foods such as sugar, salt, and fat trigger a response in the brain leading to binge eating, pervasive thoughts of food, and ultimately, obesity.

intention effects Inability to stick to one's intended routine; in the case of exercise dependence, intention effects are evidenced by exceeding the amount of time devoted to exercise or consistently going beyond the intended amount.[17]

laxatives Products used to soften stool and aid the body in excretion.

muscle dysmorphic disorder A form of body dysmorphic disorder in which a person engages in excessive amounts of resistance training in an effort to be "big."

night eating syndrome Characterized by recurrent episodes of eating after awakening from sleep or excessive food consumption after the evening meal.

orthorexia nervosa A pattern of disordered eating characterized by a preoccupation with eating an extremely healthy diet.[10]

osteoporosis Weakening of the bones, which can lead to bone fracture of the hip, spine, and other skeletal sites.

passive dehydration Dehydration resulting from fluid and food restriction.

pica A feeding disorder in which an individual has a strong desire to eat non-food items, such as dirt or clay; most frequently occurs in childhood in response to nutritional deficiency.

purging disorder Condition in which a person engages in recurrent purging behavior to influence weight or shape, such as self-induced vomiting, misuse of laxatives, diuretics, or other medications, in the absence of binge eating.

restricting type of anorexia nervosa A subtype of anorexia nervosa; during the last 3 months, the individual has not engaged in recurrent episodes of binge eating or purging behavior.

rumination A feeding disorder in which a person regurgitates (vomits) food that was just eaten and chews and swallows it again.

secondary adipositas athletica A term used to describe athletes who do not purposefully want to gain fat mass, but just want to get "bigger"; increased adiposity is an unintended consequence.

subthreshold anorexia nervosa See *atypical anorexia nervosa*.

subthreshold binge-eating disorder A condition in which all of the criteria for binge-eating disorder are met, except that the binge eating occurs, on average, less than once a week and/or for fewer than 3 months. See *eating disorder not elsewhere specified*.

subthreshold bulimia nervosa A condition in which all of the criteria for bulimia nervosa are met, except that the binge eating and inappropriate compensatory behaviors occur, on average, less than once a week and/or for fewer than 3 months.

tolerance An individual becomes accustomed to the current amount of exercise and must increase the amount of exercise in order to feel the desired effect, be it a "buzz" or sense of accomplishment, in the case of exercise dependence.[17]

weight cycling Rapid fluctuations in weight, generally used in sports when an athlete loses weight to qualify for a certain weight class, then regains the weight immediately after the weigh-in.

withdrawal In the absence of exercise the person experiences negative effects such as anxiety, irritability, restlessness, and sleep problems, in the case of exercise dependence.[17]

INTRODUCTION

Eating and exercise disorders can be found in gyms and fitness centers in small towns, suburbs, and major cities throughout the country. They manifest as the super-slim college student who works out at the gym every day at 5:00 a.m. and 6:30 p.m.—times far enough apart that no one would notice the combined 3-plus hours spent running on the treadmill each day. They are also seen in the normal-weight, healthy-appearing woman who is frequently heard vomiting in the bathroom or the weight lifter who never misses a day at the gym. They pervade locker rooms, fields, courts, and gymnasiums, affecting more than one-fourth of competitive female athletes.[1]

When faced with a client who demonstrates signs or symptoms of an eating disorder, many health professionals do not know how to best proceed: Confront? Refer? Ignore? While the situation is never easy to address, this chapter aims to help health professionals develop a systematic and productive method for helping members and clients who may suffer from, or be at risk for, an eating or exercise disorder.

UNDERSTANDING EATING AND EXERCISE DISORDERS

Eating and exercise disorders confuse and astonish many people. Just eat. Take a day off from working out. Choose foods in moderation to avoid a binge. It sounds easy enough. Why, then, does anorexia nervosa have the highest mortality rate of any psychiatric disorder, with nearly one-fourth of those deaths resulting from suicide?[2] While the precise causes of eating and exercise disorders remain somewhat elusive, advances in the understanding of these conditions provide a wealth of information for health professionals to consider when interacting with and trying to help people who have or are at risk for eating and exercise disorders. Recognizing the social, psychological, and physiological complexities of these disorders helps make it clear why the simple solutions do not work (see Myths and Misconceptions).

EATING DISORDERS

Historically, eating disorders have predominately affected Caucasian teenage females. However, the demographics have changed considerably over time with an increasing number of males, minorities, and preadolescent girls and boys affected.[3] While the causes of eating disorders are not well understood, most experts believe that certain societal pressures combine with a genetic predisposition for behavioral rigidity and perfectionism to trigger a cascade of thoughts and behaviors that can ultimately manifest as an eating disorder.[3]

The two most well-known and carefully defined eating disorders are **anorexia nervosa** and **bulimia nervosa.** Other diagnoses that are classified as Feeding and Eating Disorders in the *Diagnostic and Statistical Manual of Mental Disorders, 5th edition (DSM-5)* include the feeding disorders **pica** and **rumination**, which typically affect children and will not be discussed further here, and the eating disorders anorexia nervosa, bulimia nervosa, avoidant/restrictive, binge eating, and feeding or eating disorder not elsewhere classified.

Previous editions of the DSM manuals were frequently criticized because the majority of people with eating disorders did not meet the strict diagnostic criteria for anorexia nervosa or bulimia nervosa, and instead were diagnosed with partial syndromes or an **eating disorder not otherwise specified** (ED NOS). *DSM-5* attempts to address those issues with updated diagnostic criteria, but many individuals with eating disorders will continue to fall under the nonspecific category, which now is referred to as *eating disorder not elsewhere classified*. Athletes, especially those in weight-conscious sports such as gymnastics, running, wrestling, and dancing, are at particularly high risk of developing these partial syndromes. Regardless of the specific diagnosis, all individuals with eating disorders suffer considerable psychological and physical consequences.

Myths and Misconceptions

Eating Disorders and Food

The Myth

Eating disorders can be cured by simply eating more food (in the case of anorexia nervosa) or eating less food (in the case of bulimia nervosa and binge eating).

The Logic

Eating and exercise disorders are preventable problems that can be resolved completely by istening to one's body: eat when hungry, stop when full. The body has a physiological need for an appropriate amount of food—eat too little and it grumbles uncomfortably, eat too much and risk a belly ache. The treatment for eating disorders is straightforward and, therefore, why should they be so difficult to cure?

The Science

The cause of eating disorders is multifactorial and includes an interaction between genetic factors, environmental triggers, and personal experience. The manifestations of eating disorders —namely dysregulation in food intake—are symptoms of deeply rooted psychological distress. Advising a person who has an eating disorder to just eat more or less does not address the cause of the disorder and thus, alone, does not represent an effective treatment. To be effective, treatment for eating disorders should involve a physician to evaluate for medical problems resulting from poor nutritional status, a registered dietitian to develop an appropriate eating plan, a mental health professional to provide therapy and support to help get to the underlying causes of the disordered eating, and, in most cases, integral involvement of the affected person's close family.

Anorexia Nervosa

Stephanie is a 17-year-old female who recently visited her doctor with the chief complaint of "irregular periods," with her last menstrual period 3 months ago. The doctor's note states that the patient had been seen 6 months previously with a height of 66 inches and weight of 135 pounds (BMI 21.8). At this visit, the patient's weight had dropped to 115 pounds (BMI 18.6). On further questioning, Stephanie shared that she had been trying to "eat healthier" and cut snacks and calorie-containing drinks from her diet. She also adopted an exercise program. Despite repeated efforts to collect specific information about her diet and exercise history, the doctor reports that Stephanie evaded the questions and became defensive. Stephanie's mother shared her concern that for the past 3 months Stephanie has avoided family meals, is constantly weighing herself (though she does not allow anyone near her when she does this), and had notable weight loss. The physician expressed concern that Stephanie may be suffering from anorexia nervosa and proceeded to coordinate a multidisciplinary treatment team including a therapist, registered dietitian, psychiatrist, and herself, the primary care physician, for further evaluation and treatment. With the patient's mother's permission, the physician also initiated contact with the patient's school and the director of the fitness facility where Stephanie is a member.

Stephanie's case provides a classic example of an early presentation of anorexia nervosa. Although it usually affects teenage girls and young women, a growing number of men and middle-age women are diagnosed with anorexia nervosa, the most deadly of the eating disorders. In establishing a diagnosis of anorexia nervosa, a physician refers to *DSM-5* to see if the patient meets diagnostic criteria. In the case of anorexia nervosa, the criteria include:[4]

1. Restriction of energy intake leading to a significantly low body weight for age, sex, developmental trajectory, and physical health.
2. Intense fear of gaining weight or becoming "fat," or persistent behavior that interferes with weight gain, even though at a significantly low weight.
3. Disturbance in the way in which one's body weight or shape is experienced, undue influence of body weight or shape on self-evaluation, or persistent lack of recognition of the seriousness of the current low body weight.

Anorexia nervosa is further classified into two subtypes:

Restricting Type: During the last 3 months, the individual has not engaged in recurrent episodes of **binge eating** or purging behavior (i.e., self-induced vomiting or the misuse of **laxatives**, **diuretics**, or **enemas**).

Binge-Eating/Purging Type: During the last 3 months, the individual has engaged in recurrent episodes of binge eating or purging behavior (i.e., self-induced vomiting or the misuse of laxatives, diuretics, or enemas).

This definition is updated from the previous diagnostic criteria, which required four strict criteria: refusal to maintain body weight of at least 85% of expected weight; intense fear of gaining weight or becoming fat; body image disturbances including a disproportionate influence of body weight on self-evaluation; and the absence of at least three consecutive menstrual periods (**amenorrhea**).[5]

The causes of anorexia nervosa are multifactorial and not fully understood. A combination of genetic predisposition; personality traits of perfectionism and compulsiveness; anxiety; family history of depression and obesity; and peer, cultural, and familial ideals of beauty interact to trigger anorexia nervosa in some individuals. The most severe potential consequences of the disorder include osteoporosis, miscarriage and low infant birth weights, abnormalities in cognitive functioning, suicide, and death from starvation or heart arrhythmias.[2,6] While many people with anorexia nervosa are resistant to change and may need inpatient treatment in a psychiatric hospital, full recovery of body weight, growth, menstruation, and normal eating behavior and attitudes regarding food and body shape occurs in 50% to 70% or more of treated adolescents.[6] Only 25% to 50% of adults with anorexia nervosa severe enough to require hospitalization fully recover.[6]

Bulimia Nervosa

Tanya is a 22-year-old collegiate soccer player. She has a muscular build and BMI of 25. Her roommate, who is also a soccer player, recently confronted Tanya after she heard her inducing vomiting after the two consumed a large pizza together. While Tanya seemed content while they were eating, afterwards she expressed feelings of guilt for having eaten so much and worried that she was going to "become fat." When Tanya's roommate confronted her, Tanya denied having ever induced vomiting in the past. Wanting to protect her friend but also unsure what to do, Tanya's roommate confided in their assistant coach her concern that Tanya may be showing signs of bulimia nervosa.

Bulimia nervosa is more difficult to identify than anorexia nervosa because people with bulimia nervosa are often normal weight or sometimes overweight. Bulimia nervosa is diagnosed when the following criteria are met:[4]

1. Recurrent episodes of binge eating. An episode of binge eating is characterized by:
   - Eating, in a discrete period of time (e.g., within any 2-hour period), an amount of food that is definitely larger than most people would eat during a similar period of time under similar circumstances; AND
   - A sense of lack of control over eating during the episode (e.g., a feeling that one cannot stop eating or control what or how much one is eating)
2. Recurrent inappropriate compensatory behaviors in order to prevent weight gain, such as self-induced vomiting; misuse of laxatives, diuretics, or other medications; fasting; or excessive exercise.
3. The binge eating and inappropriate compensatory behaviors both occur, on average, at least once per week for 3 months.
4. Self-evaluation is unduly influenced by body shape and weight.
5. The disturbance does not occur exclusively during episodes of anorexia nervosa.

One percent to 5% of women (usually in their late teens to early twenties) suffer from bulimia nervosa.[7] Importantly, anorexia nervosa and bulimia nervosa often co-exist with one another and are caused by many of the same complex social, familial, and personality factors.

Binge-Eating Disorder

Steven is a 25-year-old engineer with a BMI of 35. He recently joined his local YMCA to begin an exercise program to help him lose weight. Recognizing that he needs help to achieve his goals, he hired a health coach. During the initial evaluation, he shared that at least two nights per week while watching his favorite 30-minute sitcoms on TV he eats a frozen pizza, about six cookies, and a bag of chips. He acknowledged that he wishes that he didn't do this and that he feels disgusted with himself afterwards. The health coach noted that Steven frequently stated, "I wasn't even hungry!" when describing the episodes. These episodes usually happen when he is alone. He does not engage in any compensatory behaviors afterwards.

Steven's history should raise suspicion for binge-eating disorder. **Binge-eating disorder** falls along the continuum of **disordered eating** with anorexia nervosa and bulimia nervosa (Fig. 15-1). Binge-eating disorder is characterized by repeated overconsumption of large amounts of food in a short period of time. The condition frequently co-occurs with mental health disorders such as anxiety and depression and is highly associated with obesity.[8] Some people associate binge-eating disorder with **food addiction**, though the physiological basis for each is a source of ongoing research.[9] Concerned, Steven's health coach referred him to a mental health professional for evaluation and therapy.

For the diagnosis of binge-eating disorder, the person must meet the following criteria:

1. Recurrent episodes of binge eating.
2. The binge-eating episodes are associated with three (or more) of the following:
   - Eating much more rapidly than normal
   - Eating until feeling uncomfortably full
   - Eating large amounts of food when not feeling physically hungry
   - Eating alone because of feeling embarrassed by how much one is eating
   - Feeling disgusted with oneself, depressed, or very guilty after overeating
3. Marked distress regarding binge eating is present.
4. The binge eating occurs, on average, at least once a week for 3 months.
5. The binge eating is not associated with the recurrent use of inappropriate compensatory behavior and does not occur exclusively during the course of bulimia nervosa or anorexia nervosa.

Several clues that a client may have one of the named eating disorders—anorexia nervosa, bulimia nervosa, or binge-eating disorder—are listed in Box 15-1.

Box 15-1. Signs and Symptoms of Anorexia Nervosa, Bulimia Nervosa, and Binge-Eating Disorder

Anorexia nervosa: extreme thinness; excessive exercise; fine, soft hair; easily broken bones; obsessiveness; cognitive impairment; depression; low self-esteem; extreme perfectionism; self-consciousness; self-absorption; ritualistic behavior; amenorrhea.

Bulimia nervosa: "chubby cheeks" from swollen parotid glands; eroded dental enamel; scars on back of fingers and hands from repeated self-induced vomiting; irregular menstruation; loss of normal bowel function; acid reflux; depressed mood; anxiety; alcohol and drug use; low self-esteem; irritability; impulsive spending; shoplifting; sexual impulsivity; concentration and memory impairments.

Binge-eating disorder: no definitive physical cues; repeated overconsumption of large amounts of food in a short period of time; mental health disorders such as anxiety and depression; eating when full or not hungry; eating until uncomfortably full; feeling ashamed or guilty about eating habits; feeling isolated; losing and gaining weight repeatedly, also called yo-yo dieting.

Avoidant/Restrictive Food Intake

Stephanie is an underweight 12-year-old female who participates on the middle school tennis team. Stephanie's coach has noticed that Stephanie never wants to eat any of the snacks available for the team before meets and after practices. In hopes that she will find something that Stephanie does like, the coach asks Stephanie's parents what types of snacks Stephanie would eat. Stephanie's parents share that Stephanie has severely picky eating habits and will eat only very bland, smooth foods. They also share that Stephanie was recently diagnosed with iron-deficiency anemia, calcium deficiency, and vitamin B12 deficiency, and was subsequently diagnosed by her physician with **avoidant/restrictive eating disorder**.

Avoidant/restrictive eating disorder is a new diagnosis in *DSM-5* that, for the first time, gives a named psychiatric diagnosis for what is essentially severe picky eating to the extent that it causes nutritional deficiency. It primarily affects children, though it is not limited to children.

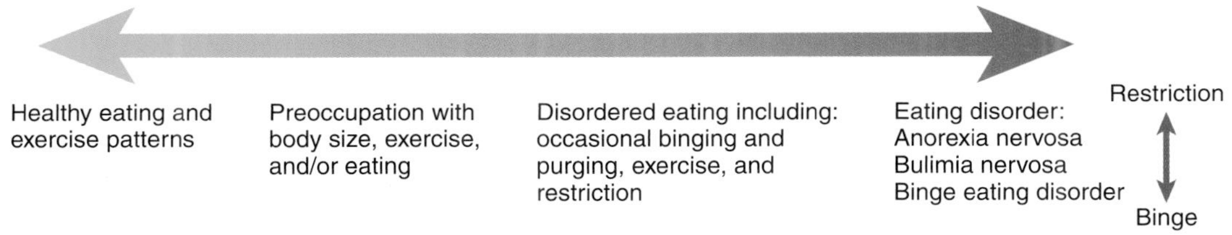

Figure 15-1. The continuum of disordered eating. Disordered eating falls on a continuum from severe restriction and anorexia nervosa to massive overeating and binge-eating disorder. While most people with disordered eating do not meet criteria for the named eating disorders, they still face severe psychological and physical consequences.

The criteria for diagnosis[4] include:

1. Eating or feeding disturbance manifested by persistent failure to meet appropriate nutritional and/or energy needs associated with one or more of the following:
   - Significant weight loss (or failure to gain weight or faltering growth in children)
   - Significant nutritional deficiency
   - Dependence on enteral feeding or nutritional supplements
   - Marked interference with psychosocial functioning
2. There is no evidence that lack of available food or an associated culturally sanctioned practice is sufficient to account for the disorder.
3. The eating disturbance does not occur exclusively during the course of anorexia nervosa or bulimia nervosa, and there is no evidence of a disturbance in the way in which one's body weight or shape is experienced.
4. The eating disturbance is not better accounted for by a concurrent medical condition or another mental disorder. When occurring in the context of another condition or disorder, the severity of the eating disturbance exceeds that routinely associated with the condition or disorder and warrants additional clinical attention.[4]

There are three main subtypes of avoidant/restrictive food intake eating disorder. The first describes individuals who do not eat enough/show little interest in eating. An example may be a child who simply refuses to eat, despite cajoling from a parent or attempted accommodation of food preferences. This pattern of avoidant intake also commonly presents in older adults. A second type describes individuals who only accept a limited diet in relation to sensory features. For example, a person may refuse to eat lumpy foods. The third type describes individuals whose food refusal is related to an aversive experience. This might occur in a person who experienced foodborne illness after consuming a particular type or types of food.

Other Eating Disorders

Importantly, just because a person may not meet the strict criteria to be diagnosed with a named eating disorder, individuals with severe dietary restriction, pervasive behaviors and thoughts about food, and subclinical forms of the mentioned disorders should trigger concern and be helped similarly to those with a diagnosed disorder. *DSM-5* categorizes these conditions as "atypical, mixed, or below-threshold conditions"; "other specific syndromes not listed in *DSM-5*"; and "insufficient information/other feeding or eating condition not elsewhere classified."

Atypical, Mixed, or Below-Threshold Conditions

A large portion of "other" eating disorder diagnoses are "subthreshold" cases of anorexia nervosa and bulimia nervosa, in which the individual meets some but not all of the necessary criteria. These conditions include:

- **Subthreshold or atypical anorexia nervosa** in which all of the criteria for anorexia nervosa are met, except that, despite significant weight loss, the individual's weight is within or above the normal range.
- **Subthreshold bulimia nervosa** in which all of the criteria for bulimia nervosa are met, except that the binge eating and inappropriate compensatory behaviors occur, on average, less than once a week and/or for fewer than 3 months.
- **Subthreshold binge-eating disorder** in which all of the criteria for binge-eating disorder are met, except that the binge eating occurs, on average, less than once a week and/or for fewer than 3 months.

Other Specific Syndromes Not Listed in *DSM-5*

Other disordered eating patterns are mentioned in *DSM-5* but diagnostic criteria are not defined or described. The specifically mentioned disorders include:

- **Purging disorder** in which a person engages in recurrent purging behavior to influence weight or shape, such as self-induced vomiting and/or misuse of laxatives, diuretics, or other medications, in the absence of binge eating.
- **Night eating syndrome** is characterized by recurrent episodes of eating after awakening from sleep or excessive food consumption after the evening meal. To have this disorder, the person must have awareness and recall of the eating, and the night eating cannot be better accounted for by external influences such as changes in the individual's sleep/wake cycle or by local social norms. The night eating is associated with significant distress and/or impairment in functioning. The person typically feels guilty and shameful during and/or after the repeated nighttime binges. The disordered pattern of eating cannot be better accounted for by binge-eating disorder, another psychiatric disorder, substance abuse or dependence, a general medical disorder, or an effect of medication.

Insufficient Information/Other Feeding or Eating Condition Not Elsewhere Classified

This is a residual category for clinically significant problems meeting the definition of a feeding or eating disorder but not satisfying the criteria for any other disorder or condition.

One emerging pattern of disordered eating that may fit this category is **orthorexia nervosa**. Although not mentioned in any diagnostic manual and barely making an appearance in the scientific literature, orthorexia nervosa has been described as a pattern of disordered eating characterized by a preoccupation with eating an extremely healthy diet.[10] First described in 1997 by an alternative medicine physician named Steven Bratman, orthorexia nervosa may start as an admirable desire to attain a state of optimal health but can evolve into a psychological crutch to exert control, escape from fears, improve self-esteem, create an identity, and search for spirituality. While not inherently undesirable, this way of eating can become problematic if a person becomes obsessive and begins to spend inordinate amounts of time thinking about food and planning meals, develops guilt with minor lapses in adherence, or uses the diet as a coping mechanism to avoid life challenges.

Signs that a person may have developed eating habits and mentality on the orthorexia nervosa spectrum include multiple yes answers to the following questions:

- Do you wish that occasionally you could just eat and not worry about food quality?
- Do you ever wish you could spend less time on food and more time on living and loving?
- Does it sound beyond your ability to eat a meal prepared with love by someone else—one single meal—and not try to control what is served?
- Are you constantly looking for the ways foods are unhealthy for you?
- Do love, joy, play, and creativity take a backseat to having the perfect diet?
- Do you feel guilt or self-loathing when you stray from your diet?
- Do you feel in control when you eat the correct diet?
- Have you positioned yourself on a nutritional pedestal and wonder how others can possibly eat the food they eat?[11]

Many people have argued that an attention to healthy eating is a positive development that more people should follow and that orthorexia nervosa is not in fact a true pathological condition (see Communication Strategies).

SPEED BUMP

1. Define and describe the signs and symptoms of the major eating disorders.

EXERCISE DISORDERS

In the pursuit to achieve an ideal body type, some people adopt severe exercise habits, which may or may not be accompanied by disordered eating patterns.

COMMUNICATION STRATEGIES

The Debate: Is a Commitment to Healthy Eating Pathological (i.e., Should Orthorexia Nervosa Be a Psychiatric Diagnosis?)

The Case

Bill is a 60-year-old man who underwent a major life transformation 10 years ago. At the age of 48, Bill's younger brother died abruptly from a heart attack. His brother was of a normal weight, but a notoriously lousy eater, frequently consuming nutrient-poor food that was high in salt and trans fat. Bill, who was overweight and sedentary at the time, decided that he needed to turn his life around so that he could see his grandchildren grow up and enjoy his retirement. He committed to eat better and be more active.

Over the years, Bill's commitment to healthy eating and exercise has become increasingly vigilant. He follows a strictly vegetarian diet and shuns processed food completely. He eats at least nine servings of fruits and vegetables every day and maintains a thriving home garden. He spends at least 60 minutes per day engaged in moderate to vigorous physical activity. He prides himself in sharing that he has not missed a day of working out for at least 30 minutes for the past 5 years. When he did miss a workout 5 years ago, he says that he felt depressed, out of energy, and developed a physical craving for exercise.

Bill has successfully maintained a weight loss of 40 pounds for the past 8 years. He takes no medications and suffers from no chronic health problems.

The Prompt

Using Bill as a case example, debate whether orthorexia nervosa should be considered a psychiatric disorder. Divide into three groups. Each group will have 15 minutes to prepare the following:

1. The first group should develop a convincing argument of why Bill is a model of health, and thus, why the condition that Bill manifests–orthorexia nervosa–should not be a clinical diagnosis.
2. The second group should develop a convincing argument of why Bill may suffer a pathological condition and thus, why orthorexia nervosa should be considered a psychiatric disorder.
3. The third group will serve as judges and should develop criteria by which to judge the presentations.

Continued

COMMUNICATION STRATEGIES—cont'd

Reconvene for the debate. Each team should select three representatives to engage in a debate. The debate will take 30 minutes. The members of each team can choose who will give: (1) the opening speech, (2) cross-examination of the other side, and (3) closing remarks. Proceed as follows:

1. Group 1 presents opening speech (5 minutes)
2. Group 2 presents opening speech (6 minutes)
3. Group 1 presents a cross-examination (6 minutes)
4. Group 2 presents a cross-examination (6 minutes)
5. Group 1 provides closing argument (3 minutes)
6. Group 2 provides closing argument (4 minutes)

The judges have 5 minutes to ask questions. Each judge then places a vote. Tally the numbers to choose a winning team.

Muscle Dysmorphic Disorder

While people with anorexia nervosa and sometimes bulimia nervosa engage in excessive amounts of exercise in an effort to lose weight and achieve an elusive state of thinness, people with **muscle dysmorphic disorder** engage in excessive amounts of resistance training in an effort to be muscular and "big." Similar to people with anorexia nervosa and bulimia nervosa, people with muscle dysmorphic disorder are preoccupied with their bodies—and their perceived imperfections. Bodybuilders have long recognized this disorder, which they term "bigorexia" and "reverse anorexia."[12] One study of 85 competitive and 48 noncompetitive weight-training athletes found that those athletes at greatest risk of muscle dysmorphia were most likely to be male competitive athletes focused on strength training to improve appearance.[13]

Muscle dysmorphic disorder is a subcategory of the general category of **body dysmorphic disorder** in *DSM-5*. Body dysmorphic disorder is diagnosed when the following criteria are met:[4]

1. Preoccupation with one or more perceived defects or flaws in physical appearance that are not observable or appear slight to others.
2. At some point during the course of the disorder, the person has performed repetitive behaviors (e.g., mirror checking, excessive grooming, skin picking, or reassurance seeking) or mental acts (e.g., comparing their appearance with that of others) in response to the appearance concerns.
3. The preoccupations cause clinically significant distress or impairment in social, occupational, or other important areas of functioning.
4. The preoccupations are not attributable to another medical condition.
5. The appearance preoccupations are not better accounted for by concerns with body fat or weight in an eating disorder.

DSM-5 allows a psychiatrist to specify if the person has the muscle dysmorphia form of body dysmorphic disorder, which is described as the belief that one's body build is too small or is insufficiently muscular.

Approximately 100,000 people, mostly men, meet the formal criteria for muscle dysmorphic disorder.[14] The health risks associated with muscle dysmorphic disorder are substantial. One study comparing men with muscle dysmorphic disorder versus men with other forms of body dysmorphic disorder found that those with muscle dysmorphic disorder were more likely to lift weights excessively (71% versus 12%), diet (71% versus 27%), exercise excessively (64% versus 10%), experience poorer quality of life, attempt suicide (50% versus 16%), and have or develop a substance abuse disorder (86% versus 51%), including anabolic steroid abuse (21% versus 0%).[12] In fact, muscle dysmorphic disorder is known to be a substantial risk factor for anabolic steroid use.[15]

Exercise Dependence

Exercise dependence describes the condition in which a person is preoccupied with exercise and training to the extent that the person engages in excessive levels of exercise, resulting in negative physiological and psychological consequences.[16] This condition has also been termed exercise addiction, excessive exercise, obligatory exercise, compulsive exercise, and exercise abuse.

Exercise dependence is not an official diagnosis listed in *DSM-5*, but could fit into the *DSM-5* category of "behavioral addiction" (though gambling is the only behavioral addiction specifically described in the manual). *DSM-5* criteria for substance dependence may be adapted to better describe exercise dependence and provide a meaningful way to differentiate an avid exerciser from a person with an unhealthy obsession. The following criteria adapted from the criteria to diagnose other forms of addiction were proposed by researchers Hausenblaus and Downs:[17]

- **Tolerance**: increasing the amount of exercise in order to feel the desired effect, be it a "buzz" or sense of accomplishment.

- **Withdrawal:** in the absence of exercise the person experiences negative effects such as anxiety, irritability, restlessness, and sleep problems.
- **Lack of control:** unsuccessful attempts to reduce exercise level or cease exercising for a certain period of time.
- **Intention effects:** unable to stick to one's intended routine, as evidenced by exceeding the amount of time devoted to exercise or consistently going beyond the intended amount.
- **Time:** a great deal of time is spent preparing for, engaging in, and recovering from exercise.
- **Reduction in other activities:** as a direct result of exercise, social, occupational, and/or recreational activities occur less often or are stopped.
- **Continuance:** continuing to exercise despite knowing that this activity is creating or worsening physical, psychological, and/or interpersonal problems.

About 3% of the general population suffers from exercise dependence.[18] Studies suggest that rates among certain groups such as ultramarathoners,[19] sports science students,[20] and other recreational and elite athletes are much higher.[21] For example, in one study of Parisian fitness club members, over 42% of the members met the criteria for exercise dependence.[22] In a study of elite Australian athletes, researchers found that 34% of the athletes met the criteria. These athletes had a higher body mass index, more extreme and maladaptive exercise beliefs, higher reported pressure from coaches and teammates, and lower social support compared to the athletes without exercise dependence.[21] Many studies have found that exercise dependence is associated with perfectionism, obsessive-compulsiveness, and anxiety; it is indirectly related to self-esteem.[16]

Exercise dependence presents in two forms: (1) primary exercise dependence, which results when a person participates in excessive amounts of physical activity due to the craving for exercise and its accompanying physiological and psychological effects, and (2) secondary exercise dependence, in which a person exercises excessively to achieve some other means, such as weight loss in a person with an eating disorder[23] (Box 15-2).

Box 15-2. A Case Study: Did Ultramarathoner Micah True Suffer From Exercise Dependence?

Micah True, the real-life character in Christopher McDougall's best-selling book *Born to Run*, was a renowned ultrarunner from Boulder, Colorado. True lived an adventurous and exotic life—his life story includes days filled with activities such as cave dwelling near sacred shrines in Hawaii and years-long sabbaticals to places like remote northwestern Mexico, where he lived in an adobe hut and logged 5,000 miles of running per year.

True developed his passion for running as an adult. After a failed relationship, he turned to trail running to find solace. He traveled around the world to experience grueling 100-mile plus runs where he engaged with the local people and explored nature. He described himself "as a trail-running bum," similar to a surfing bum or a climbing bum. In a *Washington Post* article, McDougall explained ". . . when you get him out for a run, his entire personality transformed. He ran with a smile on his face."[39]

True, who was 58 years old, was last seen alive in late March 2012 when he left for a 12-mile run in the Gila National Forest in New Mexico, a pit stop on a road trip to Phoenix. Five days later he was found dead with his legs dangling in a stream. Though the autopsy was inconclusive, True was found to have idiopathic cardiomyopathy, an enlargement and dysfunction of the heart that occurred for an unknown reason. The autopsy report noted that True did not have a regular physician and studies such as an electrocardiogram or blood pressure readings were unavailable. They concluded that his cardiomyopathy likely caused a cardiac arrhythmia during exercise that led to his death.[39]

Question

Do you believe Micah True suffered from exercise dependence? Identify the characteristics of True that would support your opinion.

SPEED BUMP

2. Define the major exercise disorders.

ATHLETES: A VULNERABLE POPULATION FOR EATING AND EXERCISE DISORDERS

Athletes face pressure to excel in their sport. Many times the opportunity for maximal performance corresponds to the achievement and maintenance of a certain body size, especially in high-intensity sports or those that focus on aesthetics, such as figure skating, gymnastics, running, swimming, and wrestling. The pressure to attain a certain body size may cause the athlete to become preoccupied with food and eating, leading to restriction of food.

Anorexia Athletica

Anorexia athletica was first described in the early 1990s by researchers who recognized the increased rates of eating disorder-like traits among athletes.[26] The term came to refer to a below-threshold eating disorder mostly affecting competitive athletes in sports that value low body weight, such as ski jumping, road cycling, climbing, gymnastics, and long-distance running,[24] and is typically associated with excessive exercise.

The definition and diagnosis of anorexia athletica are not consistent, well described, or mentioned in *DSM-5*. However, athletes with anorexia athletica tend to have many of the following characteristics:[25,26]

1. Intense fear of gaining weight or becoming "fat" even though he or she is at least 5% below expected body weight.
2. Low weight attained through excessive exercising, caloric restriction, or both.
3. Binging, self-induced vomiting, and/or use of laxatives or diuretics.
4. High achievement orientation, perfectionism, and obsessive-compulsive tendencies

While the research aimed at understanding rates of anorexia athletica is limited, studies suggest that about 6% of female athletes in aesthetic sports meet clinical criteria for the disorder.[27,28]

Female Athlete Triad

Participation in ample physical activity and consumption of a nutrient-dense and healthful diet are defining features of a healthy lifestyle. Oftentimes athletes are the model citizens of excellent health. However, a sizeable number of athletes have taken healthful habits to an extreme such that they become pathological and detrimental to overall health and well-being. Whether done inadvertently or purposefully, approximately 25% of elite female athletes in endurance sports, aesthetic sports, and weight-class sports suffer from disordered eating and some variation of the **female athlete triad**.[27]

The female athlete triad is characterized by amenorrhea (at least 3 months without a menstrual period), **osteoporosis** (weakened bones and increased risk of fracture), and disordered eating. The path from optimal health to full manifestation of the triad exists along a continuum (Fig. 15-2). The triad results when an athlete burns more calories than she consumes, creating a state of decreased **energy availability.** This can happen when an athlete increases her physical activity without appropriately increasing caloric intake or if she restricts her caloric intake. When this happens, the body attempts to restore energy balance by using less energy for growth, reproduction, and various other important body functions. Menstruation halts and hormonal imbalance ensues, which often leads to decreased bone strength and increased risk of fracture.

Athletes at highest risk for low energy availability are those who restrict caloric intake, exercise for prolonged periods, are vegetarian, and limit the types of foods that they eat. In fact, dieting is widely considered to be a precursor to disordered eating. Athletes at highest risk for dieting behaviors tend to include early start of sport-specific training, sudden increase in training volume, traumatic events such as injury or loss of a coach, and a host of other environmental and social factors including low self-esteem, family dysfunction, abuse, personality, and genetics.[29] Evaluating the Evidence features

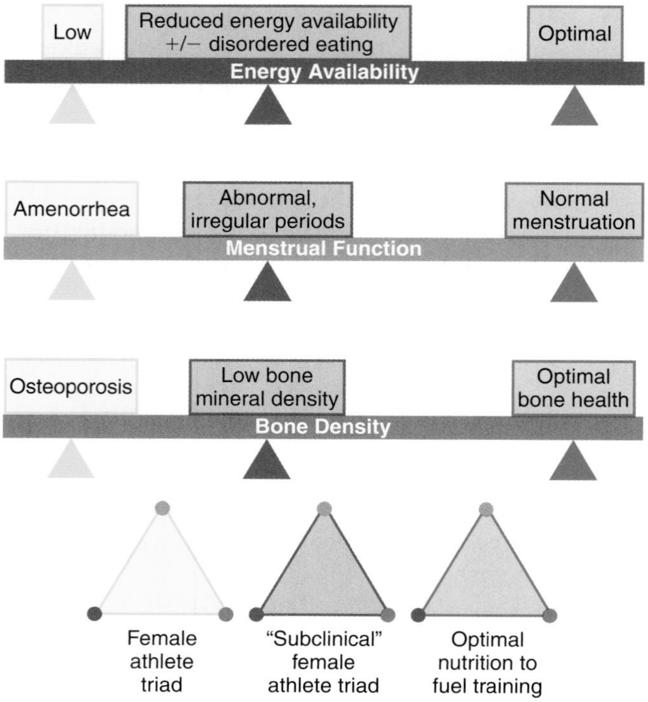

Figure 15-2. The female athlete triad exists on a continuum. The female athlete triad consists of decreased energy availability, which leads to amenorrhea and osteoporosis. However, the condition is not "all or nothing." Many athletes exhibit parts of the female athlete triad or subclinical forms of the triad. This figure shows the continuum of each component of the triad in isolation (the three sets of straight lines) and then in combination (the three joined triangles).

the American College of Sports Medicine's position statement on the female athlete triad to describe the purpose, benefits, and cautions of position statements issued by professional organizations.

SPEED BUMP

3. Define the female athlete triad and its consequences on health and performance.

Weight Cycling

Certain athletes in sports that require frequent weigh-ins and weight qualifications to compete in a particular weight class are at risk for **weight cycling.** Weight cycling refers to rapid fluctuations in weight, which can be due to fluid restriction and use of diuretics and other efforts to lose weight through decreased body water, or restrictive dieting, which can lead to large weight losses that are rapidly regained when the restriction stops.

While the research on weight cycling in athletes is limited and dated, several studies have attempted to evaluate performance and health risks and benefits from this practice.[30-33] Most of the studies focus on wrestlers, a particularly high-risk population for weight cycling due to the requirement that athletes weigh-in

EVALUATING THE EVIDENCE

The Position Stand

The American College of Sports Medicine published a position stand on the female athlete triad.[29] A committee of six people with advanced degrees in medicine, nutrition, and exercise science and who are recognized experts in their fields drafted the statement, the aim of which was to provide recommendations for primary care professionals on the screening, diagnosis, prevention, and treatment of "the triad."

Each clinical recommendation in the position paper is followed with a statement on the strength of the scientific evidence, which informed the statement. The recommendations are graded as an A, B, or C:

A. Consistent and good quality evidence for clinical outcomes on mortality, morbidity, symptoms, cost, and quality of life.
B. Inconsistent or limited quality of evidence for clinical outcomes on mortality, morbidity, symptoms, cost, and quality of life.
C. C1: evidence based on biochemical, histological, physiological, and pathophysiological outcomes; or C2: evidence based on case studies, consensus, usual practice, and opinion.

Table 15-1 restates several of the clinical recommendations of this paper along with the ratings of evidence.

Table 15-1. Female Athlete Triad Recommendations and Evidence

STATEMENT	CLINICAL EVIDENCE RATING
Clinical Recommendations for Screening and Diagnosis	
Screening for the triad should occur at the preparticipation exam or annual health screening exam	C2
Athletes with one component of the triad should be assessed for the others	C2
Athletes with disordered dieting should be referred to a mental health practitioner for evaluation, diagnosis, and treatment	C2
To diagnose functional hypothalamic amenorrhea, other causes of amenorrhea must be excluded	B
Bone mineral density should be assessed after a stress or low impact fracture and after a total of 6 months of amenorrhea, oligomenorrhea (menstrual cycles longer than 35 days), or disordered eating or eating disorders	C2
Clinical Recommendations for Treatment	
Multidisciplinary treatment for the triad disorders should include a physician (or other health-care professional), a registered dietitian, and for athletes with disordered eating or eating disorders, a mental health practitioner	C2
The first aim of treatment is to increase energy availability by increasing energy intake and/or reducing energy expenditure	C1
Athletes without eating disorders or disordered eating should be referred for nutritional counseling	C2
Athletes practicing restrictive eating behaviors should be counseled that increases in body weight may be necessary to increase bone mineral density	C1
Treatment of eating disorders and disordered dieting includes nutritional counseling and individual psychotherapy; cognitive behavioral, group therapy, and/or family therapy may also be used	B
Athletes with disordered eating or eating disorders who do not comply with treatment may need to be restricted from training and competition	C2

Continued

Continued

EVALUATING THE EVIDENCE–cont'd

Table 15-1. Female Athlete Triad Recommendations and Evidence–cont'd

STATEMENT	CLINICAL EVIDENCE RATING
Oral contraceptives should be considered in an athlete with amenorrhea over age 16 if bone mineral density is decreasing with nonpharmacological management, despite adequate nutrition and body weight	C2

CRITICAL THINKING QUESTIONS:

What are the strengths and limitations of organizational position stands?

Which of the statements in Table 15-1 are directly relevant to the health professions field you plan to choose? Why might a health professional choose to follow or not follow recommendations from a position stand?

Most of the evidence ratings for the statements in Table 15-1 are in the C category. Why do you think that there is not more A-level evidence?

prior to competition. A wrestler who does not "make weight" will be disqualified or must wrestle at a higher weight class. As a result of this high pressure to achieve a certain weight, wrestlers aggressively attempt to ensure qualification in their weight class. Historically, the most common strategy has been active and passive dehydration. **Active dehydration** results from increasing exercise and heat exposure, and **passive dehydration** results from fluid and food restriction. This focus on cutting weight in the days to hours prior to competition negatively impacts a wrestler's ability to ingest sufficient carbohydrates and gradually taper exercise intensity—two essential components for optimal performance.[33] In an effort to curb these unsafe weight-cutting strategies, organizations such as the National Collegiate Athletic Association (NCAA) have established several rules for wrestlers, including that an athlete compete at or above his or her "certified" weight and that specific gravity of urine be checked when establishing a wrestler's certified weight classification.

In studies of the general population, most of whom are overweight and sedentary, weight cycling has been linked to high blood pressure, high cholesterol, gallbladder disease, long-term weight gain, and increased depression.[34] However, these studies are not conclusive and any long-term effects are not well described or understood. Furthermore, the long-term effects of weight cycling on athletes are, for the most part, unknown.

Adipositas Athletica

A minority of athletes strive to gain fat mass to increase their competitiveness in their sport. Recently, researchers have coined the term **adipositas athletica** to describe athletes who try to gain body fat to increase insulation or increase body energy stores.[35] For example, open-water long-distance swimmers need at least 25% body fat to protect them against hypothermia and its associated compromise in muscular strength and efficiency. Other less-conventional athletes such as transcontinental skiers strive to put on fat mass to sustain an ample supply of energy to fuel the extreme expedition. Some athletes do not purposefully want to gain fat mass, but they overall just want to get "bigger," whether the increased mass comes from muscle or fat is not necessarily important to them. This is known as **secondary adipositas athletica**. These athletes may participate in sports that value massive body size such as sumo wrestling, football linemen, and martial arts, where there is no upper limit to the highest weight class. While a large body mass may prove beneficial for the short-term, the long-term complications can be severe (see the section on obesity in Chapter 12).

PREVENTING EATING AND EXERCISE DISORDERS IN HIGH-RISK POPULATIONS

Health professionals who work with young people, athletes, and others at risk for eating disorders play a critically important role in helping to prevent the onset of an obsession with weight, body image, and exercise. Special considerations for adolescents, a particularly vulnerable population, are noted in Box 15-3. Athletes, especially those in weight-conscious sports, also are at high risk for the development of disordered eating patterns.

The National Eating Disorders Association (www.nationaleatingdisorders.org) offers the following tips

Box 15-3. Adolescents and Eating Disorders

The majority of eating disorders affect adolescents—the stage in normal growth and development when the effects of eating disorders are most severe and disruptive. An adolescent athlete who severely restricts caloric intake is at high risk of suffering long-term physiological consequences from low energy availability for growth, menstruation, and development of peak bone mass. The psychological factors contributing to the development of eating disorders and as a consequence of chronic malnutrition and the typical secrecy that accompanies the disorder increase a teen's risk of long-term mental health problems, poor school performance, impaired relationships with friends and family, and self-injurious behavior.[3] However, with long-term treatment and therapy, the prognosis of eating disorders is much better for teenagers than adults. In one study of 95 people who had been hospitalized for anorexia nervosa as adolescents and were followed for 10 to 15 years, over 85% had achieved partial or complete recovery, and none had died. But the median time to partial recovery was nearly 5 years. Full recovery occurred for most after around 6.5 years.[38]

Health professionals who work with teenage athletes will most certainly encounter clients who suffer from signs and symptoms of eating disorders. It is essential to be prepared in advance for the appropriate action steps to get the teenager needed treatment and services. The American Academy of Pediatrics encourages pediatricians to keep several considerations in mind when working with adolescent clients.[3] These considerations, adapted to fit within the scope of practice of an allied health professional, are presented below:

- Allied health professionals need to be knowledgeable about risk factors, signs, and symptoms of disordered eating and eating disorders.
- When discussing with clients how to avoid or treat obesity or how to best control weight, allied health professionals should focus on healthy eating and building self-esteem in addition to controlling weight. Allied health professionals should not inadvertently encourage, endorse, or enable excessive dieting or exercise or other potentially harmful strategies used to control weight.
- Allied health professionals should refer any adolescent with concern for disordered eating or eating disorders to his or her pediatrician or primary health-care provider for a physical. The physician will plot height, weight, and BMI using gender- and age-appropriate growth charts. The physician will also assess menstrual status in girls. If concern is high for an eating disorder, the provider may initiate treatment or refer the patient for nutritional and mental health therapy.
- Allied health professionals can play a role in prevention of disordered eating and eating disorders with a focus on education, early screening, and advocacy.
- Allied health professionals should advocate for legislation and policy changes to ensure access to medical, mental health, nutritional, and care coordination for adolescents with disordered eating.

for coaches and health and fitness professionals to help prevent eating disorders:

1. De-emphasize weight. Do not weigh clients. Eliminate comments about weight, especially with those individuals you believe may be at risk for an eating disorder.
2. Do not assume that reducing body fat or weight will improve performance.
3. Help others recognize the signs of eating disorders and how to address them.
4. Provide accurate information about weight, weight loss, body composition, nutrition, and sports performance. Have a broad network of referrals (such as registered dietitians and physicians) who may also be able to help educate clients when appropriate.
5. Emphasize the health risks of low weight, especially for female athletes with menstrual irregularities (in which case, referral to a physician, preferably one who specializes in eating disorders, is warranted).
6. Avoid making any derogatory comments about weight or body composition, regardless to whom the comments are directed.
7. Do not curtail athletic performance and gym privileges to an athlete or client who is found to have eating problems unless medically necessary. Consider the athlete's physical and emotional health and self-image when deciding how to modify exercise participation level.
8. Strive to promote a positive self-image and self-esteem in clients and athletes. Carefully assess personal assumptions and beliefs.

Given the higher prevalence of eating disorders in athletes, the prevention of eating disorders among athletes requires increased vigilance. Some ways that health professionals can help to prevent eating disorders among athletes with whom they work include:

- Providing an annual education program to all athletes about the risks of disordered eating and how to adopt a healthful approach to eating and weight management

- Avoiding telling an athlete to lose weight
- Encouraging an athlete in a weight-class sport to gain strength to compete at a higher weight level if unhealthy nutrition and health practices are otherwise necessary to meet weight
- Providing education about the side effects and performance risks of undereating (such as fatigue, anemia, electrolyte imbalances, and depression)
- Providing an appropriate referral for athletes who are overweight or obese and who require healthy weight loss
- Avoiding weighing athletes for non-health-related issues
- Discouraging dieting
- Referring early to an appropriate health and nutrition professional for athletes who demonstrate concerning thoughts or behaviors around food and eating.[1,36]

SCREENING AND IDENTIFICATION OF CLIENTS WITH EATING AND EXERCISE DISORDERS

Most health professionals work with active, health conscious individuals on a daily basis and, as a result, may be instrumental in identifying, confronting, and referring clients who show signs or symptoms of an eating or exercise disorder. As such, health professionals should assess for eating and exercise disorders through a systematic screening process. This could include conducting an annual questionnaire with athletes such as the SCOFF questionnaire,[37] asking pertinent nutrition and physical activity-related questions, and carefully monitoring for symptoms of disordered eating or exercise. Questions focus on the client's attitudes and behaviors related to eating and exercise; for example, if the client has lost a significant amount of weight in the last 3 months, makes herself vomit if she feels overly full, believes she looks fat when she is thin, uses laxatives or other medications to try to lose weight, or overexercises to control weight. Those clients who demonstrate signs of disordered eating or exercise should be sensitively confronted by the health professional with the best rapport with the individual.

One approach to confronting clients who appear to be at risk for an eating disorder is aptly called the CONFRONT approach, which is highlighted in Box 15-4. When planning this confrontation, keep in mind the following "don'ts": *don't* oversimplify; *don't* diagnose; *don't* become the person's therapist; *don't* provide exercise advice without first helping the individual get professional help; and *don't* get into a battle of wills if the person denies having a problem.

Box 15-4. The Plan: CONFRONT, From the National Association of Anorexia Nervosa and Associated Disorders

Confronting an individual with a suspected eating disorder is a challenging, sensitive, and potentially volatile undertaking. In addition to the concern that the person may get angry, deny that there is a problem (and perhaps there really is not a problem?), or distance himself or herself, many people struggle to find the right words and approach to be perceived as helpful rather than antagonistic and paternalistic. To help when first approaching someone with a suspected eating disorder, the National Association of Anorexia Nervosa and Associated Disorders advocates a strategy called CONFRONT:[40]

C—Concern. Share that the reason you are approaching the individual is because you care about his or her mental, physical, and nutritional needs.

O—Organize. Prepare for the confrontation. Think about who will be involved, where is the best place, the reason for the concern, the best approach to talk to the person, and the most appropriate time.

N—Needs. What will the individual need after the confrontation? Have referrals to professional help and/or support groups available should the individual be ready to seek help.

F—Face the confrontation. Be empathetic, but direct. Be persistent if the individual denies having a problem.

R—Respond by listening carefully.

O—Offer help and suggestions. Be available to talk and provide other assistance when needed.

N—Negotiate another time to talk and timeframe in which to seek professional help, preferably from a physician who specializes in eating disorders.

T—Time. Remember that the individual will not change immediately. Recovery takes time and patience.

The most important "next step" after confronting a client who demonstrates signs or symptoms of an eating or exercise disorder is referral to the client's physician for evaluation, diagnosis, and treatment. Treatment options may range from regular follow-ups with the primary care physician, dietitian, and mental health professional to intensive day-therapy programs and inpatient hospitalization on an eating disorder ward for the most severe cases. Most individuals with eating disorders eventually recover, though the process is long and intense. One study followed 95 people who were hospitalized for anorexia nervosa as adolescents for 10 to 15 years. The median time to partial recovery was 57 months, while the median time to full recovery was 79 months.[38]

TRAINING A CLIENT WITH AN EXERCISE OR EATING DISORDER

In addition to being a source of help and empathy, health professionals—in particular exercise professionals—can play an important role in developing or implementing structured exercise programs for people recovering from eating and exercise disorders who have already sought help from a qualified medical professional. An important first step is to develop a partnership with the client's treating physician. Seek medical clearance and general recommendations from the client's treating physician regarding the maximal duration and intensity of exercise. Note that individuals with a BMI of less than 20 may not receive clearance to exercise until they gain a specified amount of weight. When working with the client, emphasize the positive psychological and health benefits of appropriate exercise and minimize focus on appearance and weight. As with all clients, strive to develop a balanced and well-rounded program that includes cardiovascular training, resistance training, and flexibility exercises. The goal is to help the client learn how to exercise in moderation. Some programs for individuals with eating disorders will use activities such as yoga and tai chi, with the goal of helping clients to relax.

A physician and sports dietitian are particularly important members of the treatment team for an athlete who suffers from an eating disorder. The physician will carefully assess the athlete's current health status and risk of negative health outcome from continued competition. The sports dietitian will provide a nutritional assessment and a meal plan. Together the physician, dietitian, and ideally an exercise professional, will develop eating and exercise recommendations and a mental health professional will provide psychological treatment. Generally accepted criteria for the return to play after diagnosis and during treatment of an eating disorder for competitive athletes include:

- Being in treatment, complying with the treatment plan, and progressing toward treatment goals
- Maintaining a weight of at least 90% of ideal body weight with a body fat percentage of at least 6% for male athletes and 12% for female athletes, or more
- Eating sufficient calories to comply with the treatment plan

SPEED BUMP

4. Identify risk factors for developing an eating or exercise disorder.
5. Describe strategies to prevent eating and exercise disorders in high-risk populations.
6. Develop a sensitive and effective approach to confronting clients with a suspected eating or exercise disorder.

CHAPTER SUMMARY

Food and exercise for people with eating and exercise disorders take on more meaning than a necessity to nourish one's body or an activity to improve fitness, health, and quality of life. At worst, they become players in a physical and psychological war of control, compulsion, and disordered thinking. But once a problem has been identified, accepted, and evaluated by a trained medical professional, the qualified health professional can play a critical role in helping a person with an eating or exercise disorder to develop a positive and healthy relationship with food and physical activity. Just as importantly, health professionals have a unique vantage point for identifying the early course and progression of eating and exercise disorders. And perhaps, through their words and their actions, health professionals may help prevent some of them from developing.

KEY POINTS SUMMARY

1. *DSM-5* describes several classes of eating disorders including anorexia nervosa, bulimia nervosa, binge-eating disorder, avoidant/restrictive food intake, and "Other Eating Disorders/Eating Disorders Not Otherwise Specified." *DSM-5* outlines strict criteria a physician must use to diagnose these disorders. Any professional working with a person who demonstrates signs of an eating disorder should refer that person to a qualified health professional for further evaluation and treatment.
2. Muscle dysmorphic disorder is a subcategory of body dysmorphic disorder, and, in addition to several diagnostic criteria, is characterized by an individual engaging in excessive amounts of resistance training in an effort to become larger. Individuals with this disorder perceive themselves as too small or insufficiently muscular.
3. Exercise dependence is not an official diagnosis; however, it could be classified as a behavioral addiction. Exercise dependence describes the condition in which a person is preoccupied with exercise and training to the extent that the person engages in excessive levels of exercise, resulting in negative physiological and psychological consequences.[16]
4. Anorexia athletica is a sport-induced subclinical eating disorder in which an athlete has all of the following characteristics: (1) weight loss (a loss of >5% of expected body weight); (2) gastrointestinal complaints; (3) absence of medical illness or mood disorder (such as depression) explaining weight reduction; (4) excessive fear of becoming obese; and (5) restriction of caloric intake (<1,200 kcal per day). In addition, the athlete must have one of the following: (1) delayed puberty; (2) menstrual dysfunction; (3) disturbance in body

image; (4) use of purging methods; (5) binge eating; and (6) compulsive exercise.

5. The female athlete triad is a set of three conditions that can occur in female athletes: amenorrhea, osteoporosis, and disordered eating.
6. Weight cycling refers to the practice by some athletes of rapidly losing and regaining weight. They generally rapidly lose weight to qualify for a particular weight class and then regain it right after the weigh-in.
7. Health professionals play an important role in the prevention of and screening for eating and exercise disorders. If after screening for an eating disorder, such as using the SCOFF questionnaire, an individual is believed to have an eating disorder, he or she should be sensitively confronted by the health professional with the best rapport with the individual, using an approach such as the CONFRONT approach, and referred to his or her physician for further evaluation and treatment.

PRACTICAL APPLICATIONS

1. After working with a new client for several sessions, you notice that she is very focused on her weight, and you are growing concerned that she has an eating disorder due to stories she tells you about binge eating, excessive exercise following binges, and jokes about "purging." Which of the following steps would be most appropriate for a fitness professional to take with this client?
   A. Inform her that she has an eating disorder and will need a physician's referral before you can continue working with her.
   B. Design a program that helps her decrease body fat to direct her focus toward body-composition changes instead of weight loss.
   C. Express how much you care about the client and your concern that she may have an eating disorder, recommend that she meet with her physician for evaluation and guidance; and offer to be there for her
   D. Show empathy by discussing healthful eating strategies and implementing an exercise routine that will help her reach her weight-loss goals in a safe and effective manner.
2. After 3 months of training, your client has achieved rapid weight loss, is now borderline underweight, and appears increasingly concerned with her body weight and appearance. Which of the following disorders is most likely to be associated with this type of behavior?
   A. Bulimia nervosa
   B. Binge-eating disorder
   C. Anorexia nervosa
   D. Muscle dysmorphia
3. Julie, an exercise physiology undergraduate student, recently suffered a stress fracture in her left foot. She has been training to run a marathon for the past 3 months. During her doctor's visit to evaluate the fracture, her doctor expressed concern she may have an eating disorder. Which of the following conditions does Julie most likely have?
   A. Bulimia nervosa
   B. Anorexia adipositas
   C. Anorexia athletica
   D. Female athlete triad
4. Tricia exercises excessively in order to counteract the effects of what she perceives as eating too many calories on a daily basis. With which of the following conditions is this type of behavior associated?
   A. Primary exercise dependence
   B. Secondary exercise dependence
   C. Anorexia athletica
   D. Muscle dysmorphic disorder
5. A person who is undergoing treatment for an eating disorder is MOST likely to be encouraged to perform which of the following types of exercise in his or her treatment plan?
   A. Yoga
   B. Dance
   C. Circuit training
   D. Weight lifting
6. Rachel has worked her way up from a body mass index (BMI) of 16 to 18. She has undergone treatment from her physician, registered dietitian, and therapist to cope with anorexia nervosa. In general, what BMI value will Rachel have to achieve before she is allowed to begin exercise training again?
   A. 19
   B. 20
   C. 22
   D. 23
7. Which type of disorder presents with no definitive physical cues, yet might be a common condition in clients who seek out help from health professionals?
   A. Anorexia nervosa
   B. Bulimia nervosa
   C. Binge-eating disorder
   D. Avoidant eating disorder
8. Last year, Mike lost 25 pounds through eating healthy and exercising and is now in the best shape of his life. Lately, Mike's friends have commented on his preoccupation with eating an extremely healthy diet, mentioning that he doesn't have time for them anymore because it seems he is solely focused on shopping for and preparing his meals. Mike might be categorized as suffering from what condition?
   A. Orthorexia nervosa
   B. Anorexia nervosa
   C. Bulimia nervosa
   D. Restrictive eating disorder

9. What condition is most closely associated with an athlete who desires a gain in body fat mass in order to have a competitive edge in his or her sport?
   A. Anorexia athletica
   B. Orthorexia athletica
   C. Adipositas athletica
   D. Exercise dependence

10. Which of the following eating disorders is known to be the deadliest?
    A. Anorexia nervosa
    B. Bulimia nervosa
    C. Binge-eating disorder
    D. Muscle dysmorphic disorder

Case 1 Brian, the High School Basketball Player

Brian is a 15-year-old high school basketball player. He is 6′2″ and 180 pounds. Several months ago, Brian's mother pointed out to him that he needs to eat better. Around the same time, his coach told him that if he wants to play basketball in college, he has to drop at least 20 pounds. Brian took this feedback to heart and started to eat a healthier diet. He enjoyed the feeling of eating healthy and became increasingly concerned about calories, fat grams, and developed the habit of weighing himself daily. In the past 6 months, Brian has lost 25 pounds.

1. What risk factors does Brian demonstrate for developing an eating disorder?
2. What further information would you like to know about Brian and his eating and activity behaviors?
3. If you were Brian's coach, would you be concerned about Brian's behaviors? If so, how would you address your concerns? If not, why are you reassured?
4. How are eating disorders in males different than eating disorders in females?
5. What are several special considerations in teenagers with signs of disordered eating?

Case 2 Kate, the Marathon Runner

Kate is an experienced 22-year-old marathon runner who trained intensively to qualify for the Boston Marathon and successfully set a new personal record at a qualifying marathon 1 month ago. She will run the Boston Marathon in 3 months. Over the course of her training, Kate inadvertently lost about 15 pounds. She says she thinks it is because she religiously committed to a physical fitness program and after workouts never felt that hungry. She says that she would get home from a long day of work, which was followed by a training run, and at least two or three times per week, go right to bed with a small post-exercise snack but without dinner. She comes to you today as her coach and confides in you that her weight loss and feeling of guilt when she misses a workout is starting to concern her and she would like to get some help.

1. List at least four reasons that you are concerned about Kate's story. List at least four facts from Kate's story that are reassuring.
2. What disordered eating and/or exercise patterns are possibilities for Kate, based on this scenario? Based on the information presented, does Kate meet criteria for the diagnosis of any eating or exercise disorders? What further information would you like to know?
3. What is your next step in helping Kate?

TRAIN YOURSELF

1. Of the various disordered eating and exercise patterns described in the chapter, do you have or have you ever had any of the risk factors or meet criteria for any of the disorders? If yes, what did you do about it?
   * Note: If you feel you may currently be suffering from any of the eating or exercise disorders presented in this chapter, please seek help from your physician or other trusted and qualified medical professional.
2. Have you ever had to confront a friend, colleague, or client who you suspected had an eating disorder? If yes, describe your experience and lessons learned. If no, how do you think you would respond to having to confront someone who you suspect may have an eating disorder? What might be some challenges you could experience?

REFERENCES

1. Sundgot-Borgen J, Torstveit MK. Aspects of disordered eating continuum in elite high-intensity sports. *Scand J Med Sci Sports*. October 2010;20 Suppl 2:112-121.
2. Arcelus J, Mitchell AJ, Wales J, Nielsen S. Mortality rates in patients with anorexia nervosa and other eating disorders. A meta-analysis of 36 studies. *Arch Gen Psych*. July 2011;68(7):724-731.
3. Rosen DS. Identification and management of eating disorders in children and adolescents. *Pediatrics*. December 2010; 126(6):1240-1253.
4. American Psychiatric Association. *Diagnostic and Statistical Manual of Mental Disorders* (5th ed.) Washington, D.C.: Author; 2013.

5. American Psychiatric Association. *Diagnostic and Statistical Manual of Mental Disorders* (4th ed., text rev). Washington, DC: Author; 2000.
6. Yager J, Andersen AE. Clinical practice. Anorexia nervosa. *N Engl J Med.* October 6 2005;353(14):1481-1488.
7. Hudson JI, Hiripi E, Pope HG, Jr., Kessler RC. The prevalence and correlates of eating disorders in the National Comorbidity Survey Replication. *Biol Psych.* February 1 2007;61(3):348-358.
8. Wonderlich SA, Gordon KH, Mitchell JE, Crosby RD, Engel SG. The validity and clinical utility of binge eating disorder. *Int J Eat Disord.* December 2009;42(8):687-705.
9. Corsica JA, Pelchat ML. Food addiction: true or false? *Curr Opin Gastroenterol.* March 2010;26(2):165-169.
10. Bratman S. *The Orthorexia Home Page.* www.orthorexia.com; 2003.
11. Kratina K. Orthorexia nervosa. *National Eating Disorders Association;* 2006.
12. Pope CG, Pope HG, Menard W, et al. Clinical features of muscle dysmorphia among males with body dysmorphic disorder. *Body Image: Int J Res.* 2005;2(4):395-400.
13. Skemp KM, Mikat RP, Schnenck KP, Kramer N. Muscle dysmorphia: risk may be influenced by goals of the weight lifter. *J Strength Cond Res.* 2013 January 8 [Epub ahead of print].
14. Leone JE, Sedory EJ, Gray KA. Recognition and treatment of muscle dysmorphia and related body image disorders. *J Athl Train.* October-December 2005;40(4):352-359.
15. Pope HG, Kanayama G, Hudson JI. Risk factors for illicit anabolic-androgenic steroid use in male weightlifters: a cross-sectional cohort study. *Biol Psych.* 2012; 71(3):254-261.
16. Hausenblas HA, Giacobbi PR. Relationship between exercise dependence symptoms and personality. *Pers Ind Diff.* 2004;36:1265-1273.
17. Hausenblas HA, Downs DS. How much is too much? The development and validation of the Exercise Dependence Scale. *Psych Health.* 2002;17:387-404.
18. Sussman S, Lisha N, Griffiths M. Prevalence of the addictions: a problem of the majority or the minority? *Eval Health Prof.* March 2011;34(1):3-56.
19. NIH conference. Gastrointestinal surgery for severe obesity. Consensus Development Conference Panel. *Ann Intern Med.* December 15 1991;115(12):956-961.
20. Griffiths MD, Szabo A, Terry A. The exercise addiction inventory: a quick and easy screening tool for health practitioners. *Br J Sports Med.* June 2005;39(6):e30.
21. McNamara J, McCabe MP. Striving for success or addiction? Exercise dependence among elite Australian athletes. *J Sports Sci.* 2012;30(8):755-766.
22. Lejoyeux M, Avril M, Richoux C, Embouazza H, Nivoli F. Prevalence of exercise addiction and other behavioral addictions among clients of a Parisian fitness room. *Compr Psych.* 2008;49:353-358.
23. De Coverley Veale DM. Exercise addiction. *Br J Add.* 1987;82:735-740.
24. Sudi K, Ottl K, Payerl, D et al. Anorexia athletica. *Nutrition.* 2004; 20, 657-661.
25. Sundgot-Borgen J. Eating disorders, energy intake, training volume, and menstrual function in high-level modern rhythmic gymnasts. *Int J Sport Nutr.* June 1996;6(2):100-109.
26. Sundgot-Borgen J. Prevalence of eating disorders in elite female athletes. *Int J Sport Nutr.* March 1993;3(1):29-40.
27. Sundgot-Borgen J, Torstveit MK. Prevalence of eating disorders in elite athletes is higher than in the general population. *Clin J Sport Med.* January 2004;14(1):25-32.
28. Herbrich L, Pfeiffer E, Lehmkuhl U, Schneider N. Anorexia athletica in pre-professional ballet dancers. *J Sports Sci.* August 2011;29(11):1115-1123.
29. Nattiv A, Loucks AB, Manore MM, Sanborn CF, Sundgot-Borgen J, Warren MP. American College of Sports Medicine position stand. The female athlete triad. *Med Sci Sports Exerc.* October 2007;39(10):1867-1882.
30. Horswill CA. Weight loss and weight cycling in amateur wrestlers: implications for performance and resting metabolic rate. *Int J Sport Nutr.* September 1993;3(3):245-260.
31. Schmidt WD, Corrigan D, Melby CL. Two seasons of weight cycling does not lower resting metabolic rate in college wrestlers. *Med Sci Sports Exerc.* May 1993;25(5):613-619.
32. Kazemi M, Rahman A, De Ciantis M. Weight cycling in adolescent Taekwondo athletes. *J Can Chiropr Assoc.* December 2011;55(4):318-324.
33. Lambert C, Jones B. Alternatives to rapid weight loss in US wrestling. *Int J Sports Med.* August 2010;31(8):523-528.
34. Weight cycling. In: National Institute of Diabetes and Digestive and Kidney Diseases Weight-Control Information Network. Washington, DC: NIH Publication No. 01-3901; 2008.
35. Berglund L, Sundgot-Borgen J, Berglund B. Adipositas athletica: a group of neglected conditions associated with medical risks. *Scand J Med Sci Sports.* October 2011; 21(5):617-624.
36. Bonci CM, Bonci LJ, Granger LR, et al. National athletic trainers' association position statement: preventing, detecting, and managing disordered eating in athletes. *J Athl Train.* January-March 2008;43(1):80-108.
37. Morgan JF, Reid F, Lacey JH. The SCOFF questionnaire: assessment of a new screening tool for eating disorders. *Br Med J.* December 4 1999;319(7223):1467-1468.
38. Strober M, Freeman R, Morrell W. The long-term course of severe anorexia nervosa in adolescents: survival analysis of recovery, relapse, and outcome predictors over 10-15 years in a prospective study. *Int J Eat Disord.* December 1997;22(4):339-360.
39. Shapiro TR. Micah True, ultramarathon runner dead at 58. *Washington Post* 4/10/2012.
40. Confront: a plan for talking to someone who may have an eating disorder. National Association of Anorexia Nervosa and Associated Disorders. Available at: www.anad.org/wp-content/uploads/2011/12/CONFRONT.pdf.

CHAPTER 16

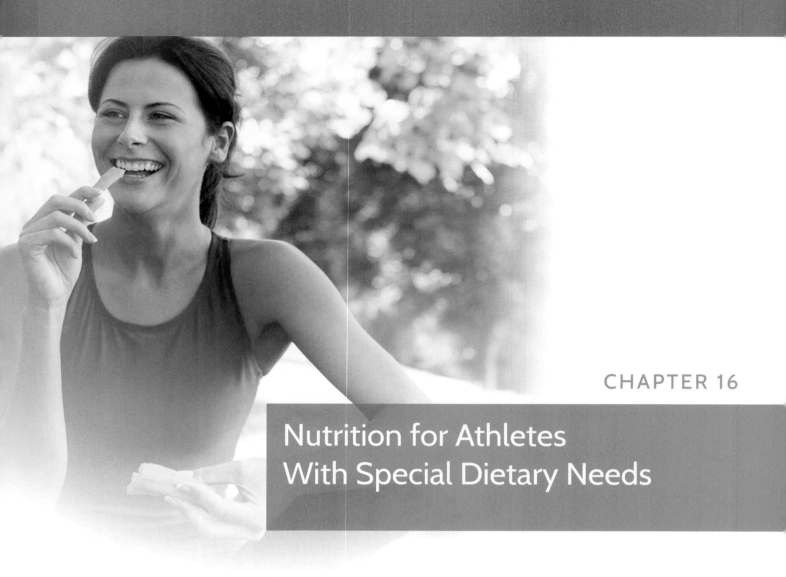

Nutrition for Athletes With Special Dietary Needs

CHAPTER OUTLINE

CHAPTER OUTLINE–cont'd

Practical Applications
Resources
References

LEARNING OBJECTIVES

After studying this chapter, the reader should be able to:

16.1 Define the types of vegetarianism.
16.2 Describe the effects of vegetarianism on athletic performance.
16.3 Explain the origin of gluten and which grains do and do not contain gluten.
16.4 Describe the effects of a gluten-free diet on athletic performance.
16.5 List the most common food allergens.
16.6 Explain the physiology of exercise-induced anaphylaxis.
16.7 Compare and contrast the Paleo diet, raw food diet, and detox diets.

KEY TERMS

anaphylactic shock The potentially life-threatening state the body enters when experiencing anaphylaxis; used interchangeably with *anaphylaxis*.

anaphylaxis A potentially life-threatening allergic reaction with a wide range of symptoms including hives, swelling, itching, and difficulty breathing and swallowing.

celiac disease A condition in which the body's immune system reacts to gluten-containing foods and initiates an allergic reaction. Inflammation of the gastrointestinal system results, and in addition to other symptoms such as abdominal bloating pain, diarrhea, vomiting, and fatigue, there is decreased absorption of nutrients by the body, which can lead to deficiencies.

detoxification Used to describe diets that attempt to purge the body of harmful 21st-century toxins including food additives, pesticides, pollutants, and other synthetic compounds in order to achieve a state of body purification.

epinephrine pen A pen-shaped applicator containing a dose of epinephrine, which is used to stop anaphylaxis, a life-threatening allergic reaction.

flexitarian diet Synonymous with the *semi-vegetarian diet*, this diet is one in which a person does not usually eat meat, fish, or poultry but will infrequently include these foods in their diet.

food intolerance A reaction to certain foods that results from a deficiency in an enzyme that is needed to break down that food. The immune system is not involved in the reaction.

food poisoning Illness that results from ingestion of toxins released by bacteria that grow on food.

gliadin A protein component of gluten, which triggers the immune system response for people with celiac disease.

gluten A protein compound that is made up of two proteins, glutenin and gliadin, and found in the grains wheat, barley, and rye.

gluten sensitivity Also known as gluten intolerance, a condition in which people appear to have a negative response to gluten-containing foods, however no allergic reaction results.

irritable bowel syndrome A gastrointestinal condition of uncertain etiology that manifests as abdominal pain and cramping, gas, bloating, and diarrhea or constipation.

lacto-ovo-vegetarian A vegetarian who consumes eggs and dairy products, but does not consume meat, poultry, or fish.

lacto-vegetarian A vegetarian who consumes dairy products, but does not consume eggs, meat, poultry, or fish.

omnivore A person who consumes both plant and animal foods.

oral allergy syndrome A condition that results when a protein in certain raw foods causes an immediate inflammatory response from the moment the food touches the mouth or skin.

ovo-vegetarian A vegetarian who consumes eggs, but does not consume meat, poultry, fish, or dairy products.

Paleo/Paleolithic diet A diet that aims to mimic what hunters and gatherers ate in the Paleolithic period over 10,000 years ago before the advent of agriculture: whole fruits and vegetables, fish, grass-fed livestock, fungi, roots, and nuts. The diet prohibits grains, legumes, dairy products, salt, refined sugar, and all processed foods.

pesco-vegetarian A vegetarian that consumes fish, eggs, and dairy, but does not consume meat or poultry.

raw food diet A diet that emphasizes intake of foods in their natural, unprocessed, uncooked form.

semi-vegetarian diet Synonymous with the *flexitarian diet*, this diet is one in which a person does not usually eat meat, fish, or poultry, but will infrequently include these foods in their diet.

vegan A person who does not include any animal products in their diet. This means they do not consume meat, poultry, fish, eggs, or dairy products.

vegetarian A person who eats a plant-based diet and does not consume meat and poultry.

INTRODUCTION

Physical therapist and elite ultramarathon runner Scott Jurek, winner of numerous accolades including finishing 165.7 miles in the 24-Hour Run (6.5 marathons in 1 day!), attributes his running success to his 100% plant-based, vegan diet. NFL player Tony Gonzalez clinched the record for all-time most receptions by a tight-end and broke the NFL career touchdown record the same year he adopted a vegan diet. Numerous other elite athletes including Olympic track star Carl Lewis, tennis champ Martina Navratilova, and power lifter Pat Reeves have chosen a vegan diet. Other Olympic athletes and super runners endorse a gluten-free eating plan, attributing the wheat-free diet to personal bests, faster recovery, and a boost in energy. The endorsements from super-athletes in contrast to the nutritional teaching that elimination of whole food groups is harmful to health and performance beg the question: Do restrictive eating patterns promote or impair optimal health and athletic performance?

A growing number of athletes have turned to specialized or restrictive eating patterns in an effort to enhance athletic performance, improve health, or both. While athletes may lead the cutting edge of nutritional trends, the special diets they adopt are not always effective, based on scientific evidence, or intrinsically safe. On the other hand, with appropriate planning, an athlete's special dietary needs or preferences can be accommodated to provide high nutritional value and contribute to optimal health and athletic performance.

VEGETARIAN DIETS

The most popular and well-understood restrictive eating plan is the **vegetarian** diet. While a vegetarian diet comes in many forms with varying degrees of restriction, it is well understood and well established that a carefully planned vegetarian eating plan can set the stage for optimal health and athletic performance.

Vegetarian diets come in a variety of forms (Fig. 16-1). A **pesco-vegetarian** diet excludes only meat and poultry. The **lacto-ovo-vegetarian** diet excludes only meat, fish, or poultry. A **lacto-vegetarian** diet excludes eggs, meat, fish, and poultry. An **ovo-vegetarian** diet

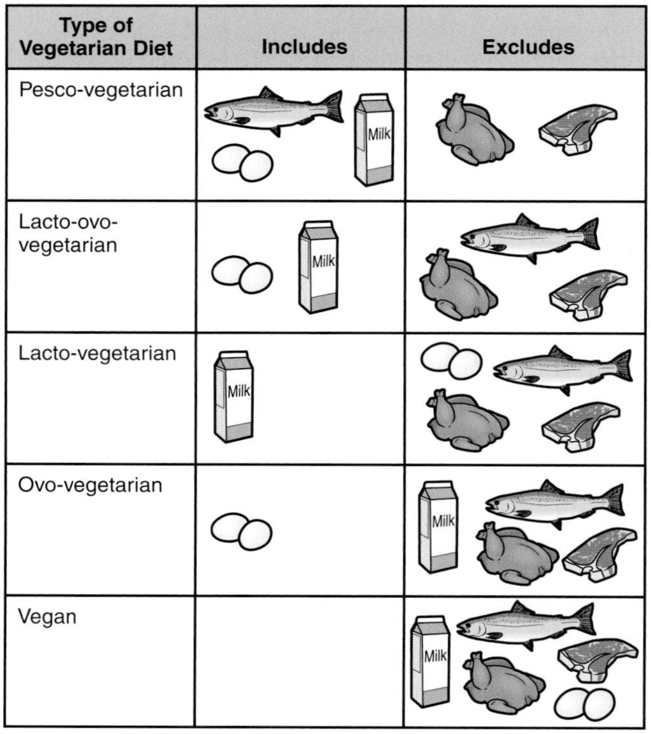

Figure 16-1. Vegetarian diets.

excludes dairy, meat, fish, and poultry. A **vegan** diet excludes all animal products and dairy such as milk and cheese.

Some people follow a **semi-vegetarian** or **flexitarian** diet in which they usually do not eat meat, fish, or poultry but will infrequently include these foods in their diet. This way of eating can be further classified as a *vegetarian-inclined* diet, in which meat alternatives are used to replace meat products for four or more meals per week, and a *health-conscious* diet, in which a person eats two to three meatless meals per week in an effort to optimize health.

Vegetarian Diets and Health

Vegetarian diets provide several health advantages. They are low in saturated fat, cholesterol, and animal protein, and high in fiber, folate, vitamins C and E, carotenoids, and some phytochemicals. Compared to **omnivores**, vegetarians have lower rates of obesity, death from cardiovascular disease, hypertension, type 2 diabetes, and prostate and colon cancer. However, if poorly planned, vegetarian diets may include insufficient amounts of protein, iron, vitamin B_{12}, vitamin D, calcium, and other nutrients.[1] Furthermore, a vegan diet may include insufficient amounts of creatine, zinc, and omega-3 fatty acids.[2,3]

In addition to ensuring adequate intake of micronutrients, vegetarians also need to carefully plan their meals and snacks to ensure optimal protein availability and adequate caloric intake. A main determinant of protein quality is whether a food contains all of the essential amino acids. Most meat-based products are higher-quality proteins because they have varying amounts of the essential amino acids, while most plant proteins are incomplete proteins because they do not contain all of the essential amino acids. Plant-based complete proteins include soy, quinoa, chia seeds, buckwheat, hemp, and flax seeds. Of note, complementary plant products such as rice and beans together provide all of the essential amino acids (Fig. 16-2). Research suggests that most vegetarians consume adequate amounts of complementary plant proteins throughout the day to meet their protein needs.[1] Thus, the complementary proteins do not need to be consumed in the same meal. See Chapter 2 for more information on complementary proteins.

Vegetarian Diets and Athletic Performance

Too few well-conducted research studies have been done to determine whether or not a vegetarian diet in itself helps or hinders athletic performance. It seems as though a well-planned vegetarian diet can set the stage for exceptional health and fitness. To ensure that the diet is appropriately planned, vegetarian athletes should consider consultation with a registered dietitian who can help to develop an individualized eating plan that will meet the athlete's unique caloric and nutritional needs.

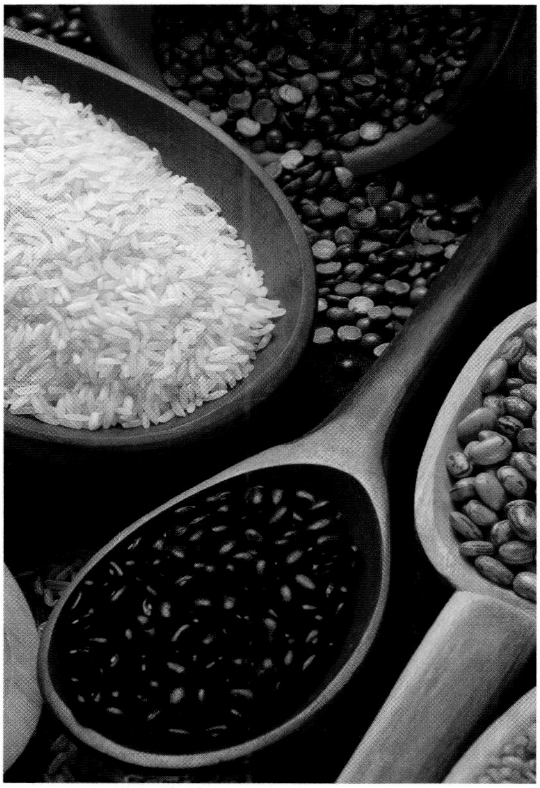

Figure 16-2. Complementary proteins.

When coaching vegetarian athletes or providing general information and tips on a vegetarian eating plan, health professionals should consider the following highlights:

Assure adequate carbohydrate and high-quality protein intake. Because carbohydrates are the preferred energy source during exercise, and vegetarian diets typically contain higher amounts of carbohydrates than omnivorous diets, a vegetarian or vegan diet could be an optimal diet for athletes. Most endurance athletes, in particular those who train longer than 60 to 90 minutes per day, are advised to consume a diet that is 60% to 70% carbohydrates to optimize glycogen synthesis.[4] A typical vegetarian diet parallels that goal with 50% to 65% of calories from carbohydrates compared to less than 50% in nonvegetarian diets.[2] The typical vegetarian diet contains about 10% to 12% of calories from protein, compared with 14% to 18% in omnivorous diets,[2] causing some to worry that vegetarians may be unable to consume adequate amounts of protein to repair damaged muscle and build muscle mass. The recommended dietary allowance (RDA) for protein is 0.8 g/kg/day. Highly trained endurance athletes may need up to 1.2 to 1.4 g/kg/day and strength athletes 1.6 to 1.7 g/kg/day,[5] though the Food and Nutrition Board of the Institute of Medicine believes that the evidence suggests athletes do not actually have increased need.[6] Legumes, dried beans, peas, nuts, soy, and meat alternatives provide ample protein, though few vegetarian foods provide all of the essential amino acids, making it necessary that vegans consume a variety of protein-rich plant foods throughout the day to meet protein requirements. Because plant proteins are not as readily digested as animal proteins, vegetarians should consume about 10% more grams of protein than the preceding recommendations.[5] That is, if an athlete consumes a 3,000-calorie diet with 10% from protein, approximately 300 calories (75 g) are from protein. A vegetarian should consume about 30 extra protein calories (8 g), for a total of 330 calories from protein. Again, a client should consult a registered dietitian for an individualized eating plan to meet these goals.

Consume enough calories. Athletes have increased energy needs due to the demands of physical activity. Depending on the duration and intensity of exercise, body composition, gender, and training regimen, a typical athlete needs to consume 2,000 to 6,000 calories per day.[2] An athlete who does not consume adequate calories to fuel exercise may suffer from low energy bioavailability, which can interfere with optimal performance, maintenance of lean tissue, and immune and reproductive functions.[5] One sign of low energy availability is unanticipated weight loss. When this occurs, some suggestions to increase caloric intake while also optimizing health include the following:

- Eat more frequent meals and snacks
- Include meat alternatives
- Add dried fruit, seeds, nuts, avocados, and other healthful calorie-dense foods to meals and snacks.

Consider creatine supplementation, if peak performance is essential. Consult a registered dietitian or physician prior to initiating supplementation. Research suggests that those who consume a vegetarian diet have decreased total muscle creatine concentration.[7] Muscle creatine stores are important for energy metabolism, in particular for exercises that are short-term and high-intensity. Vegetarian athletes may be more responsive to creatine supplementation-related improvements in sports performance compared to their meat-eating counterparts, though this is an area of ongoing investigation.[2] In any case, remember that a registered dietitian, preferably one with a focus on sports nutrition, is best equipped to discuss supplementation with a client. Recommending supplements is outside the scope of practice of most health professionals.

Prevent iron-deficiency anemia. Iron is a critical nutrient for optimal athletic performance as it is necessary for the synthesis of hemoglobin and myoglobin, iron-protein complexes that deliver oxygen from the lungs to the working muscles. Athletic training combined with low dietary intake can lead to a depletion of iron stores and subsequently hampered athletic performance, though iron-deficiency anemia is rare, affecting only about 10% of vegetarian athletes.[2] Vegetarian athletes can prevent anemia by consuming a diet rich in fortified breakfast cereals, bread, textured vegetable protein, legumes, dried beans, soy foods and meat alternatives, nuts, dried fruits, and green leafy vegetables. Vegetarian iron sources are not as well absorbed as their animal counterparts, but absorption can be enhanced by consuming a food that is high in vitamin C along with an iron-rich plant food.

Get enough zinc. Zinc is important for immune function, protein synthesis, and blood formation. It is readily lost from the body following strenuous exercise, especially in hot, humid environments. While animal sources provide the most bioavailable zinc, legumes, whole grains, cereals, nuts, and seeds are good sources. Consuming foods rich in vitamin C and soaking beans, grains, and seeds enhances absorption.

Eat fortified foods to optimize vitamin B_{12}, riboflavin, vitamin D, and calcium intake. The best sources of each of these nutrients are derived from animal products, dairy products, and eggs. However, vegans and other vegetarians can assure adequate amounts from fortified soy products, cereals, and, in the case of calcium, from low-oxalate green vegetables like broccoli, bok choy, and kale. Vitamin B_{12} is important for the normal metabolism of nerve tissue, protein, fat, and carbohydrates. It is especially important for women of child-bearing age to consume enough of the vitamin to prevent neural tube defects in a developing fetus. Riboflavin is an essential nutrient for energy production; the nutrient is stored in muscles and used most in times of muscular fatigue. Vitamin D is necessary for calcium absorption, bone growth, and mineralization. While necessary for maintaining bone structure and vitamin D metabolism, calcium is also important for blood clotting, nerve transmission, and muscle stimulation.[2] Each of these nutrients makes an important contribution to optimal athletic performance.

Vegans: Eat algae or discuss with a physician or registered dietitian the need for a supplement for optimal essential fatty acid intake. Vegan diets in particular often lack the heart-healthy, brain-protecting, omega-3 fatty acids eicosapentaenoic acid (EPA) and docosahexaenoic acid (DHA) found in fish, seafood, eggs (DHA only), and chickens fed flax or microalgae.[3] The only plant sources of DHA and EPA are microalgae, seaweed, and non-fish-oil-derived supplements. Most plant sources that contain high amounts of omega-3 fatty acids such as oils, walnuts, chia seeds, and flaxseeds, contain alpha-linoleic acid (ALA) rather than DHA or EPA. (The differences between DHA, EPA, and ALA are described in detail in Chapter 3.)

Consider periodic weight checks. Competitive athletes who regularly engage in prolonged or strenuous exercise should consider periodically monitoring weight to ensure that energy needs are being met. Many recreational athletes participate in an exercise program primarily for health benefits and weight loss rather than peak athletic performance. In these cases, weight loss may be a desired outcome. However, elite athletes will not achieve peak performance if caloric intake is insufficient to maintain weight. Be aware that frequent weight checks may be counterproductive for athletes who show signs or symptoms of eating disorders (see Chapter 15 for more information).

Avoid the female athlete triad. The female athlete triad consists of disordered eating, amenorrhea, and osteoporosis. Some athletes, especially those involved in sports with an emphasis on leanness or appearance, or who require qualification for a particular weight class, may choose a vegetarian diet to promote potentially unsafe weight loss. This may be a sign of disordered eating and may require professional evaluation. Vegetarian diets also have been associated with reduced estrogen levels and menstrual irregularities, although it is unclear whether the vegetarian diet, lower caloric intake, heavy exercise, or other factors are primarily responsible.[8] Poorly planned vegan diets are typically very low in calcium and may predispose to osteoporosis.[8] Clients who show signs of developing the female athlete triad should be referred to their primary care physician for evaluation. See Chapter 15 for more detailed information on the female athlete triad.

Suggest a checkup with the client's primary care physician. All vegetarians should periodically visit their primary care physician for a physical exam and routine blood work, which can rule out nutritional deficiencies such as iron-deficiency anemia.

Maximize training time. Train vegetarian clients for peak performance. Despite many common misconceptions about how well a vegetarian diet fuels an athlete for optimal performance, to date, all the evidence suggests that vegetarian athletes perform as well as nonvegetarians[2,4,8] (see Myths and Misconceptions). A comprehensive review of the research on vegetarian diets and athletic performance concluded that though a vegetarian diet in itself is not associated with a beneficial nor detrimental effect on physical performance capacity and, when well planned (especially important for vegan diets), it offers many benefits for athletes including high carbohydrate intake, adequate amounts of all nutrients, and long-term health benefits including reduced risk of chronic disease and decreased mortality.[4]

Myths and Misconceptions

A Vegetarian Diet Is Poorly Suited for Optimal Athletic Performance

The Myth

Vegetarian diets do not provide adequate nutrition for optimal athletic performance.

The Logic

Plant foods are for the most part low-calorie foods that do not contain all of the essential amino acids and contain iron of low bioavailability. This may result in inadequate protein intake for optimal growth and increase in muscle mass, too few calories to fuel rigorous physical activity, and inadequate iron to form hemoglobin—a molecule that is essential to deliver oxygen to working cells during physical activity.

The Science

The evidence to date supports that a carefully planned vegetarian diet can optimally fuel athletic performance as long as an athlete consumes a diet rich in complementary proteins, consumes sufficient calories to meet the body's needs, and eats iron-rich plant products in combination with a citrus food to optimize absorption.

Sources:

Craig WJ, Mangels AR. Position of the American Dietetic Association: vegetarian diets. *J Am Diet Assoc.* July 2009;109(7):1266-1282.

Venderley AM, Campbell WW. Vegetarian diets: nutritional considerations for athletes. *Sports Med.* 2006;36(4):293-305.

Rodriguez NR, DiMarco NM, Langley S. Position of the American Dietetic Association, Dietitians of Canada, and the American College of Sports Medicine: nutrition and athletic performance. *J Am Diet Assoc.* March 2009;109(3):509-527.

SPEED BUMP

1. **Define the types of vegetarianism.**
2. **Describe the effects of vegetarianism on athletic performance.**

GLUTEN-FREE DIETS

Over the past several years, a growing number of people have experimented with gluten-free diets to help alleviate symptoms like abdominal pain, cramping, and generalized fatigue. **Gluten** is present in many grains including wheat, rye, and barley. Adhering to a gluten-free diet requires diligence, as gluten is present in many foods and a completely gluten-free diet is fairly restrictive, thus increasing risk for inadequate intake of some nutrients.

In some cases, people have adopted the diet to avoid overconsumption of heavily processed, nutritionally poor foods, as many fresh foods like fruits and vegetables are gluten-free. While historically (and scientifically) a gluten-free diet has only been considered necessary for people with **celiac disease**, a condition defined by an allergy to gluten-containing products, many people who are free of celiac disease, or even **gluten sensitivity**, proclaim the benefits of a gluten-free diet. But the question that often arises is: For people who do not have celiac disease, does this restrictive eating regimen provide more benefits than risks? What is "gluten sensitivity"? Would athletes who suffer from gastrointestinal symptoms benefit from a gluten-free diet?

Celiac Disease

Nearly 1% of the population suffers from celiac disease; for unknown reasons the prevalence appears to be increasing slightly.[9] Celiac disease is characterized by an autoimmune rejection of gluten-containing foods. Gluten, present in all food products made from wheat, barley, rye, and contaminated oats, is a protein compound made up of two proteins called **gliadin** and glutenin that are joined with starch. For people with celiac disease, when the body is exposed to gliadin—the "toxic" component of gluten for people with celiac disease—it goes into immunologic overdrive. The gastrointestinal system becomes inflamed and pathological changes to the small intestine, the body's main site for nutrient absorption, ensue. When the gut is unable to absorb nutrients, common symptoms like vitamin deficiency, anemia, weight loss, and diarrhea occur. Other symptoms include abdominal pain and distention and in some cases neurological dysfunction.

Celiac disease is very difficult to diagnose and though it begins in childhood, many people do not learn that they have the disease until well into adulthood. The longer a person suffers from undiagnosed and untreated celiac disease, the more likely he or she is to develop complications such as other autoimmune disorders, osteoporosis, infertility, neurological problems, and in rare cases, cancer.[9] This is why it is very important for anyone who suffers from the symptoms of celiac disease to see a physician immediately for evaluation. Celiac disease can be diagnosed with laboratory testing and biopsy of the small intestine. The only definitive treatment for the disease is strict avoidance of gluten-containing foods.

Gluten Sensitivity (Non-Celiac Gluten Intolerance)

Gluten sensitivity, which is also referred to as non-celiac gluten intolerance in the scientific literature, is much more common and less understood than celiac disease. Gluten sensitivity occurs when the body has a pronounced response to gluten-containing foods leading to feelings of tiredness, abdominal pain, and other GI symptoms like diarrhea or constipation. Many people report experiencing these symptoms after eating gluten-containing foods (or more commonly, they report these symptoms going away after avoiding gluten), but it is not clear what causes these symptoms or the body's actual response to the gluten. While there is limited research explaining the role of gluten in causing gastrointestinal symptoms, preliminary evidence suggests that while some people without celiac disease may suffer from gluten sensitivity, the number of people with a physiological reaction to gluten is probably much smaller than the number of people who perceive benefits from a gluten-free diet[10] (see Evaluating the Evidence).

EVALUATING THE EVIDENCE

Does 'Non-Celiac Gluten Intolerance' Really Exist?

A growing number of people have adopted gluten-free diets with the belief that gluten causes fatigue and a variety of gastrointestinal symptoms including diarrhea, constipation, bloating, and cramping. Until the following study was conducted, no scientific evidence existed to support the notion of a gluten reaction in people who do not have celiac disease.

THE STUDY

Thirty-four patients who did not have celiac disease but who did have irritable bowel syndrome that improved on a gluten-free diet participated in a double-blind randomized controlled trial. Neither the participants nor the researchers recording the results were aware of who received the test item and who received the placebo. A second research party recorded the information.

The participants ate muffins and bread containing gluten or placebo over a 6-week period of time. The muffins were indistinguishable. Within the first week of the intervention and throughout the 6-week study, the participants who ate the gluten products had significantly more gastrointestinal symptoms and tiredness than the group on the gluten-free diet. The mechanisms for this difference were not elucidated.[27]

1. What conclusion do you draw from this study?
2. What are three limitations to this study?
3. What would be some cautions prior to citing this study to clients in endorsing the existence of gluten sensitivity?

The study authors couldn't understand the mechanism why the participants responded to gluten. They conducted a second study and found that, in fact, the participants had the same negative response to both whey and a control diet. This was a case of "nocebo" effect, when even a placebo makes symptoms worse. Thus, there still is no scientific evidence to support the notion of non-celiac gluten sensitivity.[10]

Gluten-Free Nutritional Considerations

Many foods contain gluten, and without appropriate dietary planning, complete elimination of gluten from the diet can lead to nutritional deficiency. The *Dietary Guidelines for Americans* recommend that most adults get anywhere from six to eight servings of grains per day. Grains are an excellent source of B-vitamins and fiber. Most standard grains such as bread, cereal, and pasta contain wheat, rye, or barley and thus include gluten. Complete elimination of gluten-containing grains *can* lead to nutritional deficiencies including B vitamins, calcium, vitamin D, iron, zinc, magnesium, and fiber. In fact, a Swedish research study of people with celiac disease who had been gluten-free for 10 years found that half of the patients had vitamin deficiencies, including low levels of vitamin B_6 or folate, or both.[11] Likewise, a survey of people on a gluten-free diet in the United States found that over half had inadequate fiber, iron, and calcium intake.[12]

While a poorly planned gluten-free diet can lead to micronutrient deficiencies, with appropriate planning, a person can safely follow a gluten-free diet without risk to nutritional quality. Thanks to the 2004 Food Allergen Labeling and Consumer Protection Act, food labels must identify if they contain any of the top eight food allergens, including wheat. Though a quick glance at the nutritional label shows that gluten is present in most foods, a growing number of either naturally or artificially gluten-free products are on the market and are clearly labeled "gluten free." Bread, pasta, cereal, and various other products that typically contain gluten have been reformulated into gluten-free products, though these products tend to cost substantially more than the gluten-containing counterpart. For people with celiac disease, the difficulty of adhering to a gluten-free diet is the price to pay for good health. The same may hold true for some people with gluten sensitivity.

Anyone considering starting a gluten-free diet should seek consultation with a physician and dietitian prior to removing gluten from the diet, as removing gluten from the diet prior to evaluation can interfere with the appropriate diagnosis of celiac disease. Most people who have celiac disease are currently undiagnosed, and for anyone with symptoms of the disease, a physician will likely want to evaluate for it. If a person sees the doctor, tests negative for celiac disease, and still would like to adopt a gluten-free diet, a registered dietitian can help plan a wholesome diet that is high in gluten-free B-vitamin- and fiber-containing foods. A list of inherently gluten-free products is highlighted in Table 16-1. It is also worth fully exploring whether it is the gluten or some other food, lifestyle behavior, or medical problem that is contributing to the gastrointestinal symptoms. Adopting a gluten-free diet is not recommended as a method to lose weight or to "become healthier." The diet is restrictive and can lead to serious vitamin deficiencies or contribute to disordered eating behaviors. And, unlike sugar and trans fat, for example, gluten itself is not inherently unhealthy.

Table 16-1. Inherently Gluten-Free Foods

GRAINS
Rice
Corn
Soy
Tapioca
Quinoa
Millet
Buckwheat
Flax
Nut flours
Uncontaminated oats
NONGRAINS
Milk
Butter
Cheese
Fruits and vegetables
Potato
Meat
Fish
Poultry
Eggs
Beans
Seeds

GLUTEN-FREE DIET AND ATHLETIC PERFORMANCE

A strenuous endurance workout demands careful nutrition planning to optimize athletic performance and minimize the gastrointestinal (GI) distress—cramps, bloating, abdominal pain, and generalized fatigue—that plagues many recreational and elite athletes. In an effort to avoid these unpleasant GI symptoms, many athletes have experimented with adopting a gluten-free diet. With scientific evidence lacking, the success (or not) of a gluten-free diet in improving athletic performance is theoretical and anecdotal. Nonetheless, if a client is contemplating going gluten-free because he or she has heard it will improve athletic performance, the athlete should first make sure that he or she understands the implications.

Many of the best sources of carbohydrates, the body's preferred energy source during intense exercise, contain gluten. Thus, anyone who adopts a gluten-free diet needs to be especially careful to make sure to eat enough gluten-free carbohydrates to fuel the exercise session. The Academy of Nutrition and Dietetics (formerly called the American Dietetic Association) recommends about 30 to 60 grams of rapidly absorbed carbohydrates per hour of intense activity.[5] Fortunately, there are many high-carbohydrate, gluten-free foods to choose from (see Table 16-1).

If an athlete experiences GI symptoms during an endurance session, it is important to investigate other potential culprits in addition to (or instead of) gluten. For example, many high-carbohydrate products have large amounts of fiber. While fiber is a nutrient that most people need to eat a lot more of for optimal health, it is also a source of GI discomfort when consumed with or soon before strenuous exercise. Other carbohydrates, such as the sugar contained in an apple, can also cause abdominal cramping in a dehydrated athlete.

Ultimately, a conscientious and nutrition-savvy athlete could successfully adopt a gluten-free eating plan to meet nutritional needs. It may be helpful to think of a gluten-free diet in a similar way as a vegan diet: because the diet is highly restrictive, people who adhere to the eating plan face potential nutrient deficits which could be detrimental to athletic performance. However, with appropriate planning, both vegan and gluten-free athletes can consume a balanced and complete diet that prepares them for peak performance. A registered dietitian with a focus on sports nutrition can help a client adopt a well-designed and individualized gluten-free eating plan to fuel optimal health and athletic performance.

SPEED BUMP

3. **Explain the origin of gluten and which grains do and do not contain gluten.**
4. **Describe the effects of a gluten-free diet on athletic performance.**

FOOD ALLERGIES

The health benefits of nuts like walnuts, pecans, and almonds dominate headlines. From preventing heart disease to building immunity, nuts are important components of a balanced eating plan. However, for the millions of Americans with food allergies, eating nuts—or other foods like shellfish and milk—can be deadly. In fact, 150 Americans die each year from food-induced **anaphylaxis**, a severe and potentially fatal systemic allergic response.[13] Another 200,000 report to U.S emergency departments with food allergy symptoms.[14] Sometimes the amount of exposure does not need to be much to cause serious harm. All it took was a kiss from a boyfriend who had eaten peanut butter to cause one Canadian teen to succumb to a fatal allergic reaction.[15]

In the United States, up to 8% of children and 4% of adults suffer from food allergies.[16] While much more common in children than adults, allergies affect people of all ages and ethnicities. Chances are good that every health professional will at some point in his or her career encounter a client, friend, or family member who suffers from a food allergy. When that happens, it will be important to recognize the most common food allergies, what causes them, how to identify and treat them, and what people with allergies (and their parents) can do to avoid experiencing harmful symptoms.

Understanding Food Allergies

The top eight most common food allergens, which account for 90% of all allergic reactions, are: milk, eggs, peanuts, tree nuts (such as almonds, cashews, and walnuts), shellfish, fish, soy, and wheat.[17] The proteins in these foods cause the bodies of millions of people to itch, break out in hives, and sometimes go into **anaphylactic shock** (Fig. 16-3). This happens because the body misinterprets the food as an invader. When the perceived "invader" enters the

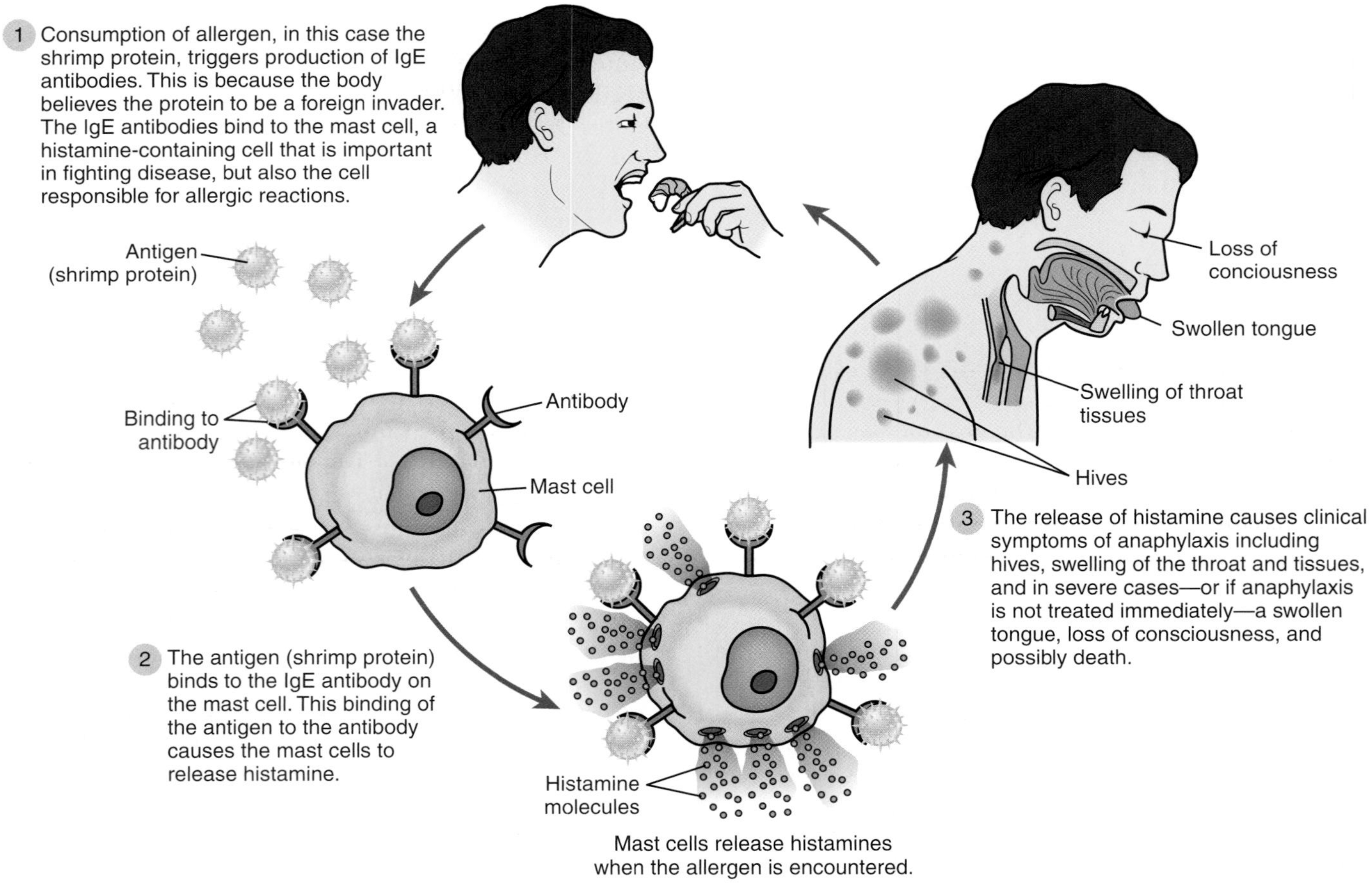
1 Consumption of allergen, in this case the shrimp protein, triggers production of IgE antibodies. This is because the body believes the protein to be a foreign invader. The IgE antibodies bind to the mast cell, a histamine-containing cell that is important in fighting disease, but also the cell responsible for allergic reactions.
Antigen (shrimp protein)
Binding to antibody
Antibody
Mast cell
2 The antigen (shrimp protein) binds to the IgE antibody on the mast cell. This binding of the antigen to the antibody causes the mast cells to release histamine.
Histamine molecules
Mast cells release histamines when the allergen is encountered.
Loss of conciousness
Swollen tongue
Swelling of throat tissues
Hives
3 The release of histamine causes clinical symptoms of anaphylaxis including hives, swelling of the throat and tissues, and in severe cases—or if anaphylaxis is not treated immediately—a swollen tongue, loss of consciousness, and possibly death.

Figure 16-3. Anaphylaxis.

bloodstream, the immune system makes an antibody called immunoglobulin E, or IgE, to kill and destroy it. With repeated exposure to the food, the antibody responds by binding to the allergen. This sets in motion a series of immunologic events including the release of histamine. Histamine is responsible for many of the harmful symptoms of food allergies including redness, swelling, itching, gastrointestinal symptoms, and hypotension. Once the body makes an antibody to a food, every time the food is eaten an immune response ensues. In the rare but deadly cases, the heart rate drops, the breathing tubes narrow, and the tongue swells, making breathing and adequate oxygenation to the body's cells a struggle. The harmful response can occur from minutes to an hour after the food is eaten.[18]

Another form of food allergy known as **oral allergy syndrome** results when a protein in certain raw foods causes an immediate inflammatory response from the moment the food touches the mouth or skin. Raw fruits and vegetables such as apples, cherries, kiwis, celery, tomatoes, and green peppers are the typical culprits, causing an itchy, tingling sensation in the mouth, lips, and throat. The reaction can also cause swelling of the lips, tongue, and throat; watery, itchy eyes; runny nose; and sneezing. Oral allergy syndrome typically affects individuals with hay fever and particularly those with spring hay fever from birch pollen and late summer hay fever from ragweed pollen. Cooking or processing easily breaks down the proteins in the fruits and vegetables that cause oral allergy syndrome and, thus, the allergic reaction does not occur with cooked, baked, or processed fruits and vegetables.[19]

It is important to differentiate a food allergy from other possible ailments such as **food poisoning**, nonfood allergy (such as pollen, dust, or dander), and especially **food intolerance**. Though both food allergy and food intolerance result from the body's inability to digest and absorb a food, their mechanisms for causing symptoms are very different. Food intolerance often results from a deficiency in an enzyme that is needed to break down a food. For example, lactose intolerance results from a deficiency in the enzyme lactase, which is necessary to digest the sugar. Undigested lactose can cause gastrointestinal symptoms such as abdominal pain, bloating, and diarrhea. Another fairly common food intolerance is fructose intolerance, or fructose malabsorption. This results from an ineffective carrier protein that impedes the absorption of fructose in the small intestine. People with fructose malabsorption suffer from gastrointestinal symptoms such as bloating, abdominal pain, vomiting, and flatulence after eating fructose-containing foods. Foods high in fructose include many fruits and some vegetables as well as processed foods containing high-fructose corn syrup. Unlike food allergy, the immune system plays no role in the dysfunction and the uncomfortable symptoms of food intolerance are not life-threatening.

Treatment, Diagnosis, and Prevention

Clearly, rapid treatment of an anaphylactic reaction is critical to preserve the health and well-being of an allergic individual. Anyone who has symptoms of anaphylaxis should be treated immediately with an **epinephrine pen**. If this is not available, it is important to call 9-1-1 and ensure that the person is transported immediately to the nearest emergency department. Either there or in the field the individual will be treated with injectable epinephrine, antihistamines, and other emergency treatments. These medicines reverse the allergic response by restoring blood pressure, blocking further production of histamine, and countering the harmful effects induced by the allergen.

After treatment of acute symptoms of an allergic reaction, the patient and allergist embark on what can either be a simple process or a prolonged journey to identify the allergen. The allergist's first objective is to get a complete history of the reaction including the onset and duration, symptoms, seasonality, suspected foods, how the food was prepared, and any other information the patient can provide. The history is followed by a complete physical exam to gather as much information about the reaction as possible. In most cases this thorough assessment will reveal a few suspect foods.

Usually the next step for people with more mild symptoms is to keep a food diary noting all of the foods eaten and whether an allergic reaction occurred. If a potential allergen is noted, it is then removed from the diet and the food diary continues. If the symptoms disappear, the diagnosis is fairly obvious, and the individual should strive to avoid the suspected allergen. If the diagnosis remains uncertain, many physicians will order a blood test to measure the level of a series of potential allergens. In other cases, a physician may refer to an allergist who can do a scratch skin test. With this test a small amount of the food is placed on the skin of the lower arm. The provider scratches this part of the arm with a needle to check for redness and swelling. If the test is positive the diagnosis is confirmed. Another test option is the gold standard for food allergy diagnosis: the double-blind food challenge. The patient swallows a capsule of a food allergen and is then watched to see if symptoms occur. Then another capsule of a different allergen is swallowed. The test is continued with the most common potential allergens. The test is double-blind because neither the patient nor the physician knows which food is in the capsule (the capsules are prepared by a third party). Though the gold standard, this test is time-consuming and impractical for many allergens. Thus, it is rarely performed. Of course, all of the preceding tests could be deadly for people with severe allergic reactions. For these individuals, diagnosis is made with a blood test that measures the presence of a food-specific antibody.

Once a diagnosis is confirmed, there is only one way to prevent a future attack: avoid the food. This is no simple task considering the widespread use of many of the most common allergens. To help ease the burden, in 2004 the FDA implemented a law requiring all food manufacturing companies to list any of the eight most common allergens included in the product and to state if the food was processed in a plant that also processes allergens where cross-contamination could occur. While this certainly will help, people with food allergies still must be vigilant. Those with severe reactions should always carry an epinephrine pen and wear a medical alert bracelet noting the allergy.

Exercise-Induced Allergies

Many myths surround food allergies. For example, it is commonly said that food allergies cause or exacerbate migraine headaches, arthritis, fatigue, and childhood hyperactivity. No credible scientific evidence exists to substantiate any of these claims. There is one myth, however, that is true—exercise can transform an otherwise benign food into a potent allergen.

Exercise-induced food allergy results when a susceptible person eats a specific food before exercising. As exercise intensity and body temperature increase, the person begins to experience itching, light-headedness, possibly hives, and sometimes even anaphylaxis. Crustacean shellfish, alcohol, tomatoes, cheese, and celery are common causes of exercise-induced food allergy reactions. Some people have this reaction to many foods, and others have it only after eating a specific food. While experiencing exercise-induced food allergy can be very frightening, it can be wholly prevented by avoiding eating suspect foods in the 2 to 3 hours before exercising.[19] While exercise-induced allergy may be the culprit behind a rapid change in clinical status and onset of unexpected symptoms during exercise, other causes, including myocardial infarction, stroke, and hypoglycemia in a person with diabetes, can cause overlapping symptoms (though these illnesses do not typically cause itching, hives, and swelling). The health professional should use professional judgment in assessing the severity of the client's symptoms and activate the emergency response system when there is any concern for a serious or compromising illness.

Be Prepared

Health professionals should be sure to maintain yearly CPR and first aid certification to be most prepared to act in case of an emergency. While food allergy management might not be a priority for most allied health professionals, anyone who works with children and teens or who trains anyone susceptible to an exercise-induced or typical food allergy may be faced with the task of recognizing and responding to a severe allergic reaction or anaphylaxis in a client. A health professional who is prepared and thinks fast could save someone's life.

OTHER SPECIAL EATING PLANS

Athletes, similar to the general population, may suffer from any of a number of ailments or chronic diseases that may require or encourage them to adopt a specialized diet. The nutritional considerations for many of these conditions, including diabetes, **irritable bowel syndrome** and other gastrointestinal disorders, cardiovascular disease, and hypertension, among others, are described in Chapter 14.

In addition to special nutrition plans described earlier in this chapter and those which accompany diagnosed conditions or diseases, some athletes may follow any of a number of other special eating plans for perceived performance or health gains. Unlike the diets described in Chapter 12, in which weight loss is the person's main motivation for starting the diet, athletes tend to adopt the eating plans described in this chapter for perceived benefits mostly unrelated to weight. A few of these diets are highlighted below.

Paleo Diet

The recent boon in backyard and community gardens, farmers markets, and availability of organic foods offers evidence of increased consumer demand for more wholesome, sustainable, and environmentally friendly foods. This growing trend to eat more fruits and vegetables and less processed foods has contributed to a surge in interest and popularity of the **Paleo diet**.

Followers of the Paleolithic diet (commonly referred to as the Paleo diet, the caveman diet, and the Stone Age diet) adopt an eating plan intended to mimic what hunters and gatherers ate in the Paleolithic period over 10,000 ago before the advent of agriculture: whole fruits and vegetables, fish, grass-fed livestock, fungi, roots, and nuts. The diet prohibits grains, legumes, dairy products, salt, refined sugar, and all processed foods.

While there is a lack of quality scientific research evaluating the merits and limitations of this eating plan, a panel of expert reviewers tasked with ranking 24 diets for *U.S. News & World Report* ranked the Paleo diet at the bottom.[20] Part of the reason for its low score was the concern that eliminating grains and dairy from the diet increases the likelihood of developing nutrient deficiencies while loading up on meat may contribute to health problems.[21] Furthermore, intake of calcium and vitamin D is particularly low for this eating plan, which is harmful to bone health.

The diet also tends to be very low in carbohydrates, which could contribute to suboptimal performance for athletes.

Raw Food Diet

The **raw food diet** emphasizes intake of foods in their natural, unprocessed, uncooked form. Raw fruits and vegetables top the list of food options. Add to that a mix of beans and legumes and the raw food diet should be a nutrient-dense and filling "perfect diet." After all, each of these foods is packed with nutrients, light on calories, and high in fiber. But a closer look reveals a more complicated, expensive, and questionable eating plan.

Beyond promoting every nutrition expert's mantra of "eat more vegetables and fruits," the standard raw food diet is true to its name—most, if not all, foods need to be raw. This means dieters are prohibited from cooking food. The only allowed "cooking" is dehydration, which requires a special machine that blows hot air through the food and increases the temperature to no more than 118°F. Because grains are indigestible raw and the diet prohibits boiling them, raw grains must be soaked overnight or allowed to sprout before consumption. Because food cannot be cooked, meat and most animal products are off limits (unless a dieter chooses to put the risk of severe foodborne illness aside and eat raw meat). For this reason, the raw food diet typically resembles a vegan diet that is free of processed and cooked food. Most raw food devotees also consume mostly organic foods to avoid exposure to pesticides and other synthetic chemicals.

Few published studies evaluate risks and benefits of a raw food diet. The limited available research suggests a variety of potential benefits such as improved LDL cholesterol and triglyceride levels,[22] weight loss,[23] improvement in fibromyalgia symptoms,[24] and decreased blood pressure,[25] as well as potential harmful effects including decreased HDL cholesterol,[22] decreased bone density,[7] and vitamin B_{12} deficiency (due to elimination of animal products).[22] Individuals who do not adopt the vegan approach but instead consume raw animal products risk serious foodborne illness. Plus, as with any restrictive diet, strict adherence to a raw food diet is challenging. The imperfect adherence, however, may be a major redeeming feature because it allows consumption of other foods and nutrients necessary for good nutrition.

Detox Diet

Detoxification, or "detox," diets aim to purge the body of harmful 21st-century toxins including food additives, pesticides, pollutants, and other synthetic compounds in order to achieve a state of body purification. These diets often promise increased energy, clearer skin, headache relief, decreased bloating, and perhaps even weight loss.

With a price tag ranging from thousands of dollars for an intensive spa-based program to a $15-book purchase or Internet subscription plus food and supplement costs, detox diets have attracted a wide variety of supporters. But beyond the testimonials and committed detox followers, many questions remain unanswered. What exactly is a detox diet, and does it really work? Do these regimens *safely* help the body to get rid of toxins of daily living better than the normal metabolic processes of the liver, kidney, skin, lymph nodes, and other body systems? Does a "toxin purge" lead to the diets' proclaimed health benefits?

The only element that all detox diets share is the goal to rid the body of toxins with some combination of fasting, food restriction, and supplementation. Most detox diets include elimination of caffeine, nicotine, and alcohol, and many restrict meat and solid foods altogether. The diets also tend to involve consumption of large amounts of liquid, fiber, and raw vegetables — ingredients that are thought to purge the gastrointestinal system of accumulated harmful substances. A variety of "cleansing boosters" such as herbal laxatives, "colonics" (also known as enemas—flushing out of the rectum and colon with water), probiotics to repopulate the natural intestinal flora, and antioxidants may be incorporated into a detox regimen. Relaxation therapies such as massage, sauna, aromatherapy baths, deep-breathing exercises, and walking are also included in some programs.

The prototypical detox diet begins with a cleansing phase, which is typically liquid-only. This is followed for 2 to 3 days before other foods such as brown rice, fruit, and steamed vegetables are added. Then about a week later, other foods may be reintroduced with the exception of red meat, wheat, sugar, eggs, and prepackaged foods. This final phase of the diet is expected to be followed indefinitely for maintenance. Of course, with no standard definition of a "detox diet," programs vary considerably.

At first glance, a detox diet may seem to make sense. In a world filled with synthetic chemicals, processed foods, pesticides, and pollutants, a thorough body cleansing via a detox diet once a year seems logical enough. But no evidence supports the notion that harmful chemicals accumulate in the body (in fact, the liver and kidneys efficiently rid the body of toxins). And even if toxins did accumulate in the body, it is unlikely that "detox" diets would get rid of them.

Toxicologists A. Jay Gandolfi, an associate dean for research in the College of Pharmacy at the University of Arizona, and Linda Birnbaum, director of the experimental toxicology division of the Environmental Protection Agency, made the following points in an article in the *Los Angeles Times:* (1) high volumes of liquid consumption could theoretically help to remove water-soluble chemicals like arsenic, but not fat-soluble chemicals (which make up most pollutants); (2) fiber consumption may help to eliminate toxic chemicals that accumulate in the liver, but not chemicals that are located in other parts of the gastrointestinal system; (3) raw vegetables have no special detoxifying properties other than that their high fiber content can further help to bulk up stools; (4) most chemicals of concern are fat-soluble and so are stored in fat.[26] The researchers note that the best way to get rid of these potential toxins is not through a detox diet, but through weight loss, as more slender people eliminate toxins more quickly than overweight and obese individuals. (Note: Though peer-reviewed journal articles, and not newspaper stories, are generally the best source of credible scientific information, in the case of detox diets, very little peer-reviewed research has been published.)

While consuming ample fiber and staying well hydrated are healthy when done in moderation and relatively harmless, use of colonics and laxatives to "purify" the digestive tract are dangerous. Their use can lead to metabolic disturbances, fainting episodes, dehydration, and muscle cramps among other complications. The more extreme programs also leave individuals protein- and nutrient-depleted. Among other consequences, this can lead to decreased lean muscle mass and slowed metabolism.

Benefits of detox diets may exist, but they likely are not due to detoxification. The decreased bloating is likely from eating less food; the clearer skin from increased hydration; and the decreased headaches from elimination of caffeine and alcohol. Improved energy levels and sense of well-being likely result from a combination of more natural food intake, the exercise and relaxation components of the program, and psychological factors.

With this said, there may be some utility in a short-term (1 to 3 days) laxative-free detox program, but not for purposes of purification. As a health-promoting practice, committing to a detox regimen helps people to stop and consider the healthy and unhealthy components of their lifestyles and make changes such as eating less, examining health habits, and omitting consumption of processed foods, nicotine, caffeine, and alcohol. Some dietitians even recommend a "gentle cleanse" to clients. That is, consuming a healthy diet of primarily fruits, vegetables, non-meat proteins, and a large volume of water, and excluding substances such as nicotine, caffeine, and alcohol.

Other Diets

This is just a sampling of many types of special eating plans that athletes may follow. Health professionals who work with active individuals are likely to encounter many more that are not discussed here. It is incumbent upon the health professional to identify reliable resources to learn more about these eating plans so as to be able to share reliable and credible information and resources with the athletes.

SPEED BUMP

5. Compare and contrast the Paleo diet, raw food diet, and detox diets.

AN APPROACH TO WORKING WITH ATHLETES FOLLOWING SPECIAL EATING PLANS

Health professionals frequently encounter competitive athletes who follow various eating plans and regimens that they adamantly endorse. In many cases, the scientific evidence to either support or reject a given eating plan is incomplete, leaving athletes and the professionals who help them to rely on informed opinions, rather than indisputable facts, to guide actions.

The key to working with athletes who follow special eating plans is to develop a consistent approach to help them optimize their nutrition and performance while respecting their beliefs. One possible approach is to:

1. Listen fully to the athlete's rationale for following the eating plan, positive and negative experiences resulting from the eating plan, adherence and commitment to the eating plan, and specific opinion of how the eating plan has or has not affected athletic performance. This process of listening and making sure that the client feels heard and understood will help to develop rapport and strengthen the relationship between the athlete and the health professional.
2. Refer the athlete to a registered dietitian who is a board-certified specialist in sports dietetics. This dietitian can work within the client's goals and beliefs to develop an individualized plan that is most likely to optimize health and athletic performance.
3. Check in. Follow up with the athlete after the nutrition consultation and learn about the recommended eating plan and approach, how the athlete feels about it, and how closely he or she is following it.

This approach will work in most situations; however, if an athlete has adopted an eating plan which is clearly dangerous, a more assertive approach, including discussing concerns with the athlete and referring to a registered dietitian and physician, may be necessary. This chapter's Communication Strategies offers tips on how to initiate a referral to a registered dietitian.

COMMUNICATION STRATEGIES

Referring to a Registered Dietitian

You have been working with an athlete who has adopted a very restrictive eating plan. You are concerned that the athlete may be at risk for nutritional deficiency. You have already shared your concern with your client, and he has agreed to visit a registered dietitian and has allowed you to share your concerns and the reason for referral with the dietitian. In this exercise you will practice initiating a referral to a qualified nutrition professional.

1. **Identify a qualified professional**. The first step to initiating a referral is to identify a nutrition professional that you trust. You may identify this person through word of mouth and a recommendation from another health professional, through the database of registered dietitians maintained by the Academy of Nutrition and Dietetics (see www.eatright.org), through the facility where you work, or other venues.
   Assume you are a health professional in your local community, or in the community in which you hope to work. Identify by name at least three potential registered dietitians to whom you might refer your client. What factors would you use to determine to whom you would consider referring your client? Example: I would ensure the registered dietitian was specially certified in sports nutrition and had experience working with athletes. In addition, I would want to make sure he or she had experience working with clients with specialized or restrictive eating plans.
2. **Establish a connection.** Before referring clients to an individual, it is helpful to establish a connection and relationship with that person. Not only does this communication help to increase the likelihood of success for your client, but it may also help to have a ready contact for future referral, and it may generate referrals to you in exchange.
   Identify at least three ways in which you might establish a connection with a local registered dietitian. Examples: Research appropriately credentialed dietitians on the Academy of Nutrition and Dietetics website (www.eatright.org) and contact them directly. Introduce yourself and find out more about them and their specialties and experience. If you work at a location that also employs dietitians, make a point of introducing yourself to your dietitian coworkers and find out more about them. Ask a colleague who works with a registered dietitian they recommend to introduce you.
3. **Make the referral.** Once you have determined to whom to refer a client, the next step is to actually make the referral. To be most effective, it is important to make your referral in writing. Your referral letter should include: (1) your name, credentials, and contact information; (2) a brief one-to two-line background about the client; and (3) the reason for referral.
   Write a brief sample referral letter to a registered dietitian for this sample client. Take the liberty to make up details for the purpose of this exercise.
   Example:
   Jane/John Doe, Athletic Trainer
   1234 Main Street
   Anywhere, Any State 00000
   (555) 555-5555
   j.doe@athletictrainingcompany.com
   Background: Client, Joe XXXX is a 22-year-old male athlete who is currently participating in competitive long-distance running. The client has recently adopted a vegan diet in hopes of improving his overall health.
   Referral: Client is following a vegan-eating plan and may not be consuming all required nutrients. Referring to ensure he is not at risk for nutritional deficiency.
4. **Follow up.** Follow up with both the registered dietitian and your client after the client has visited with the registered dietitian. You can play an important role in helping to reinforce the messages and recommendations provided by the registered dietitian and also help to monitor the client's progress. To strengthen your relationship with the registered dietitian, write a brief follow-up letter acknowledging that you appreciate the consultation, have received the recommendations, and your intended role in helping the client to achieve success with the recommendations. This follow-up letter helps to improve care for the client and also demonstrates your professionalism.
   Draft a brief follow-up letter to the registered dietitian. Take the liberty to make up details for the purpose of this exercise.
   Jane/John Doe, Athletic Trainer
   1234 Main Street
   Anywhere, Any State 00000
   (555) 555-5555

Continued

COMMUNICATION STRATEGIES–cont'd

j.doe@athletictrainingcompany.com
Dear (name of chosen dietitian),

Thank you for consulting with Joe XXXX on his current eating plan. Joe has discussed your recommendations with me, specifically the addition of a vitamin B_{12} supplement, and the increase in protein from soy products such as tofu and tempeh, as well as from beans and legumes. It is my intention to follow up with Joe in a few weeks to see how he is adhering to your recommendations, whether he is having any trouble, and to refer him back to you for a follow-up appointment so you can evaluate his progress. Thank you again for helping Joe achieve his goals of eating a vegan diet while remaining a competitive athlete.

Sincerely,
Jane/John Doe

CHAPTER SUMMARY

Many athletes may follow alternative dietary practices, whether due to a medical condition or personal preference. In most cases, with proper planning a healthful balanced diet can be maintained despite dietary restrictions. However, when poorly planned, restrictive diets can impair athletic performance and compromise an individual's overall nutritional status. The health professional can play an important role in helping clients with special dietary needs to acquire the knowledge and skill they need to make the best nutritional choices to meet their needs.

KEY POINTS SUMMARY

1. Vegetarian diets provide several health advantages. They are low in saturated fat, cholesterol, and animal protein and high in fiber, folate, vitamins C and E, carotenoids, and some phytochemicals.
2. If poorly planned, vegetarian diets may include insufficient amounts of protein, iron, vitamin B12, vitamin D, calcium, and other nutrients.[1] Furthermore, a vegan diet may include insufficient amounts of creatine, zinc, and omega-3 fatty acids.[2,3]
3. Celiac disease is characterized by an autoimmune rejection of gluten-containing foods. Gluten is a protein compound made up of two proteins called gliadin and glutenin that is found joined with starch in the grains wheat, rye, and barley.
4. Gluten sensitivity occurs when the body has a pronounced response to gluten-containing foods, leading to feelings of tiredness, abdominal pain, and other GI symptoms like diarrhea or constipation.
5. While a poorly planned gluten-free diet can lead to micronutrient deficiencies, with appropriate planning, a person can safely follow a gluten-free diet without risk to nutritional quality.
6. A food allergy is caused by the body's immune system reacting to a protein in a specific food. A food intolerance does not involve the body's immune system and results from a deficiency in an enzyme that is needed to break down a food.
7. An exercised-induced food allergy is a reaction to a food that occurs only when the food is consumed prior to exercising. As exercise intensity and body temperature increase, the person begins to experience itching, lightheadedness, possibly hives, and sometimes even anaphylaxis.
8. The Paleo diet, raw food diet, and detox diet are a few special eating plans some athletes may follow for perceived performance or health gains, as opposed to other diets described throughout the book that are followed for weight loss, or as part of the treatment for a particular chronic disease or ailment.
9. The Paleo diet is an eating plan intended to mimic what hunters and gatherers ate in the Paleolithic period over 10,000 ago before the advent of agriculture: whole fruits and vegetables, fish, grass-fed livestock, fungi, roots, and nuts. The diet prohibits grains, legumes, dairy products, salt, refined sugar, and all processed foods. While there is a lack of quality scientific research evaluating the merits and limitations of this eating plan, there is concern over the diet, as a panel of expert reviewers tasked with ranking 24 diets for *U.S. News & World Report* ranked the Paleo diet at the bottom.[20]
10. The raw food diet emphasizes intake of foods in their natural, unprocessed, uncooked form. There are both potential health benefits as well as potential health risks associated with this diet.
11. There are a variety of detox diets a client may opt to follow, each aiming to purge the body of harmful 21st-century toxins including food additives, pesticides, pollutants, and other

synthetic compounds in order to achieve a state of body purification. Some detox diets may be harmful, others can be very expensive, and some pose no apparent health risks, however, no such diet has been proven effective at "detoxifying" the body.

12. The key to working with athletes who follow a special eating plan is to develop a consistent approach to help them optimize their nutrition and performance while respecting their beliefs. However, if an athlete has adopted an eating plan that is clearly dangerous, a more assertive approach including discussing concerns with the athlete and referring to a registered dietitian and physician may be necessary.

PRACTICAL APPLICATIONS

1. Poorly planned vegetarian diets have a tendency to be low in which of the following nutrients?
   A. Omega-6 fatty acids
   B. Vitamin C
   C. Beta-carotene
   D. Vitamin B_{12}

2. Holly is an endurance runner who trains 4 to 5 days per week and typically competes in three marathons a year. She is also a vegan. What percentage of her total daily calories should come from carbohydrates?
   A. 40% to 50%
   B. 50% to 60%
   C. 60% to 70%
   D. 70% to 80%

3. Tom is a 200-pound (91-kg) bodybuilder who eats a pesco-vegetarian diet. He also supplements his daily meal plan with a smoothie that contains protein powder. According to established guidelines, what is the maximum amount of protein that Tom should eat per day?
   A. 171 grams
   B. 155 grams
   C. 144 grams
   D. 128 grams

4. Which of the following recommendations is an appropriate strategy for a vegetarian athlete who wants to increase his or her caloric intake?
   A. Add dried fruit, seeds, nuts, and avocados to meals and snacks
   B. Eat larger meals and fewer snacks
   C. Avoid meat alternatives
   D. Introduce high-calorie beverages

5. Which of the following statements about vegetarians is true?
   A. Vegetarians must consume adequate amounts of complementary plant proteins within the same meal to meet their protein needs.
   B. Iron-deficiency anemia affects approximately 30% of vegetarian endurance athletes.
   C. Vegetarian athletes should consider creatine supplementation, if peak performance is essential.
   D. Vegetarians can enhance iron absorption by consuming a food that is high in vitamin A.

6. Which of the following nutrients would most likely be deficient in a poorly planned gluten-free eating plan?
   A. B vitamins
   B. Potassium
   C. Vitamin E
   D. Phosphorous

7. Which of the following medical problems is characterized by an autoimmune rejection of gluten-containing foods?
   A. Crohn's disease
   B. Marfan's syndrome
   C. Gluten sensitivity
   D. Celiac disease

8. What condition is the result of a deficiency in an enzyme that is needed to break down a food?
   A. Food poisoning
   B. Food intolerance
   C. Food allergy
   D. Foodborne illness

9. Normally, Trisha eats a small snack about 30 minutes before exercising. Today, she snacked on a couple of slices of cheese before heading to the gym for an intense exercise session. During her workout, Trisha became light-headed and experienced itching and hives on her forearms. From what condition could Trisha be suffering?
   A. Heat exhaustion
   B. Poor histamine regulation
   C. Exercise-induced food allergy
   D. Exercise-induced inflammation

10. Which popular eating plan encourages the consumer to avoid food additives, pesticides, pollutants, and other synthetic compounds in order to achieve a state of body purification?
   A. Paleo diet
   B. Raw food diet
   C. Detox diet
   D. Gentle cleanse diet

Case 1 Kate, the Marathon Runner

Kate is an experienced 22-year-old marathon runner who recently successfully qualified for the Boston Marathon by shaving 20 minutes off of her personal record. While training for the marathon she became a vegetarian. Now she is considering eliminating all animal products from her diet and becoming a vegan.

1. What does it mean to be a vegan? List specific types of foods that are and are not consumed in a vegan diet.
2. What vitamins and minerals do vegans face increased risk of deficiency for? What are some good food sources of these vitamins and minerals that are allowable in the vegan diet? For which, if any, of the vitamins and minerals would a vegan need to take a supplement in order to avoid deficiency?
3. How does a vegan diet affect athletic performance? What are some general considerations vegan athletes should consider to optimize performance while adhering to a vegan diet?
4. Kate asks if you will help develop a vegan eating plan for her. How do you respond?

Case 2 Brian the High School Basketball Player

Brian is a 15-year-old basketball player whose mother has hired you to help him adopt a healthier eating plan and also help him optimize his fitness level in the off season. Today Brian comes to his session excited and eager to work out. However, after about 3 minutes of exercise, Brian becomes disproportionately out of breath and itchy.

1. How do you respond?
2. You learn that Brian has been trying to eat healthier and ate a lunch which included a salad with tomatoes and celery.
   a. Given this history, what is a possible cause of Brian's symptoms?
   b. How could Brian avoid this occurring in the future?
   c. What, if any, changes should Brian make in his everyday eating plan, given this event?
3. List the eight most common food allergens. For each food allergen, include several examples of foods that contain the allergen.
4. After this experience Brian shares that he is allergic to shellfish. He said that he never told you because you never asked. On further questioning he shares that he had to be hospitalized when he was 12 years old with anaphylaxis to shrimp. You ask him if he carries an epinephrine pen with him. He replies "no."
   Outline how you might proceed to discuss the management of food allergies with Brian and any further recommendations you might make.

TRAIN YOURSELF

1. Imagine you have decided to adopt a vegetarian diet.
   a. List foods that you would like to eat to form a complete protein.
   b. While you are generally satisfied with your new eating plan, you have noticed that you have decreased energy during your workouts and have unintentionally lost weight. You worry that maybe you are not eating enough calories to fuel your exercise.
      i. Describe the concept of *energy availability.*
      ii. List five nutrient-dense vegetarian foods you might eat to increase your caloric intake.

RESOURCES

Food and Nutrition Information Center, USDA. Vegetarian Nutrition. (www.nal.usda.gov/fnic/etext/000058.html). Provides the latest on vegetarianism and link to other reputable websites.

Vegan Society (vegan society.com) An educational U.K.-registered charity promoting vegan lifestyles. Provides a link for vegan and sport.

Seventh-Day Adventist Dietetic Association (www.sdada.org). An affiliate of the American Dietetic Association promoting plant-based nutrition.

VeganHealth (www.veganhealth.org). A branch of Vegan Outreach, offers links to more information about veganism and health. Includes a list of resources pertaining to veganism and athletes.

Vegetarian Resource Group (www.vrg.org). Includes a link for veganism, vegan meals, and travel.

VegRD (http://vegrd.vegan.com). Maintained by leading vegetarian researcher Virginia Messina, provides links to archived newsletters on a variety of vegan topics, including vegan foods for backpacking and vegan workout shakes.

Quick Start Diet Guide: Celiac Disease Foundation (CDF) and Gluten Intolerance Group (GIG) www.celiac.org, www.gluten.net.

Celiac Disease and Gluten-Free Diet Support Center.www .celiac.com.

Gluten Free Diet Guide for Families from the North American Society for Pediatric Gastroenterology, Nutrition, Hepatology, and Nutrition
http://naspghan.org/user-assets/Documents/pdf/diseaseInfo/GlutenFreeDietGuide-E.pdf.

REFERENCES

1. Craig WJ, Mangels AR. Position of the American Dietetic Association: vegetarian diets. *J Am Diet Assoc.* July 2009;109(7):1266-1282.
2. Venderley AM, Campbell WW. Vegetarian diets: nutritional considerations for athletes. *Sports Med.* 2006;36(4):293-305.
3. Davis BC, Kris-Etherton PM. Achieving optimal essential fatty acid status in vegetarians: current knowledge and practical implications. *Am J Clin Nutr.* September 2003;78 (3 Suppl):640S-646S.
4. Nieman DC. Physical fitness and vegetarian diets: is there a relation? *Am J Clin Nutr.* September 1999;70(3 Suppl): 570S-575S.
5. Rodriguez NR, DiMarco NM, Langley S. Position of the American Dietetic Association, Dietitians of Canada, and the American College of Sports Medicine: nutrition and athletic performance. *J Am Diet Assoc.* March 2009;109(3): 509-527.
6. *Dietary Reference Intakes for Energy, Carbohydrate, Fiber, Fat, Fatty Acids, Cholesterol, Protein, and Amino Acids.* Washington, DC: Food and Nutrition Board, Institute of Medicine; 2005.
7. Fontana L, Shew JL, Holloszy JO, Villareal DT. Low bone mass in subjects on a long-term raw vegetarian diet. *Arch Intern Med.* March 28 2005;165(6):684-689.
8. Barr SI, Rideout CA. Nutritional considerations for vegetarian athletes. *Nutrition.* July-August 2004;20(7-8):696-703.
9. Armstrong MJ, Hegade VS, Robins G. Advances in coeliac disease. *Curr Opin Gastroenterol.* March 2012;28(2):104-112.
10. Biesiekierski JR, Peters SL, Newnham ED, et al. No effects of gluten in patients with self-reported non-celiac gluten sensitivity after dietary reduction of fermentable, poorly-absorbed, short-chain carbohydrates. *Gastroenterology.* August 2013; 145(2): 320–328.
11. Hallert C, Grant C, Grehn S, et al. Evidence of poor vitamin status in coeliac patients on a gluten-free diet for 10 years. *Aliment Pharmacol Ther.* July 2002;16(7):1333-1339.
12. Thompson T, Dennis M, Higgins LA, Lee AR, Sharrett MK. Gluten-free diet survey: are Americans with coeliac disease consuming recommended amounts of fibre, iron, calcium and grain foods? *J Hum Nutr Diet.* June 2005; 18(3):163-169.
13. Sampson HA. Clinical practice. Peanut allergy. *N Engl J Med.* April 25 2002;346(17):1294-1299.
14. Clark S, Espinola J, Rudders SA, Banerji A, Camargo CA, Jr. Frequency of US emergency department visits for food-related acute allergic reactions. *J Allergy Clin Immunol.* March 2011;127(3):682-683.
15. Press TC. Girl with peanut allergy dies after kiss. *Toronto Sun* November 25, 2005.
16. *State and County Quick Facts*: U.S. Census Bureau; 2010.
17. Liu AH, Jaramillo R, Sicherer SH, et al. National prevalence and risk factors for food allergy and relationship to asthma: results from the National Health and Nutrition Examination Survey 2005-2006. *J Allergy Clin Immunol.* October 2010; 126(4):798-806 e713.
18. Keet C. Recognition and management of food-induced anaphylaxis. *Pediatr Clin North Am.* April 2011;58(2):377-388.
19. National Institue of Allergy and Infectious Diseases. Food allergy: an overview. 2010; available at: www.niaid.nih.gov/topics/foodAllergy/Documents/foodallergy.pdf Retrieved February 15, 2014.
20. *US News and World Report.* Best diets. 2013; available at: http://health.usnews.com/best-diet/best-overall-diets?page=4 Retrieved February 15, 2014.
21. Pan A, Sun Q, Bernstein AM, et al. Red meat consumption and mortality: results from 2 prospective cohort studies. *Arch Intern Med.* April 9 2012;172(7):555-563.
22. Koebnick C, Garcia AL, Dagnelie PC, et al. Long-term consumption of a raw food diet is associated with favorable serum LDL cholesterol and triglycerides but also with elevated plasma homocysteine and low serum HDL cholesterol in humans. *J Nutr.* October 2005;135(10): 2372-2378.
23. Koebnick C, Strassner C, Hoffmann I, Leitzmann C. Consequences of a long-term raw food diet on body weight and menstruation: results of a questionnaire survey. *Ann Nutr Metab.* 1999;43(2):69-79.
24. Donaldson MS, Speight N, Loomis S. Fibromyalgia syndrome improved using a mostly raw vegetarian diet: an observational study. *BMC Complement Altern Med.* 2001;1:7.
25. Douglass JM, Rasgon IM, Fleiss PM, Schmidt RD, Peters SN, Abelmann EA. Effects of a raw food diet on hypertension and obesity. *South Med J.* July 1985;78(7):841-844.
26. MacGregor HE. Purification, or just a purge? *Los Angeles Times* October 23, 2006.
27. Biesiekierski JR, Newnham ED, Irving PM, et al. Gluten causes gastrointestinal symptoms in subjects without celiac disease: a double-blind randomized placebo-controlled trial. *Am J Gastroenterol.* March 2011;106(3):508-514; quiz 515.

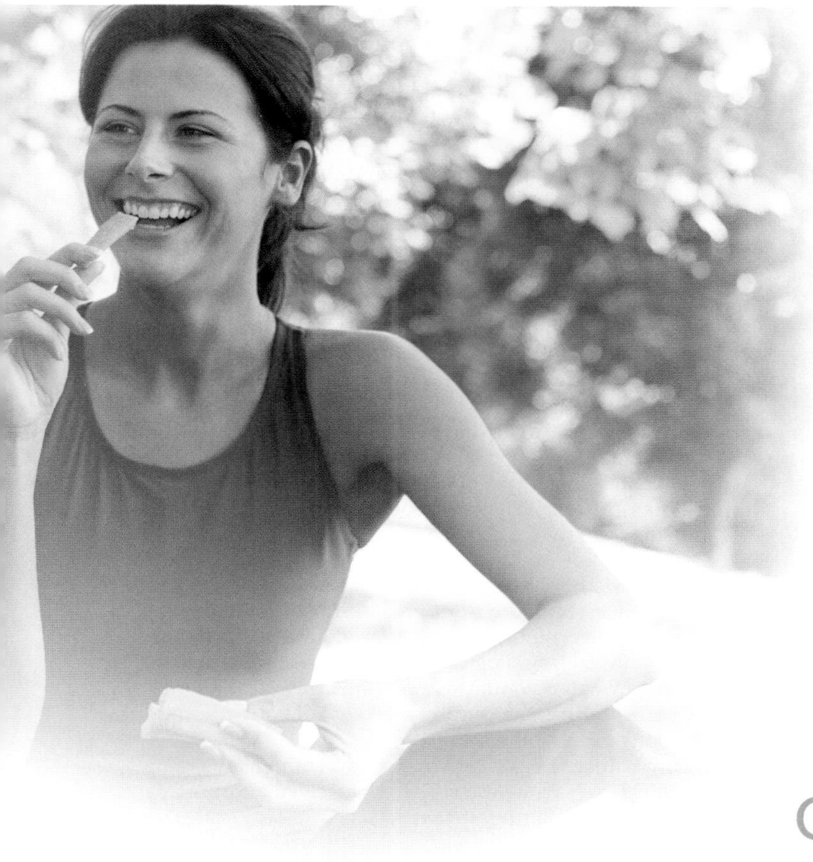

Glossary

absorption The transfer of nutrients from the digestive system into the blood supply.

acceptable macronutrient distribution range (AMDR) The range of intake for a macronutrient that is associated with decreased risk of chronic disease while providing sufficient intake of essential nutrients.

acclimatization Physiological changes that occur in response to repeated exposure to an environmental condition such as heat or high altitude.

active dehydration Dehydration resulting from increasing exercise and heat exposure.

active transport The passage of a particle from an area of low concentration to an area of high concentration made possible through the use of ATP.

acute illness Sudden onset of a time-limited ailment.

adenosine triphosphate (ATP) The body's usable energy source.

adequate intake The amount of intake believed to cover the needs of all healthy individuals in age- and gender-specific groups; used when insufficient evidence is available to establish an RDA.

adipocyte A fat cell.

adiponectin A hormone produced by fat cells; it increases insulin sensitivity and stimulates fat breakdown. Low levels may contribute to an increased risk for insulin resistance and diabetes.

adipose tissue Fatty tissue; connective tissue made of fat cells.

adipositas athletica A term describing athletes who try to gain body fat to increase insulation or increase body energy stores.

aerobic power The speed at which adenosine triphosphate (ATP) is generated; increased in endurance athletes due to metabolic adaptations.

aerobic respiration The 10-step metabolic process of breaking glucose down to intermediate pyruvate, which is converted to acetyl-coA and enters the citric acid cycle. Occurs in the mitochondria and cytoplasm in the presence of oxygen; produces a net 36 ATP.

air displacement plethysmography (ADP) (brand name is BodPod) A device that uses the displacement of air to measure body volume and density; compare to hydrostatic weighing which uses the displacement of water to estimate body composition.

alanine-glucose cycle The cycle of transporting pyruvate and nitrogen from the muscle tissues to the liver as the amino acid alanine. In the liver, the alanine unloads the nitrogen group to become pyruvate, which is converted to glucose through gluconeogenesis. This process moves the work of gluconeogenesis from the muscle to the liver.

aldosterone A hormone released by the adrenal gland that helps to maintain normal blood sodium levels by increasing the kidney's reabsorption of sodium and decreasing the amount of sodium lost in sweat.

amenorrhea A female condition defined by at least 3 months without a menstrual period.

amino acids The basic building blocks of proteins. Each amino acid has an amino- or nitrogen-containing group and a unique R chain that determines its ability to be used in various processes. Also known as peptides.

amino acid pool The amino acids available in the body to be used for protein synthesis.

amylopectin A polysaccharide, highly branched chain of glucose molecules that is easily digested.

amylose A polysaccharide made of glucose molecules bound together in a linear chain that is mostly resistant to digestion.

anabolic steroids Synthetic drugs that mimic the effect of testosterone and dihydrotestosterone in the body; cause rapid strength gains but also carry significant toxic effects; expressly prohibited in sports competition.

anabolism The state in which the body builds and creates new tissues.

anaerobic respiration The 10-step metabolic process of breaking glucose down to intermediate pyruvate and then lactic acid; occurs in the cytoplasm of cells in the absence of oxygen; produces a net 2 ATP.

anaerobic threshold (AT) Point in exercise when lactate accumulation begins; also known as lactate threshold or ventilatory threshold.

anaphylactic shock The potentially life-threatening state the body enters when experiencing anaphylaxis; also known as anaphylaxis.

anaphylaxis A potentially life-threatening allergic reaction with a wide range of symptoms including hives, swelling, itching, and difficulty breathing and swallowing.

andiuretic hormone A hormone secreted by the pituitary gland that helps to maintain blood volume in the face of dehydration by increasing water reabsorption in the kidneys and decreasing the amount of urine produced.

androgen A hormone that stimulates or produces masculine characteristics.

android body type "Apple shaped"; body tends to carry excess fat around the abdomen.

android obesity Excess weight distributed mostly in the abdomen ("apple shape").

angina Chest pain due to decreased blood flow resulting in inadequate supply of oxygen to the heart muscle.

anion A negatively charged molecule.

anorexia athletica A sport-induced subclinical eating disorder.

anorexia nervosa An eating disorder characterized by caloric restriction leading to significantly low body weight, intense fear of gaining weight or becoming fat, and preoccupation with body or inability or refusal to recognize the harm of extremely thin body size.

antibodies Proteins that fight infection.

antidiuretic hormone A hormone released by the anterior pituitary which helps to maintain blood volume in the face of dehydration by increasing water reabsorption in the kidneys and decreasing the amount of urine produced.

antioxidant A substance that prevents or repairs oxidative damage; includes vitamins C and E, some carotenoids, selenium, quinones, and bioflavonoids.

arachidonic acid A polyunsaturated omega-6 fatty acid contained within the phospholipid bilayer that, when cleaved, initiates a series of reactions leading to the formation of eicosanoids.

atherogenic dyslipidemia A triad of increased blood concentrations of small, dense low-density lipoprotein (LDL) particles, decreased high-density lipoprotein (HDL) particles, and increased triglycerides.

atherosclerosis The accumulation of fatty material on the inner walls of the arteries, causing them to harden, thicken, and lose elasticity.

atypical anorexia nervosa A condition in which all of the criteria for anorexia are met, except that, despite significant weight loss, the individual's weight is within or above the normal range.

avoidant/restrictive eating disorder A condition in which an individual restricts or limits food intake, but does not meet the criteria for other eating disorders.

beta oxidation The process in which carbon fragments are removed from the fatty acid. These carbon molecules produce acetyl Co-A, which enters the citric acid cycle and electron transport chain.

bile acids Produced by the liver and stored in the gallbladder, these acids are important in the digestion of fat. After lipid digestion, they are recycled and reused by the liver.

binge eating Eating, in a discrete period of time (e.g., within any 2-hour period), an amount of food that is definitely larger than most people would eat during a similar period of time under similar circumstances, and a sense of lack of control over eating during the episode.

binge-eating disorder A condition characterized by repeated overconsumption of large amounts of food in a short period of time.

binge-eating/purging type of anorexia nervosa During the last 3 months, the individual has engaged in recurrent episodes of binge eating or purging behavior.

bioavailability The degree to which a nutrient can be absorbed and used by the body.

bioelectrical impedance analysis An indirect measure of body composition that measures the conduction of current through muscle and fat, and inserts data into a predictive equation to estimate fat mass and lean mass.

bioenergetics The process of studying the capture, conversion, and use of energy from ATP.

body composition The proportion of fat and lean mass.

body density Calculated by dividing body weight by body volume; an intermediary to convert circumference measurements to body fat percentage.

body dysmorphic disorder A disorder in which an individual develops persistent and obtrusive thoughts and preoccupations with an imagined or slight defect in appearance.

body mass index Weight in kilograms divided by height in meters squared; a proxy for measurement of body composition.

bolus A food and saliva digestive mix that is swallowed and further digested in the stomach and small intestine.

bone age A determination of the maturation of the bones in relation to chronological age used as a marker to assess further growth potential; assessed by x-ray.

bone remodeling The continual process of bone resorption and bone formation.

bonking Athlete fatigue in which exercise intensity dramatically decreases while the athlete's perceived effort increases. Also known as "hitting the wall."

botanical See *herbal supplements*.

branched chain amino acids Essential amino acids with a branched R chain. These amino acids are metabolized in the muscle and are thought to be important in the formation of muscle mass.

brown adipose tissue Fat used to produce heat and potentially burn excess calories.

brush border The site of nutrient absorption in the small intestine. Enterocyte cells line the small intestine and have microvilli. The microvilli are closely packed together and resemble the bristles of a brush. The enterocyte cells secrete enzymes and proteins that assist with nutrient absorption.

built environment The human-made environment surrounding us, such as buildings and parks.

bulimia nervosa An eating disorder characterized by regular episodes of overeating and binge eating which is then compensated with unhealthy weight-loss strategies including vomiting, excessive exercise, or laxative abuse.

caloric deficit The net expenditure of calories created when calories expended exceed calories consumed.

calorie The amount of energy needed to increase 1 kilogram of water by 1 degree Celsius. It is used to measure the amount of energy in a food available after digestion.

carbohydrate A macronutrient made of carbon, hydrogen, and oxygen; the body's preferred energy source.

carbohydrate loading Eating pattern that consists of increasing the amount of carbohydrates consumed in the days leading up to an athletic endurance event to maximize muscle and liver glycogen stores. Typically, activity levels are decreased during this time as well.

carbonic acid An acid formed in the body that acts as an intermediate between sodium bicarbonate/hydrogen ions and carbon dioxide/water.

cardiac output (Q) The amount of blood pumped through the heart per minute (mL blood/min); calculated as stroke volume (mL/beat) × heart rate (beat/min).

cardiovascular disease A term that refers to disease of the heart and vascular system.
carnosine A dipeptide comprised of the basic amino acids alanine and histidine.
catabolism The state in which the body breaks down tissues and amino acids for fuel.
cation A positively charged molecule.
celiac disease A condition in which the body's immune system reacts to gluten-containing foods and initiates an allergic reaction. Inflammation of the gastrointestinal system results, and in addition to other symptoms such as abdominal bloating pain, diarrhea, vomiting, and fatigue, there is decreased absorption of nutrients by the body, which can lead to deficiencies.
cellulose A low viscosity starch made of long chains of glucose; a structural component of the cell wall in plants that is indigestible to humans.
Centers for Disease Control and Prevention (CDC) An agency of the federal government whose mission is to work with other health agencies to optimally promote health, prevent disease, reduce injury and disability, and prepare for and respond to health threats.
certified specialist in sports dietetics Working as a registered dietitian for a minimum of 2 years applying evidence-based nutrition knowledge in exercise and sports. They assess, educate, and counsel athletes and active individuals. They design, implement, and manage safe and effective nutrition strategies that enhance lifelong health, fitness, and optimal performance (definition from the Commission on Dietetic Registration, www.cdrnet.org).
chelation compounds A compound that consists of a molecule bonded to a single atom, usually a metal, which allows the metal to be more efficiently absorbed by the body.
cholecalciferol See *vitamin D.*
cholecystokinin (CCK) A hormone released from the small intestine in response to the presence of amino acids and fatty acids from protein and fat digestion; stimulates the pancreas to secrete enzymes, stimulates the gallbladder to contract, and slows gastric emptying through release of gastric inhibitory peptide and secretin.
cholesterol A fat-like waxy structure found in the blood and body tissues and some animal-based foods. Cholesterol is important in metabolism as the precursor to various steroid hormones. It is transported in the body via lipoproteins. Excess cholesterol can contribute to cardiovascular disease.
chylomicron A large lipoprotein particle that transports fat from digested food from the small intestine to the liver and adipose tissue.
chyme A partially digested mass of food formed in the stomach and released into the duodenum of the small intestine.
citric acid cycle A metabolic pathway involved in the chemical conversion of carbohydrates, fats, and proteins into carbon dioxide and water to generate a form of usable energy. Also known as Krebs cycle and tricarboxylic acid cycle.
cofactor A substance that needs to be present in addition to an enzyme in order for a chemical reaction to occur.
cold diuresis Increased urine production and excretion that occurs in extreme cold as a result of peripheral vasoconstriction, high blood sugar, and decreased renal reabsorption of water.
colonic bacteria Benign bacteria that colonize the large intestine (the colon) of the human gut.
complementary protein Combining two or more limiting proteins to form a complete protein.
complete protein A food item that contains all of the essential amino acids.
complex carbohydrates Oligosaccharides and polysaccharides; multiple monosacchariedes joined by glycosidic bonds; takes more time to digest than a simple carbohydrate.
contamination Inadvertent tainting of a supplement with trace amounts of another supplement without the knowledge of the manufacturer or consumer.
continuance Continuing to exercise despite knowing that this activity is creating or worsening physical, psychological, and/or interpersonal problems.
coronary heart disease The major form of cardiovascular disease that results when the arteries supplying the heart muscle (coronary arteries) are narrowed or completely blocked by deposits of fat and fibrous tissue.
creatine phosphate An important source of stored energy; its breakdown to creatine plus a high energy phosphate can rapidly fuel the first 5 to 10 seconds of exercise.
cross-bridge cycle The process whereby a series of molecular actions cause myosin and actin to combine and produce muscle contraction.
Current Good Manufacturing Practices (CGMPs) Regulations that ensure that dietary supplements made in the United States and abroad are consistently produced and of acceptable quality by creating manufacturing standards for all companies that test, produce, package, label, and distribute supplements in the United States.
daily value (DV) The recommended level of intake for a nutrient.
DASH eating plan Dietary Approaches to Stop Hypertension; an eating plan that is high in fruits and vegetables and low in sodium, which has been found to reduce blood pressure in people with hypertension as well as provide countless other benefits.
deamination The process of removing a nitrogen group from an amino acid.
decisional balance The weighing of pros and cons when considering a behavior change.
dehydration A state of decreased total body fluid, which is categorized as mild (<2% loss of body weight), moderate (2% to 7%), and severe (>7%).
denaturation The process of unfolding a protein by destroying its quaternary, tertiary, and secondary structure.
detoxification Used to describe diets that attempt to purge the body of harmful 21st-century toxins including food additives, pesticides, pollutants, and other synthetic compounds in order to achieve a state of body purification.
dietary fat Fat consumed in the diet; in contrast to fat produced in the body.
dietary fiber Nondigestible carbohydrates and lignins that are obtained naturally from plant foods.
Dietary Guidelines for Americans Published every 5 years, these federally released guidelines provide evidence-based nutrition information and advice for people age 2 and older. They serve as the basis for federal food and nutrition education programs.
dietary reference intake (DRI) A collective term used to refer to several types of reference values: recommended dietary allowance (RDA), estimated average requirement (EAR), tolerable upper intake level (UL), and adequate intake (AI).
dietary supplement A product (other than tobacco) that functions to supplement the diet and contains one or more of the following ingredients: a vitamin, mineral, herb or other botanical, amino acid, dietary substance that increases total daily intake, metabolite, constituent, extract, or some combination of the above ingredients.
Dietary Supplement and Health Education Act (DSHEA) Federal regulation that oversees supplement production, marketing, and safety; treats supplements more like food than medicine with limited oversight and accountability.
digestion The process of breaking down food into units small enough for absorption.
digestive system The network of organs and tissues that break down and absorb food and rid the body of waste. Primary organs and tissues are: mouth, esophagus, stomach,

small intestine, large intestine, and anus. Accessory organs are: liver, pancreas, and gallbladder.

dipeptide Two amino acids connected by a peptide bond.

disaccharide A simple carbohydrate; two monosaccharides bound together. Maltose, sucrose and lactose are all disaccharides.

disordered eating Eating patterns that are considered to be irregular, especially when compared to a normal, healthy individual of the same culture.

diuresis Increased urine production and excretion.

diuretics Medications or substances that lead to increased water loss from the kidneys.

doping The act of ingesting a substance banned by the World Anti-Doping Agency in an effort to improve athletic performance.

dual-energy x-ray absorptiometry (DXA) A method of body composition assessment that maps the bone density, fat mass, and fat-free tissue mass using two low-dose x-rays from different sources that measure bone and soft tissue mass simultaneously.

duodenum The approximately 1-foot long first portion of the small intestine where the majority of chemical digestion of food occurs.

eating disorder not elsewhere specified Eating disorders that do not meet the strict diagnostic criteria to be classified as more specific disorders.

ectomorph Body type characterized by thinness with lean muscles, fast metabolism, and difficulty gaining weight.

eicosanoids Locally acting hormones that are made from omega-3 and omega-6 fatty acids and play roles in inflammation, fever, regulation of blood pressure, blood clotting, immunity, control of reproductive processes and tissue growth, and regulation of the sleep/wake cycle.

electrolytes Minerals that exist as charged ions in the body and are extremely important for normal cellular function.

electron-transport chain The process of stripping NADH and FADH of their hydrogen molecules through a series of chemical reduction-oxidation reactions, which ultimately powers the conversion of ADP plus Pi to ATP and provides energy to the working cell.

empathic statements Statements that express an attempt to understand what another person is experiencing.

empty calories Calories that provide little to no nutritional value; also referred to as SoFAS (solid fats and added sugar) in the *Dietary Guidelines for Americans*.

emulsify To break lipids into small droplets to facilitate fat digestion and absorption.

encephalopathy Loss of normal function of brain tissue, which may result from a wide variety of conditions including hyponatremia.

endomorph Body type characterized by a slow metabolism and propensity to gain fat.

endurance sports Sports and activities lasting 30 minutes or more.

enema A procedure to flush out the colon and rectum using liquid applied through the anus.

energy availability The energy available in the body to fuel physical activity and energy-requiring body functions. Determined by the relationship between the calories consumed in the diet and the calories expended in physical activity.

energy balance The relationship of calories consumed with calories expended.

energy drinks Beverages containing caffeine or other supplements in addition to carbohydrates; potential risks outweigh benefits in children.

energy expenditure The amount of calories burned by the body in a 24-hour period.

enriched food A food to which specific nutrients, such as B vitamins and iron, are added to replace nutrients lost during processing.

enzymes Proteins that speed up the rate of chemical reactions.

epinephrine pen A pen-shaped applicator containing a dose of epinephrine, which is used to stop anaphylaxis, a life-threatening allergic reaction.

epiphyses Growth plates; closure signifies the cessation of further linear growth.

equal nitrogen balance The state in which the amount of nitrogen (via protein) consumed is equal to the amount of nitrogen excreted in feces, urine, and skin; a healthy adult is typically in equilibrium.

ergogenic A substance that increases athletic performance.

esophagus A muscular tube extending from the mouth to the stomach.

essential amino acid An amino acid that cannot be made by the body and must be consumed in the diet.

essential fat The fat required for normal body functioning including that of the brain, nerves, heart, lungs, and liver; typically 3% to 5% in men and 10% to 15% in women.

essential fatty acids Fats that are not produced by the body and must be consumed in the diet; linolenic and linoleic acids.

estimated average requirement An amount of nutrient known to be adequate to meet nutritional needs in 50% of an age- and gender-specific group.

estrogen A female sex hormone secreted by the ovaries that stimulates or produces feminine sexual characteristics, aids in bone formation, and plays a role in amenorrhea and the female athlete triad; typically refers to estrogen, estradiol, estrone, and estriol.

euhydration A state of "normal" body water content; the perfect balance between "too much" and "not enough" fluid intake.

excess post-exercise oxygen consumption (EPOC) The elevated oxygen consumption after high-intensity exercise has stopped.

exercise dependence The condition in which a person is preoccupied with exercise and training to the extent that the person engages in excessive levels of exercise, resulting in negative physiological and psychological consequences.

exercise immunology The study of the effects of exercise on the immune response.

exercise-related transient abdominal pain (ETAP) Abdominal pain of uncertain etiology that occurs during physical exercise; more common in novice athletes and individuals who have rapidly increased exercise intensity or duration.

exertional hyponatremia Abnormally low blood sodium level that results from excessive intake of low-sodium fluids during prolonged endurance activities.

facilitated diffusion The passage of a particle from an area of high concentration to an area of low concentration with a protein carrier.

fat adaptation Increasing dietary fat consumption in an effort to increase fatty acid oxidation during exercise with the intent of sparing glycogen stores.

fat loading A strategy of progressively increasing percentage of fat intake to increase fatty acid oxidation and thus preserve glycogen stores for prolonged exercise.

fat-soluble vitamins Vitamins that are stored in and absorbed by fat; vitamins A, D, E, and K.

fatty acids Long hydrocarbon chains with varying degrees of saturation with hydrogen.

Federal Trade Commission (FTC) The government agency tasked with the job of preventing unfair methods of competition and enforcement of "unfair and deceptive acts or practices," such as misleading advertisements.

feeding or eating disorders not elsewhere classified Eating disorders that do not meet the strict diagnostic criteria to be classified as more specific disorders.

female athlete triad A syndrome characterized by an eating disorder (or low energy availability), amenorrhea, and decreased bone mineral density.

ferritin The storage form of iron.

field methods Techniques allied health professionals commonly use to measure body composition.
flavin adenine dinucleotide (FADH) A hydrogen-carrying molecule that enters the electron transport chain to produce 2 ATPs per molecule of FADH.
flavonoid Antioxidant found naturally in many fruits and vegetables.
flexitarian diet Synonymous with the *semi-vegetarian diet*, this diet is one in which a person does not usually eat meat, fish, or poultry but will infrequently include these foods in their diet.
food addiction A controversial concept; may occur in certain individuals in which consumption of highly palatable foods such as sugar, salt, and fat trigger a response in the brain leading to binge eating, pervasive thoughts of food, and ultimately, obesity.
Food and Drug Administration (FDA) An agency within the Department of Health and Human Services which, among other functions, monitors food and drug safety, oversees nutrition labeling, regulates tobacco products, and provides the public with credible health information.
food frequency questionnaire A method used to identify typical eating habits, which is composed of a checklist of foods and beverages with a section for the client to mark how often each of the listed foods are eaten.
food intolerance A reaction to certain foods that results from a deficiency in an enzyme that is needed to break down that food. The immune system is not involved in the reaction.
food poisoning Illness that results from ingestion of toxins released by bacteria that grow on food.
food record A written report of all of the foods consumed in a pre-defined period of time, usually 3 days with at least 1 weekend day. Also includes the time of day, mood, and level of hunger when consuming each food.
fortified food A food to which specific nutrients not inherently available in that food are added, such as vitamin D in milk.
fructooligosaccharide A category of oligosaccharides that are mostly indigestible, may help to relieve constipation, improve triglyceride levels, and decrease production of foul-smelling digestive byproducts.
fructose The sweetest of the monosaccharides, found in varying levels in different types of fruits.
functional anemia Low iron ferritin levels in the context of normal hemoglobin concentration.
functional fiber Nondigestible carbohydrates that have been isolated from foods and added to food products, and have a potentially beneficial effect on human health.
functional foods Defined by the Academy of Nutrition and Dietetics as any whole, fortified, enriched, or enhanced food that has a potentially beneficial effect on human health beyond basic nutrition.
galactose A monosaccharide, a component of lactose.
gallbladder An accessory organ of the gastrointestinal system that releases bile to aid in fat digestion.
gastric bypass A weight-loss procedure in which a surgeon reduces the stomach to about the size of an egg and then reattaches it to the small intestine, thereby "bypassing" most of the stomach.
gastric emptying The process by which food is emptied from the stomach into the small intestine.
gastric inhibitory peptide Protein that is released from the small intestine and functions to slow digestion by inhibiting gastric acid secretion and stimulating insulin release.
gastric lipase Enzyme released from the stomach that works with lingual lipase to digest short- and medium-chain fatty acids into partial glycerides and free fatty acids.
gastrin Hormone that prepares the stomach for food digestion; secreted by the stomach and stimulates pepsin release.
ghrelin The "hunger hormone"; a hormone released by the stomach in response to low energy levels in the body, which signals hunger.
gliadin A protein component of gluten, which triggers the immune system response for people with celiac disease.
glucagon A hormone secreted by the pancreas that stimulates glucose release from the liver when blood glucose levels are low.
glucocorticoid A classification of hormones released from the adrenal cortex that protect against stress or contribute to protein and carbohydrate metabolism; the most important is cortisol.
gluconeogenesis The production of glucose from precursors such as proteins or fats in the liver.
glucose The predominant monosaccharide in nature and the basic building block of most other carbohydrates.
gluten A protein compound that is made up of two proteins, glutenin and gliadin, and found in the grains wheat, barley, and rye.
gluten sensitivity Also known as gluten intolerance, a condition in which people appear to have a negative response to gluten-containing foods; however, no allergic reaction results.
glycemic index A measurement of the amount of increase in blood sugar after eating particular foods.
glycemic load A measure of a consumed carbohydrate's overall effect on blood glucose levels; equal to the glycemic index multiplied by the number of grams consumed divided by 100.
glycerol A molecule containing three carbon atoms and three OH molecules; creates an osmotic gradient in the circulation favoring fluid retention, which subsequently reduces fluid excretion from the kidneys and decreases urination; supplement is banned by the World Anti-Doping Agency.
glycogen A polysaccharide that is a highly branched chain of glucose molecules. The chief carbohydrate storage material in animals formed and stored in the liver and muscle.
glycogenolysis The process of breaking down glycogen into glucose molecules.
glycosidic bond A link between two sugar molecules. The two molecules share an oxygen atom.
gravitational sport A sport in which the force of gravity combined with an athlete's body mass impacts performance; examples include long-distance running, road cycling, and ski jumping.
gynoid body type "Pear shaped"; body tends to carry excess fat around the hips and thighs.
gynoid obesity Excess weight distributed mostly in the abdomen ("apple shape").
health claim A statement that suggests that a supplement may help to diagnose, prevent, mitigate, treat, or cure a specific disease.
health history questionnaire A form that aims to gather information about an individual's past medical history and family history to assess a client's health risk and determine need for evaluation by a medical professional.
Health Insurance Portability and Accountability Act (HIPAA) Federal legislation that requires express written permission from a patient or client authorizing sharing of health information among health professionals and institutions.
health screening A systematic assessment of a client's health history and risk factors to identify clients who may require evaluation by other health professionals before beginning a nutrition or activity program.
healthy diet score An indication of how well a person follows a healthy eating plan characterized by large amounts of fruits and vegetables, fish, and whole grains and low amounts of sodium and sugar-sweetened beverages.
heat cramps (exercise-associated muscle cramps) Muscle spasms resulting from loss of large amounts of water and electrolytes during physical exertion; typically affect the abdomen, arms, and calves.

heat exhaustion A heat-related illness that occurs after prolonged exposure to heat without adequate replacement of fluids and electrolytes; symptoms include heavy sweating, fatigue, and vomiting. Heat exhaustion is less serious than heat stroke.

heat stroke A severe heat-related illness with extreme overheating resulting from prolonged exposure to heat without adequate replacement of fluids and electrolytes; symptoms include lack of sweating, strong and rapid pulse, disorientation, and loss of consciousness; often fatal without rapid treatment.

heme iron Iron bound within the iron-carrying proteins of hemoglobulin and myoglobulin complex found in meat, fish, and poultry.

hemoglobin An iron-rich protein of red blood cells that carries oxygen to working cells.

herbal supplements Plant-derived substances used for medicinal purposes.

high density lipoprotein (HDL) Lipoprotein that contains approximately 50% protein and carries excess cholesterol from the bloodstream to the liver where it can be prepared for excretion; also known as good cholesterol.

high viscosity fiber See *soluble fiber.*

"hitting the wall" Athlete fatigue in which exercise intensity dramatically decreases while the athlete's perceived effort increases. Also known as bonking.

hormones Chemicals released by the body that affect other parts of the body; many banned synthetic hormones mimic the muscle-building effects of natural hormones, such as growth hormone, erythropoietin-stimulating hormone, and gonadotropins, which trigger increased testosterone production.

hydrogenation The process of adding hydrogen atoms to unsaturated fats. This process eliminates double bonds and turns fatty acids into partially or completely saturated fats.

hydrostatic weighing Also known as underwater weighing and hydrodensitometry; measures body composition by comparing the weight of a person in water and on land.

hyperglycemia An abnormally high level of glucose (sugar) in the blood.

hyperhydration Hydrating above currently optimal levels. By consuming large amounts of fluids prior to exercise, the athlete increases fluid reserves and delays the onset of dehydration.

hyperinsulinemia An abnormally high level of insulin in the blood.

hyperplasia Abnormal increase in the number of cells.

hypertonic fluids Fluids that contain sodium and other electrolytes in higher concentrations than in blood.

hypertrophy Abnormal increase in size; excessive growth.

hypoglycemia Low blood glucose (≤70 mg/dL); characterized by symptoms such as tiredness, weakness, shaking, fast heart rate, and feeling nervous.

hyponatremia An abnormally low concentration of blood sodium (less than 135 millimoles per liter (mmol/L)) which, when severe, can lead to brain swelling and death.

hypothalamus A portion of the brain responsible for regulating body temperature, among many other functions.

hypothermia Condition in which core body temperature falls below 35°C (95°F), the minimal temperature necessary for normal metabolism and body function.

ileum The final portion of the small intestine, which is approximately 12 feet in length; where absorption of vitamin B_{12}, bile salts, and digestive products not already absorbed in the jejunum occurs.

immunonutritional support The use of nutrient intake or supplementation to attenuate immune changes and inflammation following intensive exercise or injury.

inadvertent doping When an athlete tests positive for a banned substance due to accidental ingestion, often as a result of contamination of an allowed substance.

incomplete protein A food item that does not contain all of the essential amino acids.

indirect calorimetry A noninvasive study that estimates energy needs based on the use of oxygen and production of carbon dioxide.

insoluble fiber Fiber that does not bind with water and adds bulk to the diet (includes cellulose, hemicellulose, and lignins found in wheat bran, vegetables, and whole grain breads and cereals); important for proper bowel function and reducing symptoms of constipation.

insulin A hormone secreted by the pancreas that is required for the transport of glucose from blood into tissues.

insulin resistance The cells respond inefficiently or ineffectively to insulin.

intention effects Inability to stick to one's intended routine as evidenced by exceeding the amount of time devoted to exercise or consistently going beyond the intended amount.

intermediate density lipoprotein (IDL) Lipoprotein that is composed of cholesterol, triglycerides, and protein, and results from the degradation of very low density lipoprotein; transports cholesterol throughout the body.

iron deficiency A type of anemia caused by inadequate intake of iron that leads to decreased oxygen-carrying capacity due to decreased production of iron-requiring, oxygen-carrying hemoglobin.

iron deficiency anemia A condition resulting from too little iron in the body, which decreases hemoglobin concentration and thus impairs oxygen delivery to cells.

iron depletion A state of decreased body stores of iron but normal levels of iron in the red blood cells; if not corrected, progresses to iron deficiency anemia.

irritable bowel syndrome A gastrointestinal condition of uncertain etiology that manifests as abdominal pain and cramping, gas, bloating, and diarrhea or constipation.

isotonic fluids Fluids in which electrolyte content equals that of blood.

jejunum The middle portion of the small intestine, which is approximately 8 feet in length; where much of food absorption occurs.

Krebs cycle See *citric acid cycle*.

laboratory methods Techniques to measure body composition that generally are measured in a research or laboratory setting; methods include hydrodensitometry, air displacement plethysmography, isotope dilution, and dual-energy x-ray absorptiometry

lactase The enzyme required to digest lactose.

lactate A salt of lactic acid produced in the body.

lactate threshold Point in exercise when lactate accumulation begins. Also known as anaerobic threshold or ventilatory threshold.

lactic acid A metabolic byproduct of anaerobic glucose metabolism.

lacto-ovo-vegetarian A vegetarian who consumes eggs and dairy products but does not consume meat, poultry, or fish.

lactose A disaccharide made of glucose and galactose; the principal sugar found in milk.

lactose intolerance A condition in which a person does not make enough of the enzyme lactase required to break down the sugar lactose, resulting in gastrointestinal symptoms such as abdominal cramps, bloating, diarrhea, and flatulence when lactose is ingested.

lacto-vegetarian A vegetarian who consumes dairy products but does not consume eggs, meat, poultry, or fish.

large intestine Connects the small intestine to the anus; absorbs most of the fluid from waste products and serves as a storage site for fecal waste; includes three portions: the cecum, colon, and rectum.

laxatives Products used to soften stool and aid the body in excretion.

lecithin A phospholipid that breaks down into glycerol, stearic acid, phosphoric acid, and choline; a major component of HDL.

leptin A hormone produced by adipose tissue that suppresses appetite and increases energy expenditure; levels increase with increased fat storage.

lifestyle changes Changes made to daily routines or habits; in this instance changes are made to create a healthier lifestyle.

lingual lipase An enzyme released from the mouth that begins to break short- and medium-chain fatty acids into partial glycerides and free fatty acids.

linoleic acid See *omega-6 fatty acids.*

linolenic acid See *omega-3 fatty acids.*

lipids A fat or fat-like substance used in the body or bloodstream.

lipogenesis The production of fat from excess carbohydrates, protein, or fat that is consumed beyond what the body immediately can use for energy, structural support, or glycogen storage.

lipoprotein Compounds found in the bloodstream consisting of simple proteins bound to lipids including cholesterol, phospholipids, and triglycerides. Lipoproteins transport cholesterol and other lipids to and from various tissues.

lipoprotein lipase An enzyme that facilitates transport of lipid from a lipoprotein in the blood into the adipocyte or other tissue.

liver A large vital organ inside the body which plays a major role in metabolism including protein synthesis, glycogen storage, and production of chemicals necessary for digestion; other functions include detoxification and purification and breakdown of red blood cells.

low density lipoprotein (LDL) Lipoprotein that is composed of over 50% cholesterol; transports cholesterol and triglycerides from the liver and small intestine to cells and tissues; high levels are a proven cause of atherosclerosis.

low viscosity fiber See *insoluble fiber.*

lymph A mixture of proteins and fat transported from tissues to the bloodstream. Lymph helps to fight infection.

lymphatic system A network of organs, lymph nodes, lymph ducts, and lymph vessels that produce and transport lymph.

maltose A disaccharide of two glucose molecules bound together; found in malt beverages, chocolate malts, and beer.

master athletes Adult competitive athletes ranging in age from 30 to over 85 years.

medical nutrition therapy Nutritional assessment, one-on-one counseling, and therapy intended to treat a specific illness or disease; should only be administered by a registered dietitian.

mesomorph Body type characterized by an athletic and muscular physique.

metabolic fatigue The fatigue that occurs when the substrates for energy production are used up. Early on in a strength workout this could be from the depletion of creatine phosphate stores, while later fatigue results from impaired energy production from glycogenolysis and anaerobic glycolysis.

micelle A compound similar to a soap sud that has a hydrophobic (water-averse) inside and a hydrophilic (water-loving) outside.

micronutrient A nutrient that is needed in small quantities for normal growth and development; includes vitamins and minerals.

mineralocorticoid A steroid hormone that regulates fluid and electrolyte retention and excretion by the kidneys; typically refers to the hormone aldosterone.

mitochondria Organelles known as the "power plant" of the body's cells; the location where most ATP production occurs.

monosaccharide The simplest form of carbohydrate (glucose, galactose, and fructose); it cannot be digested any further.

monounsaturated fatty acid A type of unsaturated fatty acid that has one double bond between carbon atoms; includes oleic acid, the main component of olive oil.

motivational interviewing A communication technique in which the client and coach work together to help the client develop a plan of action for behavior change.

multi-component model A reference method of assessing body composition that bases an estimate of fat and lean mass on measurements from several methods; the four-component equation is the leading reference method. The variables include body volume, total body water, bone mineral, and body mass.

muscle dysmorphic disorder A form of body dysmorphic disorder in which a person engages in excessive amounts of resistance training in an effort to be "big."

muscle protein breakdown The rate of breakdown of muscle tissue into component amino acids.

muscle protein synthesis The rate of production of muscle tissue from the amino acid pool.

myocardial infarction The medical term for heart attack, which occurs when blood flow to a portion of the heart muscle is severely restricted or stopped, resulting in inadequate oxygen supply and decreased ability of the heart to pump.

myoglobin An oxygen- and iron-binding protein found in muscle and cardiac tissue which delivers oxygen to the working muscle cells.

near-infrared interactance (NIR) Estimates body composition using the optical densities of skin, fat, and lean tissue as an infrared light probe is reflected off bone and back to the probe.

negative energy balance When fewer calories are consumed than expended; leads to weight loss.

negative nitrogen balance The state in which the amount of nitrogen (via protein) consumed is less than the amount of nitrogen excreted in feces, urine, and skin. During this time the body is breaking down muscle protein to support other metabolic functions. Negative nitrogen balance occurs during times of high stress such as infections, trauma, or starvation.

net protein balance The balance that exists between muscle protein synthesis and muscle protein breakdown.

neuromuscular fatigue Incompletely understood phenomena of a decrease in athletic performance with intensive activity to fatigue at some point in the pathway from initiation of exercise in the cerebral cortex to activation in the muscle cell.

neutral energy balance When the number of calories consumed is equal to the number of calories expended.

nicotinamide adenine dinucleotide (NADH) A hydrogen-carrying molecule that enters the electron transport chain to produce 3 ATPs per molecule of NADH.

night eating syndrome Characterized by recurrent episodes of eating after awakening from sleep or excessive food consumption after the evening meal.

nitrogen balance The amount of nitrogen (via protein) consumed compared to the amount of nitrogen excreted. This provides information as to the person's metabolic state, muscle synthesis, muscle degradation, or equilibrium.

nitrogen balance studies Tests that measure the amount of nitrogen in the urine, which provide an indication of whether too much, too little, or enough protein is being consumed.

nonessential amino acid An amino acid that can be made by the body.

nonessential fat Triglycerides and other fatty tissue stored in muscle, around vital organs, and within subcutaneous tissue.

nutrient density An indicator of nutritional value of a food based on the levels of vitamins and minerals compared with the number of calories.

nutrition assessment Evaluation of nutrition status and nutritional needs.

older adult Defined by the Older Americans Act as a person older than 60 years.

oleic acid A monounsaturated fatty acid that occurs naturally in many animal and vegetable oils; improves cardiovascular health when used as a substitute for saturated fat and refined carbohydrates.

oligosaccharide A complex carbohydrate, a chain of approximately 3 to 10 monosaccharides.

omega-3 fatty acids Named for the position of their first double bond; alpha linolenic acid (ALA) is an essential polyunsaturated fatty acid that can be converted to eicosapentaenoic acid (EPA) and docosahexanoic acid (DHA); found in flaxseed, walnuts, dark green leafy vegetables, egg yolks, and cold water fish like tuna, salmon, mackerel, cod, crab, shrimp, and oysters. ALA, EPA, and DHA can be converted to eicosanoids.

omega-6 fatty acids Named for the position of their first double bond. Linoleic acid is an essential polyunsaturated fatty acid that can be converted to eicosanoids; found in sunflower, safflower, corn, and soybean oils.

omnivore A person who consumes both plant and animal foods.

open window of impaired immunity A period of time lasting 3 to 72 hours in which athletes who engage in intensive training are at particularly increased risk of infection.

oral allergy syndrome A condition that results when a protein in certain raw foods causes an immediate inflammatory response from the moment the food touches the mouth or skin.

orthorexia nervosa A pattern of disordered eating characterized by a preoccupation with eating an extremely healthy diet.

osteopenia A condition in which bone density is lower than normal; a precursor to osteoporosis.

osteoporosis Weakening of the bones, which can lead to bone fracture of the hip, spine, and other skeletal sites.

ovo-vegetarian A vegetarian who consumes eggs but does not consume meat, poultry, fish, or dairy products.

oxidation The process of binding oxygen to a molecule.

oxidative phosphorylation Process in which energy from electrons passed through the electron transport chain is captured and stored to produce ATP.

oxygen-carrying capacity The body's ability to get the oxygen that is breathed in from the environment into the lungs and bloodstream; affected by two main factors: (1) the ability to adequately ventilate the alveoli in the lungs, and (2) hemoglobin concentration in the blood.

oxygen deficit Oxygen shortage in cells which occurs with anaerobic activity.

oxygen delivery The ability of the body to transport oxygen from the lungs to the mitochondria of the working cells; the amount delivered is a function of cardiac output.

oxygen extraction The ability to transfer oxygen from the blood to the working muscle cells.

Paleo/Paleolithic diet A diet that aims to mimic what hunters and gatherers ate in the Paleolithic period over 10,000 years ago before the advent of agriculture: whole fruits and vegetables, fish, grass-fed livestock, fungi, roots, and nuts. The diet prohibits grains, legumes, dairy products, salt, refined sugar, and all processed foods.

pancreas A vital organ that is both a digestive organ, secreting pancreatic juice containing digestive enzymes that assist the absorption of nutrients and the digestion in the small intestine, and an endocrine organ that releases important hormones including insulin, glucagon, and somatostatin.

partially hydrogenated oil An oil in which the double bonds of an unsaturated fatty acid have been chemically manipulated to create a saturated fatty acid.

passive dehydration Dehydration resulting from fluid and food restriction.

passive diffusion See *simple diffusion*.

peak growth velocity The period in early adolescence in which a child experiences the fastest rate of growth.

pepsin The stomach acid responsible for initiating the digestion of proteins.

peptide bonds The connections between amino acids.

peptide YY An appetite suppressant released by the small intestine.

percent daily value The percentage of recommendations for key nutrients based on a 2,000-calorie diet.

periodized nutrition program A nutrition program in which calorie and macronutrient intakes vary based on the training regimen. Energy and nutrient needs are highest during peak training, somewhat decreased during taper and competition, and much lower during the transition and rest phase.

periodized training program An exercise training program that is separated into phases (periods) that vary in intensity and volume to maximize performance.

peristalsis The process by which muscles in the esophagus push food to the stomach through a wave-like motion.

pesco-vegetarian A vegetarian who consumes fish, eggs, and dairy but does not consume meat or poultry.

pharynx The portion of the respiratory system extending from the base of the skull to the esophagus (the throat).

phosphagen system The energy system used when there is an immediate energy need, generally within the first 30 seconds to 1 minute of exercise. Utilizes creatine phosphate to produce ATP.

phospholipid A compound with a modified glycerol backbone and two fatty acids. The molecule is water-soluble at one end and water-insoluble at the other end. These compounds form the cell-membrane structure phospholipid bilayer.

phytochemicals A variety of compounds found in plants that may have potential health benefits in humans.

pica A feeding disorder in which an individual has a strong desire to eat non-food items, such as dirt or clay; most frequently occurs in childhood in response to nutritional deficiency.

polypeptide A chain of many amino acids connected by peptide bonds.

polysaccharide A complex carbohydrate, long chain of monosaccharides. There are three categories: starch, fiber, and glycogen.

polyunsaturated fatty acids A type of unsaturated fatty acid that has two or more double bonds between carbon atoms; includes the essential fatty acids omega-6 and omega-3 fatty acids; improves heart health when used to replace saturated fats.

portal circulation Circulatory system that takes nutrients directly from the stomach, small intestine, colon, and spleen to the liver.

positive energy balance When more calories are consumed than expended; leads to weight gain.

positive nitrogen balance The state in which the amount of nitrogen (via protein) consumed is greater than the amount of nitrogen excreted in feces, urine, and skin. During this time the body is building muscle protein; this occurs during pregnancy, infancy, childhood, adolescence, recovery from illness, and in response to resistance training.

postural hypotension The pooling of blood in the legs and inadequate blood supply to the upper body, causing dizziness, weakness, and collapse; often occurs with dehydration and heat stress and may be confused with heat stroke.

power A measure of force (strength) and speed.

power output The amount of force generated in a specified period of time.

power-to-weight ratio The amount of force generated divided by body mass, or force adjusted by weight; a high ratio especially benefits athletic performance in gravitational sports like long-distance running and road cycling.

pregnancy-induced anemia The low red blood cell count that occurs during pregnancy due to increased blood volume and lag in increased red blood cell production; a normal phenomenon.

probiotics Bacteria that can be consumed in foods or supplements that help to keep a healthy balance of gut organisms.
prohormone A precursor to a hormone.
protein digestibility corrected amino acid score (PDCAAS) A measure of protein quality that compares the essential amino acid composition of a reference protein with the test protein; the FDA- and WHO-endorsed method of measuring protein quality.
proteolysis The process by which proteins are broken down into simpler, soluble compounds.
proteolytic enzymes Enzymes made in the pancreas and released into the small intestine to break peptide bonds between amino acids during digestion.
provitamin Inactive vitamin that can be converted to an active vitamin with enzyme activation.
purging disorder Condition in which a person engages in recurrent purging behavior to influence weight or shape, such as self-induced vomiting, misuse of laxatives, diuretics, or other medications, in the absence of binge eating.
qualified health claims A health claim on a packaged food that is supported by scientific research that attests a relationship between a substance and its ability to reduce the risk of a disease or health-related condition.
quasi-vitamins Similar to vitamins in having important roles in the normal functioning and health of the body, but currently there are no known human requirements.
quercetin A flavonoid that may help to protect from illness and enhance healing from injury.
rapport Relationship of trust and respect.
raw food diet A diet that emphasizes intake of foods in their natural, unprocessed, uncooked form.
reactive hypoglycemia Also known as rebound hypoglycemia; the drop in blood sugar that results from a surge in insulin. Theoretical concern when eating shortly before exercise because carbohydrate load and onset of exercise both cause an increase in insulin.
recommended dietary allowance (RDA) The amount of nutrient known to be adequate to meet the nutritional needs of nearly all healthy persons.
reference methods The most accurate, but least practical, methods used to measure body composition; infrequently used in practice or in research studies of body composition; includes CT scan, MRI, and multi-component models.
reflecting An active listening technique in which the listener states his or her understanding of a statement that the speaker has made.
registered dietitian A health professional with specialized training in nutrition who has completed the minimum requirements for the credential including a bachelor degree, completion of an accredited program in nutrition, and 1,200 hours of an approved supervised internship in nutrition, and passed a national examination. The registered dietitian is an expert in nutrition and is qualified to provide individualized nutrition assessment and recommendations, and to provide medical nutrition therapy.
reliability The reproducibility of a measure.
resistin A hormone secreted by adipose tissue that decreases cell sensitivity to insulin.
respiratory quotient (RQ) The amount of carbon dioxide, the end product of metabolism, produced by the body divided by the amount of oxygen consumed. Also called respiratory exchange ratio (RER).
resting energy expenditure (REE) The number of calories expended at rest to maintain normal vital function. Also referred to as resting metabolic rate (RMR).
restricting type of anorexia nervosa During the last 3 months, the individual has not engaged in recurrent episodes of binge eating or purging behavior.
rhabdomyolysis Breakdown of skeletal muscle tissue and release of contents into the bloodstream that sometimes leads to kidney failure; caused by dehydration and heat stress.
rumination A feeding disorder in which a person regurgitates (vomits) food they have just eaten and chews and swallows it again.
SAID principle The training principle of "specific adaptation to imposed demands"; when the body is placed under stress, it starts to make adaptations to improve its functioning in the future when it experiences that same stress.
saliva A secretion from the salivary glands that begins digestion; consists of water, salts, and enzymes.
sarcopenia "Muscle wasting," or a decrease in muscle mass and strength.
sarcopenic obesity Decline in skeletal muscle and strength combined with excess body fat, which is common during older adulthood.
satiety A feeling of being fully satisfied, when there is no longer a desire to eat.
saturated fatty acids Fatty acids that contain no double bonds between carbon atoms. Foods high in saturated fatty acids are typically solid at room temperature and are from animal products such as butter and lard.
screening tool A test that is useful in identifying nearly all people who have a condition, but it typically has a high "false positive" rate in that not everyone who tests "positive" actually has the condition.
secondary adipositas athletica A term used to describe athletes who do not purposefully want to gain fat mass but just want to get "bigger"; increased adiposity is an unintended consequence.
semi-vegetarian diet Synonymous with the *flexitarian diet*, this diet is one in which a person does not usually eat meat, fish, or poultry but will infrequently include these foods in their diet.
simple carbohydrate Monosaccharides and disaccharides.
simple diffusion When a substance moves from an area of high concentration to an area of low concentration without the need for a carrier protein.
skinfold calipers A hand-held device used to measure in millimeters the thickness of subcutaneous fat at standardized locations in the body.
small intestine The three-segment portion of the digestive system between the stomach and large intestine that is responsible for the majority of digestion and absorption of swallowed foods.
social-ecological model A model for health behavior change that emphasizes the development of coordinated partnerships, programs, and policies to support healthy eating and active living.
sodium bicarbonate A compound found naturally in blood and taken endogenously by some athletes as a supplement; helps to reduce muscle acidity by increasing the release of hydrogen ions from muscle cells.
SoFAS (solid fats and added sugars) A term first introduced in the 2010 *Dietary Guidelines for Americans* that refers to a food ingredient that provides little nutritional value and should be avoided. The guidelines recommend that Americans: (1) cut back on calories from solid fats and added sugars; (2) limit foods that contain refined grains, especially refined grains that contain solid fats, added sugars, and sodium; and (3) use oils to replace solid fats whenever possible.
soluble fiber A type of fiber that forms gel in water; may help prevent heart disease and stroke by binding bile and cholesterol, diabetes by slowing glucose absorption, and constipation by holding moisture in stools and softening them; includes gums, pectin, and psyllium seeds.
somatotype Body type.
sphingomyelin A class of phospholipid composed of phosphoric acid, choline, sphingosine, and a fatty acid; found in high concentration in cell membranes of nervous tissues.
sports anemia A pseudo-anemia characterized by low hemoglobin concentration due to increased plasma volume

in response to exercise; the actual total hemoglobin content is normal and the athlete does not have true anemia.

sports drinks Beverages containing carbohydrates, protein, or electrolytes.

stages of change Also known as transtheoretical model, a theory of behavior change which posits that people progress through a series of stages as they ready themselves to make a behavioral change, such as modification to nutrition or physical activity behaviors.

starch Plant carbohydrate found in grains and vegetables.

sterol A type of lipid. Cholesterol is the most common type of sterol. Cholesterol can be converted to steroid hormones.

stimulant A substance that activates the central nervous system and sympathetic nervous system. It increases heart rate and cardiac output as well as glucose availability, and may suppress appetite.

stomach An organ between the esophagus and small intestine that stores swallowed food, mixes the food with stomach acids, and then sends the mixture to the small intestine.

strength The production of maximal force.

strength sports Sports that require production of maximal force for optimal performance.

stroke volume The amount of blood pumped out of the heart with each heartbeat.

structure/function claims A health claim on a packaged food that describes the effect that a substance has on the structure or function of the body. An example is "calcium builds strong bones." Structure/function claims must be truthful and not misleading, but they are not reviewed or authorized by the FDA.

subthreshold anorexia nervosa See *atypical anorexia nervosa.*

subthreshold binge-eating disorder A condition in which all of the criteria for binge-eating disorder are met, except that the binge eating occurs, on average, less than once a week and/or for fewer than 3 months. See *eating disorder not elsewhere specified.*

subthreshold bulimia nervosa A condition in which all of the criteria for bulimia are met, except that the binge eating and inappropriate compensatory behaviors occur, on average, less than once a week and/or for fewer than 3 months.

successful aging Maintenance of low disease risk and cognitive and physical function.

sucrose A disaccharide formed by glucose and fructose linked together; also known as table sugar.

sugar Chemically speaking it may refer to simple carbohydrates (mono and disaccharides), or it may refer to table sugar or sucrose.

summarizing An active listening technique in which the listener paraphrases his or her understanding of what the speaker has said.

SuperTracker An online tool by the USDA that can track, analyze, and evaluate nutrition and physical activity.

testosterone A male sex hormone secreted by the testes that induces masculine characteristics and muscle-building (anabolic) effects.

three-dimensional photonic scanning Uses a low-power laser light and digital cameras to rapidly produce a 3-D digital model of the human body, which is used to approximate lean and fat mass.

TNF-alpha Tumor necrosis factor; helps to regulate fat metabolism and along with other cytokines contributes to acute inflammatory reactions.

tolerable upper intake level The maximum intake that is unlikely to pose risk of adverse health effects to almost all individuals in an age- and gender-specific group.

tolerance An individual becomes accustomed to the current amount of exercise and must increase the amount of exercise in order to feel the desired effect, be it a "buzz" or sense of accomplishment, in the case of exercise dependence.

trans fatty acid An unsaturated fatty acid in which the double bonds are in the trans configuration. A double bond in the trans configuration has the H's on opposite sides of the double bond. Some occur naturally, most are manmade. Fatty acids with trans double bonds function like a saturated fat in the body by elevating LDL cholesterol.

transferrin The protein that binds and transports iron.

triacylglycerols Stored triglycerides (fats); compound consisting of three fatty acids and one glycerol molecule.

tricarboxylic acid cycle See *citric acid cycle.*

triglycerides Three fatty acids bound to a glycerol backbone; the primary form of fat storage in the body and the composition of most fats in the food supply.

tripeptide Three amino acid chain combined by peptide bonds.

trypsin The active form of the precursor trypsinogen, which breaks down protein chains into single amino acids, dipeptides, and tripeptides.

twenty-four hour recall A method of gaining information about a client's eating habits by asking for detailed information about the foods and drinks the client consumed in the 24 hours prior to the consultation.

ultra-endurance sports A subset of endurance sports that lasts 4 hours or more.

United States Department of Agriculture (USDA) The federal department that develops and implements policy on food, farming, forestry, and agriculture, and issues dietary recommendations.

unsaturated fatty acids Fatty acids that contain one or more double bonds between carbon atoms; typically liquid at room temperature and fairly unstable, making them susceptible to oxidative damage and a shorter half life.

urea The nitrogenous byproduct of protein deamination; formed in the liver and excreted in the urine.

urea cycle A complex metabolic system that removes nitrogen from organic compounds and prepares the remaining nitrogenous structure (urea) for excretion in urine.

validity The accuracy of a measure.

vegan A person who does not include any animal products in their diet. This means they do not consume meat, poultry, fish, eggs, or dairy products.

vegetarian A person who eats a plant-based diet and does not consume meat and poultry.

ventilatory threshold (VT) Point in exercise when lactate accumulation begins. Also known as anaerobic threshold or lactate threshold.

very low density lipoprotein (VLDL) The least dense of all of the lipoproteins, carrying a greater ratio of lipid to protein than LDL; main transport mechanism for endogenously produced lipids.

villi Folds or finger-like projections of the small intestine that increase surface area for digestion and absorption.

vitamins Organic substances obtained from plant and animal foods that are essential in small quantities for normal growth and activity of the body.

VO_2 max A measure of maximal oxygen uptake; liters of O_2 consumed per kilogram of body weight per minute.

waist circumference Abdominal girth measured at the level of the umbilicus; values greater than or equal to 40 inches (102 cm) in men and greater than or equal to 35 inches (89 cm) in women are strong indicators of abdominal obesity and associated with an increased health risk.

waist-to-hip ratio (WHR) Waist circumference divided by hip circumference; a number greater than or equal to 1.0 confers increased health risk; a ratio of 0.9 or less in men and 0.8 or less in women is considered safe.

water-soluble vitamins Vitamins that are readily dissolved in water and thus are not effectively stored in the human body.

weight cycling Rapid fluctuations in weight, generally used in sports when an athlete loses weight to qualify for a certain weight class, then regains the weight immediately after the weigh-in.

whey A high-quality protein; the liquid remaining after milk has been curdled and strained.

whey concentrate A whey protein supplement that is 25% to 89% protein by weight.

whey protein isolate A whey protein supplement that is 90% or more protein by weight; lactose free.

whey protein powder A form of whey protein that is 11% to 15% protein by weight; used as an additive in many food products.

white adipose tissue Storage site for triglycerides, cushion to protect vital organs, and insulation to maintain body heat.

withdrawal In the absence of exercise the person experiences negative effects such as anxiety, irritability, restlessness, and sleep problems, in the case of exercise dependence.

work-to-rest ratio The relationship of the amount of time spent in strenuous activity and the amount of time spent in rest between sets or vigorous bouts of activity.

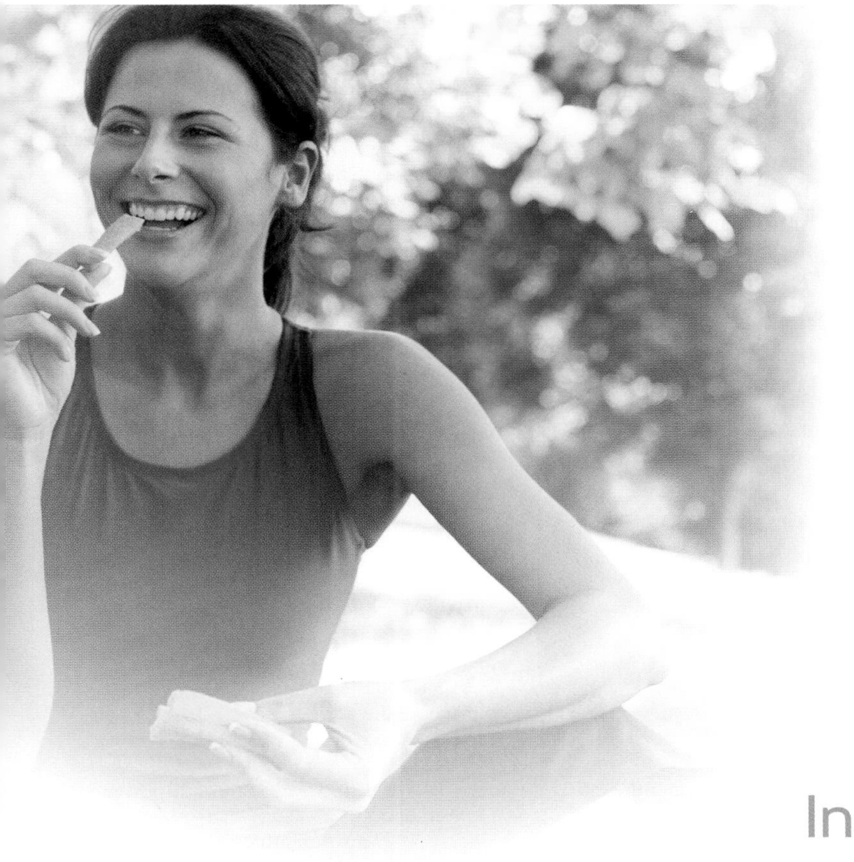

Index

Page numbers followed by *f* indicate figures; *t*, tables; *b*, boxes and boxed material.

F

G

H

M

Q

R

W

X

Y

Z